KINESIOLOGY

Kinesiology is the study of human movement and the body's response to exercise. It is an examination of systems, factors, and principles involved in human development within the context of society. Relevant fields in the study of kinesiology include anatomy, physiology, biomechanics, motor learning and control, and sport psychology and sociology.

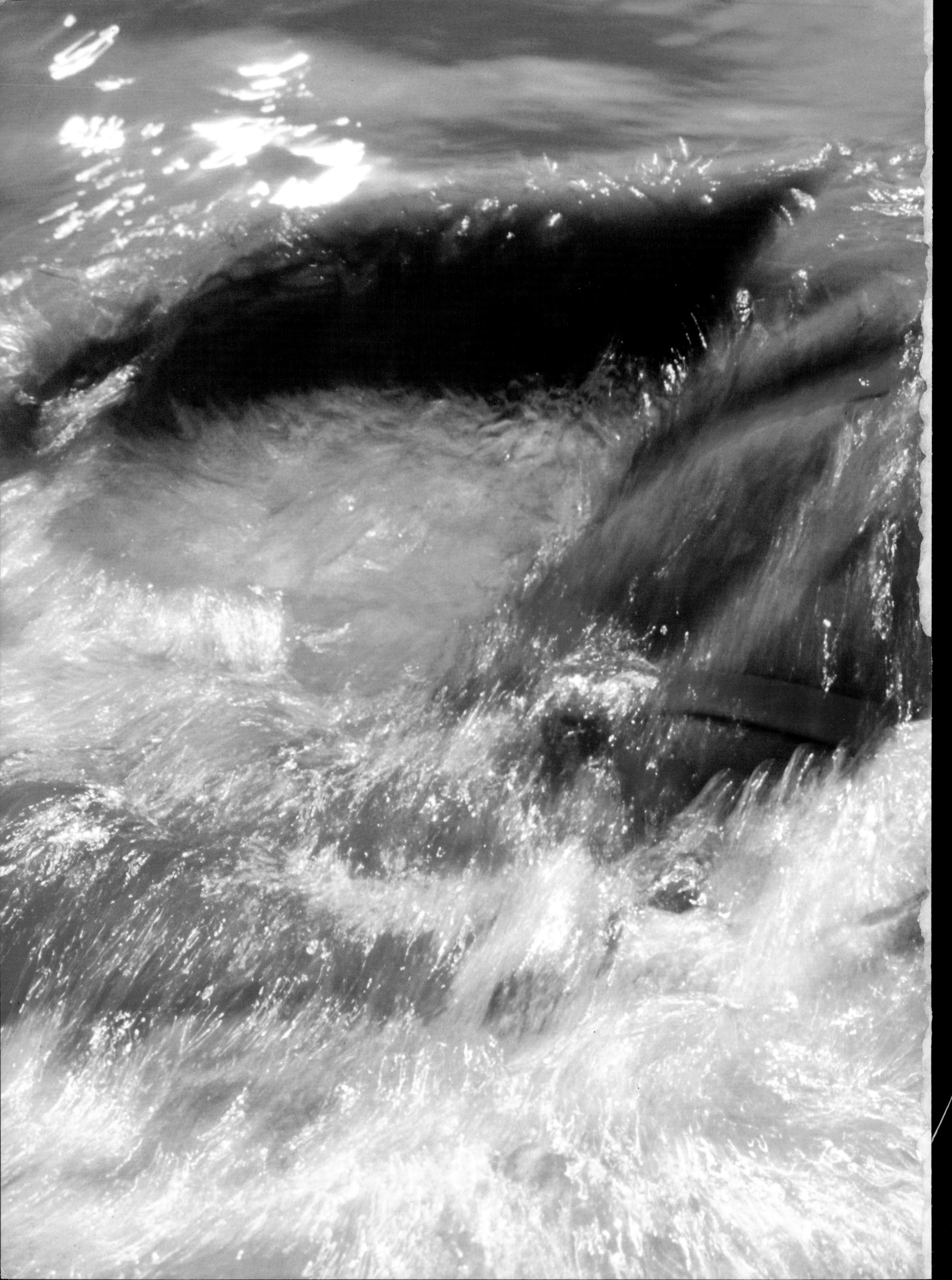

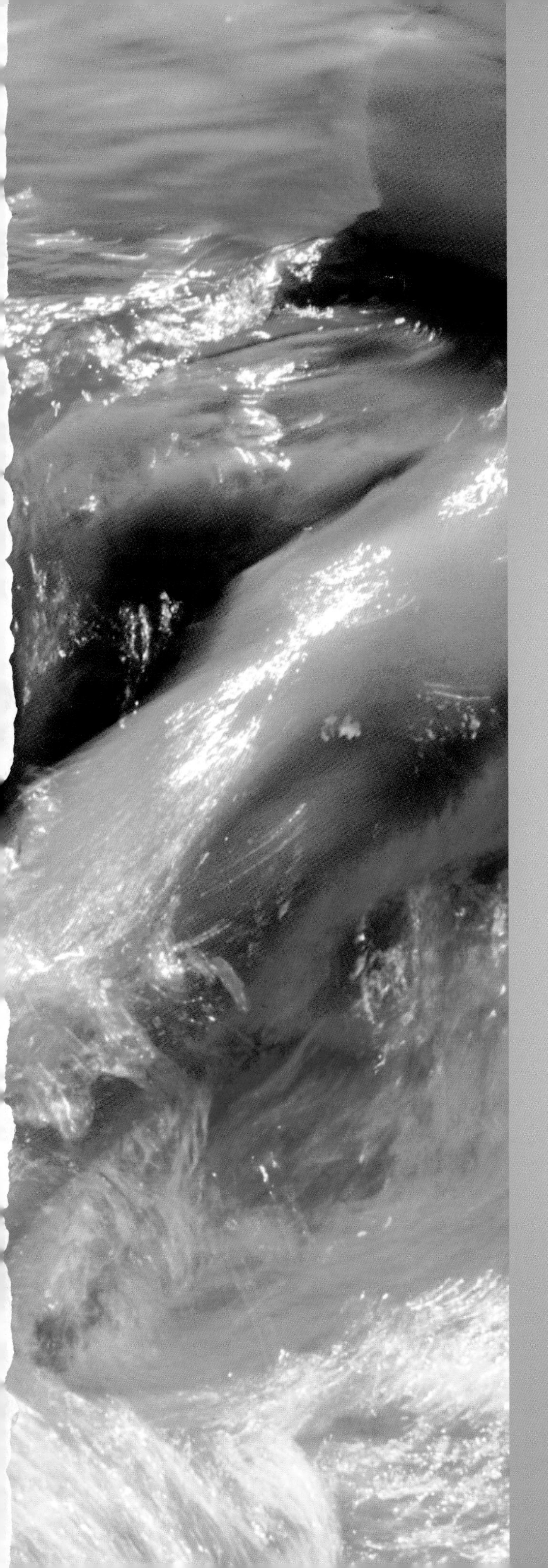

INTRODUCTION TO KINESIOLOGY
A BIOPHYSICAL PERSPECTIVE

P. Klavora, PhD
Professor Emeritus
University of Toronto

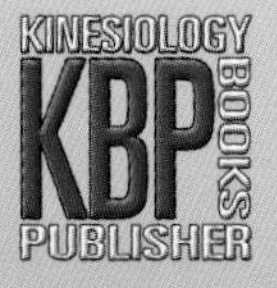

Kinesiology Books Publisher
A division of Sport Books Publisher

Design by My1 Designs

Library and Archives Canada Cataloguing in Publication

Klavora, Peter
Introduction to kinesiology : a biophysical perspective / Peter Klavora.

Includes bibliographical references and index.
ISBN 978-0-920905-27-2

1. Kinesiology--Textbooks. I. Title

QP303.K58 2008 612.7'6 C2008-903841-X

Copyeditor: Patricia MacDonald
Proofreader: Patricia MacDonald

Distribution worldwide by
Kinesiology Books Publisher
212 Robert Street
Toronto ON M5S 2K7
Canada

www.kinesiology101.com
E-mail: kbp@kinesiology101.com
Fax: 416-966-9022

Contributing Authors

This book was written first and foremost with the student in mind. It was completed with the efforts of kinesiology professors and graduate students from various universities across Canada and the United States. It was important that this book be user-friendly, and this collaborative effort among students and professors allowed this text to achieve a degree of accuracy and clarity while remaining sensitive to the needs of students. Because the student writers had fresh experiences with the subject matter and were still familiar with what it meant to be a young student with a keen desire to learn, their input was invaluable in the process of completing this text. All along during the preparation of this text, several teachers and students provided valuable feedback at various levels. The result is a book that makes expert knowledge about topics and issues in physical and health education available to students – an engaging and palatable resource for students and teachers alike.

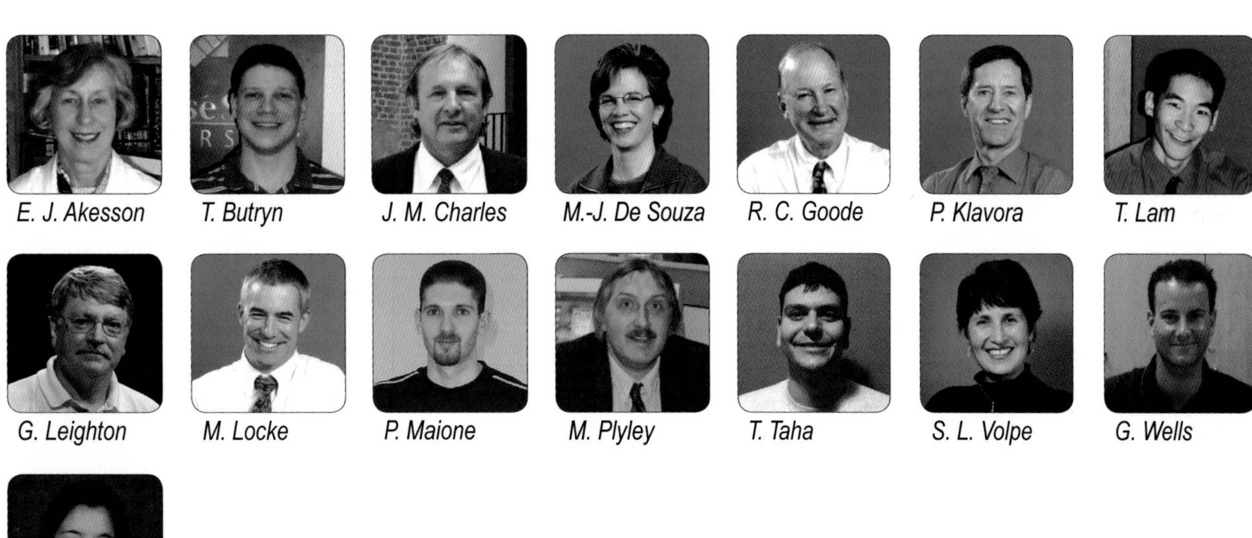

E. J. Akesson — T. Butryn — J. M. Charles — M.-J. De Souza — R. C. Goode — P. Klavora — T. Lam

G. Leighton — M. Locke — P. Maione — M. Plyley — T. Taha — S. L. Volpe — G. Wells

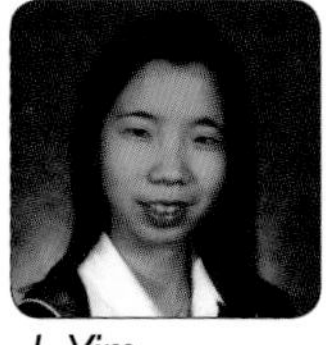

I. Yim

Authors

Akesson, B., Prof. Emerita, University of BC (2)
Butryn, T., PhD, San José State University (9)
Charles, J. M., PhD, The College of William and Mary (1)
Klavora, P., PhD, University of Toronto (5, 7, 10-13)
Lam, T., BPHE, D.C., University of Toronto (3)
Leighton, G., BA, GDJ, University of Minnesota (16)
Locke, M., PhD, University of Toronto (7, 12, 15)
Maione, P., BPHE, University of Toronto (14-15)
Taha, T., PhD, University of Toronto (9)
Tupling, S. PhD, University of Toronto (8)
Volpe, S. L., PhD, University of Pennsylvania (14-15)
Wells, G., PhD, University of Toronto (4-6)
Yim, I., BPHE, University of Toronto (7, 13)

Contributors

De Souza, M.-J., PhD, Pennsylvania State University (15)
Goode, R. C., PhD, University of Toronto (12)
Plyley, M., PhD, Brock University (4-6)

Academic Reviewers

Goodman, J., PhD, University of Toronto (12)
Lockwood, K., PhD, Brock University (8)
Rogers, C., PhD, University of Saskatchewan (14, 15)
Su, J., M.D., Dip. Sport Med. (3)
Thomas, S., PhD, University of Toronto (4-7)
Wolfe, E., PhD, OISE, University of Toronto (8)

Contents

UNIT 4: Fitness and Health *255*

APPENDIX: Career Opportunities in Kinesiology *379*

Foreword

Imagine that you are sitting at home on a Saturday night and have just tuned in to the basketball game. What do you see? Players running back and forth at break-neck speed? Fancy footwork and a great move to elude a defensive player? A three-point shot that drops through the net with an audible "swish"? Perhaps you even notice the crowd cheering, the head coach appearing just a little more at ease, or the athletes offering encouragement to their teammates.

The more you watch, the more you appreciate the remarkable amount of action in an average basketball game. While that may be obvious, something even more remarkable is perhaps less obvious. Although records, awards, and titles may be the simple goals of any basketball player, what goes on inside an athlete such as LeBron James is much more complex and fascinating than meets the eye.

The mark of any champion can be found in his or her perseverance and dedication to training for excellence. As a young child, James amused himself for hours at a time with a miniature ball and hoop. But how did this very basic activity contribute to his outstanding ability on the court? How did simple childhood play maintain and improve his skill level throughout the crucial stages of growth and development? Further, what is the best way to train? Would James be the success he is today if he had used a different training regimen?

Another quality that champion athletes possess is the ability to overcome adversity. In 2003, speedskater Cindy Klassen sliced open her right forearm in a training accident, severing tendons, a major artery, and a nerve. Amazingly, she began training again only two months after reconstructive surgery. Less than three years later, at the 2006 Torino Olympics, Klassen won five medals, making her the most decorated athlete of the Games.

What was going on in Klassen's mind when doctors told her she might never regain full use of her hand? What was going on within her body as she gracefully powered her way around the Olympic speedskating oval? How did she ensure she had enough energy to compete in five events? Are we all capable of that level of endurance, or did Klassen possess a unique supernatural trait? And where did she find the energy to pace herself for a 5,000-meter race?

This raises a range of other questions – where did this energy come from? Was it derived from the food she ate? How did her body store and allocate energy to support long, tiring races? Where did she find the burst of energy for a sprint to the finish line?

Successful performances also require some degree of muscular training. What muscles did James develop to make him a fast and agile runner? Do these muscles bear unusually large amounts of stress? Basketball players are particularly prone to ankle injuries; what is it about the sport that makes its athletes so vulnerable? Do drugs or treatments exist that may prevent such mishaps? And while we are on the topic of drugs, how do steroids and other substances influence athletic performance? Does an athlete's requirements for training change with drug use?

Maybe an athlete's ability has little to do with years of practice. Certain laws of physics can be applied to sport, so it may be that Klassen knew something about biomechanics that gave her a competitive advantage. Maybe she understood the proper technique to maximize skating efficiency while minimizing fatigue. After all, principles of biomechanics have been used by sport scientists for many years in sports such as gymnastics, pole vaulting, and cycling.

In a league full of talented defensive players, how does James manage to score so many points? Was he lucky enough to be born with remarkable shooting accuracy, or did he have to develop this ability? As an outstanding individual player, James's talents are not limited to his phenomenal physical skills: he also has exceptional vision. His ability to read the play and anticipate how it will unfold helps him unleash his trademark passes. What goes on in his mind to make him always conscious

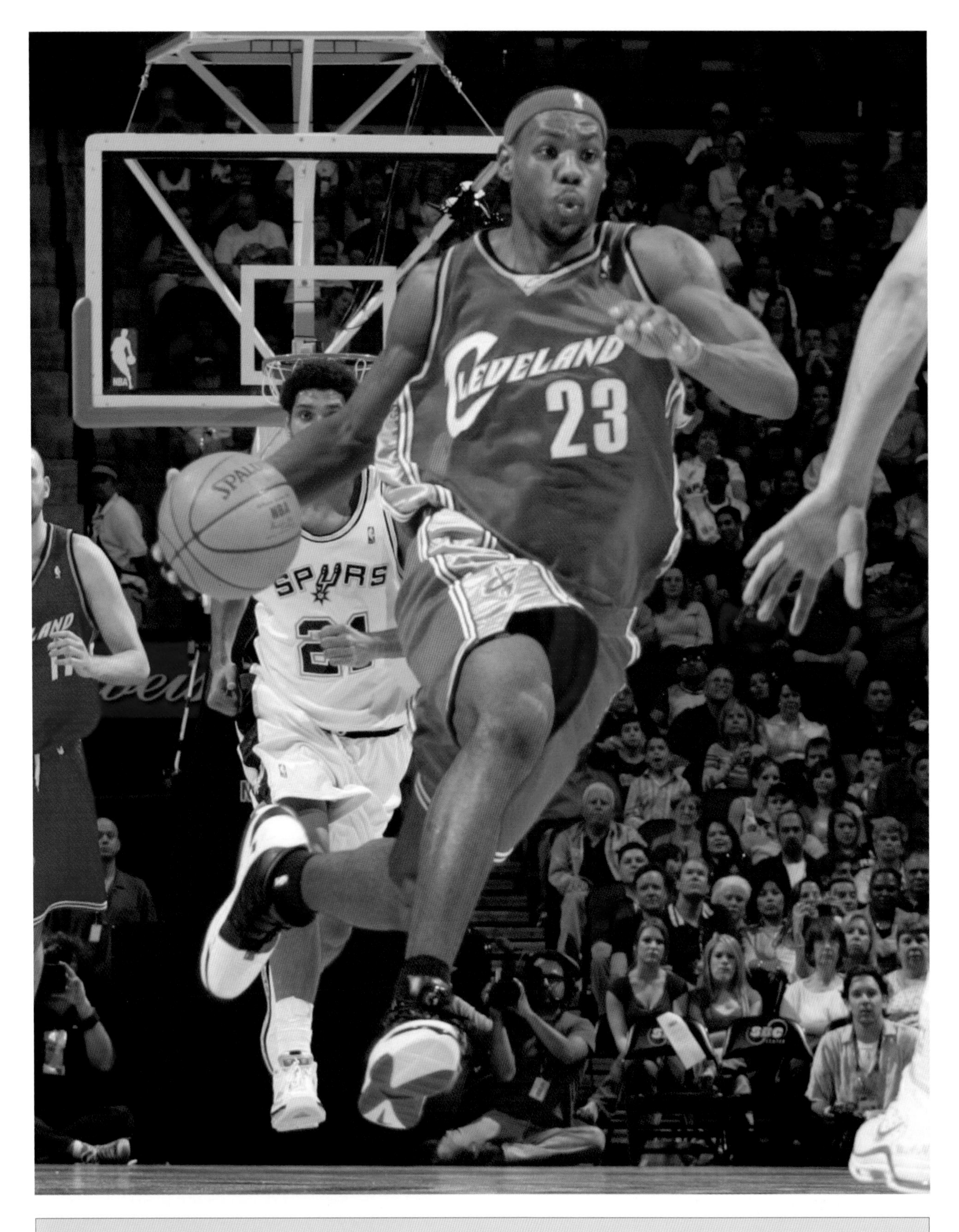

LeBron James made the jump to the NBA out of high school and quickly proved that he belonged. Touted as the next basketball superstar, the 2003-2004 rookie of the year has lived up to expectations. His court vision and superior passing skills should translate into many outstanding seasons in the years to come.

of every player on the court? Does James ever get nervous or lose his focus?

There must be days when athletes just don't feel they can perform up to their potential. Every athlete is prone to such doubts over a career. But how was Klassen able to stay motivated to train and return to form after a serious injury? What does it take to remain competitive year after year with the same focus and drive? How does James rise to the occasion in a big game while others wilt under the pressure? With the salaries that many professionals are bringing in these days, the motivation to perform might be found in their back pockets.

When you review the number of games a basketball player plays in a season, year after year, with different teams and different teammates, the question arises: How do they stay "up" for every game? Does James ever relax and perform only marginally? Did Klassen have physiological characteristics that allowed her to endure more pain than the average person? Did her experience and years of training help her overcome an injury that could have ended another skater's career?

What made the difference for these two athletes? Their personality characteristics certainly helped both rise to stardom in their respective sports – time after time they excelled against the best competitors the world could offer. What made the difference? Was it because they could afford the best coaches, trainers, and equipment?

This brings up the issue of money. Where do astronomical sums of cash fit into the broader picture of sport? Do large salaries make players excessively greedy, to the point that they are willing to strike, risking the loss of an entire season of play? Does this change how the fans perceive players? Does this aspect detract from the beauty and tradition of sport by placing it in the hands of capitalism and big business?

And speaking of fans, how do we, as spectators, view sport, and how does it affect our lives? Every North American has certainly had some degree of exposure to basketball, soccer, and other sports. Increasingly, as women and minorities seek the opportunity to play, and as citizens' coalitions band together to prevent televised violence, sport has become a focus of political and social issues.

As you can see, a single glimpse into the world of sport can generate discussion over a variety of subjects. And that, specifically, is the purpose of this textbook. The chapters that follow expose you to a variety of perspectives associated with physical and health education. You are most likely familiar with the sporting and physical activity aspects of these courses; however, this course is designed to provide a unique opportunity for students to apply sports-related ideas to associated areas including medicine, sociology, physics, and business.

With the expansion of your knowledge in these areas, you should be motivated to strive for a higher quality of life through your own level of physical fitness. Rather than simply tell you that healthy living is desirable, we will show you why. For this reason, the following chapters are structured so that you have the opportunity to apply the knowledge you learn.

A devastating injury could not prevent speedskater Cindy Klassen from reaching the pinnacle of her sport. This gutsy, determined athlete is a world record holder, a world all-around champion, and an Olympic gold medalist.

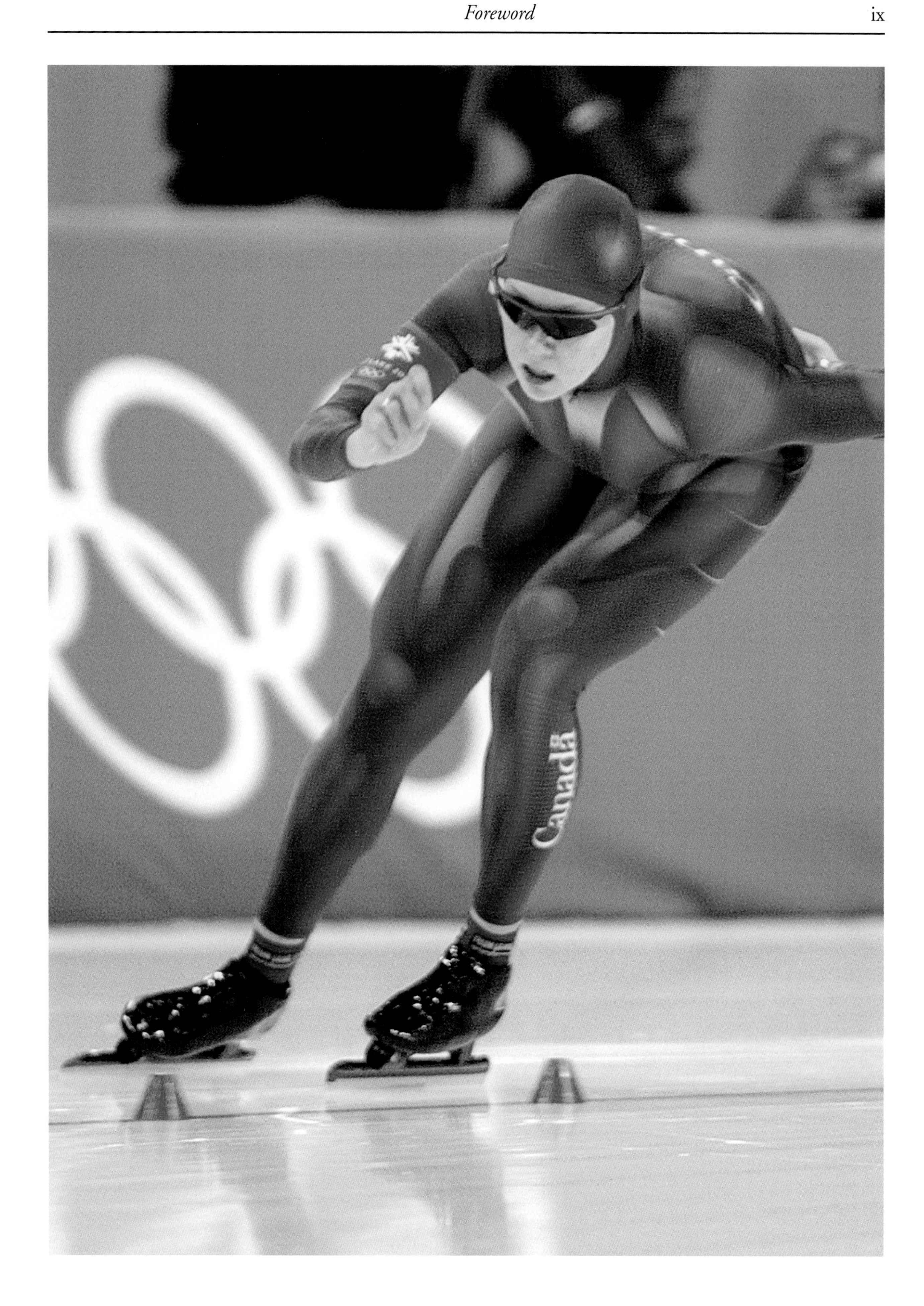
Canada

In This Chapter:

CHAPTER 1

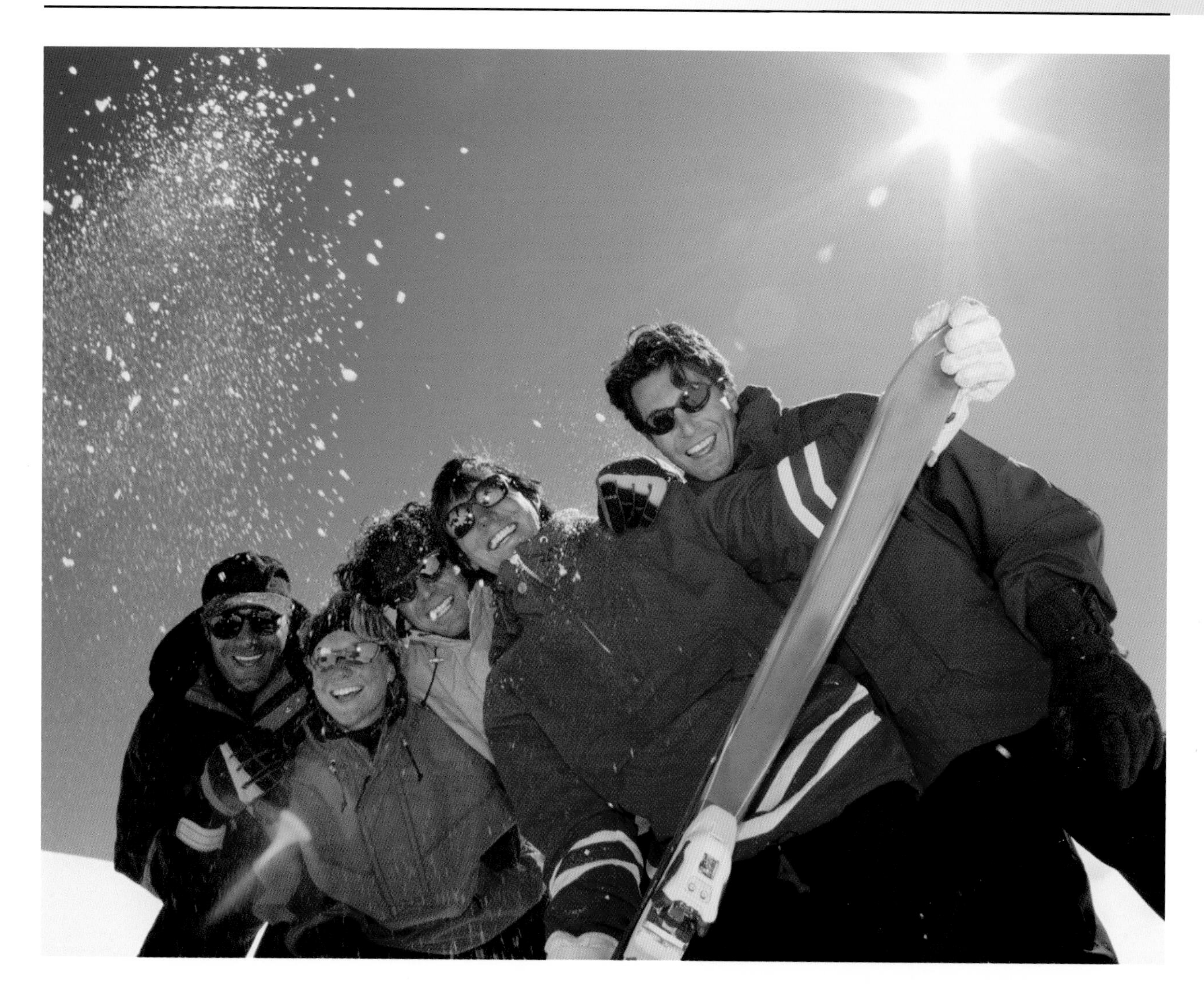

Introduction to Kinesiology

After completing this chapter you should be able to:

- explain the meaning, significance, and scope of the focus of kinesiology;
- explain the choice of kinesiology as the preferred name for our field;
- describe the spheres of scholarly study that constitute kinesiology;
- experience the meaning of kinesiology in your own life.

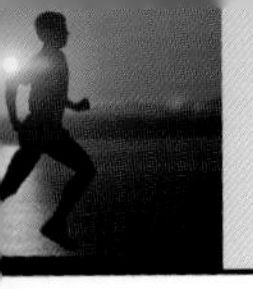

Studies in kinesiology, or the science of human movement, not only accommodate a range of educational purposes but also have a very personal impact. From the moment we wake up in the morning to the moment our heads hit the pillow at night, we perform hundreds of different movements and engage in a wide array of physical activities. Human movement affects our personal health, wellness, and physical achievements in distinct ways, providing a unique opportunity to explore and interact with the world around us.

In fact, issues related to health and human movement have become primary concerns of all societies today. From health promotion to human performance, the highly interdisciplinary field of kinesiology provides a natural springboard for students interested in discovering and unraveling the complexities of human movement.

The popularity of kinesiology reflects its wide scope and significance as an emerging field of study. But to understand where we are going, we have to understand where we came from. This chapter will help you understand how the discipline of kinesiology has evolved and will discuss why it has taken its current form and focus.

Definitions and Dimensions

Kinesiology Defined

Kinesiology is the new and exciting field of study of human movement. The meaning of kinesiology was best defined in 1990 by the American Academy of Physical Education when it resolved to identify a common name and focus in order to describe the academic discipline and to unite the field. Through this action, the Academy hoped to settle the following problems facing the emerging academic field of study:

- More than 100 different names were being used for academic programs and administrative units related to the study of human movement.
- The basic conceptual framework of this body of knowledge varied greatly from university campus to campus.
- The multitude of degree titles, program names, and administrative rubrics produced confusion regarding the nature of the study of movement, even among academicians who work in the field.

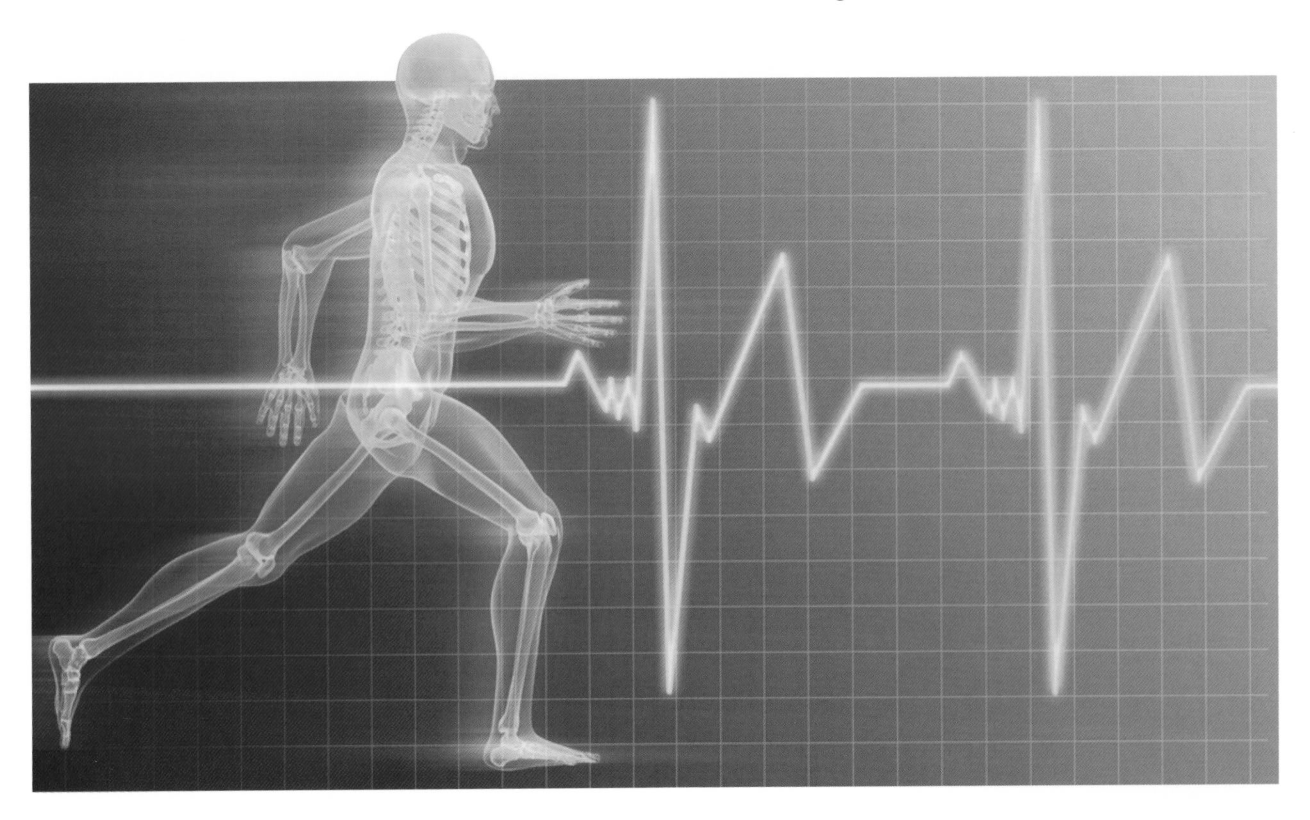

The American Academy of Physical Education believed that a nationally accepted name and definition of the body of knowledge would provide a stronger sense of purpose, higher visibility in the academic community, and a greater understanding of the discipline by the public, so it crafted the following resolution:

> Be it resolved that the American Academy of Physical Education recommends that the subject matter core content for undergraduate baccalaureate degrees related to the study of movement be called Kinesiology, and that baccalaureate degrees in the academic discipline be titled Kinesiology. The American Academy of Physical Education encourages administrative units, such as departments or divisions, in which the academic study of Kinesiology is predominant, to adopt the name Kinesiology. Finally, in any situation in which an administrative unit feels comfortable in describing the totality of its components by the title of the body of knowledge, the Academy recommends that this descriptor be Kinesiology.

This statement by the Academy was a long time coming; the leaders of the field had been discussing definitions and dimensions throughout the preceding century. As long ago as 1893, Thomas Wood suggested, in his address to the International Congress of Education, that "the term physical education is so misleading, and even misrepresented, that we look for a name which shall represent fairly the real idea of the science." In 1964, Franklin Henry, one of the founding fathers of our academic study, recognized that a schism was developing between disciplines claiming to study human movement: "There is an increasing need for the organization and study of the academic disciplines herein called physical education. As each of the traditional fields of knowledge concerning man becomes more specialized, complex, and detailed, it becomes more differentiated from physical education."

The Scope of Kinesiology

One of the underlying reasons that the confusion about definitions and dimensions went on for so long is the extraordinary breadth and scope of academic approaches and professional purposes that have both defined and divided programs through the years. The ways that changes in the structure and purpose of higher education have led to the modern approach to social, cultural, behavioral, and biophysical perspectives of kinesiology are discussed later in this chapter (see the section on spheres of scholarly study) and throughout the book. Despite (and because of) years of intense – and sometimes tense – discussions among the leaders of the evolving field about the form it should take and the name it should be given, the field has continued to flourish.

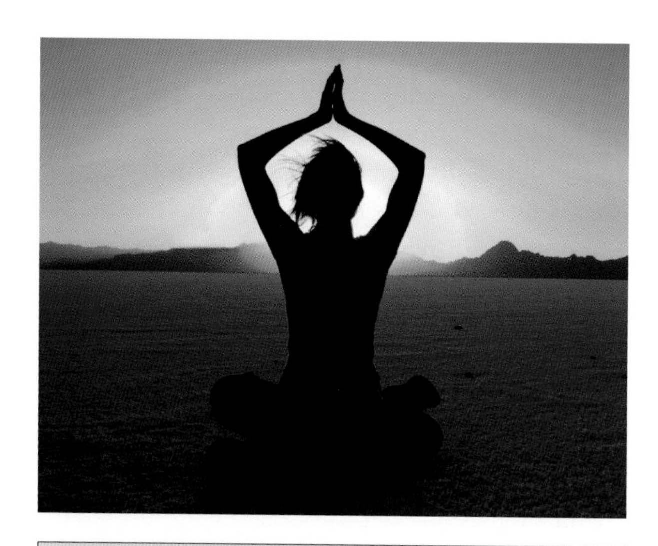

Figure 1.1 A primary reason for the popularity of kinesiology is the increasing recognition of the importance of health-related and skill-related human movement.

A primary reason for the popularity of kinesiology is the increasing recognition of the importance of health-related and skill-related human movement. Because health and human movement are so closely linked, the study of human movement naturally links with a concern for health. The correlation between being physically active and being healthy is proven. Physical activity of various types is valued not only for its preventive capacities but also as a form of treatment for many conditions. Of course, it has always been the basis of physical therapy, but physical activity is also recommended as part of the remedial protocol for many lifestyle diseases in the Western medical establishment and as a form of health promotion through such activities as tai chi and yoga in the Eastern tradition (Figure 1.1).

The biophysical bases of movement to which you will be introduced in this book are essential prerequisites for professions in human movement and health enhancement. It is no accident that graduates of kinesiology programs are in great demand in health-related and medical professions as well as in performance-enhancement and teaching settings. Health in kinesiology is more **proactive** and preventive than the **reactive** forms of medicine that focus exclusively on the treatment of disease. Health encompasses the dynamic, constantly changing process of trying to reach one's potential; **wellness** goes one step further to combine health and happiness in a balanced state of well-being.

Skill-related performance is an important star in the constellation of kinesiology practice. It includes athletic movement that may involve varying degrees of vigor and may invoke both fine and gross motor skills. It fluctuates along a continuum of organization, from the creative freedom of play to the more structured modes of organized competitive sport played at every level by people of all ages with varying degrees of seriousness. Competition is a variable concept that may range from team sports, where groups of people compete against each other in such popular pastimes as football and basketball, to a range of individual challenges (Figure 1.2), including

- one versus self – contests motivated by a desire for personal challenge;
- one versus another – individual sport contests, such as tennis;
- one versus many – activities such as marathon running and triathlons;
- one versus standards – of distance (jumps, throws) or time (time trials); and
- one versus nature – conquering the elements (e.g., rock climbing).

When combined into one program of study, health-related movement and skill-related physical activity provide considerable scope for study and a broad array of potential professions in and through kinesiology.

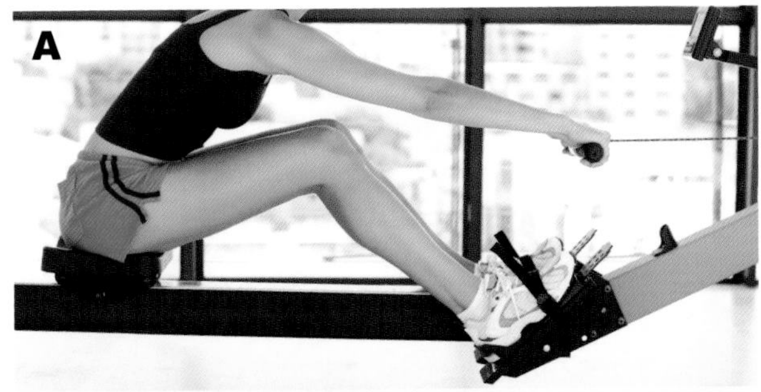

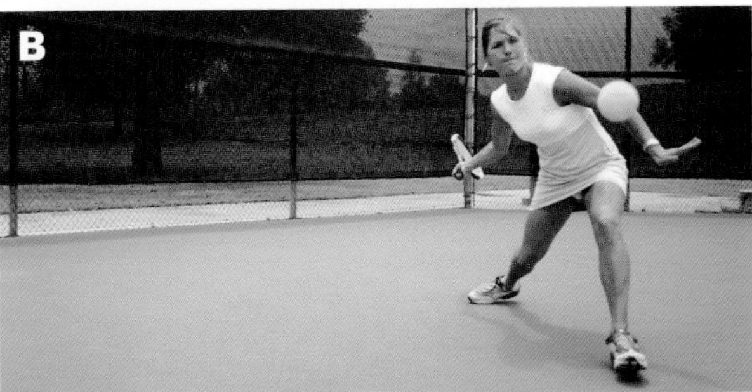

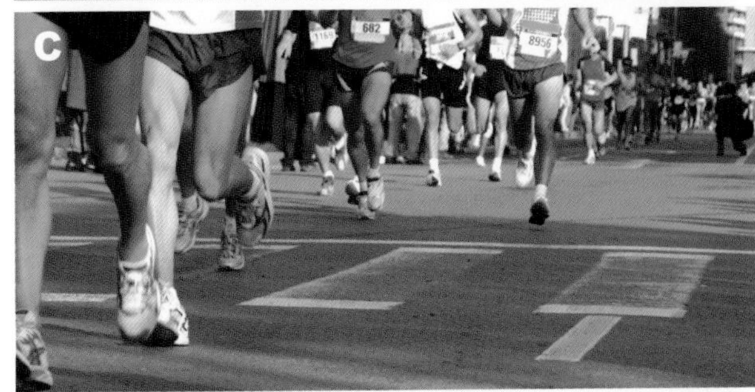

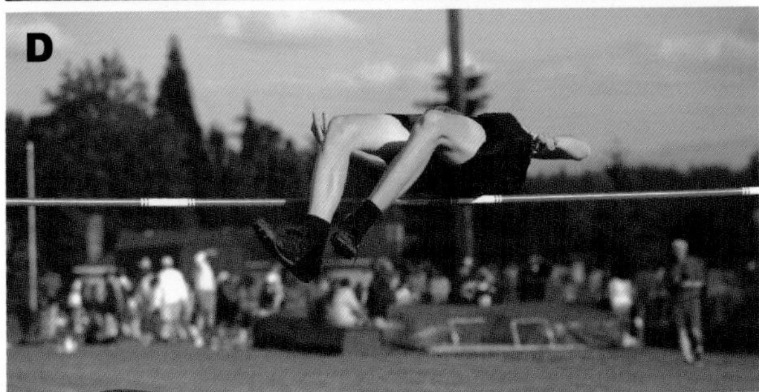

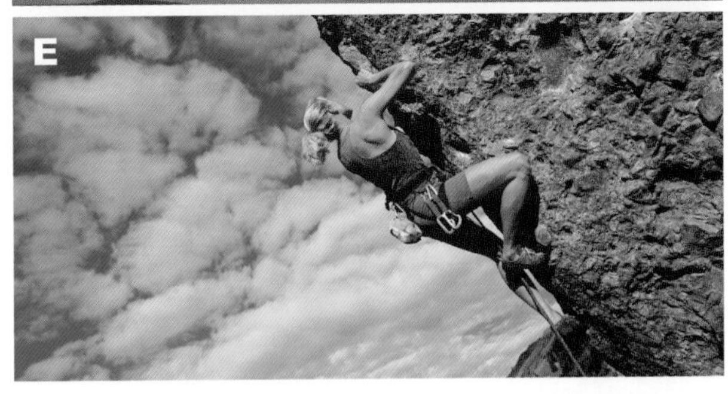

Figure 1.2 Competition is a variable concept that includes a range of individual challenges including **A.** One versus self. **B.** One versus another. **C.** One versus many. **D.** One versus standards. **E.** One versus nature.

The Significance of Kinesiology

Human movement has potential as the focus of our studies because it is eminently researchable and because performance and health enhancement are topics of great interest to us individually and to the larger global community today. The field lends itself readily to both descriptive and prescriptive research methodologies. Building from the description of the current state of affairs (*what is*), we can proceed to study, research, and prescribe *what might be* (e.g., how could performance be enhanced). Human movement is also highly accessible to research from a wide range of social, cultural, behavioral, and biophysical disciplines, so it is an attractive focus from a variety of perspectives.

Kinesiology has the potential to help answer many of the major questions facing the global community. It is hard to name other academic fields that address topics of such significance as personal, public, and environmental health; teaching and learning based on motor development and skill acquisition; and performance at every level up to elite sport. Issues abound in high-level athletic performance, and the research conclusions can have great significance in a cultural phenomenon of intense public interest. Professional sports culminating in such popular events as the Olympic Games and World Cup soccer grip the attention of nations.

Kinesiology also has a focus of considerable scholarly significance in sport because of organized sport's cultural impact. Influenced by media coverage of sport and by concern for their own health, people of all ages, of every skill level, and in the full range of physical conditions are active in sports. Similarly, the focus on health and wellness, prevention of lifestyle diseases, and promotion of lifespan well-being has never been as pronounced or as widespread as today. The biophysical bases of our field, such as exercise physiology, biomechanics, and nutrition, attract many to kinesiology, as does the scope for sociocultural, behavioral, and philosophical analysis afforded by the full range of human movement action in society today. Consequently, kinesiology is becoming the choice of an ever-increasing cadre of students, who ultimately swell the ranks of such movement-related professions and health-related careers as teachers and coaches, researchers and professors, physicians and physical therapists (Figure 1.3; also see Chapter 16).

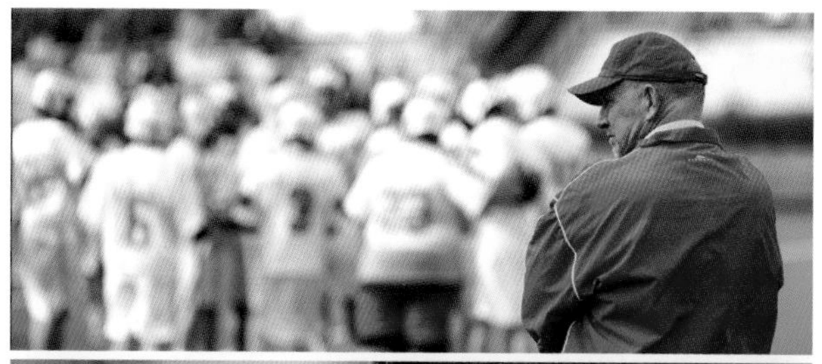

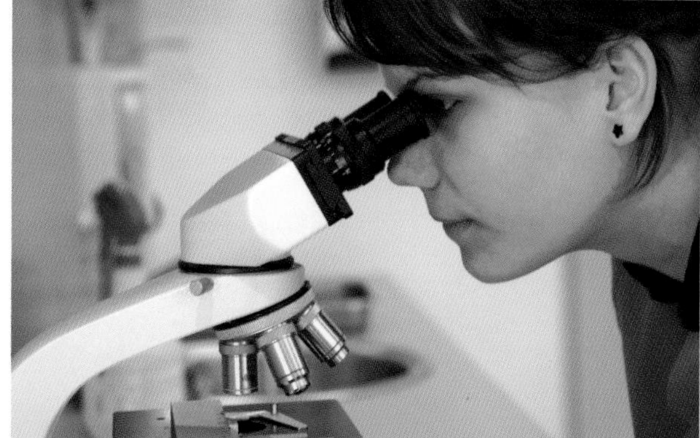

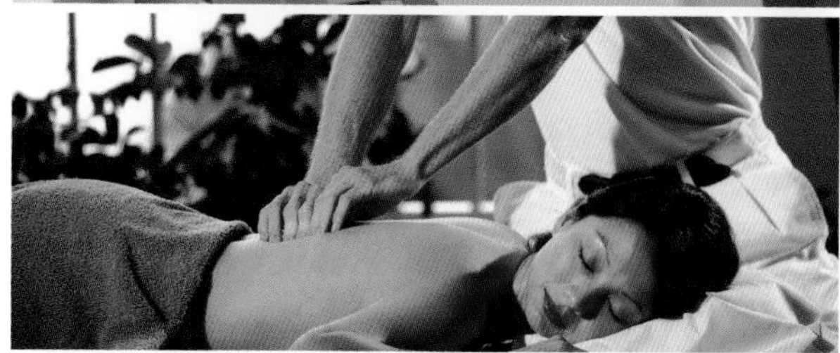

Figure 1.3 An ever-increasing number of students are choosing to pursue movement-related professions and health-related careers as the focus on health and wellness has grown.

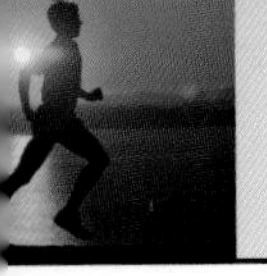

The Name Game

The Importance of Finding the Right Name

Through words we communicate our understanding of reality. Unlike numbers, which might have the same meaning to all, words are loaded with alternative interpretations, hence the frequency of misunderstandings in daily dialogue. The choice of words is a political act; the outcome of an interaction depends on the appropriateness of their selection. Similarly, the choice of labels to introduce and define ourselves, and most importantly to describe our field of study, has drastic consequences. It immediately implants images of what we do and who we are. We can wear the right label proudly, as a badge of respectability, or we can expend time and effort dispelling negative connotations from the minds of our audience if we pick an inappropriate term. Acceptability, credibility, and viability ride on our choice. Centrality in an organization (such as a university), funding for research, and our upward professional mobility are affected by how we project ourselves and how others view the reputation of our field.

The Contenders in the Name Game

Many names have been tried through the ages, some of which are preferred over kinesiology in particular institutional settings.

Physical Education

The most widely used name for our field throughout history has been **physical education**, sometimes joined by health, recreation, and dance to form HPERD departments. In some universities and in some societies other than North America, physical education might still be the best choice, particularly when the sole mission of that program is to prepare teachers of physical education for the public school system. However, a consensus seems to be forming in North American higher education that physical education is no longer the most appropriate descriptor for most programs, primarily because the field of study has undergone a curriculum metamorphosis in the latter part of the 20th century. The title *physical education* fails to adequately describe either the focus of study or the change in approach (Figure 1.4). Since the initiatives of Franklin Henry, the field has gradually been shifting toward a more scholarly, research-oriented, disciplinary approach. Forty years later the reality of kinesiology is far removed from stereotypes of physical education. Changing these stereotypes is problematic, because they are deeply rooted in traditional associations with the following:

- Activity programs encountered in K-12 that are devoid of academic content and rarely linked to the intellectual mission of the school.
- High school and college athletics programs that may, or may not, be based on the development of student-athletes. On the one hand, you would expect an individual who excels in athletic performance to gravitate toward the department that studies human movement. Many of these student-athletes excel in all spheres of learning and are so well rounded that they become leaders of the field, but some are

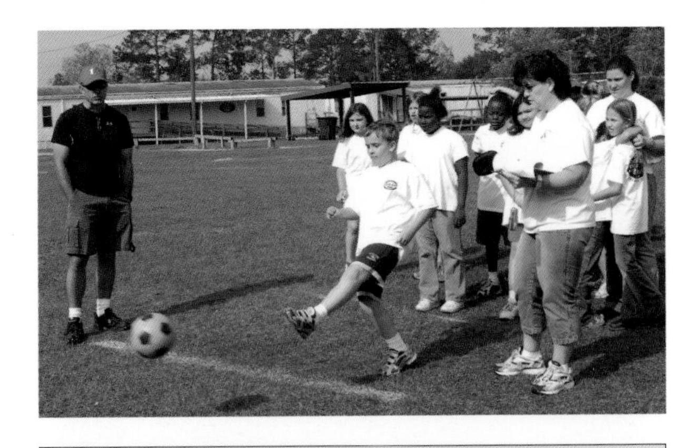

Figure 1.4 Although physical education has been the most widely used name for the field throughout history, this name may still be appropriate only for programs focusing on preparing teachers of physical education for the public school system.

marginal students with high athletic talent but low scholarly expectations. All too frequently in the past, teacher-coaches who taught physical education would "take care of" such athletes in the classroom, providing passing grades to ensure athletic eligibility regardless of academic performance. The damaging "easy major" stereotype that runs counter to the modern-day reality of academic excellence, terminal degrees, and cutting-edge research lingers on despite the best efforts of physical education reformers to eradicate them.

- One exclusive mission: the preparation of school teachers. Recently, the focus of professional preparation has broadened to encompass an array of alternative opportunities. The label *physical education* suggests one future career and one only, which complicates the lives of students who have chosen to study human movement in order to embark on professional pathways in fields far removed from teaching, such as health care or research.
- Labels that are limited and limiting. The word *physical* is too narrow to be used in the title. In a world of dichotomies, physical tends to suggest that the study of human movement is not intellectual, mental, or spiritual. Similarly, *education* is unnecessary and redundant in a university setting: Other departments do not add education to their titles (history education or mathematics education). And, once again, the word *education* is misleading in that it narrowly points toward a teaching degree in a setting where students are preparing for many other careers.

Other Names

Other names exist to describe the study of human movement. Many of them incorporate the words *exercise*, *sport*, *fitness*, and *human movement*, usually in combination with *science*, *studies*, or, less frequently, *arts*. The problem with such titles is their constricting capacity; such labels as exercise science by definition limit the focus of the program (to exercise) and eliminate alternative methodological approaches (except science). Because the label *physical education* is laden with stereotypes and entrenched in public misperception, and to avoid overly elaborate and complex titles such as human movement and sport studies, many academic units have opted to adopt the name change resolution proposed by the leaders in the field and reinforced when the American Academy of Physical Education changed its own name to the American Academy of Kinesiology and Physical Education.

Why Is Kinesiology the Name Game Winner?

Because it FITS best, where **FITS** stands for **F**ocus of study, **I**ntuitively appropriate, **T**reats all approaches equally, and **S**ounds right (Figure 1.5).

Focus of Study Above all, the name of the department should evoke the *focus of study* of that unit. The word *kinesiology* does just that; its roots can be traced back to ancient Greek terminology to literally mean the study of (*logy*) human action (*kin*). Consequently, this title clearly presents the central topic of human movement and represents all of the facets of this focus through a nonspecific umbrella term that covers exercise, fitness, sport, health, leisure, recreation, and play in a way that

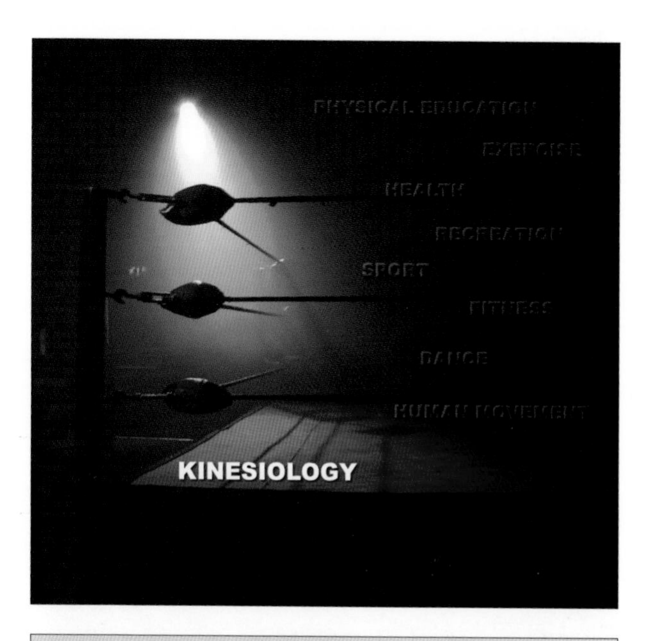

Figure 1.5 Of all the contenders in the name game, kinesiology has been thrust into the spotlight because it FITS.

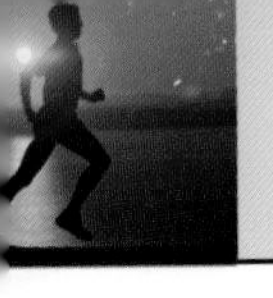

is broad and neutral, allowing its practitioners to study all aspects of human movement from the perspectives of the arts and sciences.

Intuitively Appropriate The title kinesiology is *intuitively appropriate* and meaningful to academia and society. Unlike many of the improvised proposals, kinesiology seems valid and familiar to the college community and the general population as it has been associated with the study of physical activity in higher education for at least a century, initially as a title for biomechanics and more recently as an umbrella term for the study of human movement.

Treats All Approaches Equally Kinesiology *treats all approaches equally*. The neutrality of *logy*, meaning the study of, provides leeway for a range of methodological approaches to human movement. Beneath this term, natural science, social science, and humanities approaches are all permissible, as opposed to the restrictive titles that legitimate only one focus and one approach, such as sport science.

Sounds Right It *sounds right* in that it draws on the historic roots of the word, it evokes the mission of the field, and the word has obvious academic linkage, sounding much like other science and social science departments (e.g., biology, sociology, psychology, anthropology). Although it evokes the "feel" of these department names, it is unique, which allows it to remain independent and intact rather than subsidiary to another field. It is brief and avoids the problem of patchwork titles designed to be all-inclusive that combine several different areas of study into one long department name. At the same time it covers all the bases and offers opportunities for greater cooperation, collaboration, and integration between a true community of scholars in the field.

Spheres of Scholarly Study

The Diversity of Higher Education

For any field of scholarly study to be universally accepted in a nation's higher education system, it must be able to fit into a wide range of college and university models from community colleges to research universities, from technical colleges to liberal arts universities. Although the basic building blocks of the academic field may remain constant, the design and function of the curriculum should vary with the mission of the university if the academic field is going to be a good fit in that institution. As it has expanded from teacher training settings to all of the other types of universities and colleges, the emerging field of kinesiology has broadened its appeal in recent years.

Training Physical Education Teachers

The traditional mission of training physical education teachers remains intact and strong in schools

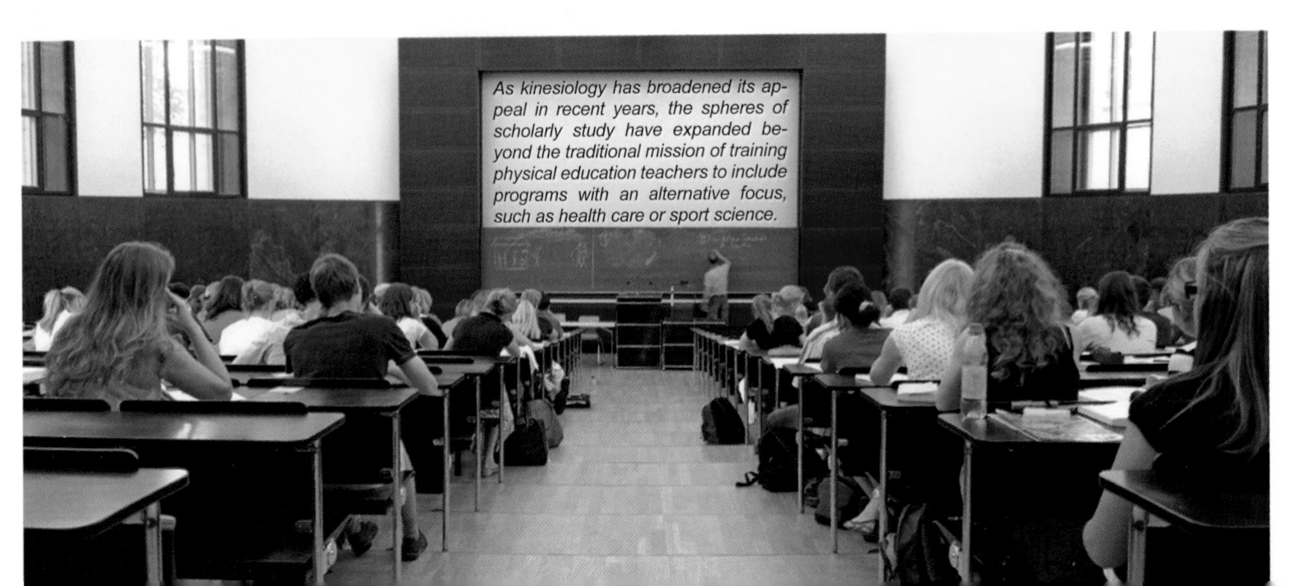

As kinesiology has broadened its appeal in recent years, the spheres of scholarly study have expanded beyond the traditional mission of training physical education teachers to include programs with an alternative focus, such as health care or sport science.

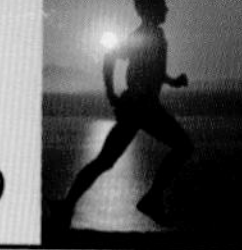

of education, but the study of human movement has also taken hold in settings where teacher preparation is not a priority but where there is an alternative focus, such as health care or sport science.

Even schools of education are introducing more comprehensive and broad-based training for future teachers. The face of teacher education is changing to include more substantive and relevant academic subject matter, a more rigorous general education and subject matter preparation, and more sophisticated clinical aspects of teacher preparation programs interspersed throughout the professional component of the program. In many cases, student teachers who would previously have obtained their teaching certification through a four-year program combining academic subject matter and professional methodology courses will now complete a four-year subject-based undergraduate degree before proceeding to complete their education certification in a fifth year.

Beyond the Gym

Through the years, the percentage of kinesiology programs preparing students for professions other than education and in the liberal arts has grown, and as they have taken on the shape and mission of their parent institutions, they have flourished, in part because professions such as medicine, law, and business are changing to seek people with more than basic technological capability. They want to attract more comprehensively educated individuals to populate their professions. For example, medical schools are seeking more broadly trained college graduates with a background in the humanities and in the social as well as the natural sciences – individuals who have a common foundation of knowledge, skills, values, and attitudes and a sound general liberal arts and science baccalaureate education.

To be acceptable within the university community, kinesiology must be seen to contribute to the mission of undergraduate education, as interpreted by each particular institution of higher learning, in a unique and important way. This is even true in a liberal arts university, where programs of study are not focused on professional preparation for any particular vocation, but where the ideal of learning is the acquisition of knowledge as its own reward. A liberal education is not directly linked to the job market in the narrow vocational sense of developing professional competencies; rather, a liberal education is a liberating experience. It allows faculty and students to develop critical consciousness and cultural awareness through teaching and learning, research, and publication. Yet liberal education is not divorced from the professions. The fundamental knowledge about human movement, considered in its broadest context, provides an invaluable foundation for professional training. It facilitates the growth of the independent learner, one who has learned to think and to reason and to compare and to discriminate and who will consequently be an asset in any job market and in all future professional and life changes.

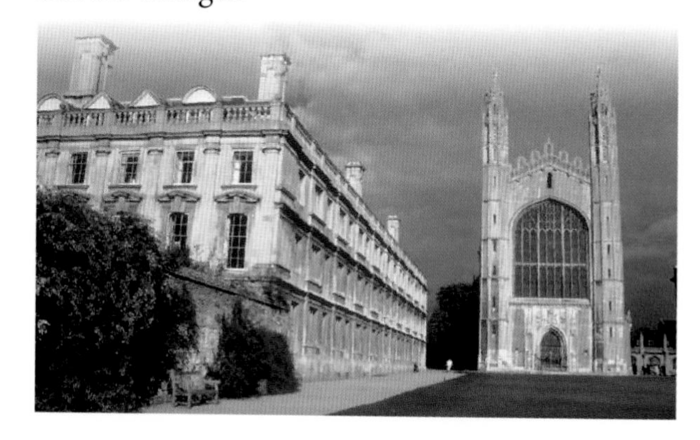

The Inclusiveness of Kinesiology

Kinesiology is not a one size fits all approach to the study of human movement. It is malleable enough that it can be modified for different purposes, in part because it is organized horizontally (as well as vertically) on a cross-disciplinary basis to include **exercise physiology**, **motor learning**, **motor development**, **biomechanics**, and the roles of athletics, dance, and other physical activities in our culture. By its very nature, kinesiology is an ideal foundational component of the undergraduate experience.

Human movement is an ever-present phenomenon in that everybody moves, so it is a good starting point for study because we

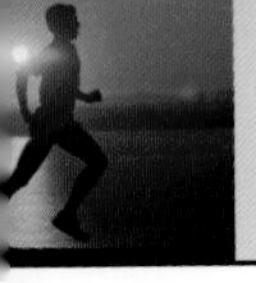

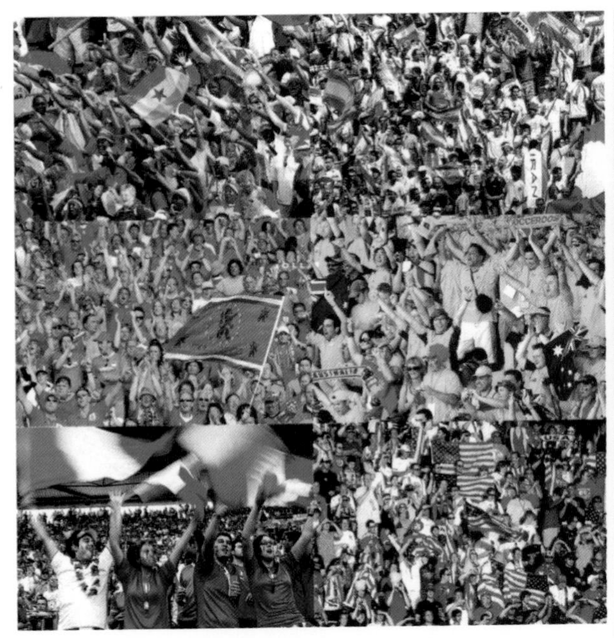

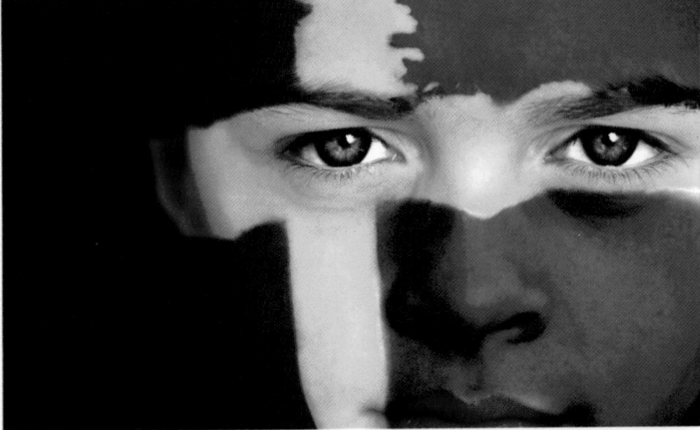

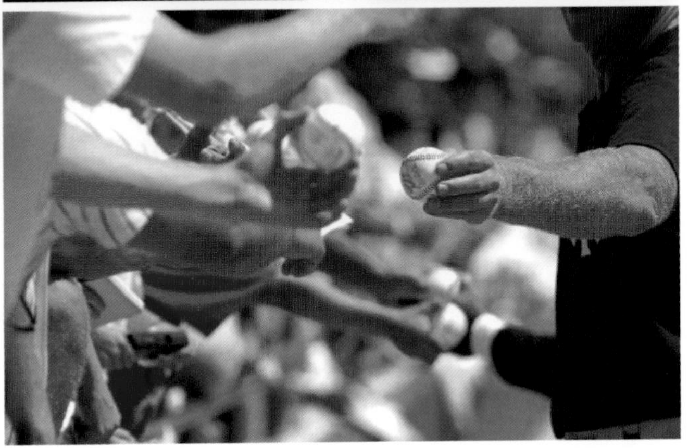

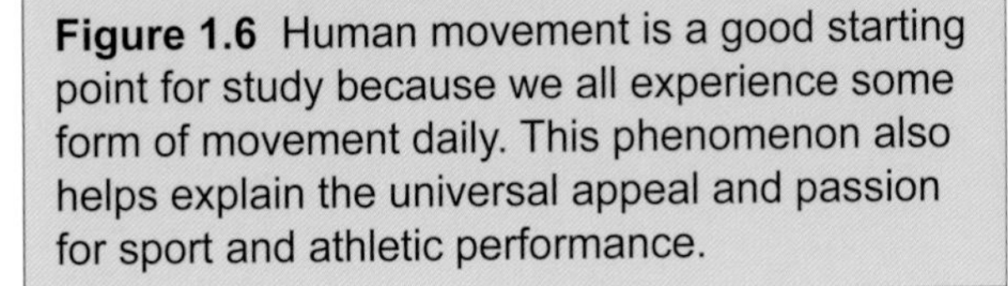

Figure 1.6 Human movement is a good starting point for study because we all experience some form of movement daily. This phenomenon also helps explain the universal appeal and passion for sport and athletic performance.

all experience our bodies daily. One form of movement – sport – is extraordinarily popular, to the extent that it is almost a universal language with a shared vocabulary that stimulates passionate and enthusiastic interaction (Figure 1.6). The widespread participation, the abundance of information and statistics, and the cultural meanings of sport fuel a significant research agenda. Consequently, the study of athletic performance is an appealing, attractive focus. Similarly, the link between health and human movement is particularly attractive to individuals who are interested in disease prevention and health promotion. Kinesiology has a clearly defined central focus as its exclusive academic terrain and is constantly evolving to provide access to a variety of rewarding careers.

Kinesiology approaches human movement from diverse perspectives, thus exposing students to an array of teaching styles and ways of thinking because of the range of concepts from the humanities, social sciences, and natural sciences and the practical experience of movement skills in the curriculum. Human movement is, by definition, a dynamic phenomenon that can be understood through both intellectual abstraction and experience. A range of experiential teaching and learning conditions may be developed within the context of kinesiology. Each of these might be designed not only to educate students in the use of their bodies but also to use physical activity to illuminate the theoretical concepts that underlie the study of human movement and to prepare students for the physical challenges of their future professions.

The Value of Our Knowledge Bases

With appropriate prerequisites from the traditional disciplines in the humanities and the physical, biological, and social sciences, a core curriculum has traditionally been planned that systematically presents nine areas of knowledge in the study of human movement: human anatomy/function; physical growth and motor development; biomechanical aspects of movement; exercise physiology; behavioral and neuromuscular control of movement; motor skill acquisition; psychological factors in movement, exercise, and sport; sociocultural factors in movement, exercise, and sport; and history/philosophy of movement, exercise, and sport.

The academic study of human movement has changed in both form and function. Professional opportunities are changing radically, and disciplines tend to take their shape from the changing face and needs of society. For example, as changing health needs and biotechnology come to the forefront, more emphasis might be placed in the kinesiology curriculum on cell physiology/tissue system physiology, anatomy, biomechanics, neuroscience/motor control, motor learning, social psychology, anthropology of human movement, and philosophic thought, particularly ethics. The units outlined in *Foundations of Kinesiology* will focus on the biophysical perspective of human movement.

Experiencing the Body of Knowledge

Personal Applications

The reason that so many students are selecting kinesiology as their primary area of study and that scholars are finding it to be a fruitful avenue of research is no mystery. Human movement is so topical that it is "*now*," its serious scholarly study is *new*, and the outcome of kinesiology is significant *new knowledge now*. What sets kinesiology apart from other subject fields in higher education is the personal impact of the study of human movement. Where else can you experience the body of knowledge so profoundly? As you read *Foundations of Kinesiology*, you will realize how meaningful these concepts and experiences can be in your **OWN** lives.

Human movement affects everyone's personal health and performance. It has powerful potential in our lives, in our cultures, and beyond, yet it is something we all own in our own unique ways. The significance of **OWN**ership in the context of the meaning of movement is that it helps us define **O**urselves, it contributes to our **W**ell-being, and it is a medium to display and enhance our **N**atural talents.

Defining forms of human movement in discrete categories, using such tactics as the OWN approach, is valuable in helping to isolate different aspects, but the methodology should not obscure the malleability of movement. All forms of human movement interlock and sometimes interlace; they touch each other, sometimes overlap, and even merge. It is conceivable that during a given activity an individual may move from one realm to another freely and frequently, from health-related activity that might also be categorized as athletic performance even as it leads to self-definition and self-actualization.

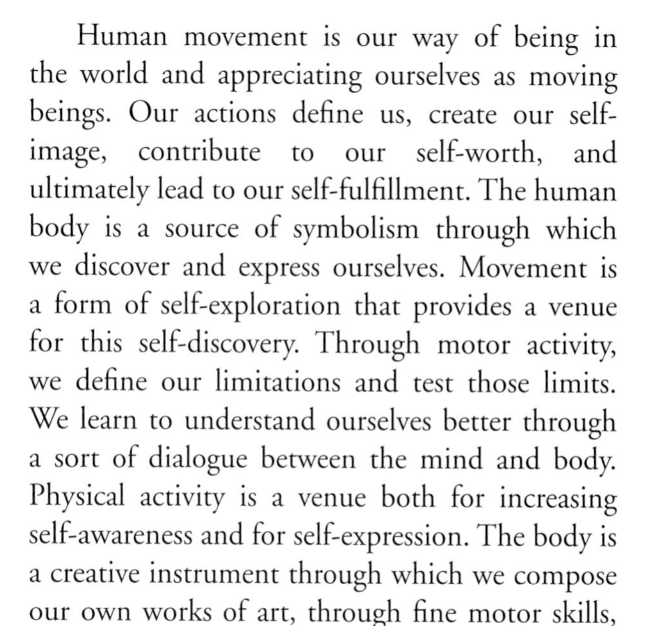

Human movement is our way of being in the world and appreciating ourselves as moving beings. Our actions define us, create our self-image, contribute to our self-worth, and ultimately lead to our self-fulfillment. The human body is a source of symbolism through which we discover and express ourselves. Movement is a form of self-exploration that provides a venue for this self-discovery. Through motor activity, we define our limitations and test those limits. We learn to understand ourselves better through a sort of dialogue between the mind and body. Physical activity is a venue both for increasing self-awareness and for self-expression. The body is a creative instrument through which we compose our own works of art, through fine motor skills, such as those necessary for brush strokes and sculpting, or the precise movements of ballet and formal gymnastics. Alternatively, creativity may be expressed in the free-flowing form of contemporary dance, outdoor adventure activities, or spontaneous play. Body language is an essential piece of the jigsaw of how we interact and express ourselves beyond the realm of our athletic endeavors; it also supplements our verbal communication in daily interaction. Personal meanings can be expressed even when we are deprived of words, thanks to human movement that we develop into a language of the body to enable communication.

Kinesiology has unique personal application in the realm of well-being and human movement. No other subject field in a university has such immediate personal impact as the study of health-related human movement. In many cases, academic subject fields are detached from the lived reality of a student, whereas kinesiology has immediate bearing on lifestyle and well-being (Figure 1.7). Since Western society entered the era of lifestyle disease, our choices and habits tend to lead alternatively to well-being or such modern-day killers as obesity, heart disease, and cancer. In this medical milieu, it is critically important to be well informed. The independent learner in university becomes the independent decision maker in life. Kinesiology prepares students to wisely make those lifestyle choices that will help determine their future quality of life.

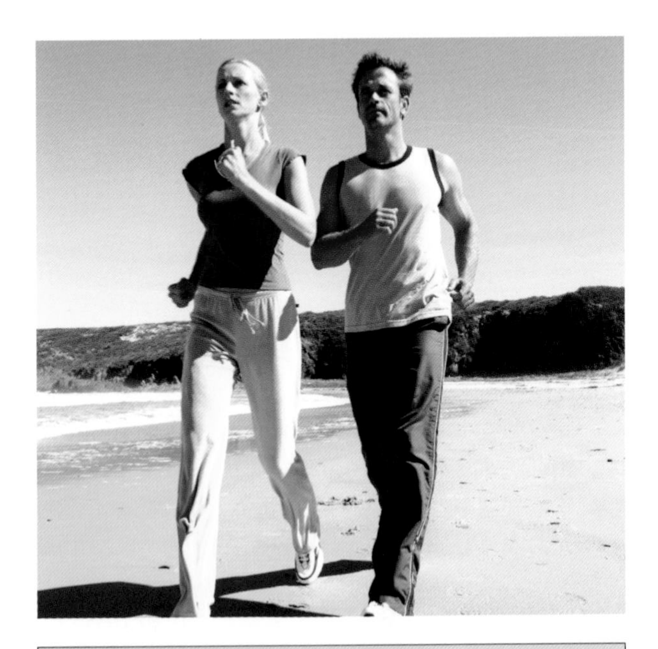

Figure 1.7 No other subject field in a university has such immediate personal impact as the study of health-related human movement, especially since our lifestyle choices and habits directly affect our quality of life.

Natural talent enhancement is an enticing feature of kinesiology. Many students are attracted to the study of human movement because they love to move, they enjoy athletic activity, and they either want to enhance their own performance or share in the enterprise of studying and improving the athletic performance of others. Kinesiology is the field of study that gives athletically inclined individuals direct access to cutting-edge research and state-of-the-art equipment. Performance using natural talents transcends the playing field. It embraces every venue where physical skill is a prerequisite for success.

The knowledge and skills acquired through kinesiology will enhance the unique performance needs of all: the artist as much as the athlete, the sculptor as much as the skater. It extends beyond the demands of athleticism and artistry to incorporate the physical challenges of the workplace: the skills of physical therapy or athletic training, of medicine or mountain rescue. Motor development and motor learning, anatomy and physiology, and adapted and even physical activity classes can enhance natural talent for people of all skill levels, regardless of physical condition, special needs, or age. The activity service program can be truly self-serving in that it can be designed to help all students develop the skills and natural talents they will need in their future work and play. Kinesiology therefore has extraordinary personal meaning and universal applicability for all students who have a desire to enhance their own natural talents.

Public Implications

Health and human movement are central concerns of all societies today. Education and the dispersal of knowledge can lead to the eradication of many modern-day diseases across the globe. From issues of public health to the condition

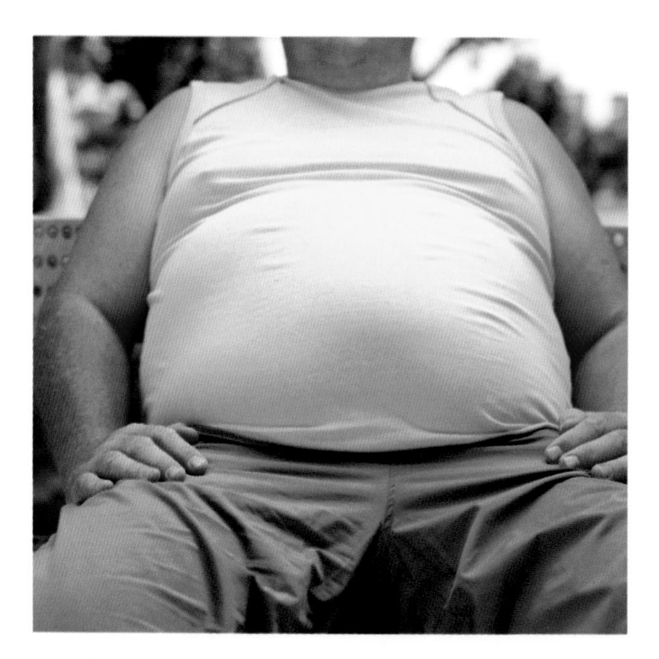

Figure 1.8 Kinesiology students will leave university armed with the knowledge and skills that are necessary to combat the multitude of lifestyle-related diseases and to promote healthy active living.

of the environment, how we understand and tackle the pressing health-related issues of our day will affect the well-being and economy of a nation. Kinesiology is a natural stepping stone for students who want to make a difference through the transmission of health-related learning. They will leave the university armed with the knowledge and skills that are necessary to combat lifestyle-related diseases and to promote health and enhance human performance, such as informed analyses of the cause and prevention of obesity, heart disease, cancer, and AIDS and research-based programs of exercise and nutrition (Figure 1.8).

Similarly, conceptual and experiential fluency in the fundamentals of skill enhancement will be extraordinarily valuable in tomorrow's world, where public demand for quality human performance shows no signs of abating. From the highest level of sport to the daily routine of activity, people expect improvement and success. The public implication of kinesiology is that its skills and knowledge are the foundation of the enhanced movement of the world population, so the professional promise is exciting.

Professional Promise

Driven both by the opportunities of the marketplace and by changing perceptions of the importance of the study of health-related movement, the core curriculum in kinesiology is changing. More emphasis is being placed on understanding human movement and learning about the fundamental qualities of movement for its own sake and for the sake of promoting health and human movement in society. In this way, each aspect of kinesiology is presented in the broader context of the study of human movement, and students become liberally educated as they absorb specialized information that will be useful in their professional futures without ever losing sight of the bigger picture.

A modern university is much more than a diploma factory; its intent is to create independent learners. In each class offered in a kinesiology curriculum, students will encounter liberal learning skills in varying ways. For example, critical thinking skills are emphasized heavily in philosophy classes, whereas biomechanics classes lean more heavily on scientific and quantitative modes of enquiry. Kinesiology grounded in these scientific bases of human movement is an excellent undergraduate springboard to the biophysical medical and allied health professions, particularly those that use physical activity, play, and exercise as therapy, and to the research and development of human performance, motor development, and physical activity and sport in society. The increasing choice for students created by a broadening of approaches and missions in kinesiology in recent years has led to a wider range of professional promise and a very bright future.

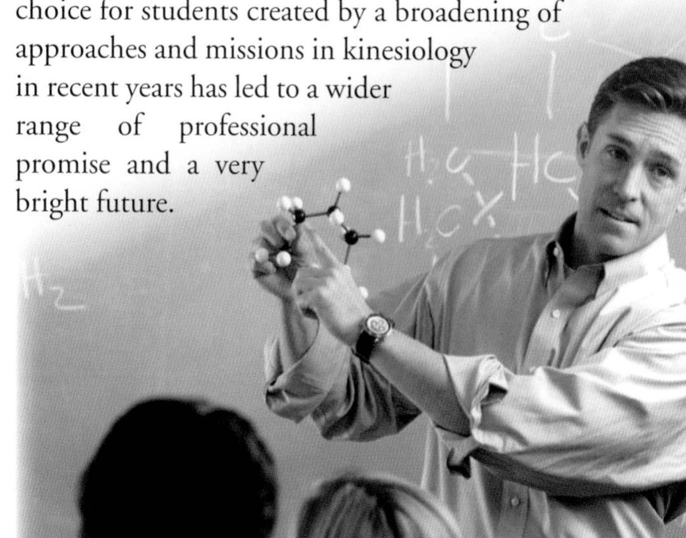

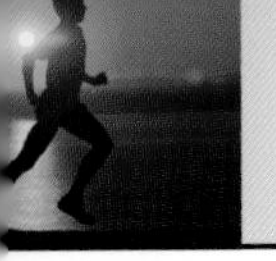

What the Future Holds

The emerging field of kinesiology is relatively new, malleable, and volatile, so ideas abound about what direction the field should take in the future, most particularly in *Quest*, the scholarly journal of the National Association for Kinesiology and Physical Education in Higher Education. The purpose of this journal is to stimulate professional development by publishing articles about issues that are critical to kinesiology in higher education; much of the groundbreaking discussion of this topic can be found in its pages (or online at www.HumanKinetics.com/Quest).

A review of this scholarly literature confirms that the highway ahead does not guarantee smooth passage, the quality of the programs will be uneven, and travelers may experience bumps along the way relative to the name and nature of the field. The name game will continue unabated. Even as the National Research Council has recently recognized kinesiology as a legitimate field of scientific study, academic units on many campuses will cling to alternative titles that are considered to better describe the approach at that university. The diversity of names reflects the potential fragmentation of the field, most particularly the division between approaches that emphasize the subdisciplines, professional preparation, and motor performance.

Typically, the subdisciplinary approach is heavily scientific and research oriented; the professional approach is premised on the preparation of physical education teachers; and the motor performance approach places a high premium on sport, exercise, and physical activity performance classes. The subdisciplinary approach has many advantages, most particularly the high regard of the college community, but when taken to an extreme, it creates division and isolation within a department. In a worst-case scenario, the corporate identity of the department is threatened. Professional preparation and physical activity are forced to take a back seat, while the scientists work alone in their laboratories, neither comprehending the research of colleagues ensconced in their own silos (silos are the vertical structures that hold the subdisciplines, such as biomechanics, physiology, motor control, sport psychology, and philosophy, and that tend to divide them from each other), nor caring about the contribution of the professional

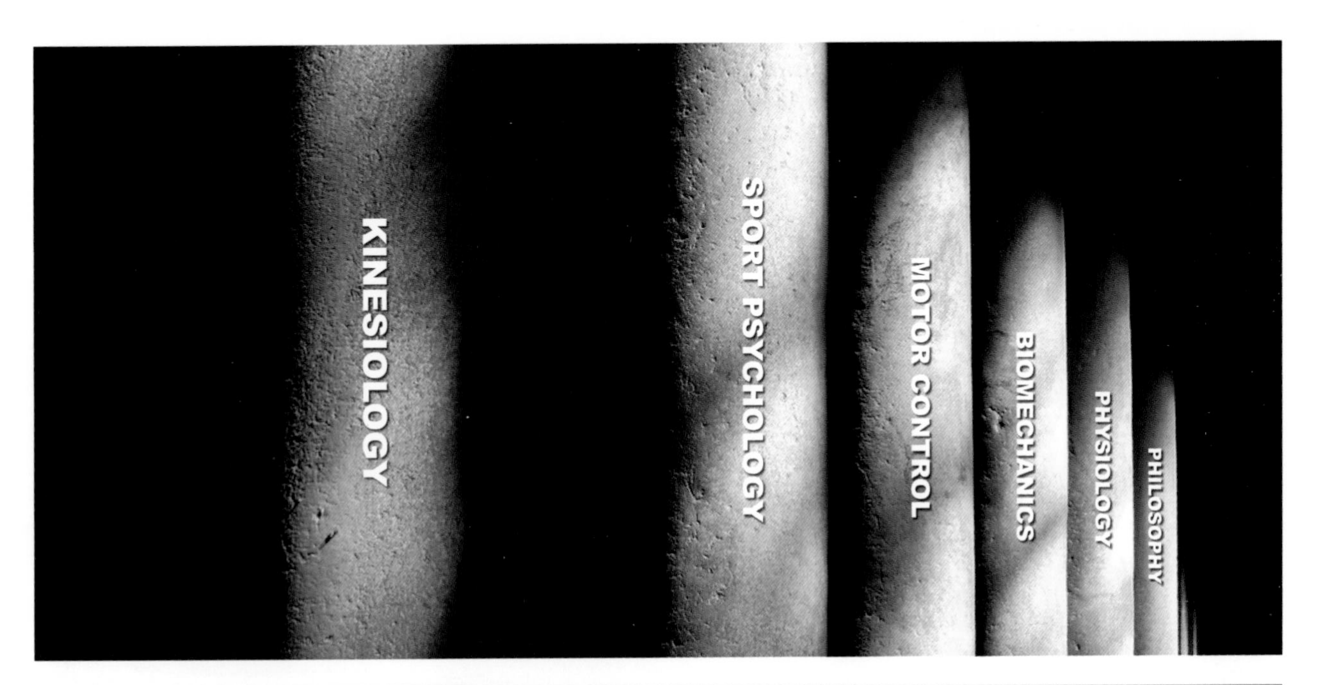

Figure 1.9 Although the subdisciplinary approach has its advantages, it can create division and isolation within a department when taken to an extreme.

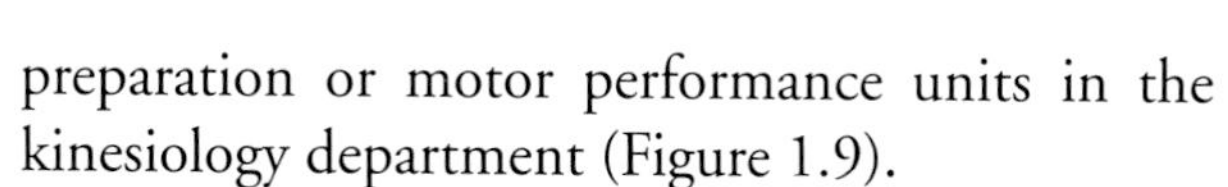

preparation or motor performance units in the kinesiology department (Figure 1.9).

In a penetrating paper published in the November 2007 edition of *Quest*, Scott Kretchmar, a leading philosopher in the field, suggests a new paradigm for the future of kinesiology in which silo-limited research is rejected in favor of thematic, cross-disciplinary work that focuses on a problem from multiple perspectives at once.

New ways of looking at the field are necessary to understand the vibrant interconnections of the multifaceted study of health and human movement. A hope for the future is that this new emphasis on collaborative research will tend to create bridges within departments between pure and applied, theory and practice, science and everything else.

Summary

In this chapter, we review the evolution of kinesiology – how and why it has taken its current form and focus – and we make reference to some of the individuals who have been most influential in defining its current shape.

The study of health and kinesiology is very popular because of the increasing recognition of the importance of health-related and skill-related human movement and because it has the ability to accommodate a range of educational purposes. Human movement, performance, and health enhancement are researchable from a wide range of social, cultural, behavioral, and biophysical perspectives, which makes kinesiology of great interest to us individually and to the larger global community.

Kinesiology focuses on scholarly disciplinary knowledge and prepares professionals for a range of health and human movement fields. It can be structured as a preprofessional program leading to any number of health- and human movement-related fields and as a liberal arts major with clear and viable professional applications.

Key Terms

biomechanics
exercise physiology
kinesiology
motor development
motor learning
physical education
proactive health
reactive health
wellness

Discussion Questions

1. Why was it necessary to find a common name and focus for the academic field of human movement?
2. Discuss the relationship between health, human movement, and kinesiology.
3. Briefly describe five types of individual competition in sport.
4. Explain why the name *physical education* is both limiting and misleading.
5. Describe how the name *kinesiology* evokes the focus of study of the field.
6. Why is the study of sport and athletic performance so appealing?

7. Identify the nine areas of knowledge that represent the core curriculum of human movement.

8. Briefly discuss the relationship between human movement and our sense of self.

9. How does a degree in kinesiology prepare graduates to tackle health-related issues in our society?

10. Identify the biggest disadvantage of the subdisciplinary approach. How will collaborative research solve this problem?

UNIT 1

Anatomical Kinesiology

- Human Anatomy: The Pieces of the Body Puzzle
- Out of Harm's Way: Sports Injuries

In This Chapter:

CHAPTER 2

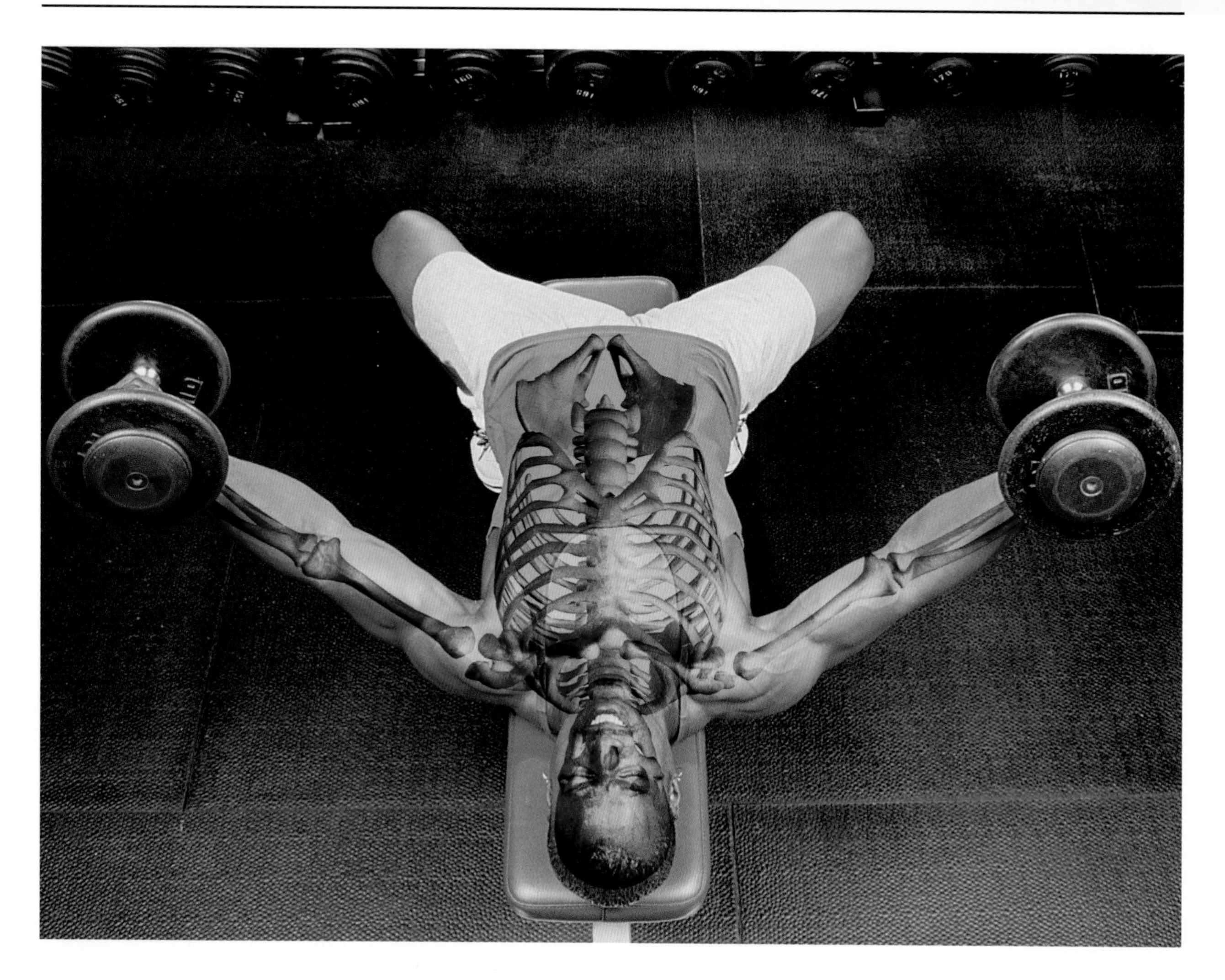

Human Anatomy: The Pieces of the Body Puzzle

After completing this chapter you should be able to:

- demonstrate an understanding of the basis for anatomical description and analysis;
- use correct anatomical terminology when describing the human body and performance;
- describe the various parts of the skeletal and muscular systems and the ways in which they relate to human performance;
- demonstrate an understanding of the organization and complexity of human anatomy.

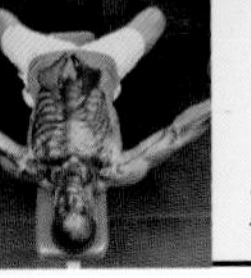

The human body has fascinated the human mind for centuries. What enables us to run, jump, and throw? How are we able to move our fingers with such remarkable dexterity? What are the structures that allow us to perform the myriad of tasks we do? The study of the structures that make up the human body, and how those structures relate to each other, is called **human anatomy**. Questions concerning human anatomy continue to capture the curiosity of human beings worldwide because it is a subject that binds all humans together. An understanding of how our bodies are structured to perform is important if we are to gain our full potential, especially in the world of sport and physical activity.

It is important to realize that structure often determines function; the structures of the human body are well designed for efficient movement. You have probably marvelled at the strength of the human skeleton that is able to withstand great impact and stress, not to mention its light weight that allows movements to be swift and active. The human body is undoubtedly a strong, flexible, well-oiled machine, able to move and perform with astonishing efficiency (Figure 2.1). But what structures allow some power lifters to lift weights two or three times their own body weight? How does Tyson Gay run a distance of 100 meters under 10 seconds?

In fact, how are we able to stand upright and move against gravity and other forces? The science of anatomy attempts to shed light on these and other questions, as well as to provide answers based on the complex and intricate structure of the human body.

Many systems make up the human body. Some of them are the respiratory, urogenital, cardiovascular, nervous, endocrine, digestive, and musculoskeletal. The cardiovascular and nervous systems are essential to the musculoskeletal system and are presented in Chapters 7 and 11, respectively. In this chapter we will deal with the musculoskeletal system.

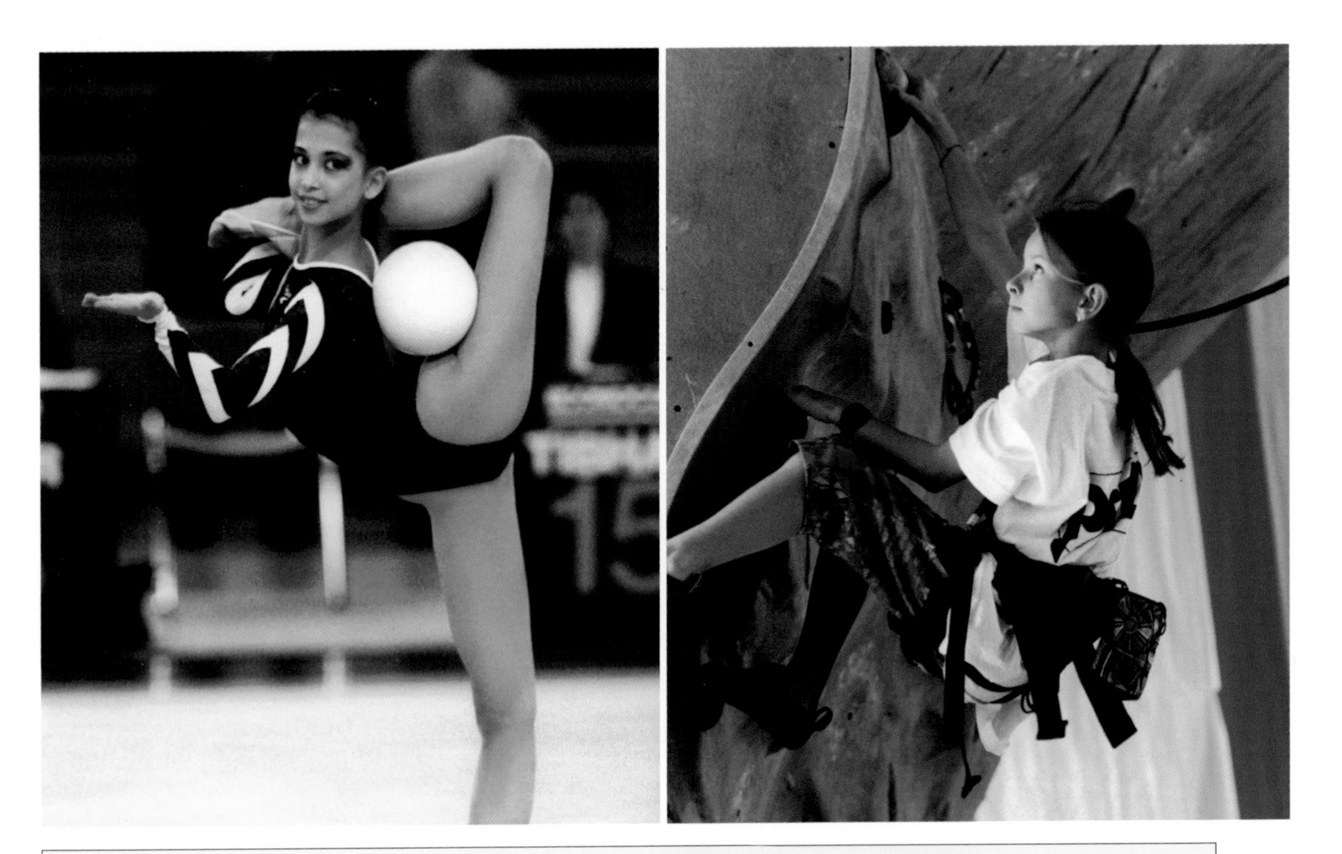

Figure 2.1 The human body is capable of moving gracefully and performing very challenging tasks.

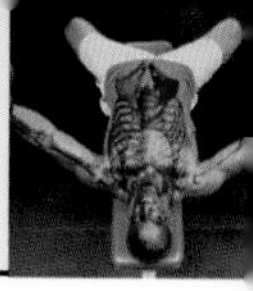

Terms and Concepts Worth Knowing

In order to describe anatomy with clarity, there is a certain language or terminology to be learned. The language of anatomy may be difficult to grasp at first because it is largely unfamiliar to you; but once you gain a general understanding of the word roots, suffixes, and prefixes commonly used in anatomy, the terminology will become increasingly meaningful. For example, if you know that *myo* refers to muscle and that *cardio* pertains to the heart, you can reach the conclusion that *myocardium* refers to the muscle of the heart. The knowledge of some basic terms and concepts is invaluable for improving your understanding of anatomy.

Front to Back

The terms "ventral" and "dorsal" were used originally to describe positions in four-legged animals. In bipedal humans (two-legged animals such as ourselves) the terms "anterior" and "posterior" are used. However, the terminology "ventral" and "dorsal" may appear in some texts.

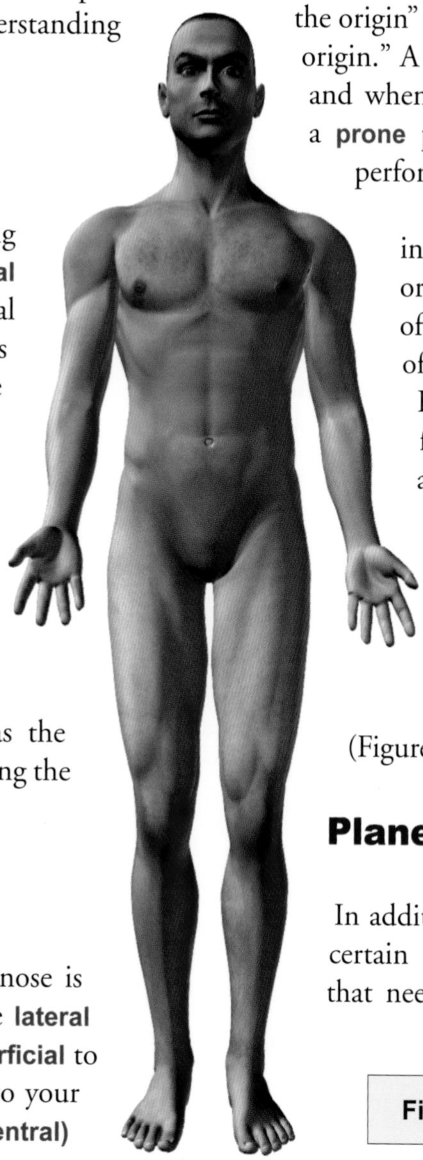

Anatomical Position

Of particular importance to studying anatomy is the basic **anatomical position**. It is used in all anatomical description, specifying the locations of specific parts of the body relative to other body parts; it can best be learned by you, the student, in the following position: standing erect, facing forward, arms hanging at the sides with palms facing forward, legs straight, and heels and feet together and parallel to each other. The anatomical position is universally accepted as the starting reference point for describing the human body (Figure 2.2).

Directional Terms

In the anatomical position, your nose is **medial** to your eyes, your ears are **lateral** to your cheeks, your skin lies **superficial** to your muscles, your heart is **deep** to your ribcage, your lips are **anterior (ventral)** to your teeth, your back is **posterior (dorsal)** to your abdomen, and your lips are **superior** to your chin. Also, the hands are **distal** to the arms, and the arms are **proximal** to the hands. The terms proximal and distal are also used to describe nerves and blood vessels, proximal meaning "toward the origin" and distal meaning "away from the origin." A person lying on his back is **supine** and when lying face down is said to be in a **prone** position (e.g., when preparing to perform a push-up).

Each of the terms described here indicates the location of a body part or position in relation to another part of the body, giving a clear indication of where body parts may be found. If you want to locate the abdomen, for example, you would say, "The abdomen is **inferior** to the thorax," rather than saying, "The abdomen is below the thorax." It is important to note, however, that directional terms are based on the assumption that the body is in the anatomical position (Figure 2.2).

Planes of the body

In addition to directional terms, there are certain planes (imaginary flat surfaces) that need to be defined and understood;

Figure 2.2 The anatomical position.

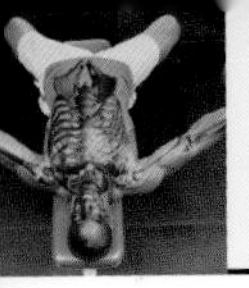

Directional Terms

Superior – *Nearer to the head*
The head is superior to the thorax.

Inferior – *Nearer to the feet*
The stomach is inferior to the heart.

Anterior (Ventral) – *Nearer to the front*
The quadriceps are anterior to the hamstrings.

Posterior (Dorsal) – *Nearer to the back*
The hamstrings are posterior to the quadriceps.

Superficial – *Nearer to the surface of the body*
The skin is more superficial than muscle.

Deep – *Farther from the surface of the body*
The heart lies deep to the ribs.

Medial – *Nearer to the median plane*
The nose is medial to the eyes.

Lateral – *Farther from the median plane*
The eyes are lateral to the nose.

Distal – *Farther from the trunk*
The hands are distal to the arms.

Proximal – *Nearer to the trunk*
The arms are proximal to the hands.

they divide the body for further identification of particular areas. These terms always refer to the body in the anatomical position. For an individual standing in the anatomical position, the point at which the median, frontal, and transverse planes intersect represents the body's center of gravity (center of mass).

The **median plane** or **midsagittal plane** is a vertical plane that bisects the body into right and left halves; the **sagittal plane** is any plane parallel to the median plane; the **frontal plane** or **coronal plane** is any vertical plane at right angles to the median plane; and the **transverse plane** or **horizontal plane** is any plane at right angles to both the median and frontal planes (Figure 2.3).

These planes can also be used to describe different movements or actions, being described as sagittal, frontal, or transverse plane movements when they occur in a plane that is parallel to one of these planes. For example, a forward roll would be considered a **sagittal plane movement** because the forward and backward motion is parallel to the sagittal plane. Other sagittal plane movements include cycling and running. Similarly, movements that are lateral, or side-to-side in nature, can be described as **frontal plane movements**; some good examples are cartwheels, jumping jacks, and side-stepping. Can you think of any activities that would be considered **transverse plane movements**? How about a twist performed by a diver, or a pirouette in ballet?

Although many movements do not occur in any one plane, large movements and movements that occur at joints can often be described as being sagittal, frontal, or transverse plane movements; therefore, these reference planes still remain useful for describing human movement.

Joint Movements

Most movements are often found in pairs: for every movement, there is generally a movement that is opposite to it. There are exceptions, but the following descriptions apply to most joints and are illustrated in Figure 2.4.

Flexion–Extension

This usually occurs in a sagittal plane. In general, **flexion** reduces the angle between two bones at a joint and **extension** increases it. Consider the elbow joint when a biceps curl is performed. Lifting the weight requires flexion (reducing the angle at the joint), while lowering the weight involves extension (increasing the angle at the joint). These terms are modified in certain actions, for example, at the ankle joint, where the terms *dorsiflexion* (motion bringing the top of the foot toward the lower leg or shin) and *plantar flexion* ("planting" the foot) are used.

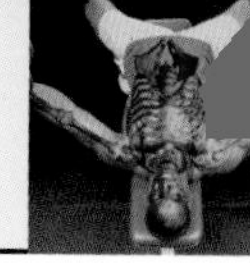

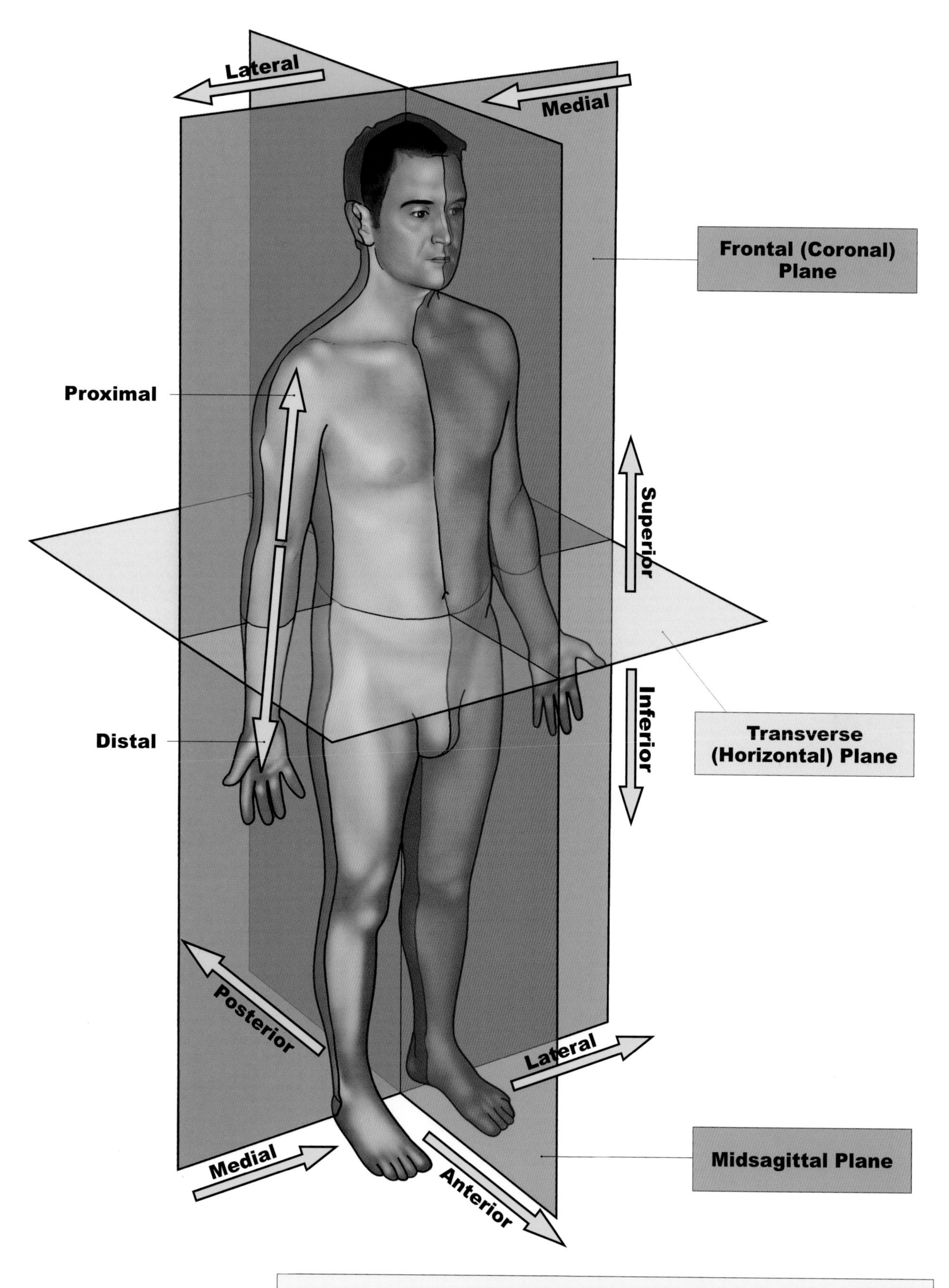

Figure 2.3 Anatomical position, directional terms, and planes of the body.

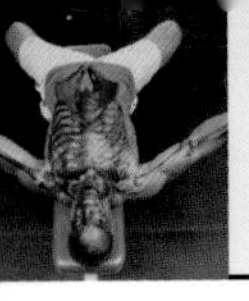

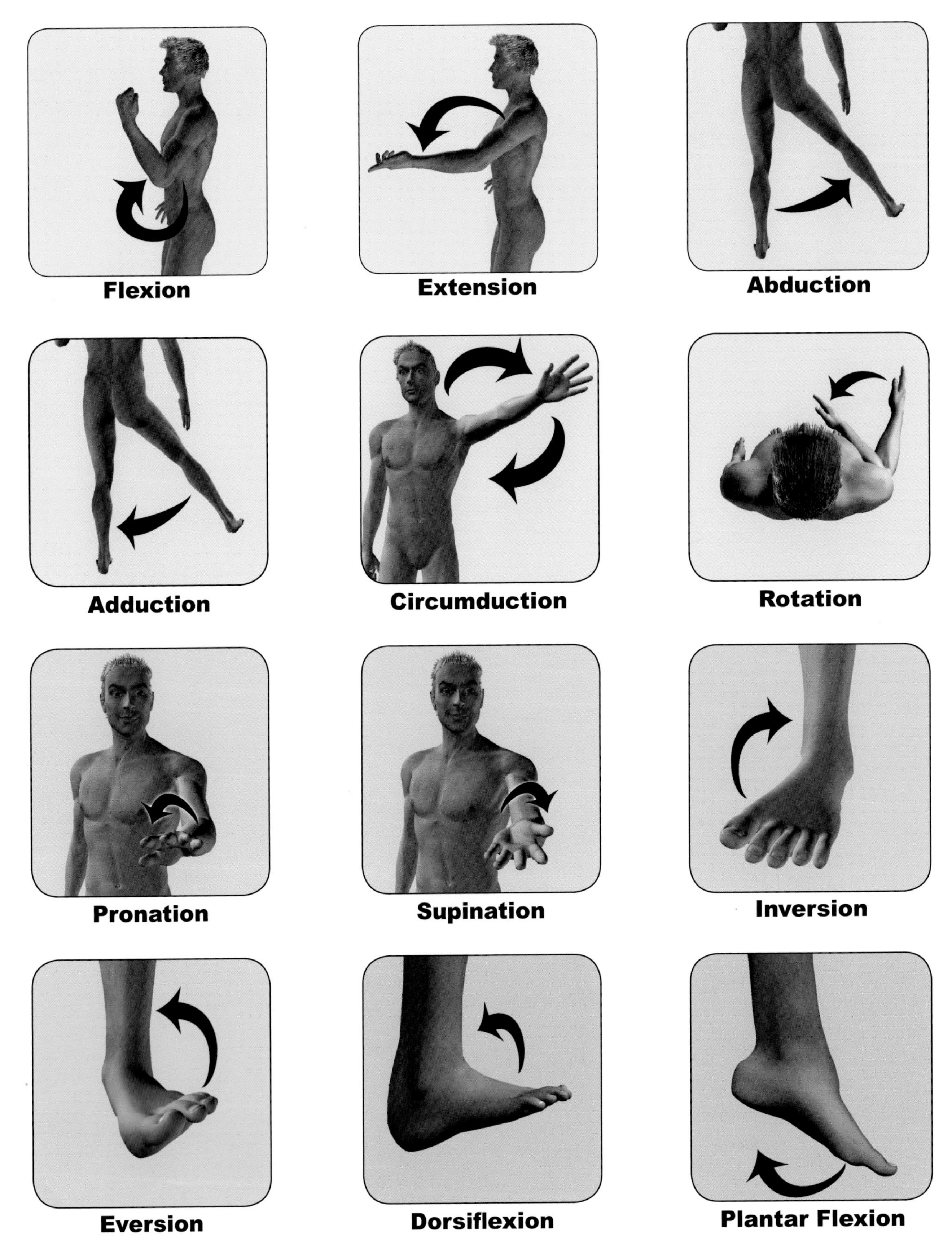

Figure 2.4 Major body movements around joints.

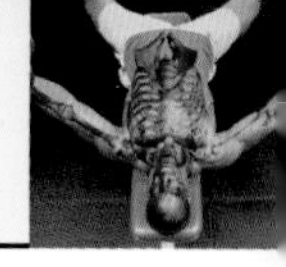

Abduction–Adduction

In general, **abduction** is movement away from the midline of the body and **adduction** is movement toward the midline of the body in the frontal plane. The motions of the arms and legs during a jumping jack are examples of these two types of movements.

Circumduction

When flexion–extension movements are combined with abduction–adduction movements, a cone of movement occurs but does not include any rotation. Tracing an imaginary circle in the air with your index finger while the rest of the hand remains stationary produces **circumduction**. The tip of your finger represents the base of the cone, while your knuckle forms the apex of this conical motion. This movement can occur at other moving body segments such as the hip and shoulder.

Rotation

A bone may also rotate along its longitudinal axis. To illustrate this action, flex your right elbow, place your left hand on your right shoulder, and now rotate your right arm so that your hand is carried toward your abdomen. This movement toward the median plane is called **medial** or **internal rotation**. When you rotate your arm back to the original position or out laterally, this is called **lateral** or **external rotation**.

Pronation–Supination

This movement is used to describe movements relative to the forearm and hand. When the palm is moved to face anteriorly, this is **supination** (you can hold a bowl of soup); when the palm is moved to face posteriorly, it is **pronation**. These actions are required when turning a door knob, opening a jar, or performing a topspin shot in tennis.

Inversion–Eversion

This movement is relative to the sole of the foot. When the sole is turned inward (as when you "go over" on your ankle) it is inverted: this movement is called **inversion**. Injuries are common at the ankle joint, occurring when the joint is severely inverted beyond its normal range of motion. When the sole is turned outward or away from the median plane of the body, it is everted: this movement is called **eversion**.

Dorsiflexion–Plantar Flexion

The movement of the ankle so that the dorsal surface of the foot moves superiorly is called **dorsiflexion**. It is the opposite of **plantar flexion**, which draws the foot inferiorly in the anatomical position. These actions occur when standing on the toes or using the pedals of a car while driving.

The Musculoskeletal System

The musculoskeletal system is composed of three distinct yet interdependent components: the bones, the joints, and the muscles. While each provides its own unique contribution, it is the interaction of these systems that allows human movement to occur. The bones form a rigid skeletal framework with numerous joints that can be moved as a result of the forces produced by the attaching muscles. As the muscles pull against the bones, the bones act as levers that can produce diverse movements in all directions. These three major components work together to make the human body strong, efficient, and capable of moving with grace.

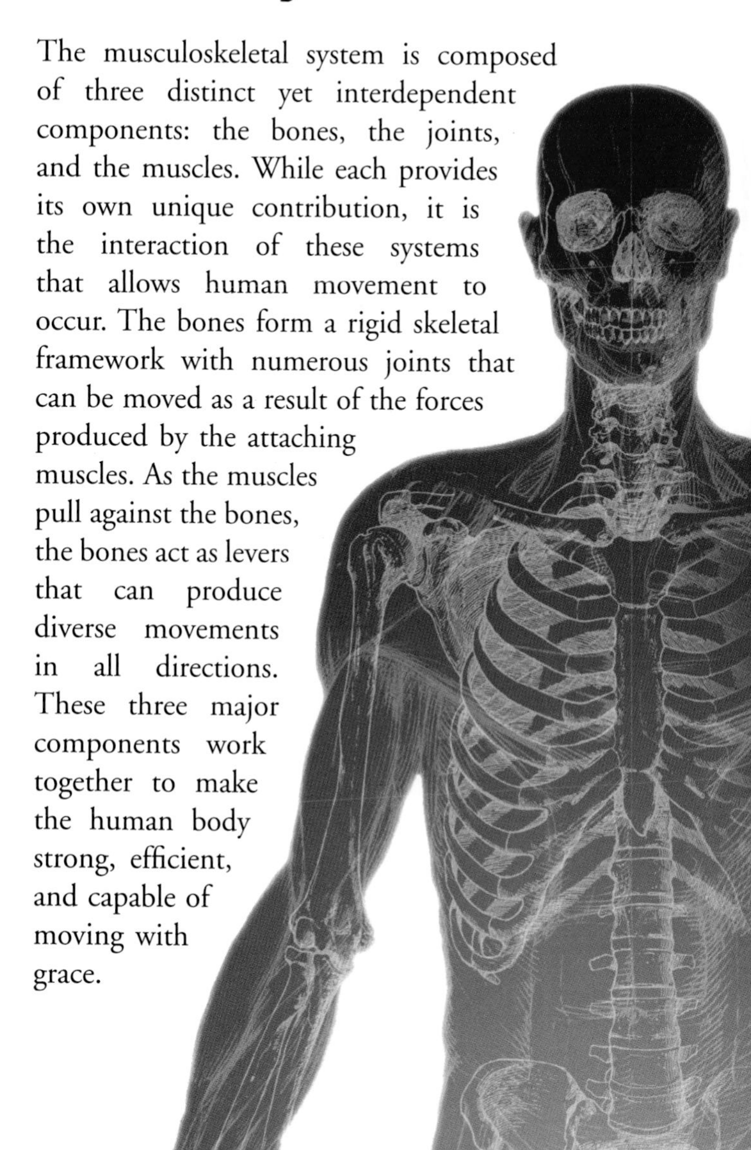

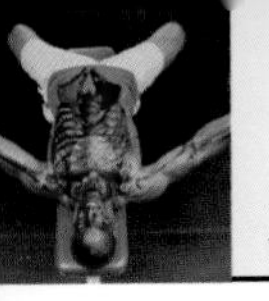

Bones of the Human Body

The bones of the human body provide the supporting framework and protection for the vital organs of the body – living tissue complete with blood supply and nerves. Remember how painful it is to hit your shin on something firm and sharp?

Bone Shape

Bone can be classified by shape as **short** (e.g., bones of the wrist and ankle), which serve as good shock absorbers; **long** (like the femur of the thigh and the humerus of the upper arm), with proximal and distal enlargements; **flat** (like the bones of the skull and scapula), which largely protect underlying organs and provide areas for muscle attachment; **irregular** (like the bones of your face and vertebrae), which fulfill special functions; and **sesamoid** (shaped like a pea and found in tendons). The structures and shapes of the bones of the human body allow them to perform specific functions more effectively (Table 2.1).

Bone Classification

The amount of mineral content in bone varies with one's age but also with the specific bone in the body. Bones that are more **porous** have a smaller proportion of calcium phosphate and carbonate, and greater nonmineralized tissue. According to the degree of porosity, bone can be classified into two general categories. Bone that has low porosity is called **cortical bone** (Figure 2.5). It is less flexible and can resist greater stress. In contrast, **spongy** or **cancellous bone** has a relatively high porosity with more nonmineralized tissue. Spongy bone has

Table 2.1 Bone classifications.

Shape	Examples	Skeleton
Long	Femur, tibia, fibula, humerus, radius, ulna, metatarsals, metacarpals, phalanges	Appendicular
Short	Carpals, tarsals	Appendicular
Flat	Scapula Clavicle Ribs, sternum Frontal, parietal, occipital, mandible	Appendicular Appendicular Axial Axial
Sesamoid	Patella	Appendicular
Irregular	Facial bones of skull, vertebrae Pelvis	Axial Appendicular

a characteristic honeycomb structure and provides more flexibility. Cortical bone is largely found in long bones (such as the bones of the arms and legs), whcih are required to be stronger to resist greater stress, while spongy bone is found where shock absorption and a better ability to change shape are important (e.g., vertebrae). Typically, long bones have a marrow cavity filled with red marrow in children and yellow marrow in adults.

Bone Composition

Bone is very strong for its relatively light weight. What gives bone this important characteristic? The major components of bone are calcium carbonate, calcium phosphate, collagen, and water. The two calcium compounds make up approximately 60 to 70 percent of bone weight, providing much of the bone's stiffness and resistance to pressing or squeezing forces. The collagen component (a protein) gives bone its characteristic flexibility and contributes to its ability to resist pulling and stretching forces. The bones of children are significantly more pliable than those of adults. With aging, collagen is lost progressively and bone becomes more brittle. Although the human body as a whole is composed of about 60 percent water, bone only contains approximately 20 percent water (20 to 25 percent of total bone weight). Consequently, bones are stronger and more durable than many other structures, such as skin.

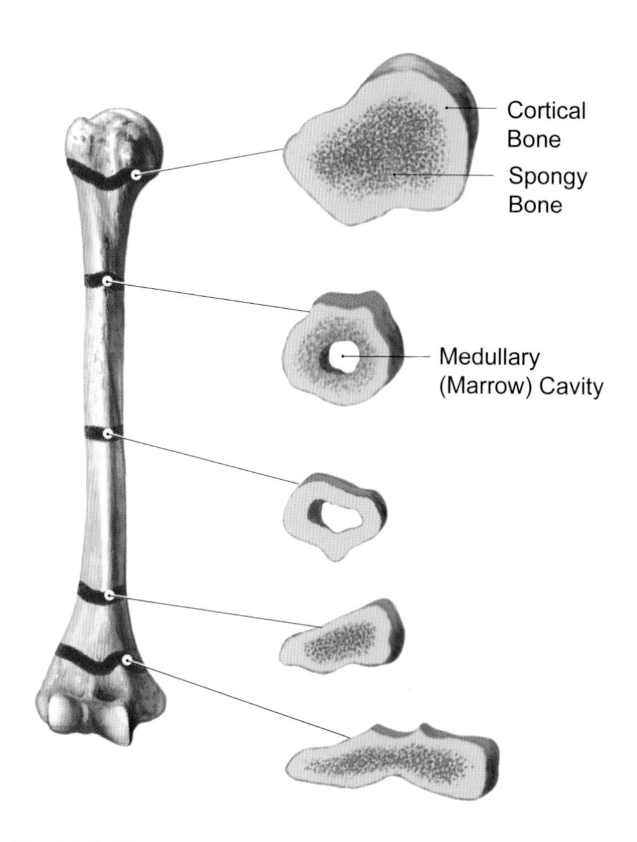

Figure 2.5 Transverse sections of the humerus, a long bone of the upper limb.

Effect of Fitness on Bone

Similar to muscles, bone also responds to the presence or absence of different forces with changes in size, shape, and density. When bones are subjected to regular physical activity and habitual loads, bones tend to become denser and more mineralized than the bones in people who are less active. This is revealed by the right-handed tennis player whose right forearm bones are denser than the left, as a result of using them more frequently. Similar changes can be found in throwers and runners in other sports. But just as forces acting on bone can increase bone density, inactivity works in the opposite direction, leading to a decrease in weight and strength. Loss of bone mass as a result of reduced mechanical stress has been noted in bed-ridden patients, inactive senior citizens, and astronauts.

The Human Skeleton

Approximately 206 bones make up the human skeleton. The skeleton (Figures 2.6 and 2.7) may be divided into axial and appendicular sections. The **axial skeleton** is composed of the skull, vertebrae, ribs, and sternum (the head, spine, and trunk), numbering 80 bones. The **appendicular skeleton** is made up of the pectoral (shoulder) and pelvic (hip) girdles and the upper (arms) and lower (legs) limbs, which are appended (hung) from the girdles. The appendicular portion of the skeleton consists of about 126 bones. While the axial skeleton serves mainly to support, stabilize, and protect vital organs of the body, the appendicular

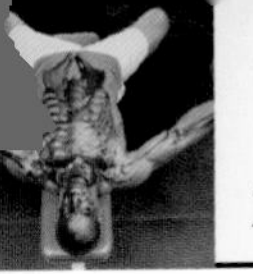

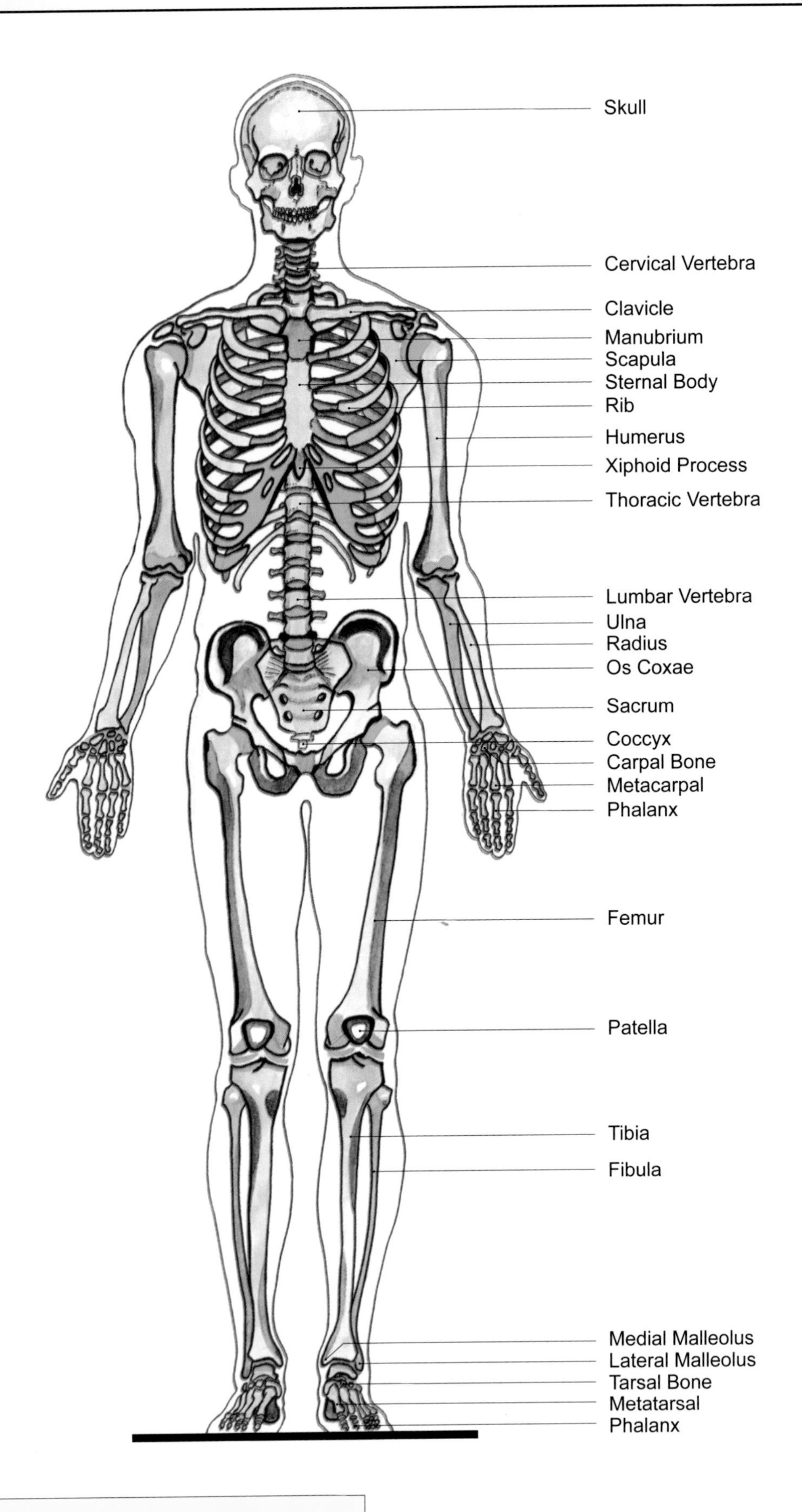

Figure 2.6 The human skeleton anterior view.

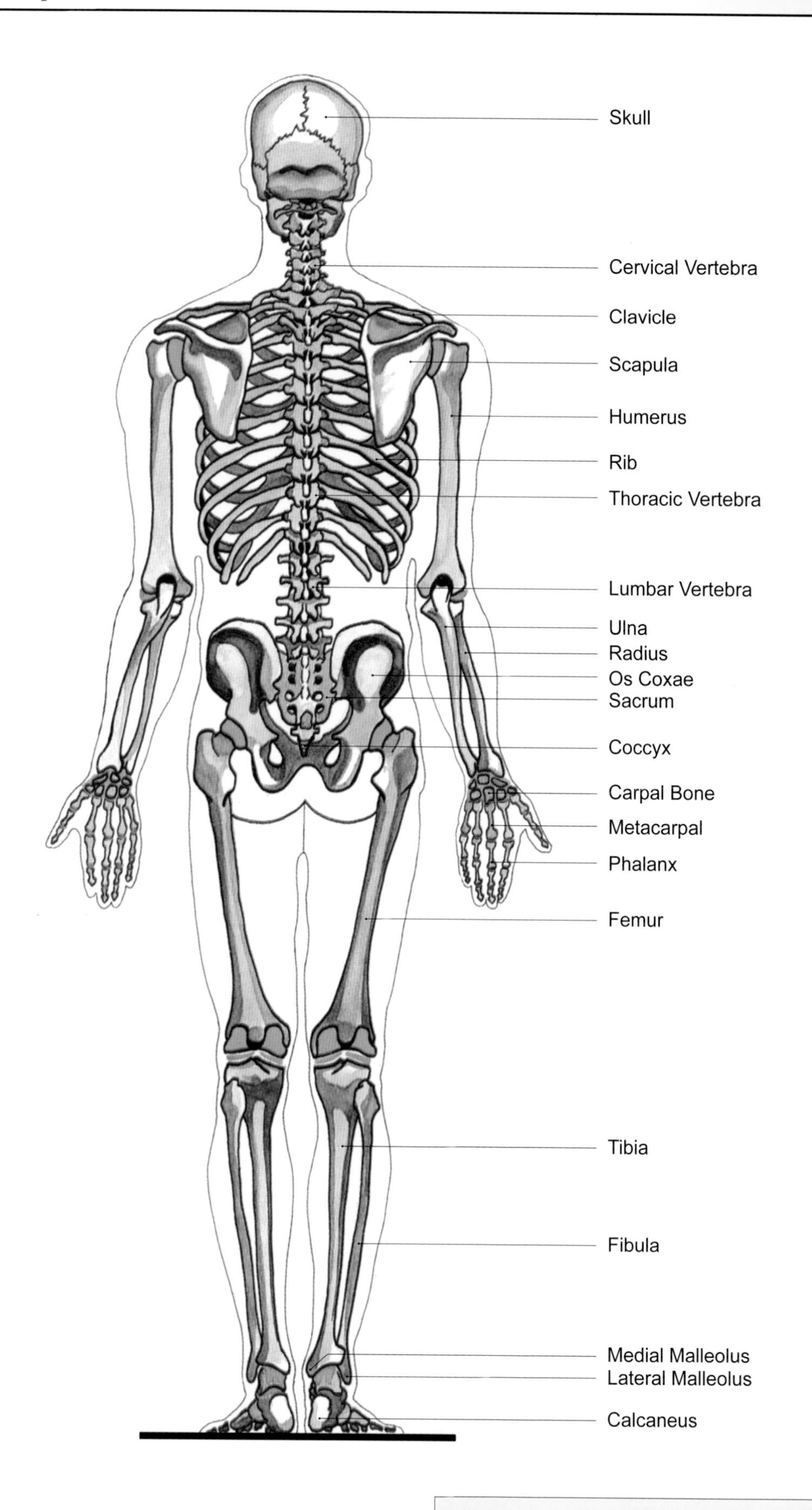

Figure 2.7 The human skeleton posterior view.

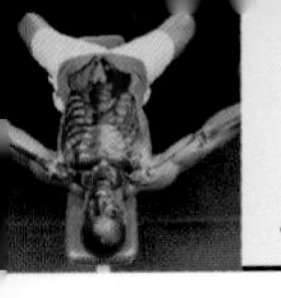

skeleton is responsible for a large portion of the movements we perform.

Axial Skeleton

Skull The skull is divided into two major parts. The curved flat bones form the **calvaria**, or vault that protects the brain and brain stem. The irregular bones of the **face** give it its individuality and provide protection for the eyes and air passages, as well as allow chewing and entry of food into the body (Figure 2.8).

Calvaria The calvaria is formed by the **frontal**, **parietal**, **temporal**, **occipital**, and **sphenoid bones**. These may be fractured by blows to the skull (Figure 2.8) (e.g., as a result of hitting the skull during a skateboarding fall). The more fragile of the calvaria bones is the temporal bone, and it overlies one of the major blood vessels supplying the membranes protecting the brain. If the temporal bone is fractured and displaced internally, it can cut the middle meningeal artery, resulting in an **epidural hemorrhage** (bleeding between the skull and the meninges, or protective covering of the brain; see Figure 2.8). This is a clinical emergency, and bleeding must be stopped as quickly as possible so that blood collecting within the vault of the skull does not compress the brain, which is soft (the consistency of toothpaste) and easily damaged – a good reason for sport helmets, if you ever questioned their necessity.

Facial Bones The facial bones (Figure 2.8) include the **nasal** (nose), **lacrimal** (for drainage of

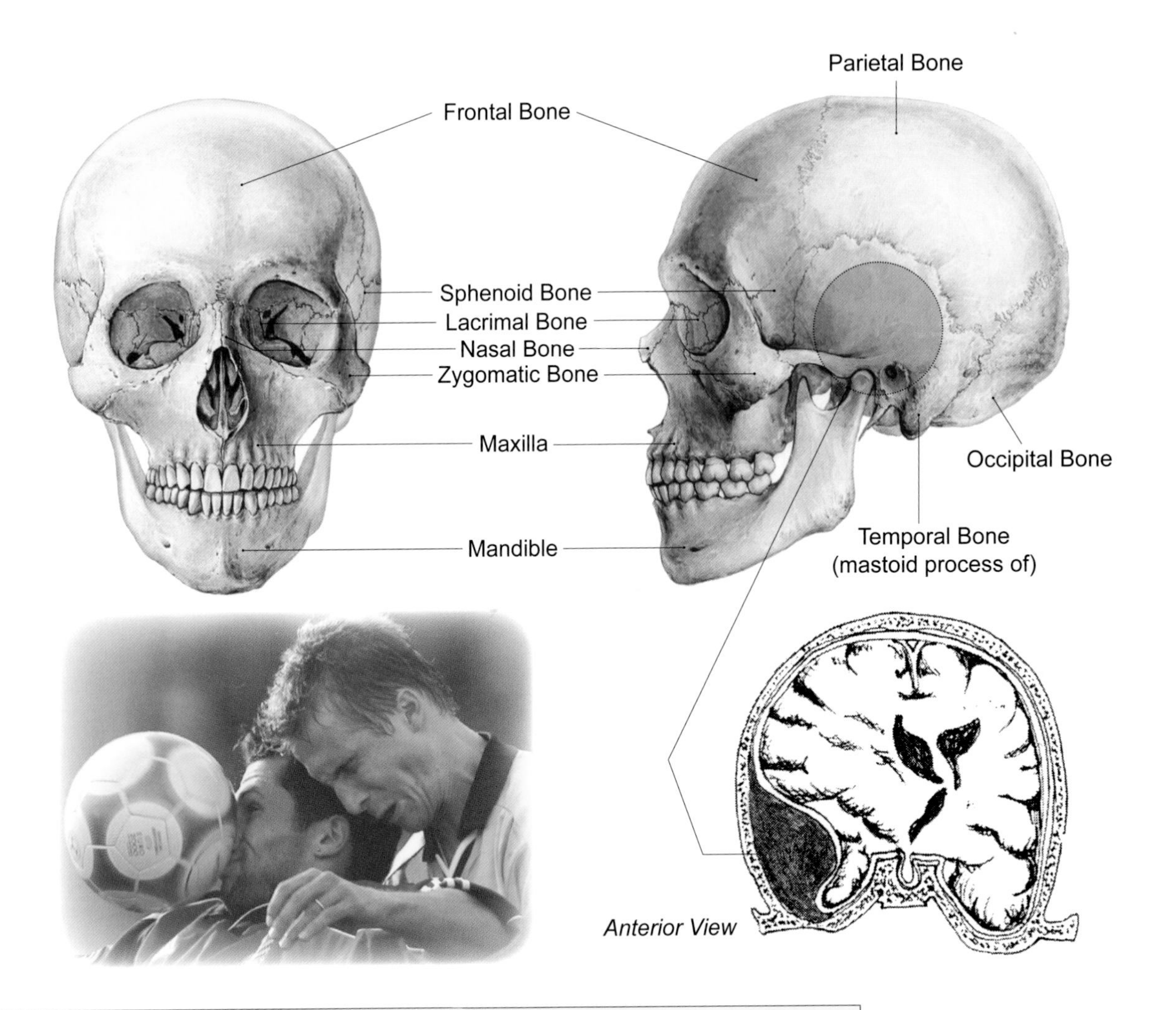

Figure 2.8 Anterior and left lateral view of the skull with epidural hemorrhage.

tears), **zygomatic** (cheek), **maxilla** (upper jaw), and **mandible** (lower jaw) **bones**. Facial bones are the ones often broken in contact sports due to rough impact. Some fractures across the maxilla (upper jaw) can leave the lower face separated from the upper face.

Vertebral Column The vertebral column (Figure 2.9) is composed of up to 35 bones: 7 **cervical** (neck) vertebrae, of which the first 2 are named the **atlas** (C1) and the **axis** (C2), 12 **thoracic** (chest) vertebrae, 5 **lumbar** (lower back) vertebrae, 1 **sacrum** (midline region of buttocks) made up of 5 fused vertebrae, and 1 **coccyx** (tail bone) made up of 4 or 5 fused vertebrae.

Vertebrae are arranged in a cylindrical column interspersed with fibrocartilaginous (intervertebral) discs, forming a strong and flexible support for the neck and trunk. The vertebral column is also the point of attachment for the muscles of the back. The column has a snakelike form when viewed from the side, with cervical, thoracic, lumbar, and sacral curves extending from the base of the skull through the entire length of the trunk. Not only does the column protect the spinal cord and nerves, it also provides essential support for the body and the ability to keep the body erect. The **intervertebral discs** absorb shock effectively when the load on the column increases and allow the vertebrae to move without causing damage to other vertebrae or to the spinal cord.

Ribs and Sternum There are usually 12 pairs of **ribs**, made up of bone and cartilage that give strength to the chest cage and permit it to expand (Figure 2.10). The ribs are curved and slightly twisted, making them ideal to protect the chest

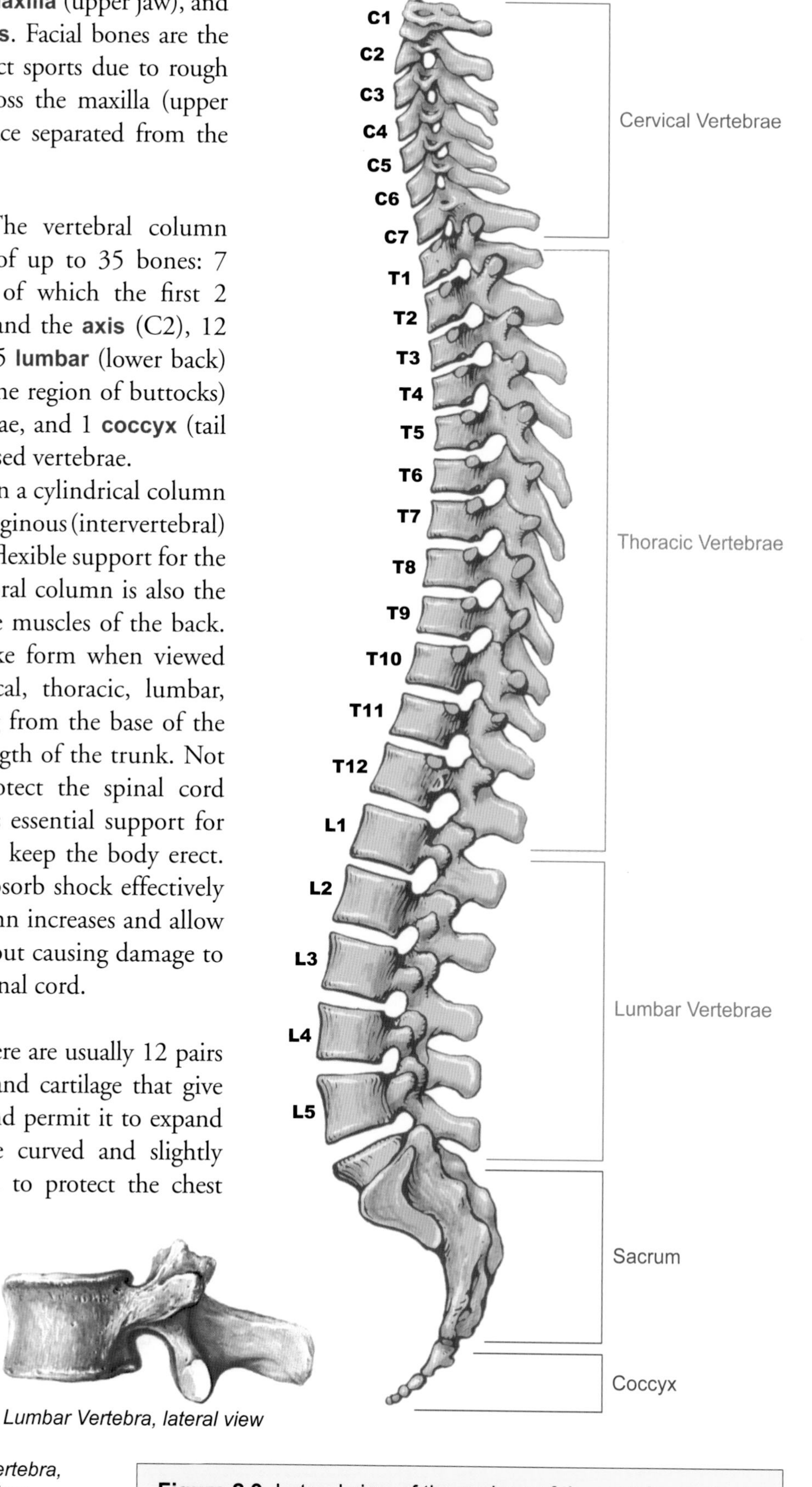

Lumbar Vertebra, lateral view

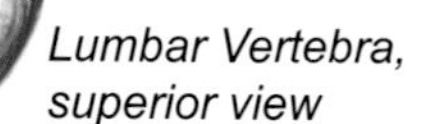

Lumbar Vertebra, superior view

Figure 2.9 Lateral view of the regions of the vertebral column.

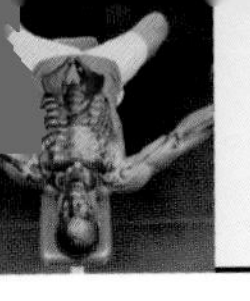

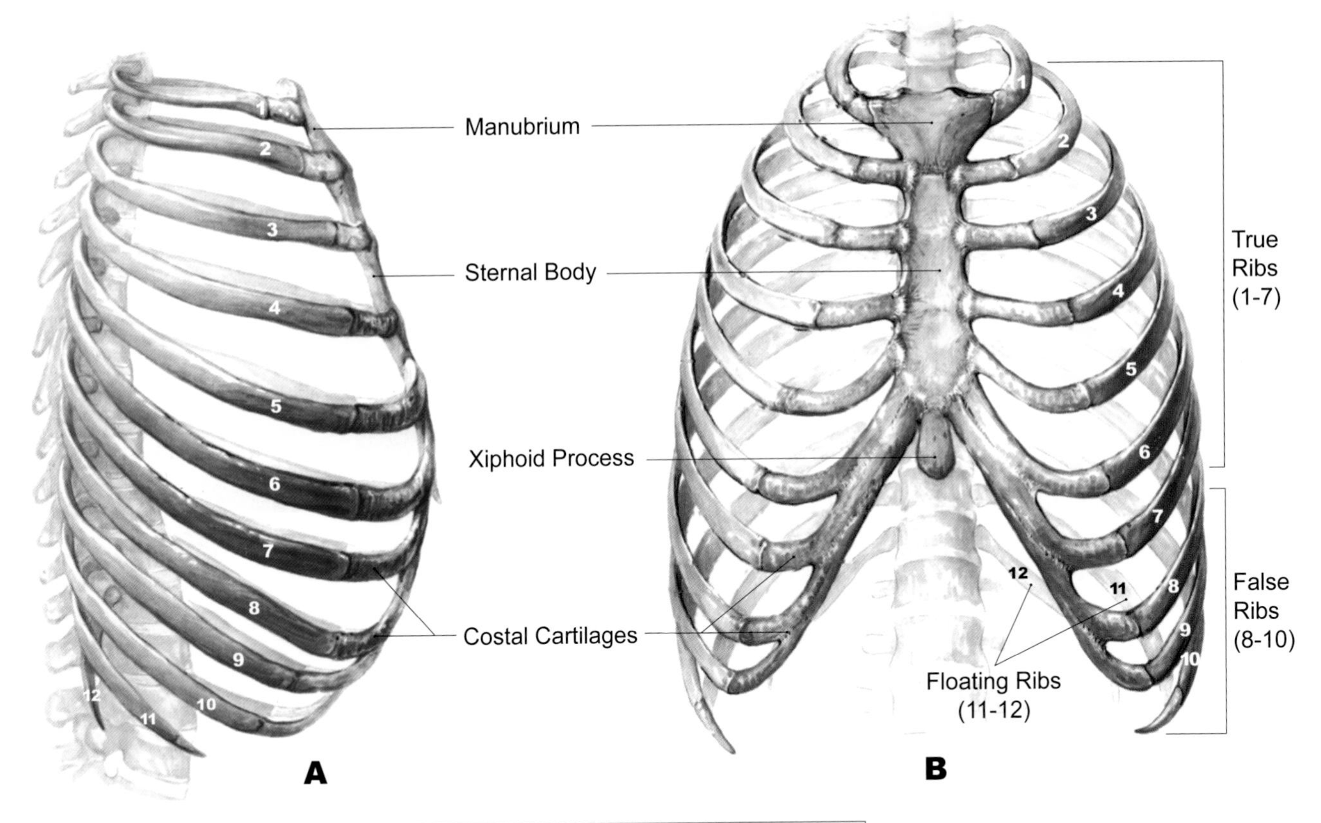

Figure 2.10 Rib cage and sternum. **A.** Lateral view. **B.** Anterior view.

area, effectively deflecting most blows that come its way. The upper 7 pairs (1 to 7) are the **true ribs** (attaching to both the vertebrae and the sternum), the next 3 pairs (8 to 10) are the **false ribs** (attaching to the sternum indirectly), and pairs 11 and 12 are **floating ribs**, so called because they attach only to the vertebral column. All 12 pairs of ribs articulate with the 12 thoracic vertebrae posteriorly.

The midline breastbone is called the **sternum**, made up of three parts – the **manubrium**, **sternal body**, and **xiphoid process**. The clavicles and ribs 1 to 7 articulate with the sternum (Figure 2.10).

Appendicular Skeleton

Pectoral Girdle The bones of the pectoral girdle are the **scapula** (shoulder blade) and the **clavicle** (collar bone) (Figure 2.11). They are held to the chest wall by many muscles that allow the upper limb great mobility. A fracture of the clavicle is very common during falls or collisions during sport or everyday activities. The *sternoclavicular joint* between the sternum and clavicle is the only bony joint between the axial skeleton and the pectoral girdle (Figure 2.15 A).

Upper Limb The arm (shoulder to elbow) bone is the **humerus**. From the elbow to the wrist the forearm is made up of the **radius** and the **ulna**, the radius being located on the thumb side of the hand. Therefore, when you pronate the forearm, the radius is actually crossing over the ulna. Try it yourself.

The **carpus** (wrist) is formed by two rows of four bones per row called **carpals** (Figure 2.11); from lateral to medial the proximal row contains the **scaphoid** (the bone most commonly fractured when you fall on the outstretched hand), **lunate**, **triquetral**, and **pisiform**; the distal row is made up of the **trapezium**, **trapezoid**, **capitate**, and **hamate** (the acronym **SLTPTTCH**, representing the carpals from lateral to medial, can be useful by remembering this sentence: *She Likes To Play, Try To Catch Her*). The distal row joins with the five **metacarpal** bones of the hand, which in turn articulate with the digits (fingers). All digits except the thumb are made up of three **phalanges** (singular = **phalanx**), *proximal*, *middle*, and *distal*. The thumb has only two phalanges, *proximal* and *distal* (Figure 2.11).

Pelvic Girdle The pelvic girdle is formed from the paired **os coxae**, or hip bones (made up of the ilium, pubis, and ischium), which join with the sacrum posteriorly and join each other anteriorly to form a basin-like girdle that supports the bladder and abdominal contents. On the lateral surface of the os coxae is a cup-shaped **acetabulum** for the head of the femur (Figure 2.12).

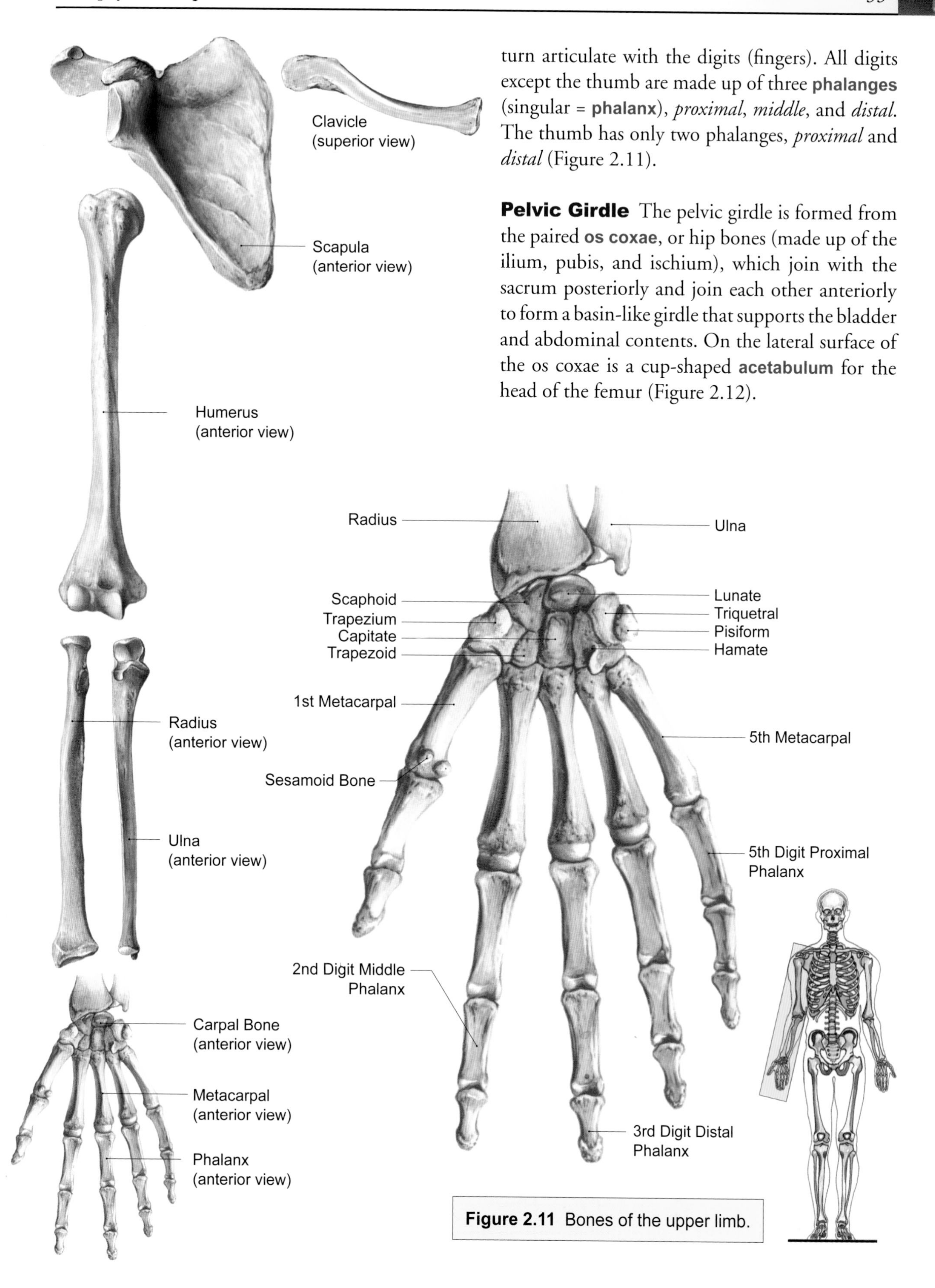

Figure 2.11 Bones of the upper limb.

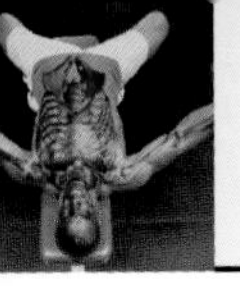

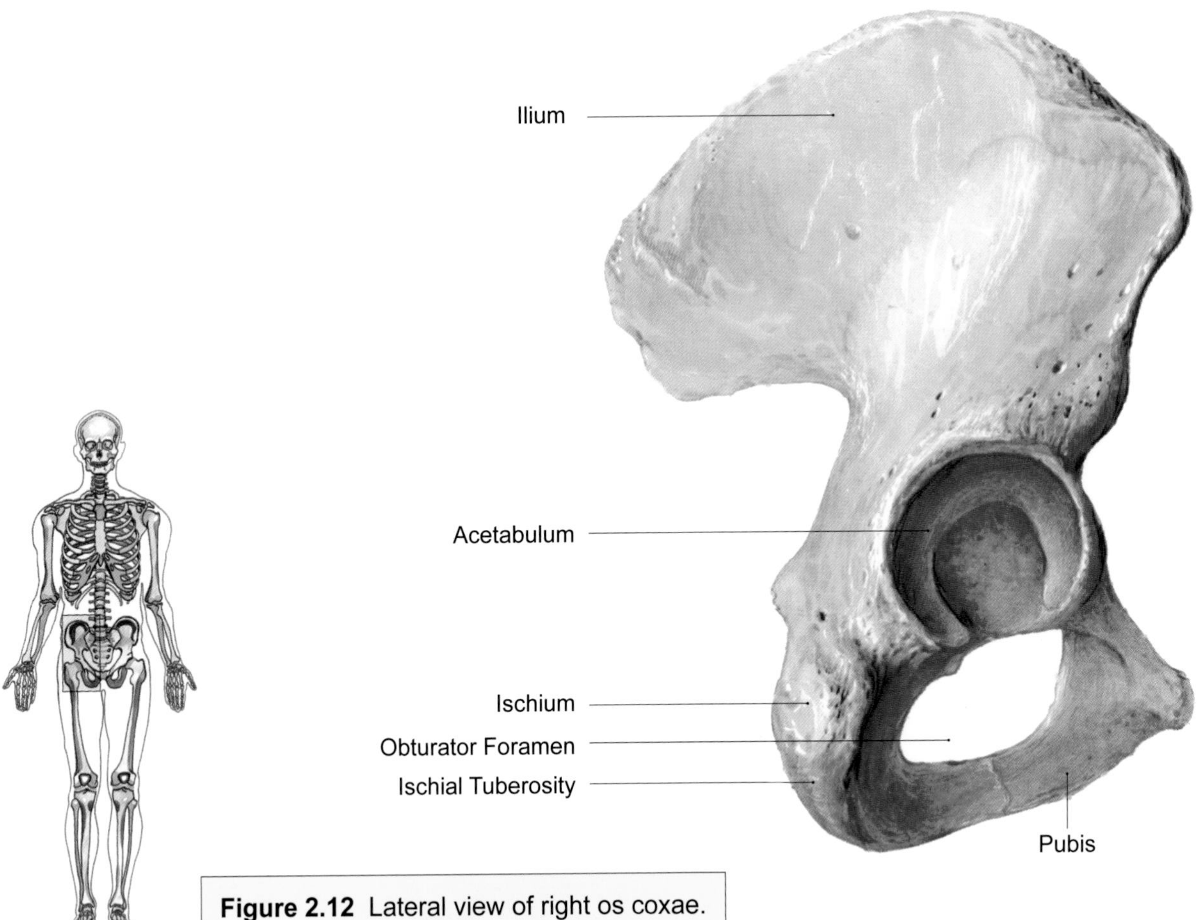

Figure 2.12 Lateral view of right os coxae.

Lower Limb The thigh (from hip to knee) bone is the **femur** (Figure 2.13). The **patella** (or kneecap) is a sesamoid bone in the tendon of the quadriceps muscles (thigh). From knee to ankle, the leg bones are the **tibia** and **fibula**. The tibia and fibula are held together very firmly by an *interosseous membrane* that provides stability and an area for muscle attachment. The distal ends of the tibia and fibula extend on the medial and lateral sides of the ankle (talus and calcaneus), forming a mortise into which the talus projects. These extensions can be felt subcutaneously and are commonly referred to as the "ankle bones" (Figure 2.13). Anatomists call them the **medial malleolus** and **lateral malleolus**.

The **tarsus** (ankle), like the wrist, is made up of several bones: the **talus**, resting on the **calcaneus** (heel bone), **navicular**, **cuboid**, and **1st (medial)**, **2nd (intermediate)**, and **3rd (lateral) cuneiforms** (*cuneiform* = wedge-shaped). The bones of the foot are the five **metatarsals**, in turn uniting with the toes. The great toe has only two phalanges while the lateral four toes have three (Figure 2.13).

Joints of the Human Body

A joint is basically the point of connection between two or more bones. The stability and integrity of joints are maintained by strands of connective tissue called **ligaments**, which hold the bones together. Joints can be generally classified by the material that joins them.

Classification of Joints

There are fibrous, cartilaginous, and synovial joints. The latter are the most common in the body and have certain typical characteristics that will be described later.

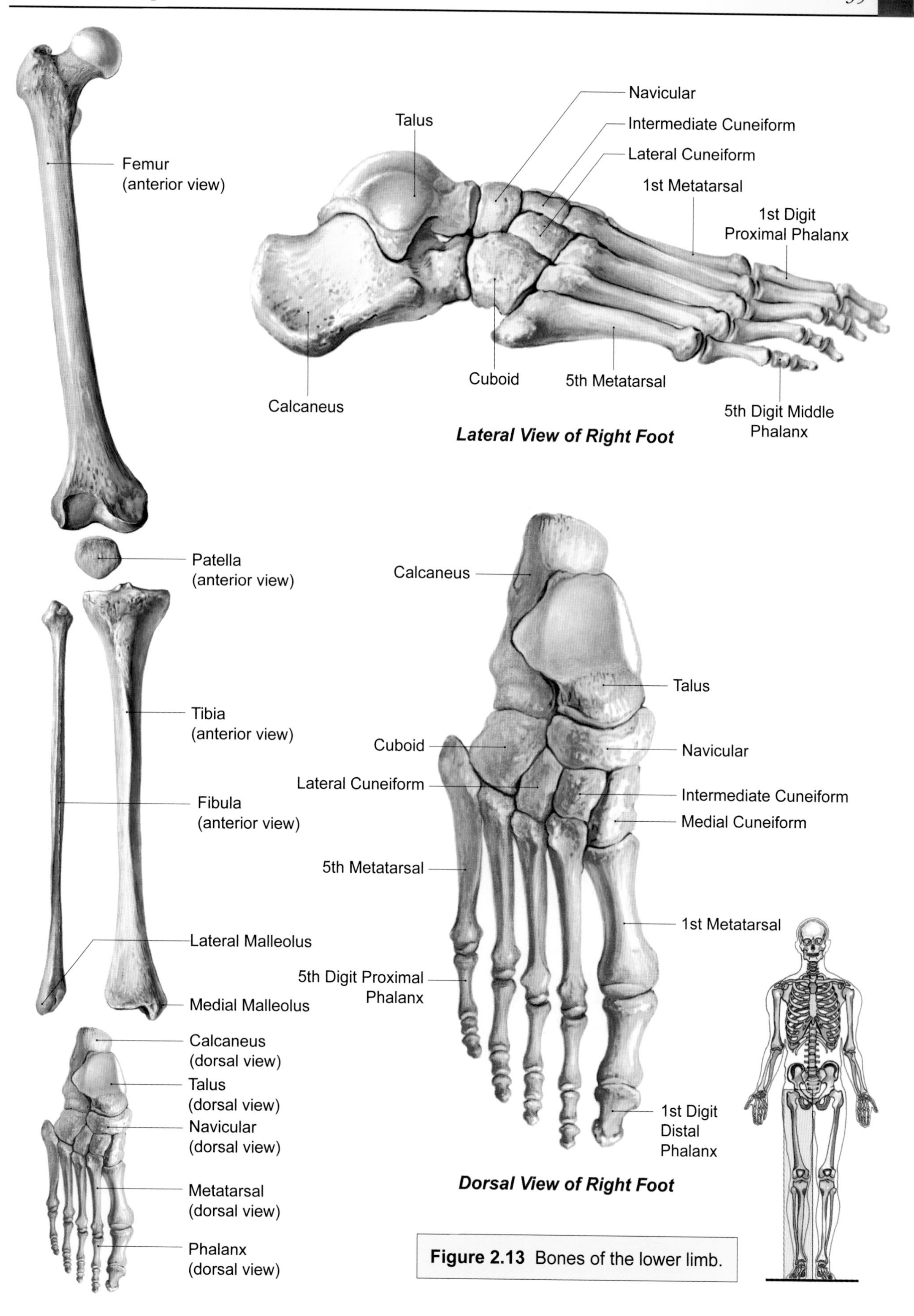

Figure 2.13 Bones of the lower limb.

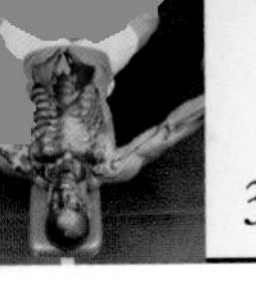

Joints may also be classified according to their motion capabilities; some allow for a great deal of movement, while others are severely restricted. The joints that exhibit the least mobility are **fibrous** and **cartilaginous**. These joints can absorb shock but permit little movement, if any (e.g., interosseous ligaments). There are also slightly movable joints that are cartilaginous and can also attenuate applied forces (e.g., *intervertebral joints* and the *symphysis pubis*). The joints that allow the greatest amount of motion are the **synovial joints**, which have only slight limitations to movement capability, making possible a wide array of movements. The characteristics of synovial joints are presented in the box on the right. The following discussion will therefore focus on synovial joints.

> **Characteristics of Synovial Joints**
>
> - There is a joint **capsule** lined with a **synovial membrane** that secretes the lubrication fluid for the joint. The capsule may or may not have thickenings called intrinsic ligaments that add support.
> - There is a joint **cavity** surrounded by the capsule.
> - There is a capillary layer of **synovial fluid** to lubricate the joint.
> - Outside the capsule and not connected to it are **extrinsic ligaments** that support the joint and connect the articulating bones of the joint.
> - Some joints have special features such as **articular discs**, **fibrocartilaginous labra** (singular = labrum) and **menisci** (singular = meniscus), and **intracapsular tendons**.

Types of Synovial Joints

Synovial joints vary widely in structure and movement capabilities and may be classified in different ways – by the movements possible at the joint or simply by the axes around which the joint can be moved. The more common classification is based on the shape of the joint (Figure 2.14).

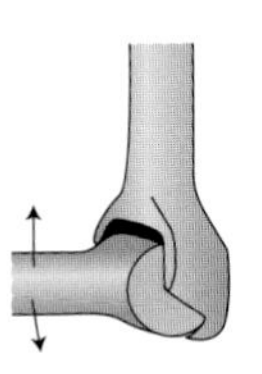

Hinge (Ginglymus) Joint This type of joint has one articulating surface that is convex and another that is concave. Examples include the humeroulnar joint at the elbow and the interphalangeal joints of the fingers.

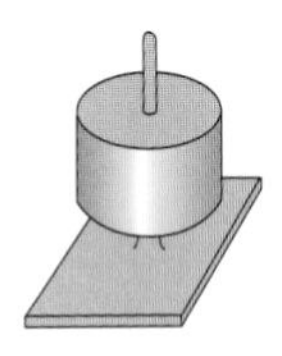

Pivot Joint In these types of joints, one bone rotates around one axis. For example during pronation–supination of the forearm, the radius rotates along its long axis and the ulna remains fixed.

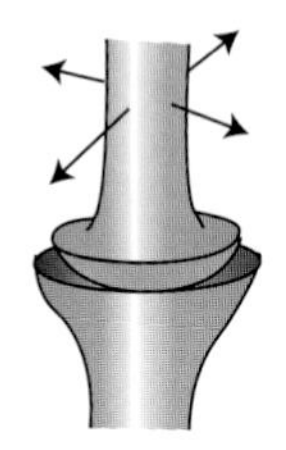

Condyloid (Knuckle) Joint The joint surfaces are usually oval, as in the joint between your third metacarpal (bone of the hand) and the proximal phalanx (bone) of your third digit. One joint surface is an ovular convex shape, and the other is a reciprocally shaped concave surface. At this joint, flexion–extension, abduction–adduction, and circumduction are all possible.

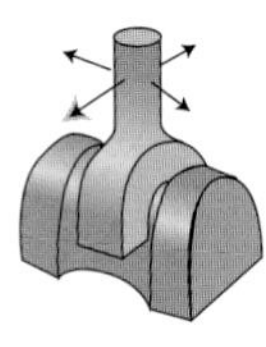

Saddle Joint The bones are set together as in sitting on a horse. This is seen in the carpometacarpal joint of the thumb. Movement capability at this joint is the same as the condyloid joint, but with a greater possible range of motion permitted.

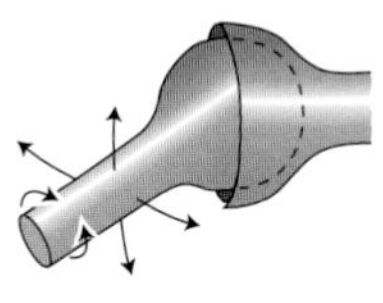

Ball and Socket Joint A rounded bone is fitted into a cuplike receptacle. This is the kind of joint found at the shoulder and the hip, where rotation in all three planes of movement is possible.

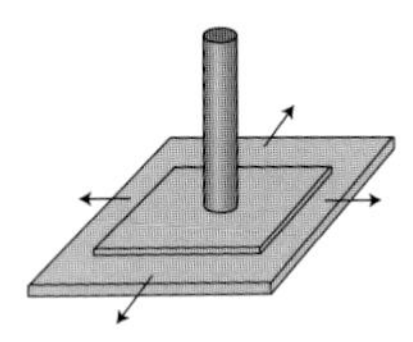

Plane (Gliding) Joint This joint permits gliding movements, as in the bones of the wrist. The bone surfaces

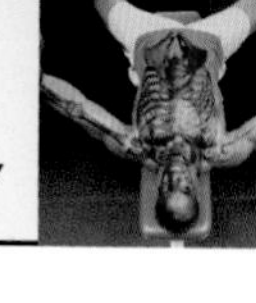

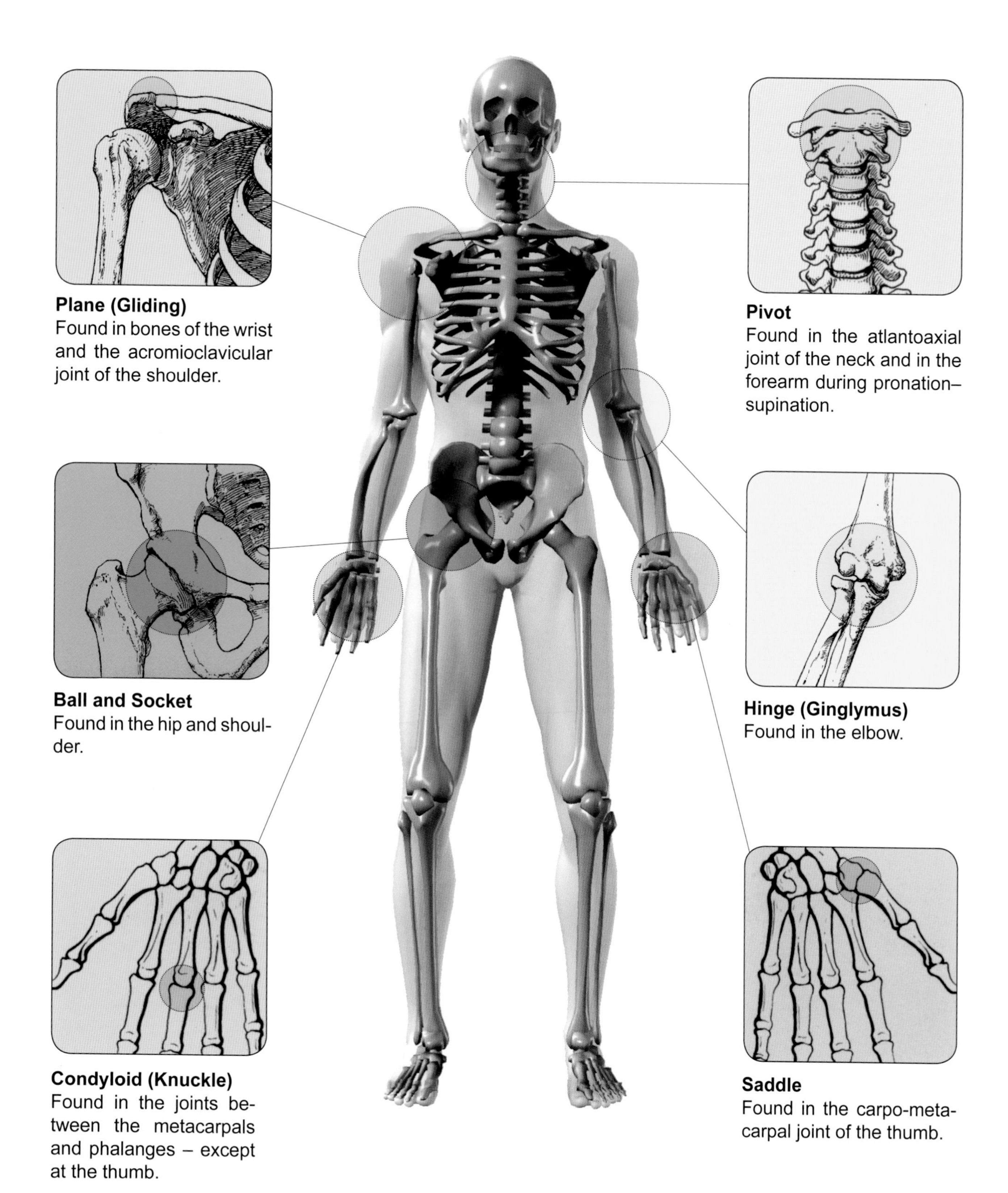

Figure 2.14 Typical synovial joints of the human body.

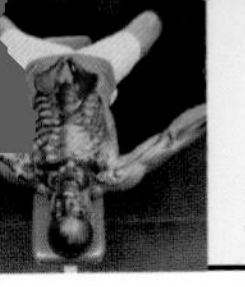

involved are nearly flat, so the only movement allowed is a gliding action. Another example of such a joint is the facet joints of the vertebrae.

The principal synovial joints of the body are presented in the following sections. While some of the terms may seem confusing, just remember that anatomical terms can be figured out by identifying the root words involved. Junctions of bones are called joints. Some fibrous joints (e.g., sutures of the skull) allow no movement, cartilaginous joints (e.g., intervertebral discs) allow limited movement, and synovial joints (e.g., elbow and wrist) allow a large range of movement. In synovial joints, bone ends are covered with smooth **cartilage**, and the entire joint is enclosed in a capsule filled with **synovial fluid**. Ligaments and cartilage provide additional support.

Joints of the Pectoral Girdle

The pectoral girdle, made up of the scapula and clavicle, has two joints. These joints are presented starting below.

Sternoclavicular Joint

This is the only joint connecting the pectoral girdle to the axial skeleton (the clavicle to the sternum). It is a true synovial joint strengthened by an intracapsular disc and extrinsic ligaments. This is important as this joint must absorb all forces

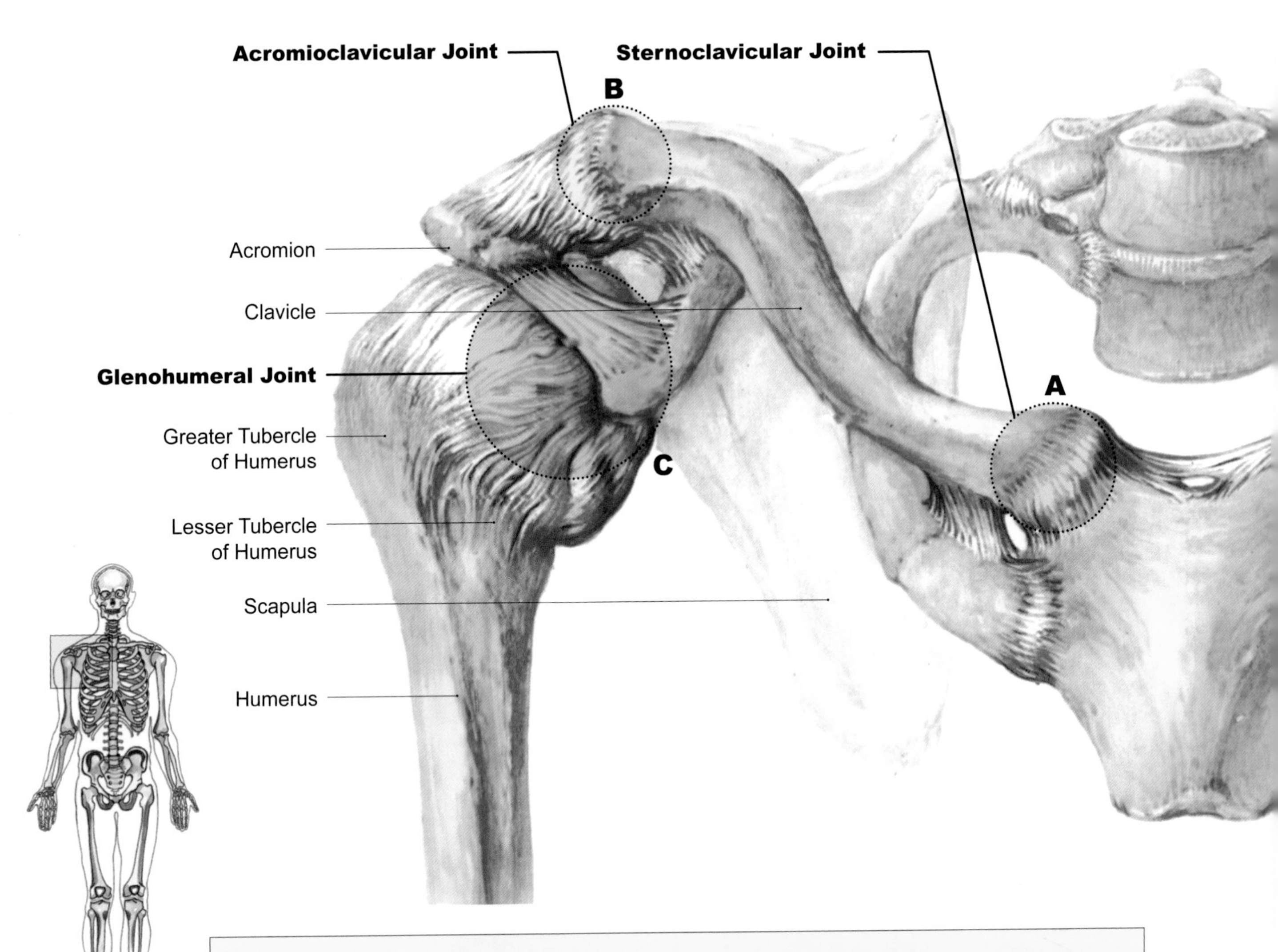

Figure 2.15 Anterior view of the right shoulder demonstrating the pectoral girdle. **A.** Sternoclavicular joint. **B.** Acromioclavicular joint. **C.** Glenohumeral joint.

transmitted to the upper limb in many activities, including many sports (Figure 2.15 A).

Acromioclavicular Joint

This joint unites the lateral end of the clavicle with the acromion process of the scapula. It is here that shoulder separations can, and often do, occur in sports such as hockey, baseball, and football (Figure 2.15 B).

Joints of the Upper Limb

Glenohumeral Joint

This is the joint between the upper limb and the scapula. Because we enjoy a wide range of movement at this joint, the compromise is a relative lack of stability. You have a large ball (of the humerus) articulating with a relatively shallow cup (of the scapula). The integrity of the joint depends on the rotator cuff muscles that **SSIT** on the greater and lesser tubercles of the humerus and cross the joint to attach to the scapula. These letters stand for the *Subscapularis*, *Supraspinatus*, *Infraspinatus*, and *Teres minor* muscles that hold the head of the humerus firmly against the *glenoid fossa* of the scapula. This area is commonly injured by water polo players (Figure 2.15 C).

Elbow Joint

There are actually three joints at the elbow: (1) the **humeroradial joint** between the capitulum of the humerus and the head of the radius (Figure 2.16 A); (2) the **humeroulnar joint** between the trochlea of the humerus and the olecranon process of the ulna (Figure 2.16 B); and (3) the **radioulnar joint** between the radius and the ulna (Figure 2.16 C). Flexion–extension occurs at the first two, and pronation–supination occurs at the radioulnar joint.

Joints of the Wrist

The distal radius articulates with the proximal row of carpal bones at the **radiocarpal joint** (between the radius and the carpals). Flexion–extension as well as abduction–adduction occur here (Figure 2.17). As well, there are **midcarpal** and **intercarpal**, **carpometacarpal**, and **intermetacarpal joints**. There are gliding joints between the bones of the

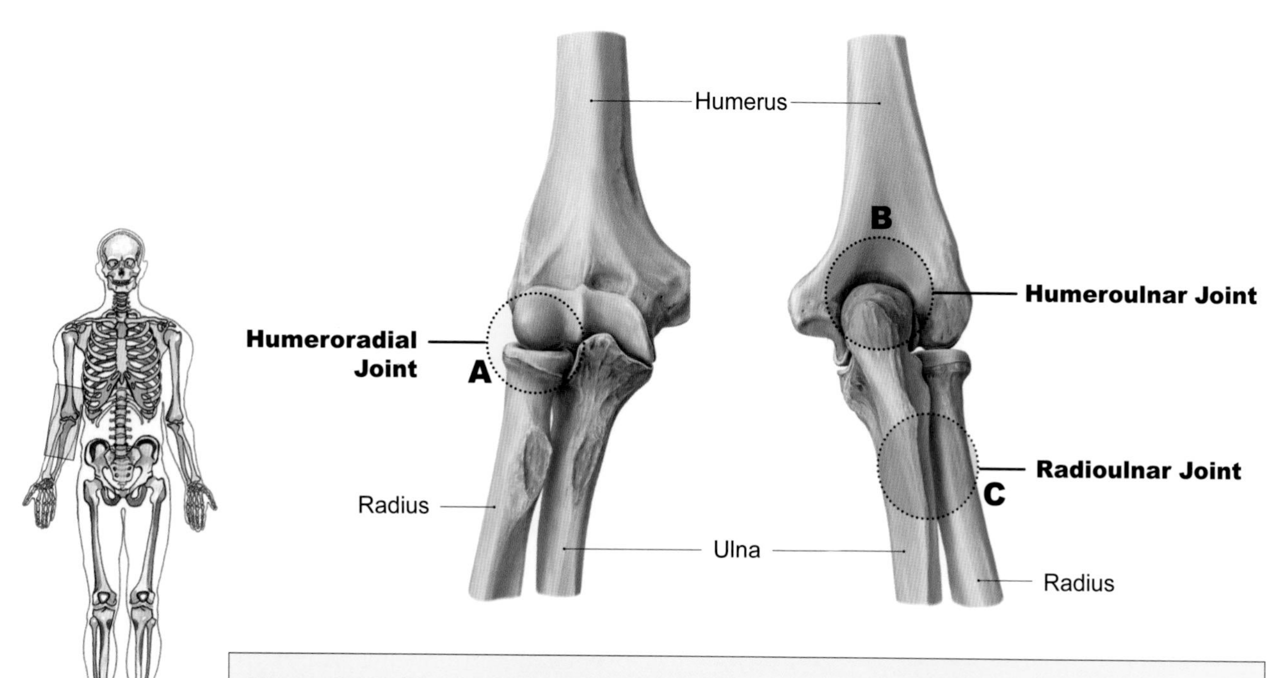

Figure 2.16 The right elbow joint. **A.** Humeroradial joint. **B.** Humeroulnar joint. **C.** Radioulnar joint.

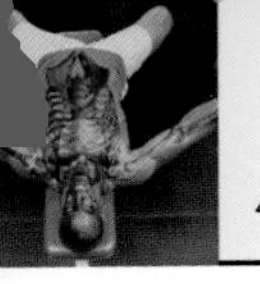

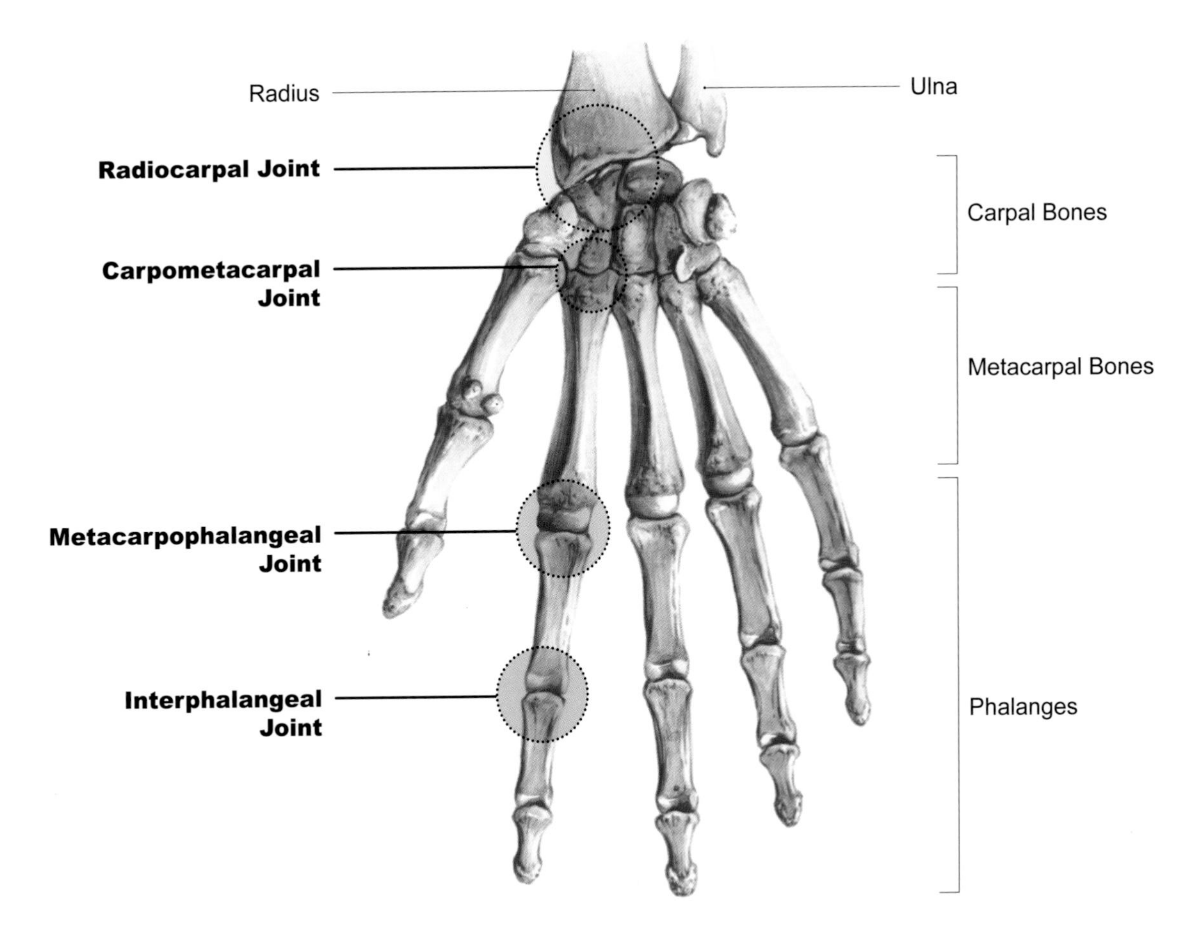

Figure 2.17 Major joints of the wrist and hand.

carpus. The metacarpal of the thumb sits in the saddle of the trapezium and lies at an angle of 90 degrees to the palm of the hand. This allows the range of movement necessary for *opposition*, the ability to touch the tip of your thumb to each of your fingertips.

Joints of the Hand

The knuckles are the **metacarpophalangeal joints** (Figure 2.17). Flexion–extension and abduction–adduction can occur here, allowing us to manipulate our hands with amazing dexterity. Between the phalanges are **interphalangeal joints** (recall that there are three phalanges per finger, while the thumb has only two) that also permit flexion–extension (Figure 2.17).

Joints of the Pelvic Girdle

The hip bones (os coxae), made up of the ilium, pubis, and ischium, together with the sacrum, form the pelvic girdle. It has two joints.

Symphysis Pubis

This is a fibrocartilaginous joint uniting the two pubic bones and completing the pelvic girdle anteriorly. It can soften just before giving birth to permit a wider opening for the baby.

Sacroiliac Joint

This joint unites the sacrum with the paired ilia (singular = ilium). It has both a fibrous and a synovial component. Minor displacement of the fibrous component can result in excruciating sacroiliac pain.

Joints of the Lower Limb

Hip Joint

Between the head of the femur and the cup (acetabulum) of the hip bone (os coxae) is the **hip** or **iliofemoral joint**. As in all ball and socket joints, movements of flexion–extension, abduction–adduction, and circumduction can take place here, allowing for the greatest range of motion and mobility (Figure 2.18).

The hip joint is the body's most stable synovial joint as it is provided with a deepened socket (via a lip, or fibrocartilaginous labrum) and intrinsic and very strong extrinsic ligaments. In contrast to the shoulder joint, another ball and socket joint, dislocation of the hip joint, even in the most aggressive contact sports, is rare. Dislocation usually occurs when someone sitting in the front seat of a car is involved in a head-on collision and the knees are driven into the dashboard. The

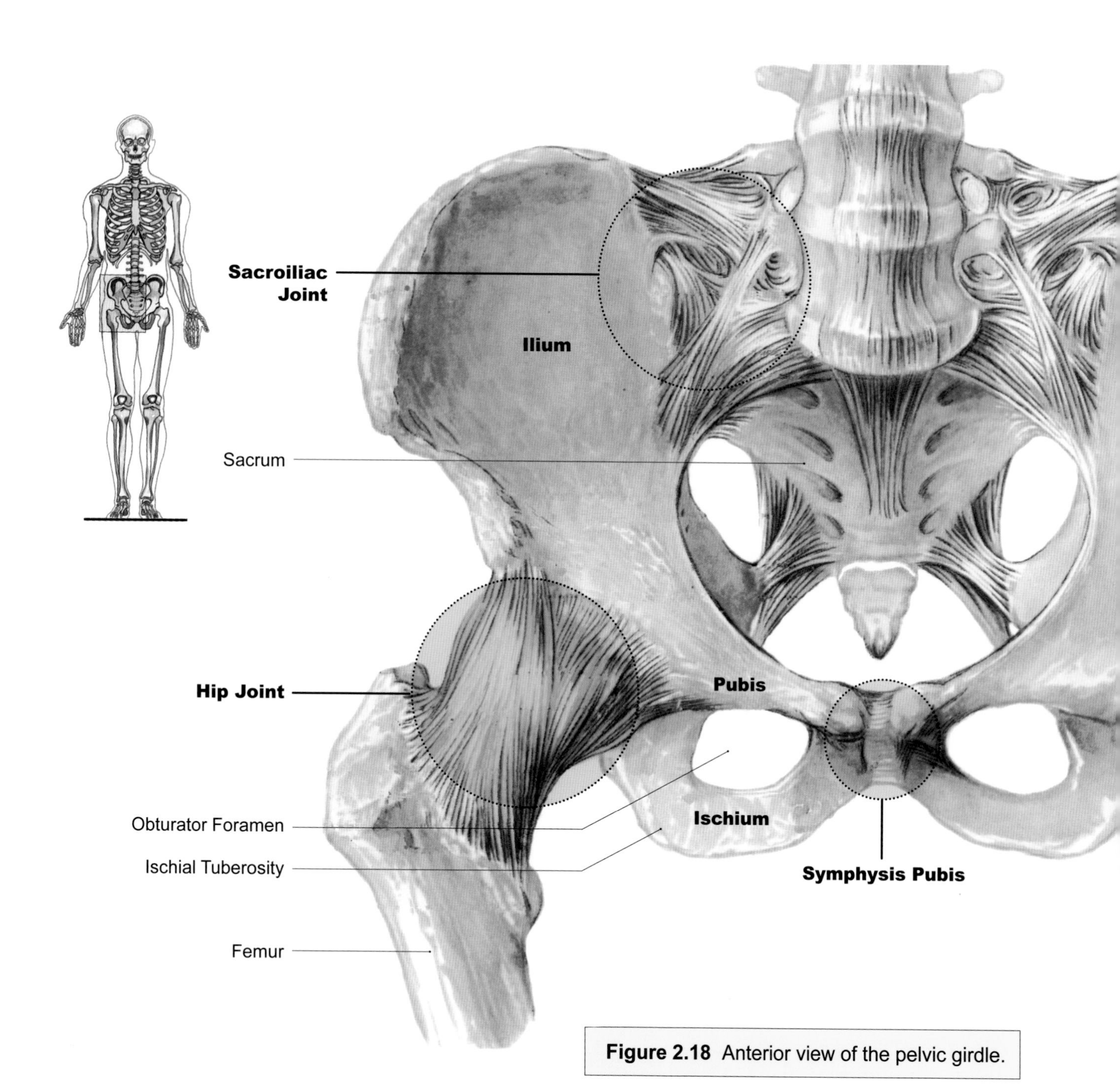

Figure 2.18 Anterior view of the pelvic girdle.

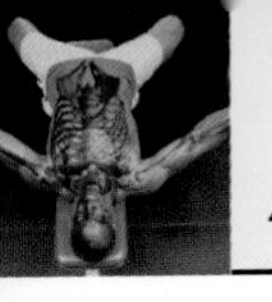

force of impact can either dislocate the head of the femur posteriorly or drive it through the posterior lip of the acetabulum.

Knee Joint

Despite its very shallow receptor surface on the tibial plateau for the medial and lateral condyles of the femur, the **knee (tibiofemoral) joint** is a relatively stable joint with an incredible range of movement (Figure 2.19). It has additional structural supports from the **menisci** (shock-absorbing fibrocartilaginous discs), **anterior** and **posterior cruciate ligaments** (in the center of the joint), **lateral** and **medial collateral ligaments** (extending from the sides of the femur to the fibula and tibia), and the musculature that surrounds it. The primary action here is flexion–extension, such as when performing a squat or jump, but when the knee is flexed, medial and lateral rotation can also occur at the joint. Try it out yourself.

When You Sprain an Ankle

As with bone and muscle, all joints have a rich nerve supply. The muscles that pass over a joint and give it movement have the same nerve supply as the joints over which they act.

Question: When a joint becomes swollen (as in an ankle sprain) what causes the swelling? Why is this painful?

Answer: Trauma causes the synovial membrane of the joint to secrete fluid. This causes the swelling that results in stretching of the joint capsule, which can activate pain receptors in the joint. When the joint becomes painful, the surrounding muscles may go into spasm. Once the inflammation is reduced, the pain will subside and the muscles will have to be remobilized with physiotherapy.

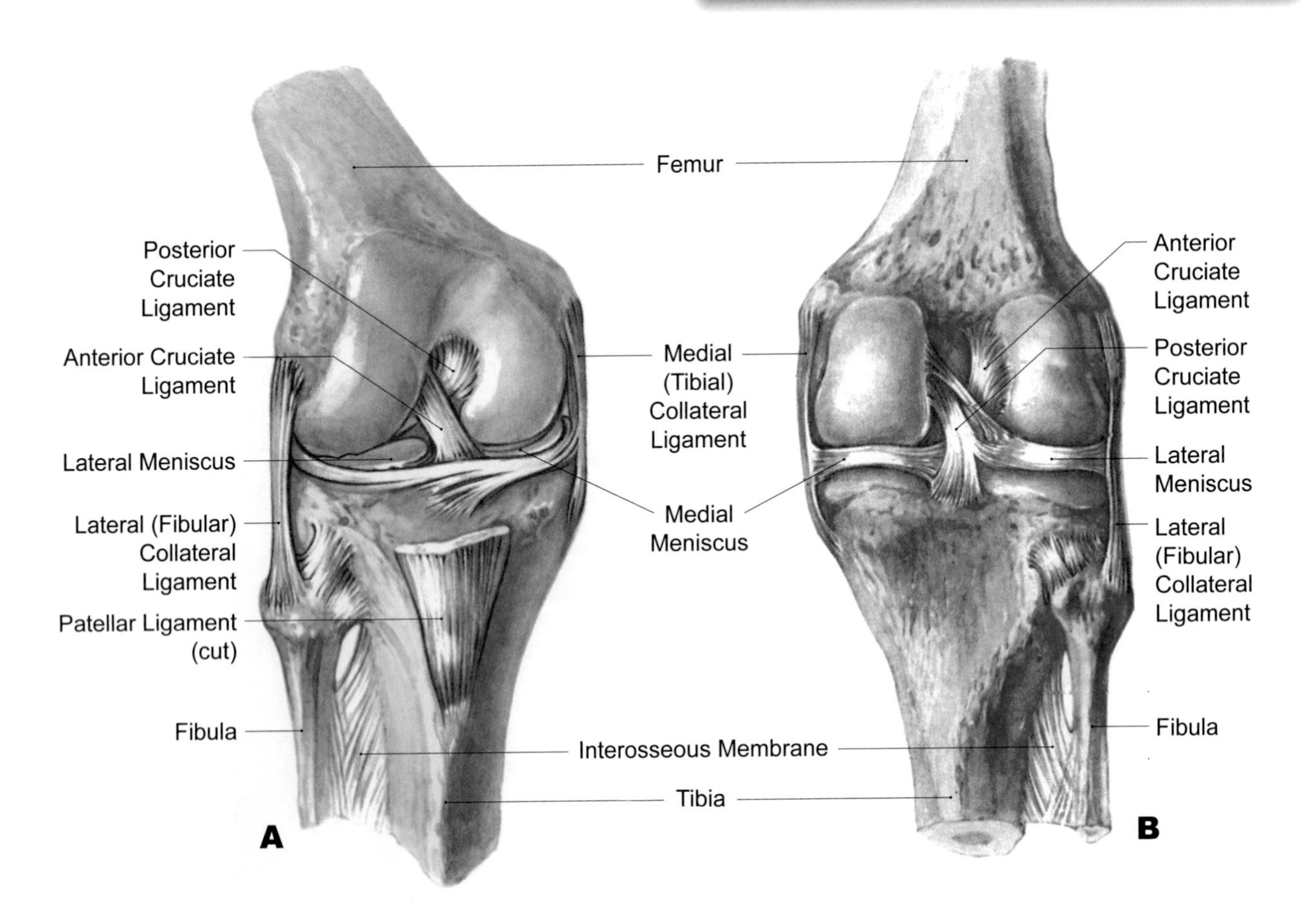

Figure 2.19 The right knee. **A.** Anterior view. **B.** Posterior view.

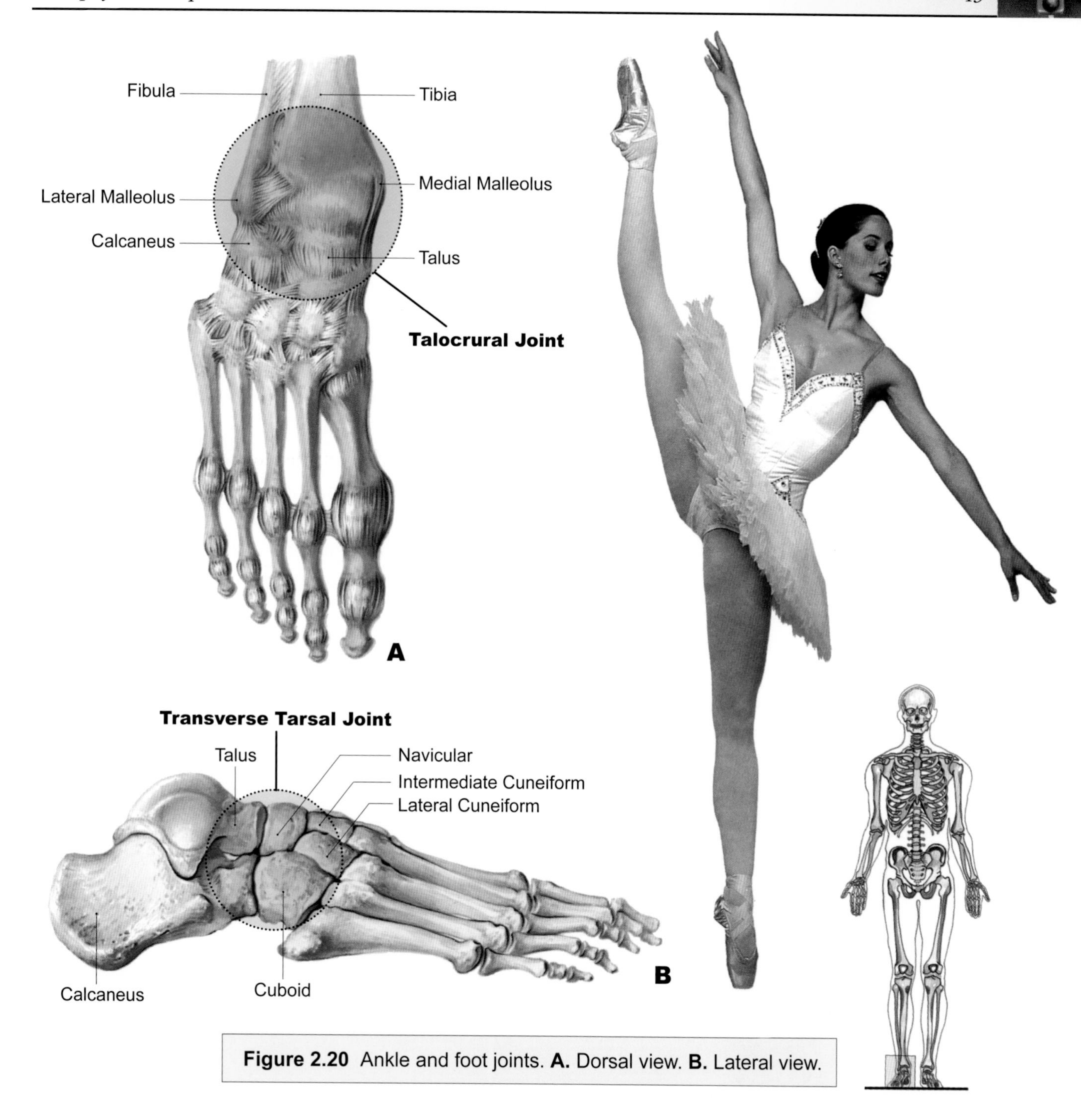

Figure 2.20 Ankle and foot joints. **A.** Dorsal view. **B.** Lateral view.

Ankle Joint

Several bones, the medial and lateral malleoli of the tibia and fibula, the head of the talus, and the calcaneus (heel bone), are involved in the **ankle (talocrural) joint** (Figure 2.20).

The talus is wedged into the mortise formed by the medial and lateral malleoli. Because the talus is wider anteriorly than posteriorly, when you dorsiflex at the ankle, you put the ankle into its most stable position. This is the reason for the forward cant in a downhill ski boot. The ankle is least stable in the "en pointe" position in ballet, putting great pressure on dancers' ligaments and tendons and increasing the risk of injury.

Foot and Toe Joints

There are two rows of tarsal bones of the **transverse tarsal joint**. Movement between the proximal and

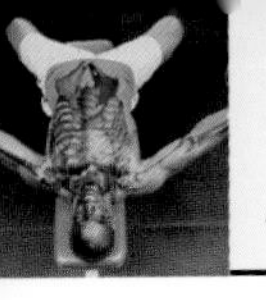

distal rows of the transverse tarsal joint is inversion–eversion of the sole of the foot. This action enables you to adjust to uneven ground when walking or running. As in the hand, there are joints between the tarsal bones, metatarsals, and phalanges. They are strengthened by plantar ligaments that aid in maintaining the arch of the foot (weakened ligaments result in "flat foot," although you may be born with flat feet that cause you no discomfort).

Muscles of the Human Body

Muscles allow the skeleton to move. Most muscles are attached from one bone to another with a joint in between. The attachment closer to the center of the body is the muscle's **origin** (also known as its *proximal attachment*). The attachment away from the center of the body is the muscle's **insertion** (also known as its *distal attachment*). The origin of the muscle is usually attached to more stationary parts, whereas the insertion is attached to more mobile structures of the skeleton. Remember, muscles can act only on the joints they cross.

There are over 600 muscles present in the human body. It would be impossible to describe here all the muscles, so keep in mind that a short section in this chapter cannot do justice to the vast number and functions of these muscles. Only the major superficial muscles will be identified (Figures 2.24 and 2.25) as they relate to the bony regions discussed in the previous section.

Muscles of the Face

Facial muscles enable you to change expression and display your emotions outwardly; but most important, they allow you to close your eyes and your mouth (Figure 2.21). Closing the eyelids, as in blinking, acts to move tears across the cornea of the eye, keeping it moistened. When the eyeball is not kept moist, it will dry out and ulcerate, leading to discomfort and irritation, even blindness. People with paralysis of facial muscles will put artificial tears in their eyes to prevent this.

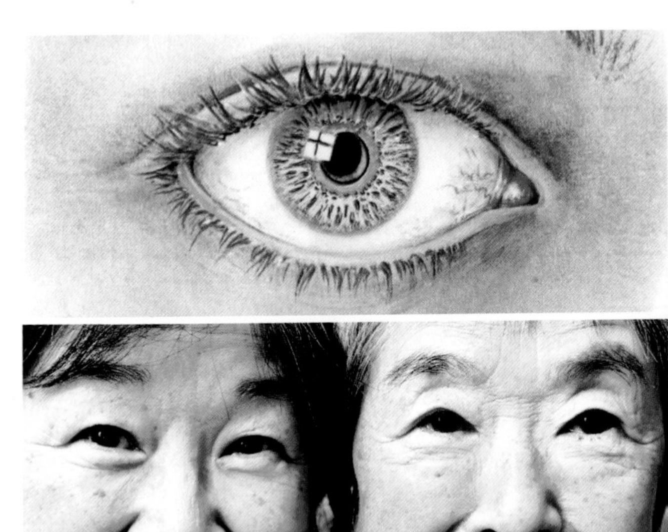

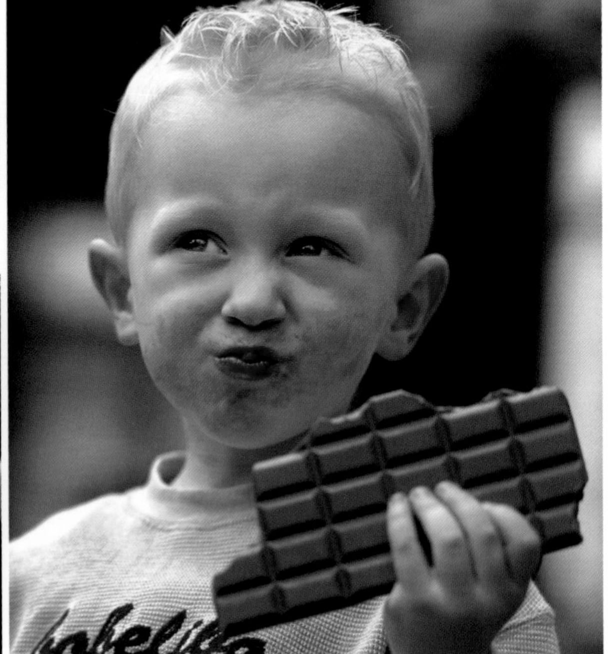

Figure 2.21 Facial muscles are essential for a variety of tasks, from smiling and blinking to chewing and speaking.

Facial muscles are also essential for opening and closing the mouth, thereby keeping food in the mouth and allowing you to move it between the teeth during chewing, to say nothing of forming words in speaking.

Muscles of the Neck and Back

The head sits on the first cervical vertebra (C1), called the atlas. To maintain this position there are muscles posterior, lateral, and anterior to the neck, or cervical, region that allow you to hold up your head and also permit a wide range of movement. Try turning your own head while keeping your shoulders in a fixed position. The most important anterior pair of neck muscles are the **sternocleidomastoids** (Figure 2.22). Acting together, they are the muscles that allow you to flex your head toward your chest. Without them you cannot get up from a supine position (lying down). Individually, each sternocleidomastoid muscle tilts the face up and toward the opposite side.

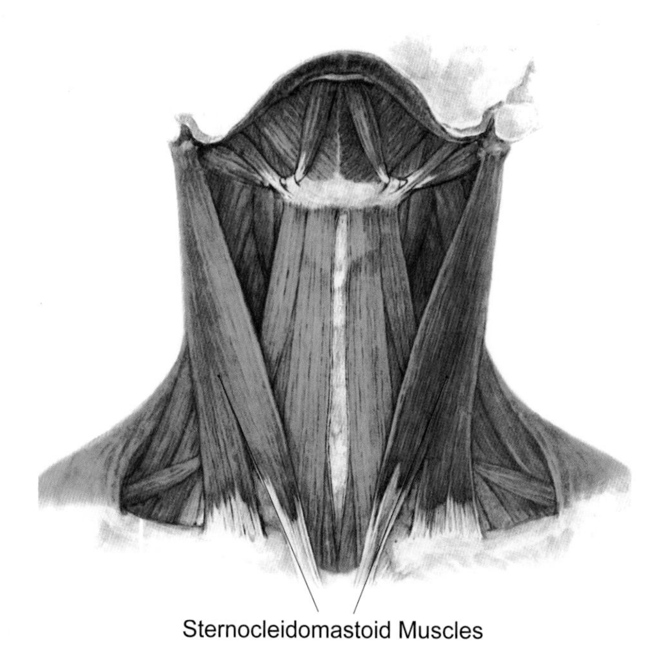

Figure 2.22 Anterior neck with sternocleidomastoid muscles.

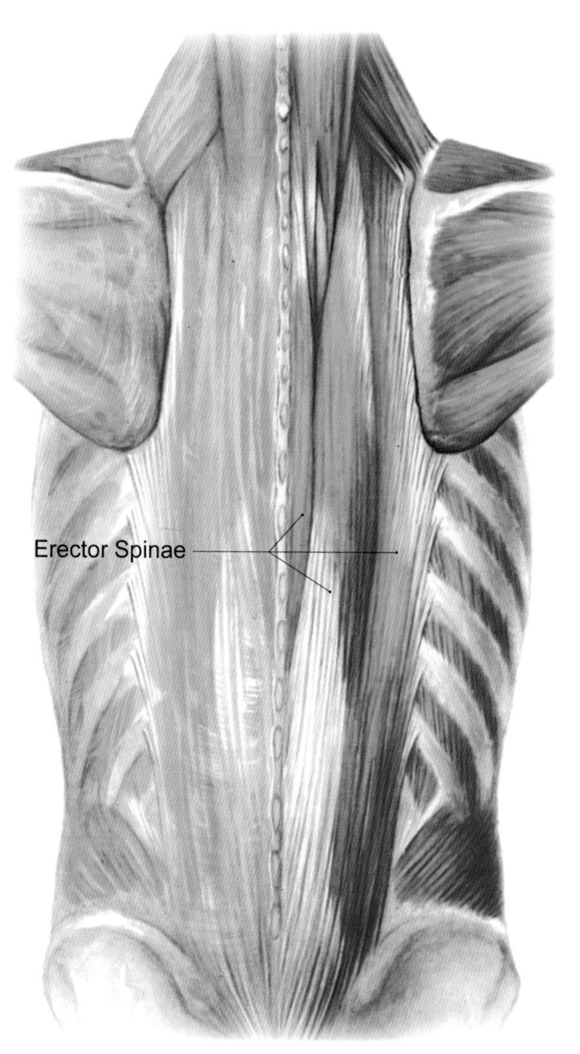

Figure 2.23 Deep posterior back muscles.

Posteriorly, there is a large muscle mass reaching in segments from the sacrum inferiorly, and to the skull superiorly, called the **erector spinae muscles** (Figure 2.23). They do what their name suggests – maintain your erect position. They are sometimes called the **antigravity muscles**. When someone faints, these muscles no longer function, and the body falls face forward to the ground. Just imagine what it would be like if we were unable to keep our bodies upright – this ability to stand erect and walk on two feet is one feature that sets us apart from most other species.

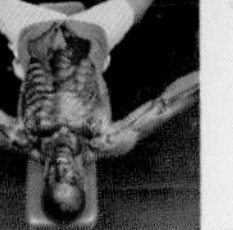

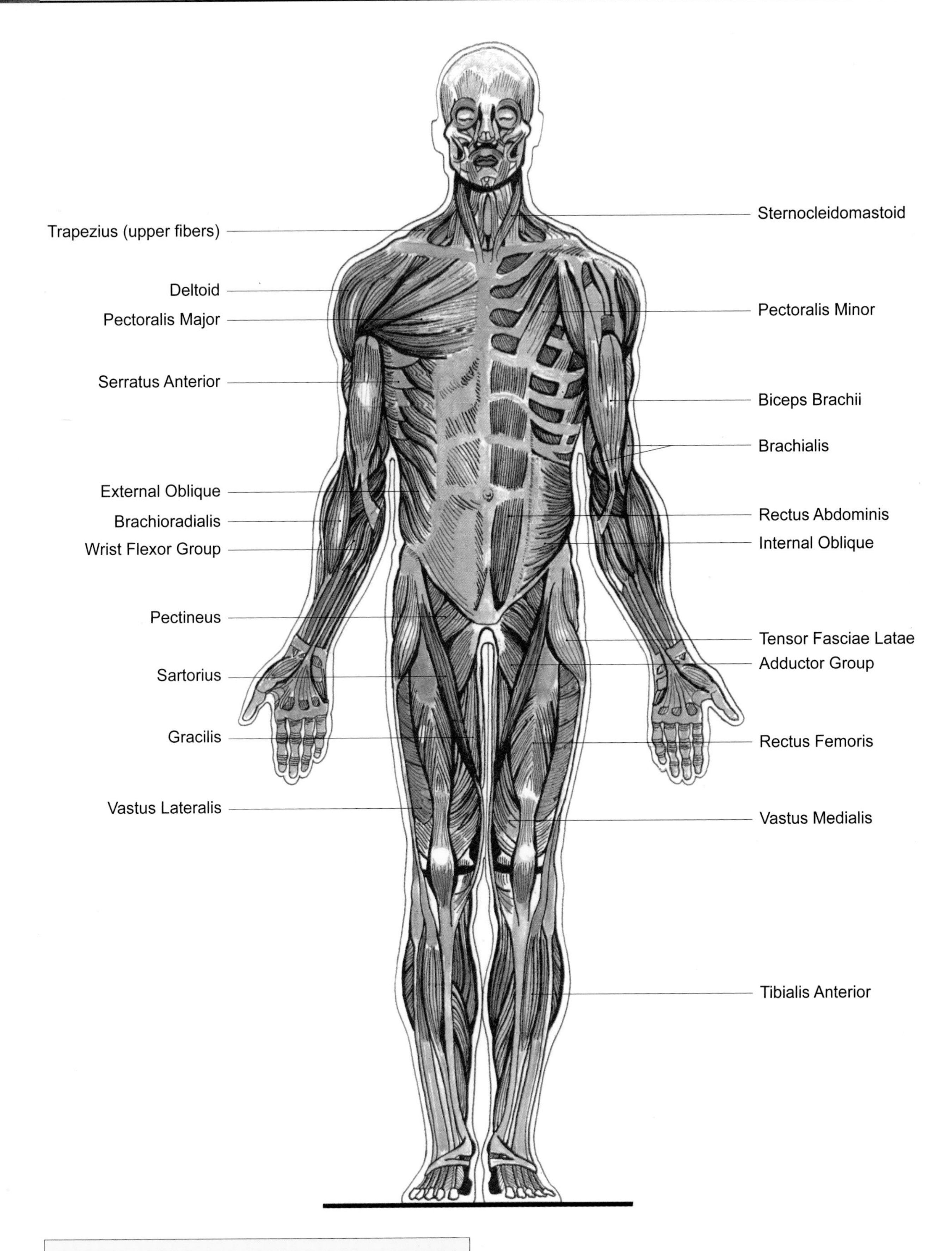

Figure 2.24 Anterior muscles of the human body.

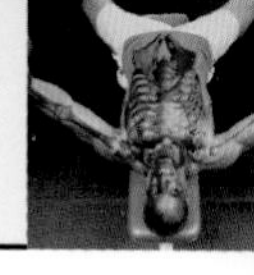

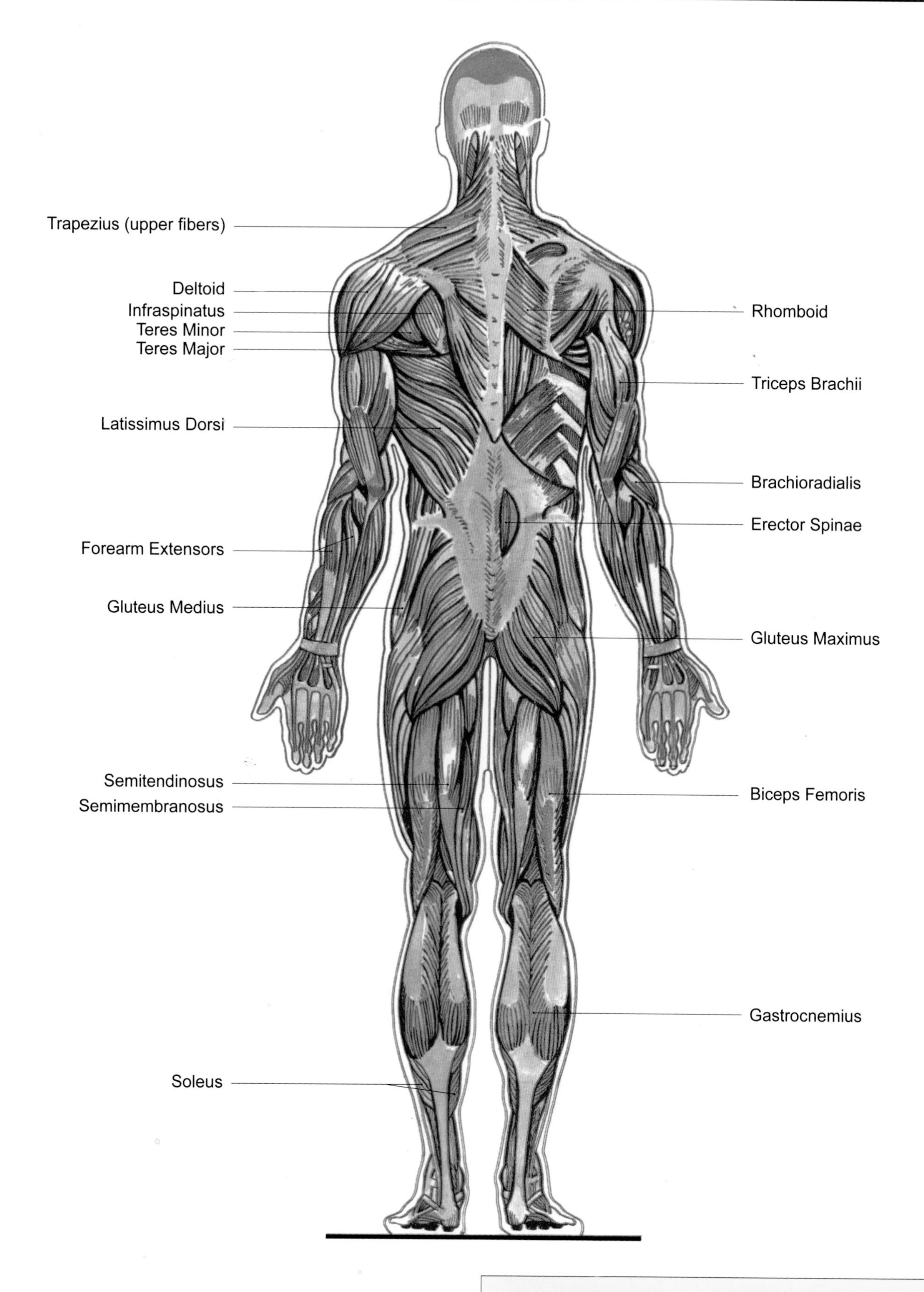

Figure 2.25 Posterior muscles of the human body.

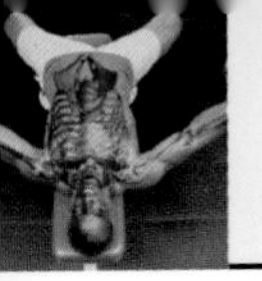

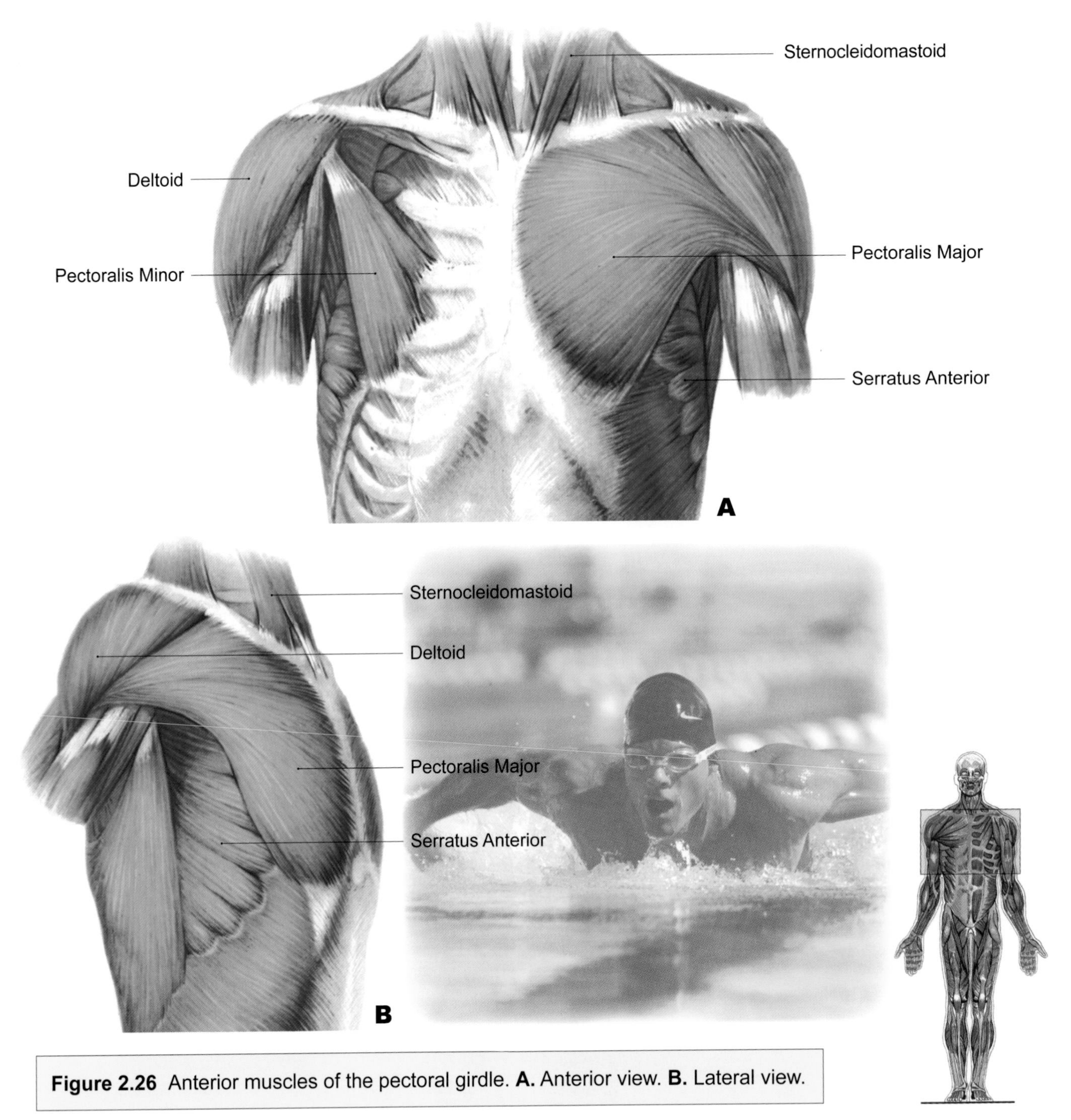

Figure 2.26 Anterior muscles of the pectoral girdle. **A.** Anterior view. **B.** Lateral view.

Muscles Connecting the Humerus and Scapula to the Axial Skeleton

Anterior and Posterior Groups

Muscles acting to hold the pectoral girdle to the chest wall can be divided into anterior and posterior groups as follows.

Anterior Group **Pectoralis major** has two heads. The clavicular head (attached to the clavicle) flexes and medially rotates the shoulder joint; the sternal head (attached to the sternum) extends the shoulder joint from a flexed position and medially rotates the shoulder joint. **Pectoralis minor** depresses and stabilizes the scapula. **Serratus anterior** steadies and holds the scapula forward (protracts it) against the chest wall (Figure

2.26). This frees the upper limb for actions such as rope climbing. These muscles as a group would also be required to perform the butterfly stroke in swimming.

Posterior Group **Trapezius** has three groups of fibers reflecting their relative positions. The *upper fibers* elevate the scapula, *middle fibers* retract the scapula, and *lower fibers* depress the scapula. **Latissimus dorsi** medially rotates, adducts, and extends the humerus, and **teres major** medially rotates the humerus (Figure 2.27).

Scapulohumeral Region

The following muscles from the scapula to the humerus act across the shoulder joint. Their primary role is to stabilize the shoulder joint to allow full use of the upper limb.

Anterior Group **Subscapularis** adducts and medially rotates the upper limb (Figure 2.27 C).

Superior and Posterior Group **Supraspinatus** initiates abduction of the upper limb at the shoulder joint. **Infraspinatus** and **teres minor** adduct and

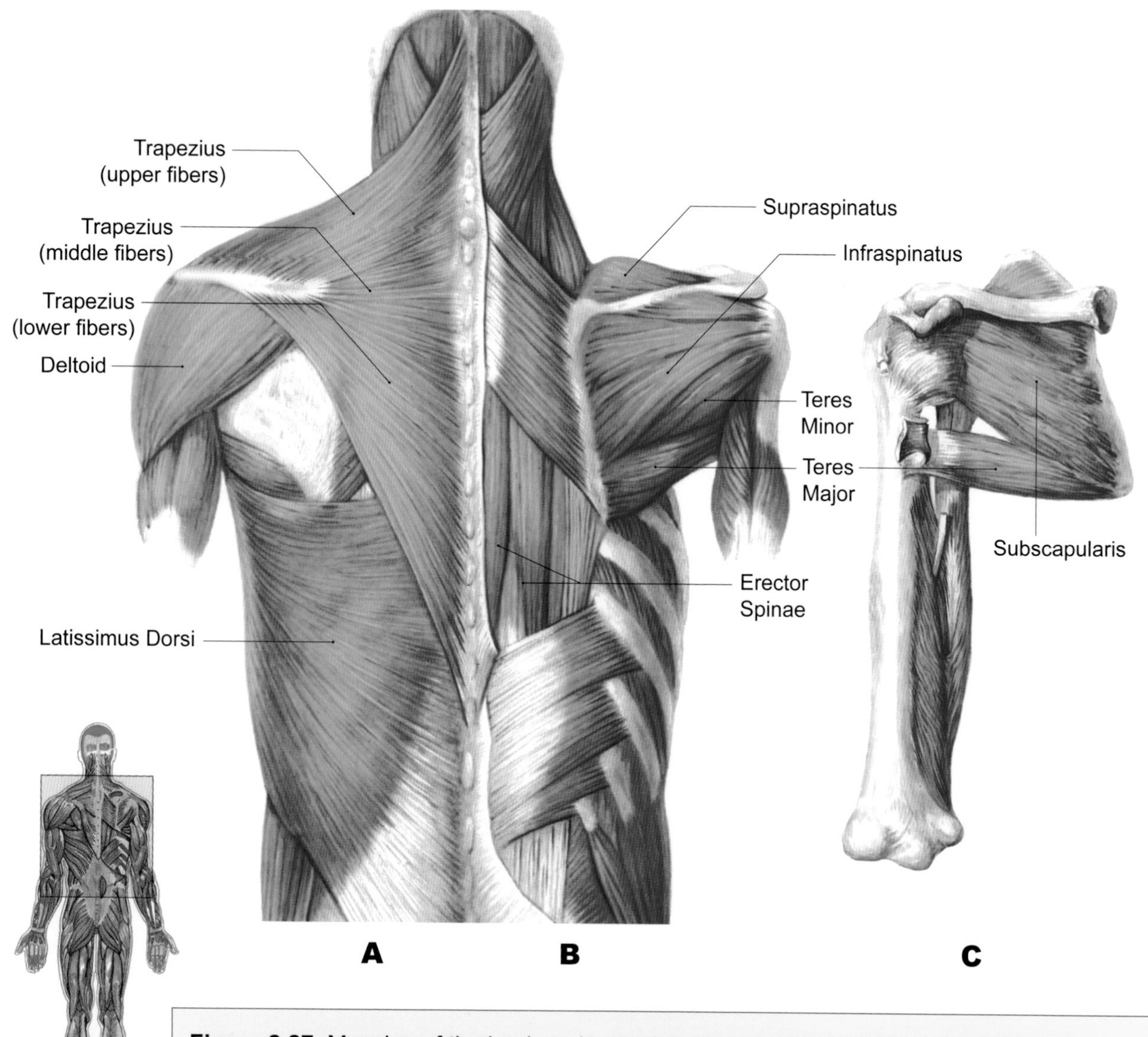

Figure 2.27 Muscles of the back and scapulohumeral region. **A.** Superficial posterior muscles of the back. **B.** Posterior muscles of the scapulohumeral region, deep and lateral to latissimus dorsi. **C.** Anterior subscapularis muscle of the scapulohumeral region.

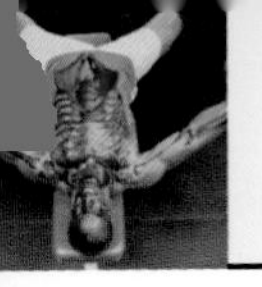

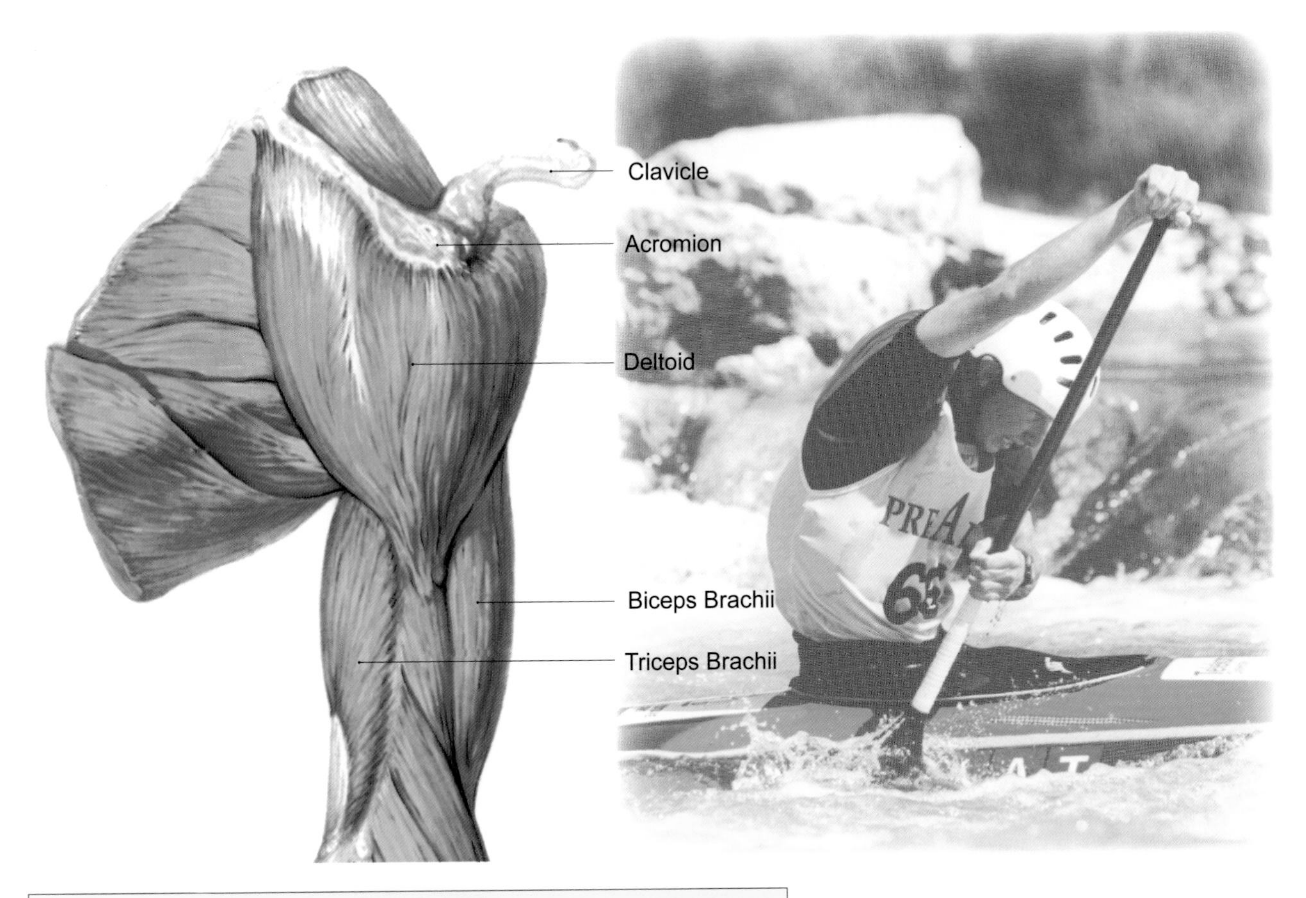

Figure 2.28 The lateral muscles of the scapulohumeral region.

laterally rotate the upper limb at the shoulder joint. These muscles, combined with subscapularis, are the **SSIT** (rotator cuff) muscles of the shoulder (Figure 2.27 B).

Lateral Group **Deltoid** has three functional groups of fibers. The *anterior fibers* flex and medially rotate the upper limb, the *middle fibers* abduct the upper limb, and the *posterior fibers* extend and laterally rotate the upper limb. All actions occur at the shoulder joint (Figure 2.28). The deltoid muscles are used extensively in paddling sports such as kayaking and canoeing.

Muscles of the Arm

Muscles of the limbs are primarily flexors or extensors. In the upper limb, the flexors are on the anterior surface of the arm, forearm, and hand, and the extensors are on the posterior surface. Some muscles from the scapula to the forearm span the arm to reach the radius and ulna of the forearm.

The muscles with proximal attachments to the humerus are divided by a strong fascial sheet of connective tissue into anterior and posterior compartments.

Anterior Compartment A muscle with two heads, both attached proximally to the scapula, the **biceps brachii** spans the arm to reach the radial tubercle of the radius. It is a powerful flexor of the elbow joint and supinator of the forearm (Figure 2.29 A). **Brachialis** is attached proximally to the anterior surface of the humerus and attaches distally to the coronoid process of the ulna. An important and powerful flexor of the elbow joint, it works along with the biceps brachii. To isolate brachialis in exercise, flex and pronate the forearm and perform repeated elbow curls.

Posterior Compartment **Triceps brachii** has three heads. The medial and lateral heads are attached to the humerus. They join with the long head from the scapula to attach distally to the olecranon process of the ulna. It is *the* powerful extensor of the elbow (Figure 2.29 B).

Muscles of the Forearm

The distal end of the humerus widens into lateral and medial epicondyles, which provide attachments for muscle groups that act on the forearm and wrist.

The forearm muscles act on the elbow, wrist, and digits (fingers and thumb). Muscles attached to the medial epicondyle of the humerus are the **flexor–pronator** group (Figure 2.29 A), while those attached to the lateral epicondyle of the humerus are the **extensor–supinator** group (Figure 2.29 B).

One muscle attached above the lateral epicondyle of the humerus is the **brachioradialis** muscle. It is on the extensor side of the humerus, but because it is positioned anterior to the elbow joint, it acts as an elbow flexor, especially when the forearm is partially pronated. You use this muscle when you shake hands with someone.

Muscles of the Hand

These muscles are divided into groups. The **thenar (palm) group** acts on the thumb and its metacarpal to abduct, flex, and oppose the thumb tip to the four remaining digits. The **hypothenar**

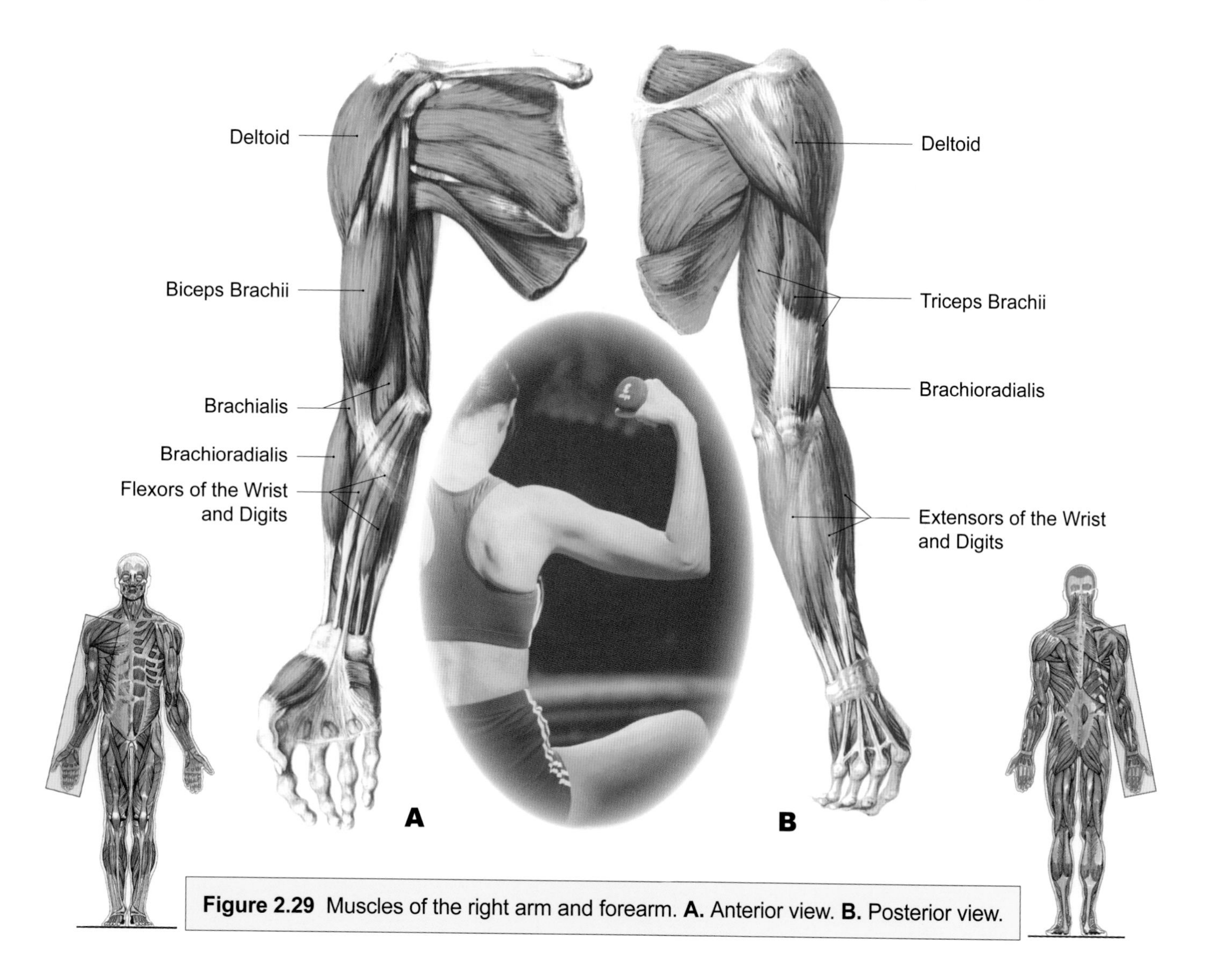

Figure 2.29 Muscles of the right arm and forearm. **A.** Anterior view. **B.** Posterior view.

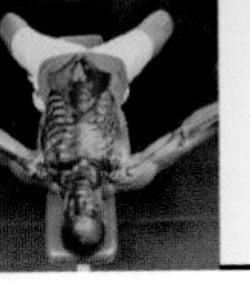

(little palm) group acts on the little finger and its metacarpal. Together the thenar and hypothenar muscles permit you to cup your hand as in holding a baseball. Between these two groups lie the **interossei** (between bones) and the **lumbrical** (earthworm) **muscles**, which are referred to collectively as the **intrinsic** (within) muscles of the hand. Together they flex, extend, abduct, and adduct the fingers, positioning the digits for fine movements.

Muscles of the Pelvic Girdle

From the bony pelvis, muscles are attached that permit a wide range of movement in the lower limb; but here, stability and transfer of weight for walking are the prime focus, not the fine discriminatory movements that are necessary with the hands and fingers. Some of the muscles acting at the hip joint come from the abdomen; others come from the sacrum and external surface of the hip bone (os coxae).

Because the hip joint is a ball and socket joint, flexion–extension, abduction–adduction, medial and lateral rotation, and circumduction can all occur here. Try it yourself. Notice, however, that the movement here is more limited than at the shoulder joint.

Anterior Group **Psoas major** (from the abdomen) and **iliacus** (from the iliac fossa of the pelvis) unite to form the **iliopsoas** muscle, which crosses the anterior aspect of the joint and is the primary flexor of the hip, allowing you to bring your thighs up to your chest or your chest to your knees (Figure 2.30).

Posterior and Lateral Group Large gluteal muscles cover the hip posteriorly. Put your hand on your hip and extend the joint. Feel the large muscle mass as it contracts. These are the three **gluteals**. The largest and most superficial posterior muscle, **gluteus maximus**, is the principal power extensor of the hip. **Gluteus medius** and **minimus** lie deep and lateral to maximus in that order and

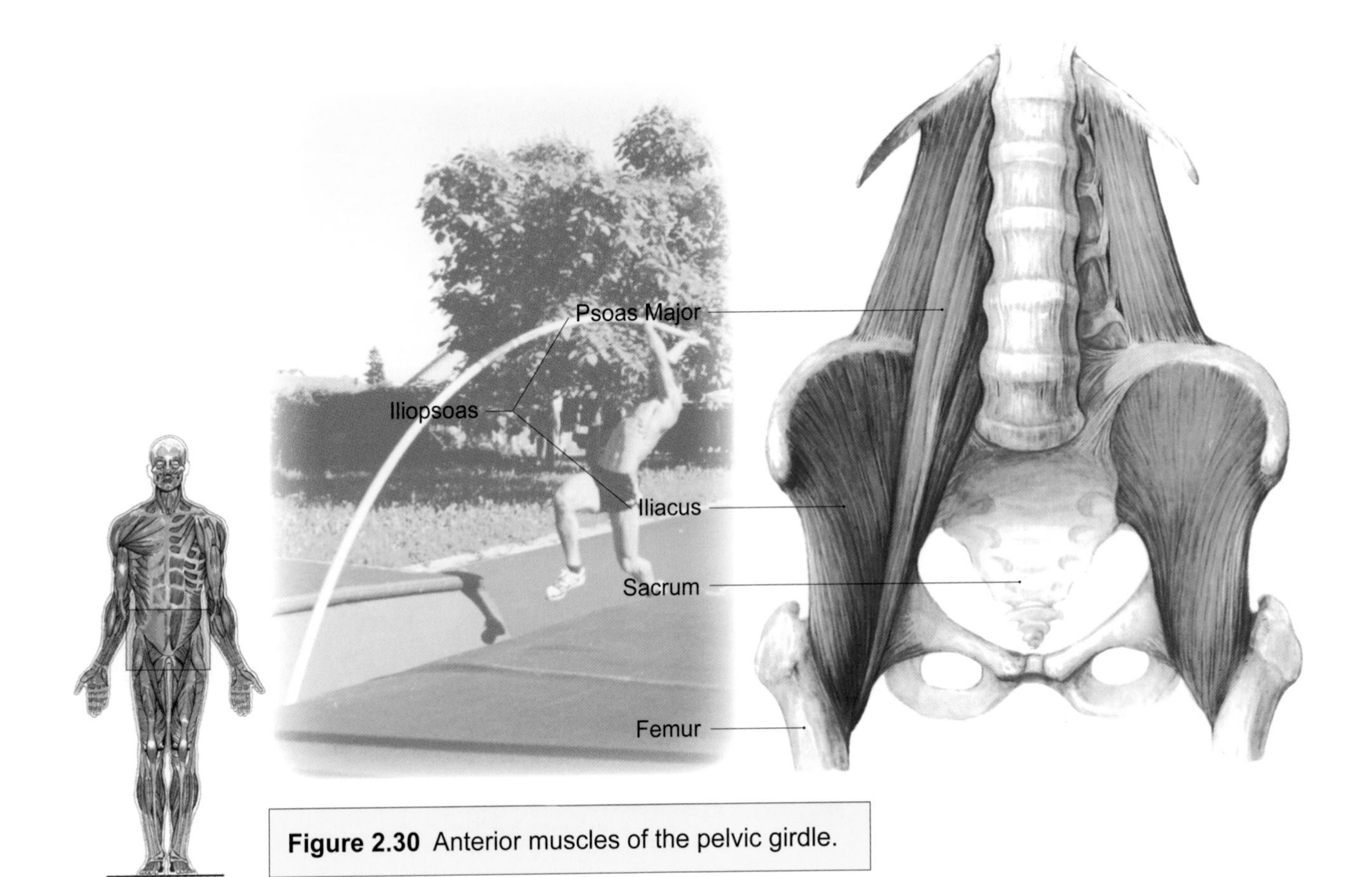

Figure 2.30 Anterior muscles of the pelvic girdle.

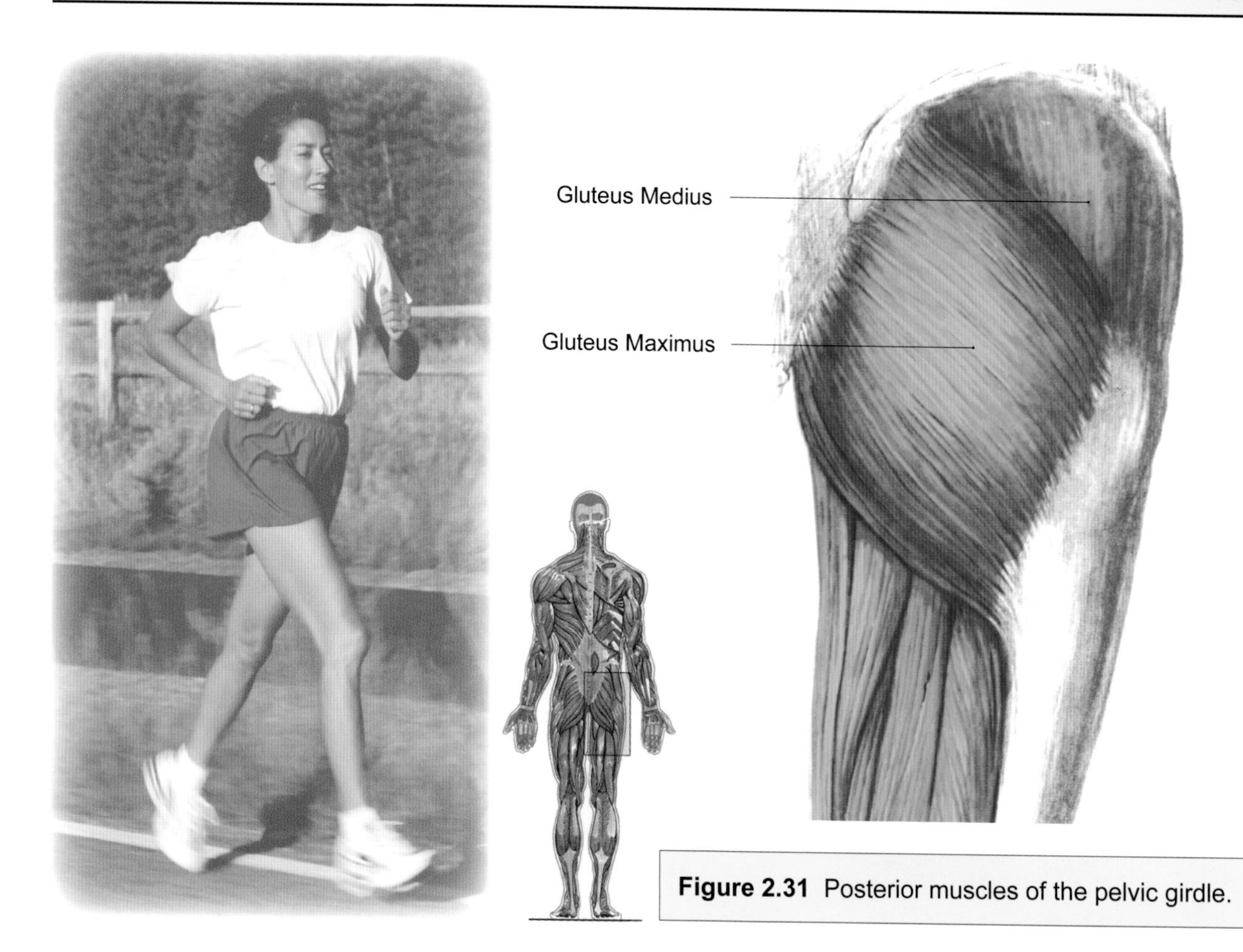

Figure 2.31 Posterior muscles of the pelvic girdle.

have a very important role – they abduct the hip (Figure 2.31). This is a very important movement in normal gait, or walking (a skill that is required for so many physical activities). Deep to gluteus maximus are six little muscles that all perform the same job: they laterally (externally) rotate the hip.

Muscles of the Thigh

The thigh is divided very conveniently into three compartments: medial, anterior, and posterior. Like the arm, most of the muscles acting in these compartments are attached proximally to the pelvic girdle. Some will attach distally to the femur; others will span the entire length of the femur and attach to the bones of the leg.

Anterior Compartment The anterior group is the extensor group, also known as the **quads** or **quadriceps**. They are the **rectus** (*rectus* = straight) **femoris**, **vastus lateralis**, **vastus intermedius**, and **vastus medialis** (Figure 2.32 A). The principal role of the quads is to extend the knee. To kick a soccer ball the knee must come into full extension for maximum distance, utilizing these leg extensors. The **sartorius** muscle lies anterior to the quads and acts to abduct and flex the thigh at the hip and to flex the knee. You use this muscle to dance the limbo or to sit cross-legged on the floor.

Medial Compartment This group of medial muscles has one primary action – to adduct the thigh toward the midline. This action prevents your leg from swinging too wide laterally as you walk. It is also the group of muscles you would use to stay on a horse. As their action implies, they are the adductor muscles, made up of **pectineus**, **adductor longus**, **adductor brevis**, and **adductor magnus** as well as **gracilis** (Figure 2.32 B).

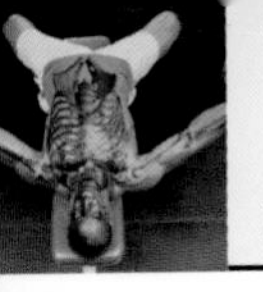

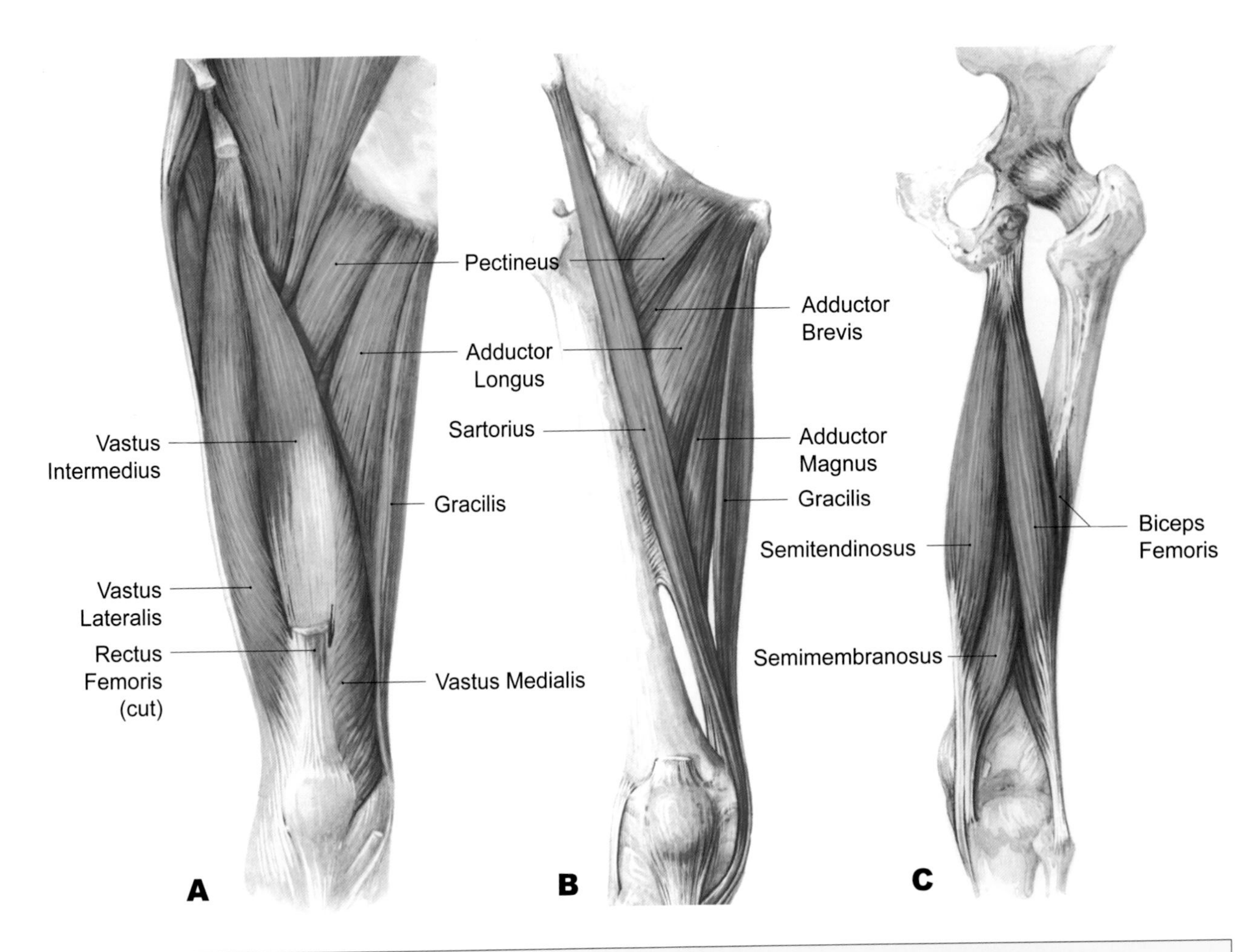

Figure 2.32 Muscles of the right thigh. **A.** Anterior compartment. **B.** Medial compartment. **C.** Posterior compartment.

Posterior Compartment The posterior group includes the muscles you know as the **hamstrings**. You may have thought the hamstrings were one muscle, but the group is actually made up of the **biceps femoris**, **semitendinosus**, and **semimembranosus** (Figure 2.32 C). Their role is to flex the knee and extend the hip with gluteus maximus. They are attached proximally to the ischial tuberosity (the bony part you sit on that gets sore when you sit on a hard chair for too long a time). Distally, the muscles cross posterior to the knee joint, with the biceps femoris attaching to the head of the fibula and the semitendinosus and semimembranosus attaching to the tibia.

Muscles of the Leg

The joints of the leg are arranged in the opposite conformation to the arm. The extensors are on the anterior surface and the flexors are located posteriorly. Let's look at the compartments.

Nature is very kind to those studying anatomy. Again, as in the thigh, the leg muscles are grouped into compartments, but here into anterior, lateral, and posterior compartments.

Anterior and Lateral Compartments

Anterior Compartment These muscles do not cross the knee joint but arise from the anterolateral surface of the tibia, from the interosseous membrane between the tibia and the fibula, and from the anterior surface of the fibula. Their tendons cross anterior to the ankle joint and go to the medial side of the foot and to the distal phalanges of the digits. They are primarily dorsiflexors of the ankle and extensors of the toes. The major anterior compartment muscle is **tibialis anterior** (Figure 2.33 A), which also functions to invert the sole of the foot. Loss of the nerve supply to these muscles results in foot drop.

Lateral Compartment There are two muscles in the lateral compartment, the **peroneus longus** and **peroneus brevis** (Figure 2.33 A). Both muscles attach to the lateral surface of the fibula and pass behind the lateral malleolus to enter the foot. Because they cross behind the ankle joint, they are plantar flexors of the ankle and evertors of the sole of the foot. For example, loss of the nerve supply to these muscles would mean you would have difficulty adapting your foot to uneven ground surfaces when running.

Posterior Compartment

Superficial Group The large muscles of the calf are formed by the **gastrocnemius** and **soleus** muscles (Figure 2.33 B). Gastrocnemius has two proximal heads attached to the medial and lateral epicondyles of the distal femur. They come together to form a large muscle belly that attaches to the back of the calcaneus (large bone of the heel) in common with the tendon of soleus as the calcaneal tendon (**Achilles tendon**). These three are the principal plantar flexors of the ankle. Often, the medial head of gastrocnemius can be partially torn away from its attachment to the

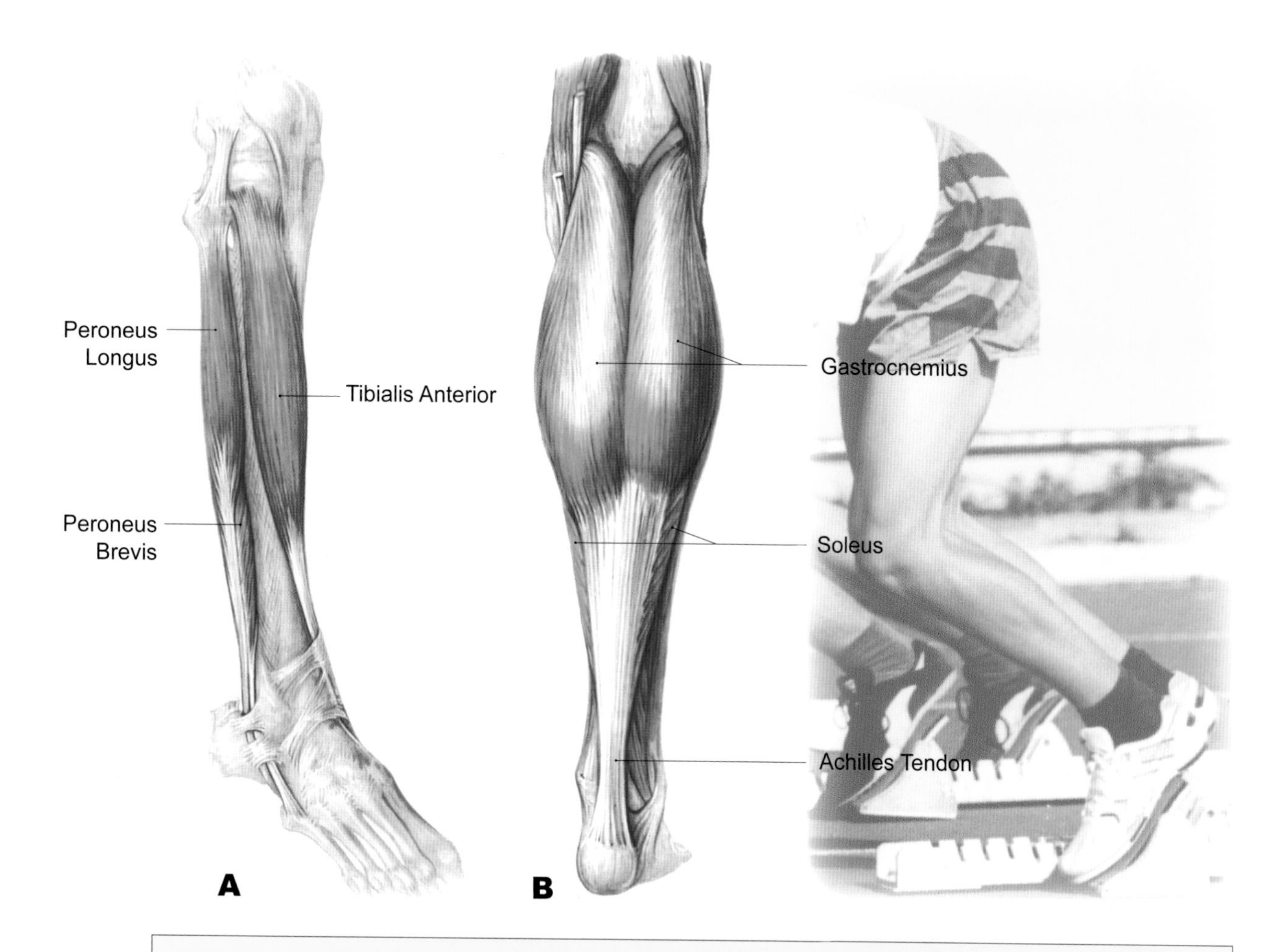

Figure 2.33 Muscles of the right leg. **A.** Anterolateral compartment. **B.** Posterior compartment.

femur (e.g., during a game of squash when you are making very sudden starts, stops, and turns); it can be very painful, but the fibers will naturally reattach during the healing process.

Deep Group The deep muscles are the ones that assist in plantar flexion of the ankle, but their primary role is flexion of the toes. Their tendons enter the foot by passing behind the medial malleolus of the tibia.

Muscles of the Foot

There are four layers of intrinsic foot muscles. Together with the bones and ligaments, they are arranged to permit the foot to support the body on uneven ground. As a group, they permit flexion, extension, abduction, and adduction of the digits. The great toe (digit 1) is the primary lever in the "push-off" in walking, running, and jumping.

Muscles of the Abdomen

The anterior abdominal wall is a plywood-like trilaminar muscular wall. The triple layer is formed by, from superficial to deep, the **external oblique**, **internal oblique**, and **transversus abdominis** muscles (Figures 2.34 and 2.35). They reach

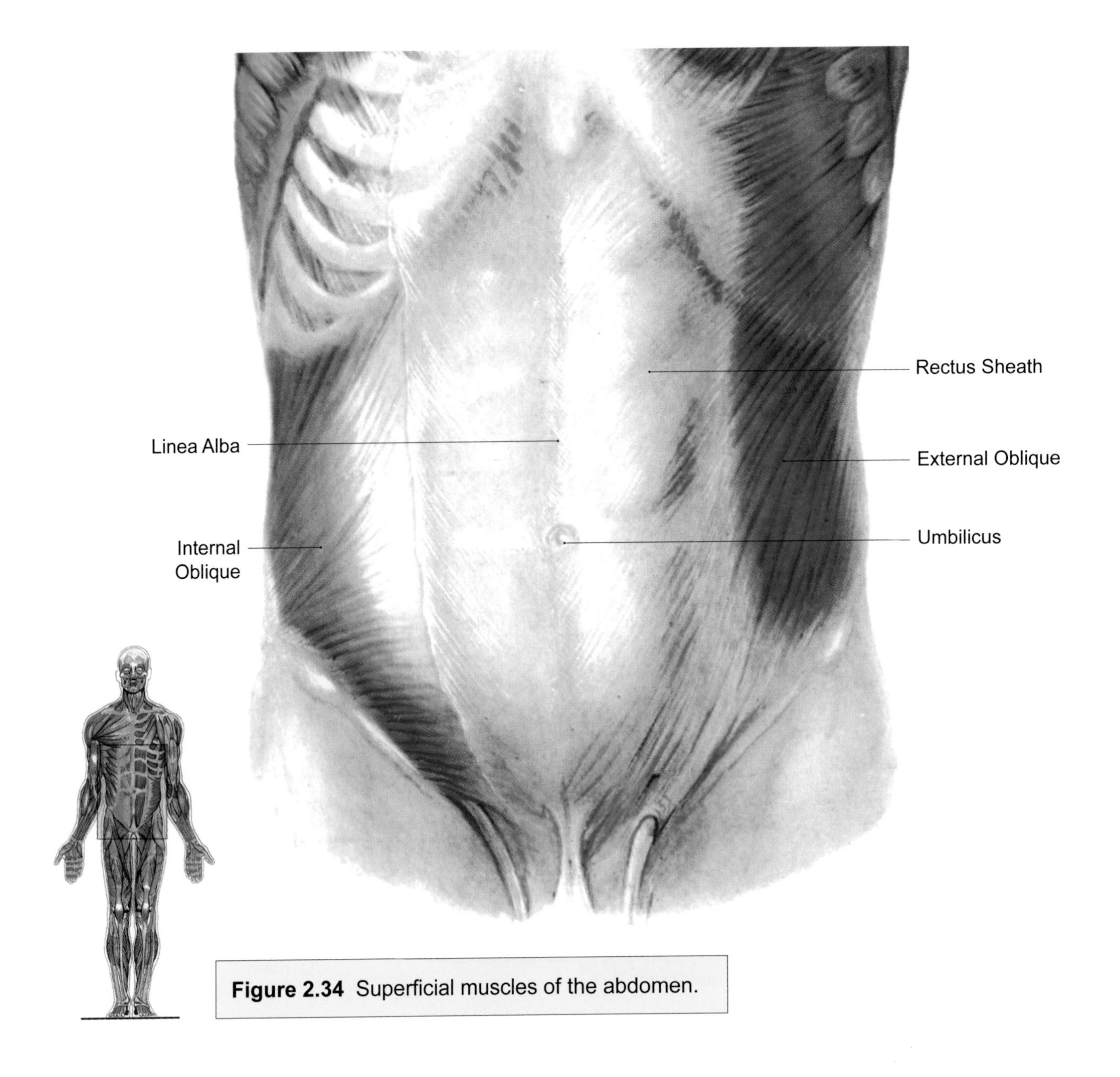

Figure 2.34 Superficial muscles of the abdomen.

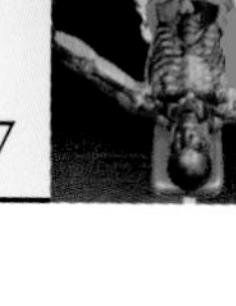

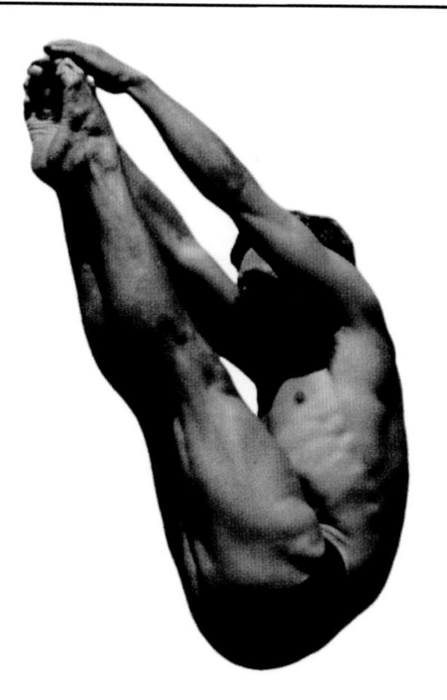

from the vertebral column, ribs, and hip bone posteriorly to meet in the midline anteriorly at the **linea alba**. As the right and left muscle groups approach each other, they envelop paired midline muscles, the **rectus abdomini** (Figure 2.35). The obliques are important in lateral bending and in rotation of the trunk (e.g., in throwing the javelin). They also permit extension of the abdomen during forced inspiration and allow the development of a pregnant uterus. They contract during forced expiration and help to expel fecal contents from the rectum. The rectus abdominis, the muscle used in sit-ups, is a powerful flexor of the anterior abdominal wall. Strengthening of the

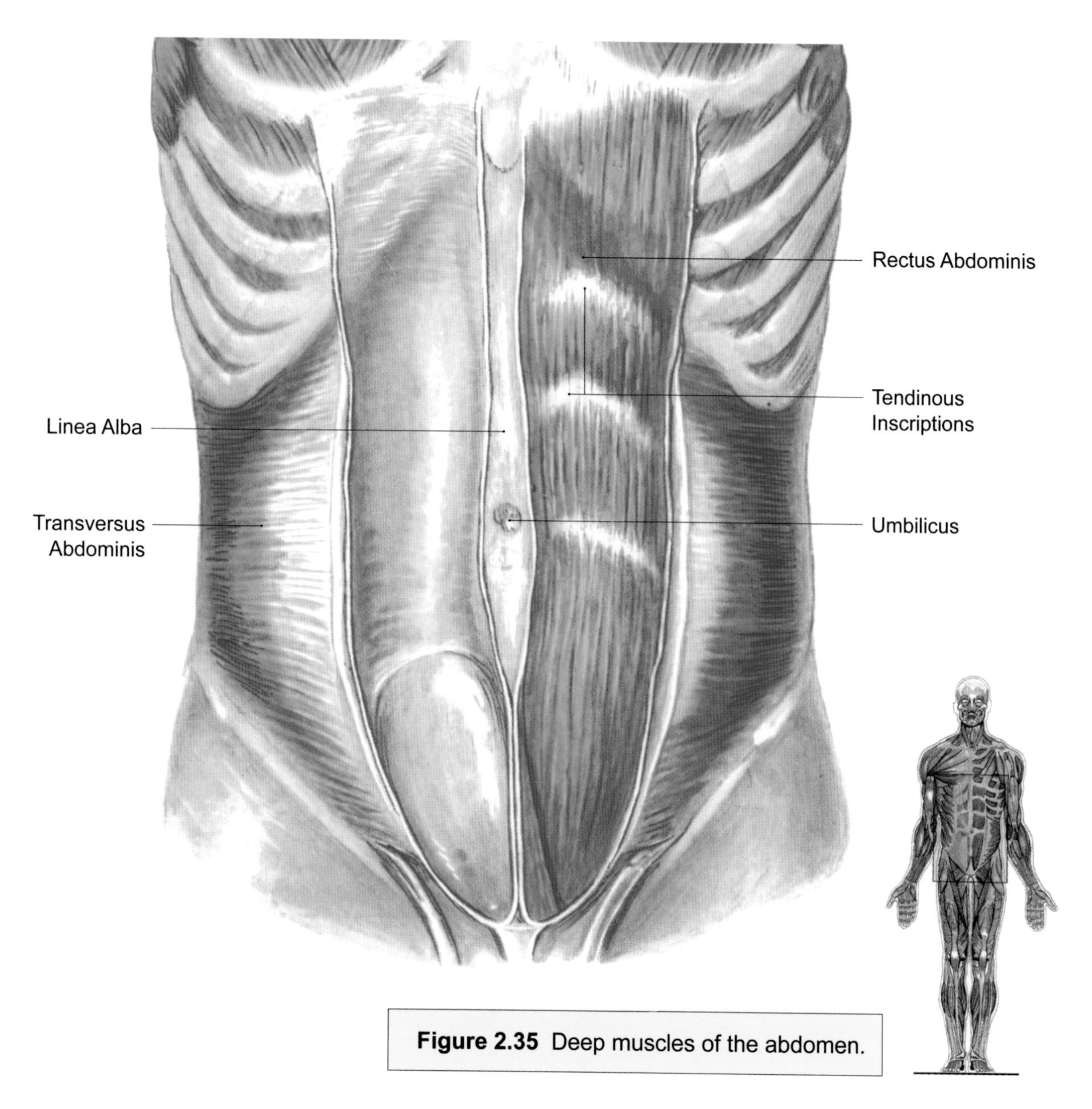

Figure 2.35 Deep muscles of the abdomen.

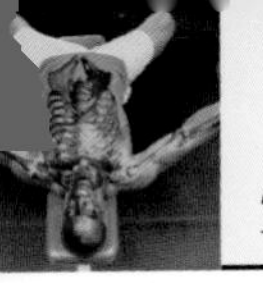

Table 2.2 Summary of major muscles and movements of the upper limb.

Joint	Action	Muscles	Sport or Activity
Shoulder	Flexion	*Pectoralis major, clavicular head *Deltoid, anterior fibers *Biceps brachii	Cross-country and downhill skiing, pull-through in freestyle swimming
	Extension	*Latissimus dorsi Teres major *Deltoid, posterior fibers Pectoralis major, sternal head	Iron cross formation in gymnastics, freestyle stroke, racket positioning in tennis
	Abduction	*Deltoid Supraspinatus	Position in takeoff in diving
	Adduction	*Pectoralis major Latissimus dorsi	Dance positions, cross-court shot in tennis
	Medial rotation	*Pectoralis major *Deltoid, anterior fibers Latissimus dorsi	Crossing one's arms, butterfly stroke in swimming, arm positioning in ballet
	Lateral rotation	*Deltoid, posterior fibers Teres minor Infraspinatus	Backstroke in swimming, lawn bowling, curling
Elbow	Flexion	Brachialis *Biceps brachii Brachioradialis	Weightlifting, shaking hands, positioning forearm to write, boxing
	Extension	*Triceps Anconeus	Pull stroke in paddling, backhand in tennis, painting a wall
Radioulnar	Pronation	Pronator teres	Volleyball spike, tennis serve, football pass
	Supination	*Biceps brachii Supinator	Fencing, volleyball serve, lawn bowling
Radiocarpal	Flexion–Extension	Forearm flexors and extensors	Baseball pitch, throwing a javelin
	Abduction–Adduction	Forearm flexors and extensors	Positioning wrist to maneuver a basketball or baseball
Metacarpo-phalangeal	Flexion–Extension	Forearm flexors and extensors	Position of wrist for throwing baseball, basketball, darts, javelin
	Abduction–Adduction	Forearm flexors and extensors Intrinsic hand muscles	Grasping a basketball or javelin, releasing a baseball or dart
Inter-phalangeal	Flexion–Extension	Intrinsic hand muscles Forearm flexors	Grasping an object (e.g., baseball, darts); releasing an object

* indicates prime movers

As you read the sports and activities listed in the table, try to imagine how the movements would be performed.

Table 2.3 Summary of major muscles and movements of the lower limb.

Joint	Action	Muscles	Sport or Activity
Hip	Flexion	*Iliopsoas Sartorius Pectineus Rectus femoris	Sprinting, climbing, gymnastics, diving
	Extension	*Gluteus maximus Semitendinosus Semimembranosus Biceps femoris Adductor magnus	Rising from a squat in weightlifting, running uphill, gymnastics
	Abduction	*Gluteus medius Gluteus minimus Tensor fasciae latae	Figure skating, gymnastics, hurdles
	Adduction	Adductor magnus Adductor longus Adductor brevis Gracilis	Equestrian events, cross-country skiing
	Lateral rotation	Obturator externus Obturator internus Piriformis Quadratus femoris	Figure skating, gymnastics, soccer
	Medial rotation	Tensor fasciae latae Gluteus medius Gluteus minimus	Gymnastics, ballet, diving
Knee	Extension	*Quadriceps femoris Tensor fasciae latae	Place kick in football, diving, gymnastics
	Flexion	*Biceps femoris *Semimembranosus *Semitendinosus Gastrocnemius Sartorius Gracilis Popliteus	Running, hurdles, rowing
Ankle	Dorsiflexion	*Tibialis anterior Extensor hallucis longus Extensor digitorum longus Peroneus tertius	Heel-toe walking, skiing
	Plantar flexion	*Gastrocnemius *Soleus Tibialis posterior Flexor hallucis longus	Push-off in sprinting, going "en pointe" in dance, gymnastics, diving
Transverse Tarsal	Inversion	*Tibialis anterior Tibialis posterior	Maintaining stability when walking on uneven ground
	Eversion	Peroneus longus Peroneus brevis	Maintaining stability when walking on uneven ground

* indicates prime movers

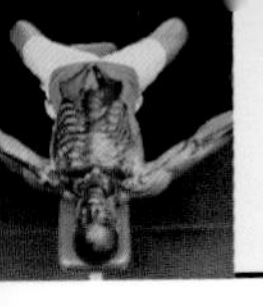

anterior abdominal wall is a very important part of back therapy, whereby the anterior wall muscles act to support the back.

Summary

Human anatomy deals with the structures that make up the human body and how these various structures are related to one another. Having knowledge of the structures of the human body and their associated functions; the major bones, joints, and muscles that allow us to move; and anatomical description and analysis is important to realizing your full potential as an individual.

The bones, joints, and muscles that make up the musculoskeletal system allow numerous movements to occur, with varying degrees of motion capabilities, strength, and flexibility. Bones provide the structural framework necessary for support, muscles supply the power, and the joints supply the mechanism that allows human movement to occur.

While the human body is highly organized, intricate, and complex, it is structured precisely to respond to the demands of the world around us with astounding efficiency. Our ability to move and perform an almost limitless number of skills can be enhanced with knowledge of anatomy; and because structure determines function, knowing our structure can go a long way in improving the functions of those structures for performance in our everyday lives.

Key Terms

abduction
adduction
anatomical position
anterior (ventral)
appendicular skeleton
axial skeleton
ball and socket joint
circumduction
condyloid (knuckle) joint
deep
distal
dorsiflexion
epidural hemorrhage
eversion
extension
flat bone
flexion
frontal (coronal) plane
hinge (ginglymus) joint
human anatomy
inferior
insertion
inversion
irregular bone
lateral
lateral (external) rotation
long bone
medial
medial (internal) rotation
median (midsagittal) plane
origin
pivot joint
plane (gliding) joint
plantar flexion
posterior (dorsal)
pronation
prone
proximal
saddle joint
sagittal plane
sesamoid bone
short bone
superficial
superior
supination
supine
synovial joint
transverse (horizontal) plane

Discussion Questions

1. Describe the anatomical position and discuss its relationship to the directional terms of the body.

2. What are the four major planes that bisect the body? Provide an example of a movement that occurs in each plane.

3. Define three types of movement and give an example of each for a specific joint in the human body.

4. List the six major types of synovial joints. Which synovial joints allow the greatest amount of movement? The least?

5. Outline the components and roles of the axial and appendicular skeletons.

6. List the five regions of the vertebral column from the most superior to the most inferior. In what region are the atlas and axis located?

7. What type of joint is the knee? What structures present at the knee provide additional support to this joint?

8. What muscles are primarily responsible for maintaining an upright posture?

9. The posterior group of leg muscles is commonly called the hamstrings. What three muscles combine to form the hamstrings? What role do they play?

10. List the four major muscles that make up the abdomen. Which layer is most superficial? Most deep? What actions do these muscles allow you to do?

In This Chapter:

CHAPTER 3

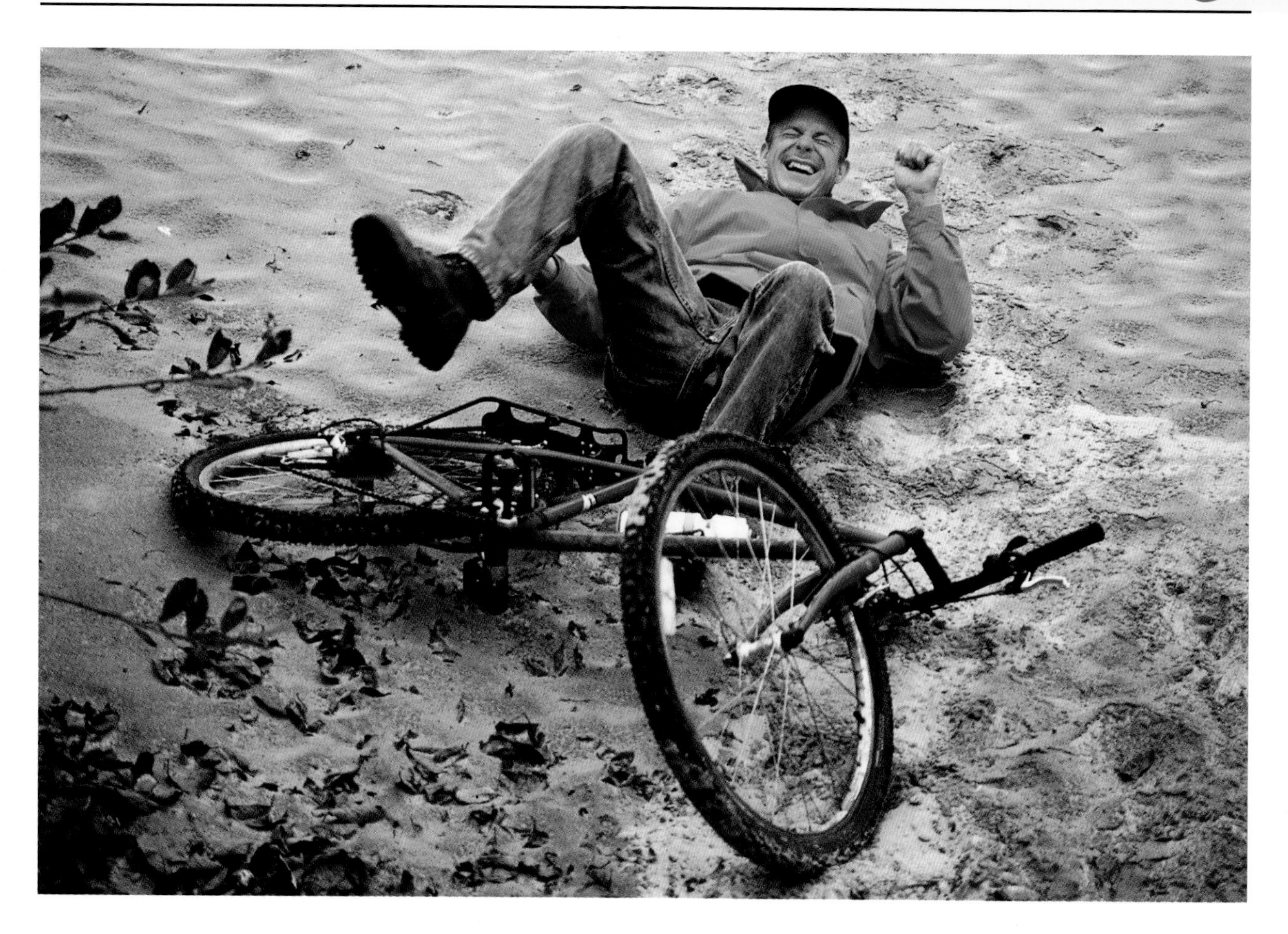

Out of Harm's Way: Sports Injuries

After completing this chapter you should be able to:

- identify the factors associated with injury prevention;
- describe the common musculoskeletal injuries;
- demonstrate an understanding of the implications of various chronic and acute injuries and how to treat them.

The human body is designed to perform a wide variety of simple and complex movements and skills. Clearly, this ability relies on all its parts working together in harmony. An injury to one body part can disrupt the harmony of the entire body. Fortunately, many injuries are preventable.

With more people participating in sports and physical activity for health, fitness, and fun, avoiding injury is a notable concern. Many people ignore the warnings and risks that accompany certain activities, believing that nothing can possibly happen to them. Even the most careful physically active person can experience a mishap, but following some specific guidelines can greatly decrease your risk of sustaining an injury. Whether you make a concerted effort to improve your skills and technique when exercising, recognize the hazards that exist around you, perform proper conditioning exercises, or demand safe and quality equipment, you can enjoy an enhanced level of safety and confidence in your physical pursuits. You must take responsibility for your own actions by making appropriate decisions that reflect your safety and personal health (Figure 3.1).

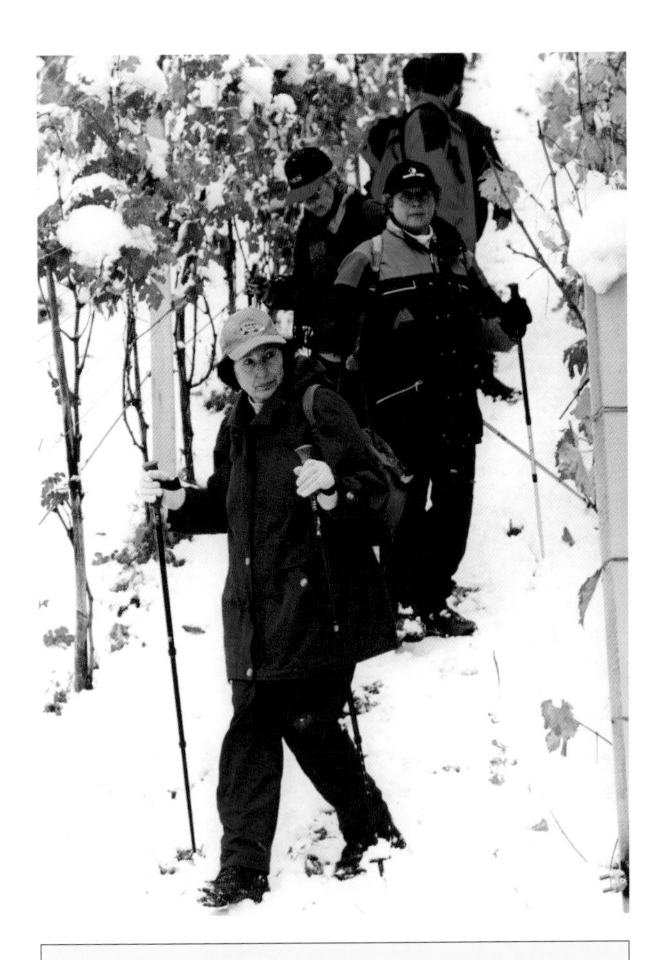

Figure 3.1 Staying fit and active throughout your life requires attention to conditioning, healthy lifestyle choices, and safety.

Despite our efforts to take all of the necessary precautions, all dangers can never be completely eliminated; accidents do happen and injuries do occur. While most injuries are minor and not life threatening, knowing what to do if an injury occurs helps you deal with the situation quickly and correctly. An injury that is not cared for properly can easily escalate into a chronic problem that may plague your efforts to lead an active life.

Biomechanical Principles of Injury

The human body is made up of tissues or groups of cells that work together to perform a particular function. The four basic types of tissue are **epithelial** (e.g., skin), **muscle**, **connective** (e.g., tendons, bones, and ligaments), and **nervous**. Each type of tissue possesses unique mechanical characteristics. For example, bones are strong and stiff, whereas tendons are flexible so that joints can be mobile.

To best understand the biomechanical characteristics of tissue, we examine its behavior under **physical load** (see box *Forces Acting on Tissue*). Under load, a tissue experiences **deformation**. This change in shape phenomenon can be visualized in the load–deformation curve in Figure 3.2.

Did You Know?

When developing a prosthesis for human parts, such as a hip joint, biomechanical engineers ensure that the prosthesis can handle loads as well as or better than the human tissue it will be replacing.

Characteristics of the Load–Deformation Curve

- Loads occurring in the elastic region do not cause permanent damage.
- Permanent deformation will occur if loads exceed the yield-level point.
- The area under the entire curve represents the strength of the material in terms of stored energy.
- The slope of the curve in the elastic region indicates the stiffness of the material. Stiffness is the resistance to deformation, where the greater the slope of the curve, the greater the stiffness of the structure.

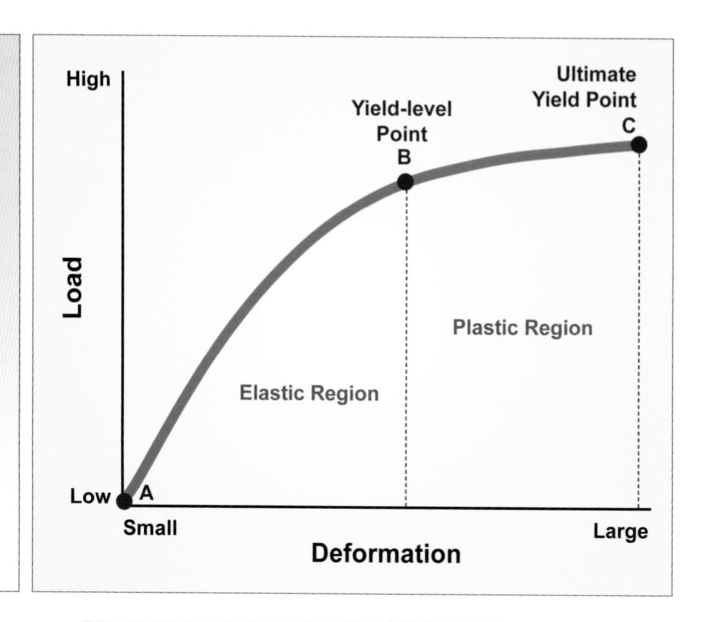

Figure 3.2 Load–deformation curve of a bone.

The A to B segment of the curve represents the **elastic region** of the tissue structure. Elasticity is the capacity of a tissue to return to its original shape after a load is removed. For example, when you push your finger into your thigh, the skin and the muscle underneath your finger become depressed. When pressure is removed, the tissues return to their original shape.

Point B on the curve (**yield-level point**) signals the **elastic limit** of the tissue, where the **plastic region** begins. In this region, increased loads cause permanent tissue deformation, resulting in micro-failure or injury to the tissue. Sprains and strains are good examples of such injuries. If the load continues to increase to the **ultimate yield point** (point C on the curve), **ultimate failure** of the tissue eventually occurs: a bone fracture or torn ligament. At this point the tissue becomes completely unresponsive to loads.

Tissue Responses to Training

Human tissue responds to training loads or stresses by becoming stronger. When training loads are at or near a tissue's *yield-level point* (Figure 3.2, point B), cells may divide to make new cells or to make proteins such as *actin*, *myosin*, *collagen*, or *elastin* to improve the mechanical properties of the tissue under **stress**. This muscle response is called the **positive training effect**.

Training overloads may cause microscopic injuries in various muscle regions, leading to sore muscles. In these situations, the muscle structures are *temporarily* weakened. It is important to let them recover before another workout. Research has shown that optimal training occurs at a level of tissue stress just below the yield-level point.

Injury Treatment and Rehabilitation

Treatment and rehabilitation are two directly linked aspects of recovery. During **treatment**, a patient receives care by a health care professional. Early and correct treatment promotes the healing process and improves the quality of the injured tissue(s), allowing the person to return to activity more quickly. **Rehabilitation** involves a therapist's physical restoration of the injured tissue along with the patient's active participation by following prescribed rehabilitation guidelines on his or her own.

Although an individualized rehabilitation

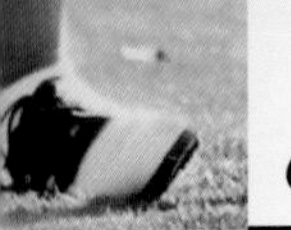

Forces Acting on Tissue

Tissue is exposed to a variety of physical stresses during physical activity. These stresses are forces and moments acting as directional loads that generate **tension** (pulling), **compression** (squeezing), **bending**, **shear**, or **torsion**.

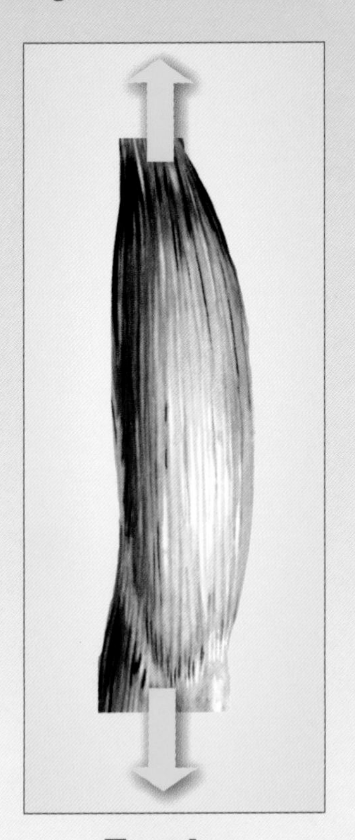

Tension

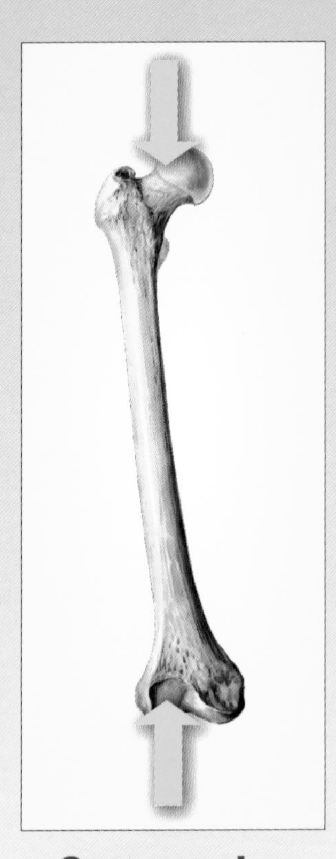

Compression

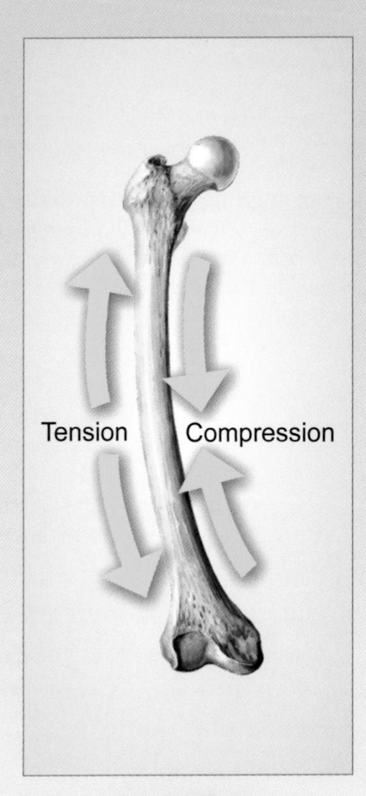

Bending

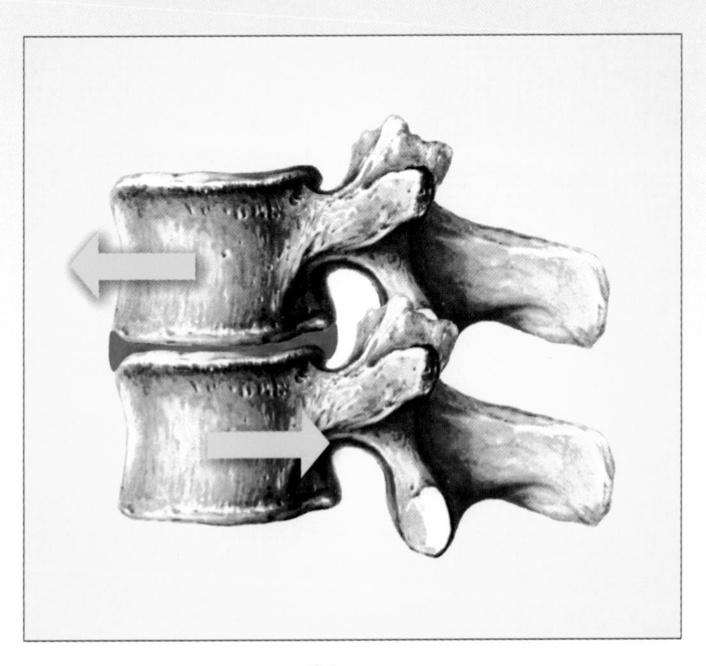

Shear

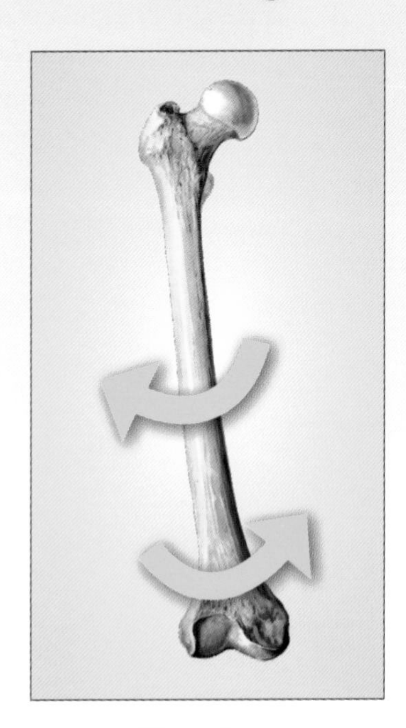

Torsion

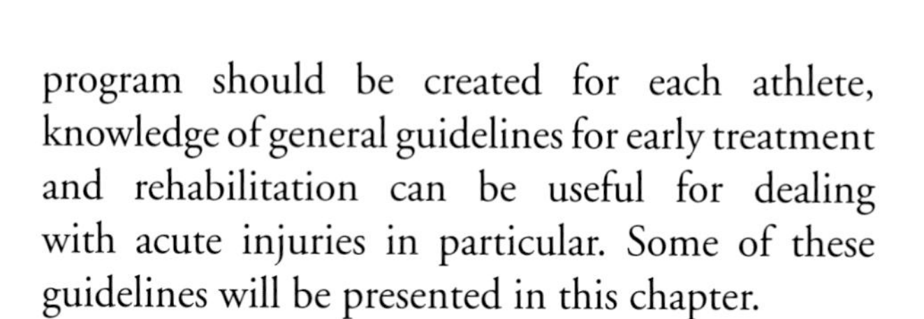

program should be created for each athlete, knowledge of general guidelines for early treatment and rehabilitation can be useful for dealing with acute injuries in particular. Some of these guidelines will be presented in this chapter.

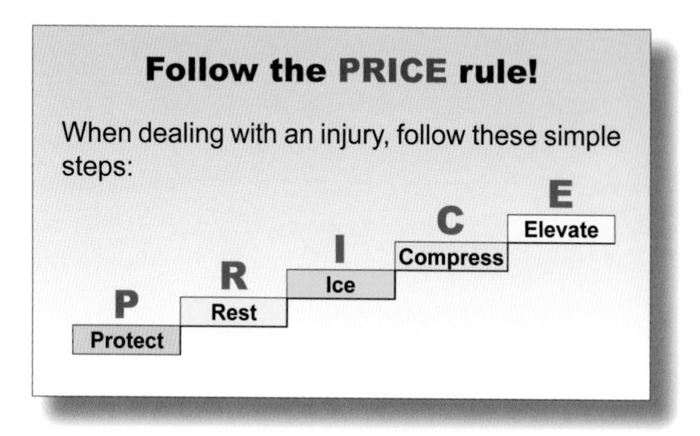

Healing Phases

The healing process begins immediately after injury and consists of three overlapping phases: the inflammatory response phase, the fibroblastic repair phase, and the maturation–remodeling phase (Figure 3.3).

Inflammatory Response Phase

The **inflammatory response phase** sets the stage for tissue repair. Inflammation begins at the time of injury, or shortly after, and may last from two to four days. The injured area may show signs of redness, swelling, pain, increased temperature, and loss of function.

To allow healing to begin, the injury must be protected and rested. **Cryotherapy** (ice or cold water immersion for 15 to 20 minutes at a time) limits the amount of swelling and decreases bleeding, pain, and muscle spasms. **Compression** is applied over the ice, usually in the form of an elastic bandage. During cold water immersion, a compression bandage can be wrapped around the injured area. Finally, the area is elevated above the level of the heart to encourage the return of venous blood to the heart, thereby helping to decrease acute swelling and bleeding.

Fibroblastic Repair Phase

The **fibroblastic repair phase** leads to scar formation and repair of the injured tissue. It begins within a few hours of injury and may last as long as four to six weeks. A delicate connective tissue called **granulation tissue** forms to fill the gaps in the injured area. Fibroblasts produce **collagen fibers**, which are deposited randomly throughout the forming scar. In this second phase, many of the signs and symptoms seen in the inflammatory response subside.

During the fibroblastic repair phase, it is important to introduce controlled rehab-specific exercises that are designed to restore normal range of motion and strength to the injured tissue, as well as stressing the tissue to promote optimal tissue response (see box *Tissue Responses to Training*). Manual massage therapy and ultrasound help break down scar tissue. Protective taping or a brace is often used during this phase of rehabilitation.

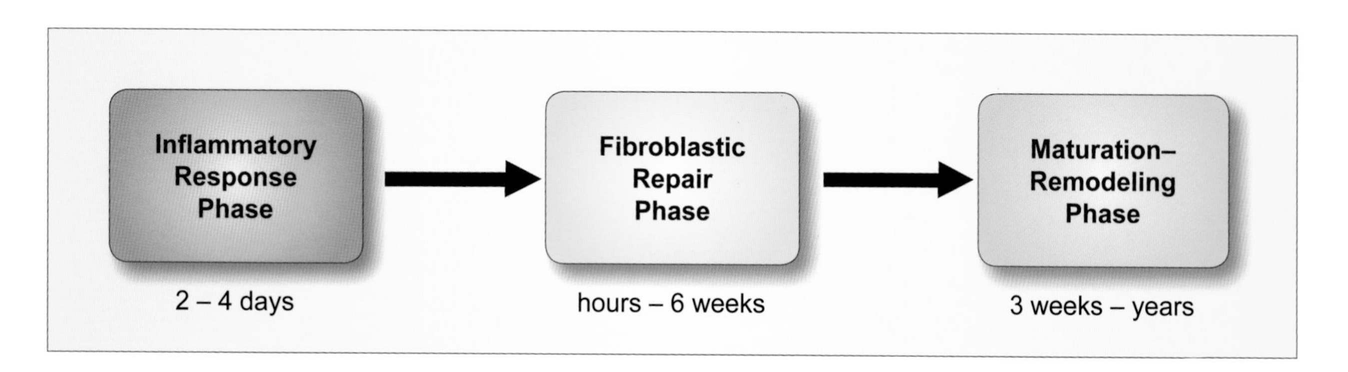

Figure 3.3 The three phases of the healing process.

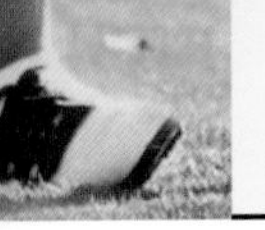

Maturation–Remodeling Phase

The **maturation–remodeling phase** is a long-term process of remodeling or realigning the scar tissue. It begins about three weeks after injury and may continue for as long as several years. Stretching and strengthening become more aggressive in this phase because the goal is to organize the scar tissue along the lines of tensile stress. Sport-specific skills and activities are usually included in rehabilitation.

Pain: Nature's Warning System

Pain is nature's way of telling us something is wrong. However, many athletes ignore pain altogether. Professional athletes in particular believe that a little pain is natural, and taking a few days off to nurse an injury makes you weak and vulnerable. As a result, they choose to mask the pain with medication, which allows them to play through an injury. While the pain may subside, the problem remains unaddressed (Figure 3.4). Continued participation will push injured tissues closer to ultimate failure, resulting in a need for surgical repair. Other serious consequences of using medication to mask pain include addiction and gastrointestinal complications.

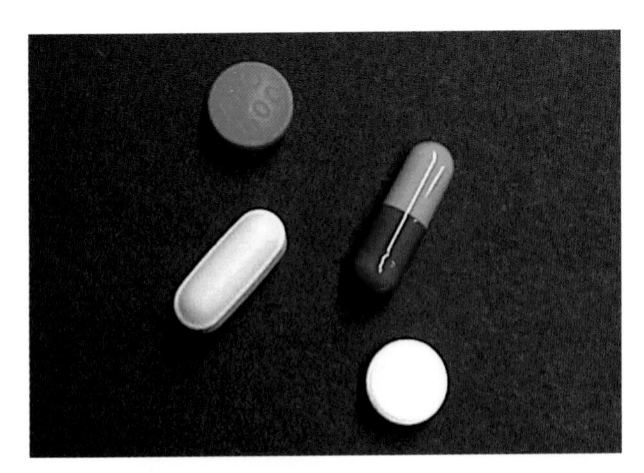

Figure 3.4 Pain medication helps reduce discomfort but fails to address the cause of the problem.

Having said that, the temporary use of certain medications to decrease pain and inflammation may be helpful and appropriate. One should always consult a physician prior to using any medication or supplement.

How long an athlete should rest an injury depends on the type and extent of the injury and also varies among individuals. Pain is one of the most important indicators of when it is best to resume play. We all feel it, we all know when it is present, and we all know when it has subsided. If it is painful to walk on a sprained ankle, whether one day after the injury or weeks later, it is simply too early to resume all-out activities. Once pain has subsided, training and competing may be introduced with caution. The load placed on an injured structure should increase gradually. Overloading an injured area, or coming back too early, can set you back longer than the original injury, and an acute injury may eventually become a chronic problem.

Soft Tissue Injuries

Contusions

When a compression force crushes tissue, a **contusion** results. Commonly called a bruise, symptoms include discoloration and swelling. What some athletes call a "charleyhorse" is a contusion injury, often to the quadriceps muscle group on the front of the thigh. While most

Myositis Ossificans

In a severe contusion, abnormal bone formation may occur. This is called **myositis ossificans**. The most common sites are the anterior and lateral thigh. A 1- to 1.5-inch (2- to 4-cm) mass is often palpable. Referral to a medical doctor is needed.

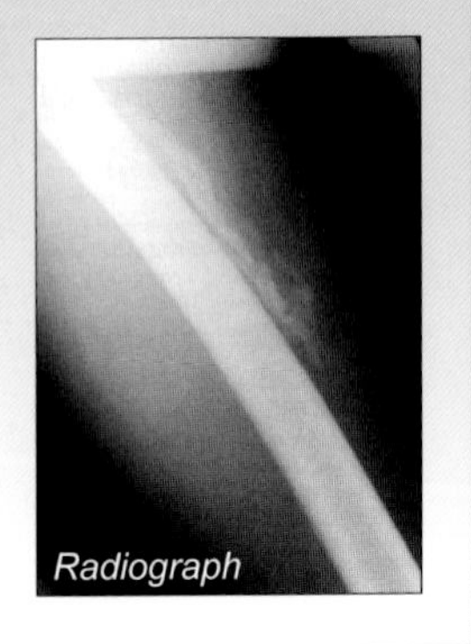

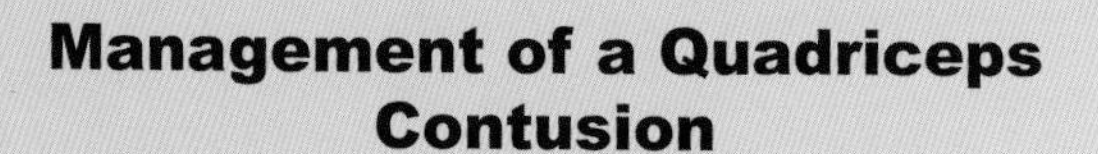

Management of a Quadriceps Contusion

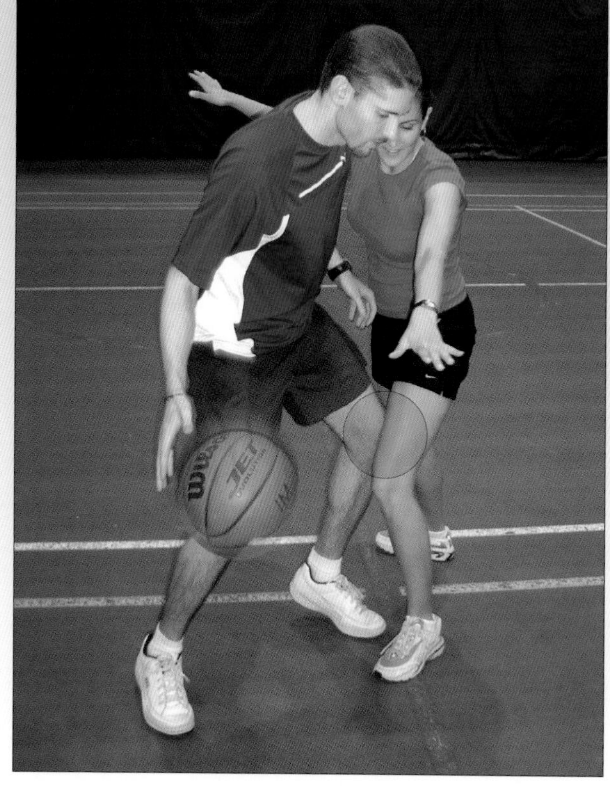

Acute Phase (first 24 to 48 hours)

- Apply ice and compression with knee flexed at 120 degrees for 20 minutes each hour for a minimum of 4 hours.
- Begin pain-free passive or active range-of-motion exercises.

Subacute Phase (2 to 5 days)

- Continue with ice and compression.
- Continue active range-of-motion exercises.
- Begin partial weight-bearing activities.

Full Weight-bearing Phase

- Continue with ice and compression.
- Range of motion should be full.
- Slowly return to previous activities, and use protective padding to prevent reinjury.
- If there is still pain seek medical attention.

These are only general guidelines. Please consult a licensed health care practitioner for further details and individual situations.

contusions are minor injuries, they can be serious and even life threatening if the tissue involved is a vital organ such as the brain or kidneys.

Strains and Sprains

A **strain** occurs when muscle or tendon tissue is stretched or torn. A **sprain** results when a ligament or the joint capsule is stretched or torn, often from twisting movements or impacts that force the affected joints beyond their normal limits. Sprains and strains are classified into three grades based on the amount of damage to the tissues and the resulting pain and loss of function (Table 3.1).

Grade three sprains and strains result in complete rupture of the tissue and often require surgery. An example is an **anterior cruciate ligament tear**. The anterior cruciate ligament (ACL) and posterior cruciate ligament (PCL) crisscross the knee joint and give the knee stability. Of the two, the ACL is weaker and more likely to tear, often when changing directions rapidly or slowing down after running or landing from a jump as in basketball. A loud popping noise often accompanies an ACL tear, which is very painful. The knee joint gives out and swells very rapidly.

Common Strains

Common muscles strained in the lower extremities include the adductors (pulled "groin"), quadriceps, hamstrings, and hip flexors (iliopsoas). In the upper extremities, muscles of the rotator cuff, which help stabilize the shoulder joint, are often vulnerable to strains.

Hamstring Strains The hamstrings are the most frequently strained muscles in the body. The main mechanism of injury is rapid contraction of the hamstring muscles in a lengthened position. Most typically, this occurs during sprinting or running (Figure 3.5).

Weak hamstring muscles compared with

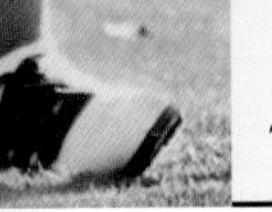

Table 3.1 Grades of strains and sprains.

Grade		Strain	Sprain
1st	Description	A few muscle fibers have been stretched or torn	Ligament has been slightly stretched or torn
	Pain	Minor pain during isometric and passive movements	Minor pain during passive movements
	Range of motion	Decreased	
	Swelling	Minor	
	Weakness	Minor	
	Disability	Little or no loss of function	
2nd	Description	More muscle fibers have been torn	Ligament has been moderately stretched or torn
	Pain	Moderate pain during isometric and passive movements	Moderate pain during passive movements
	Range of motion	Decreased	
	Swelling	Moderate	
	Weakness	Moderate	
	Disability	Moderate loss of function	
3rd	Description	Muscle is completely torn	Ligament is completely torn
	Pain	No pain during isometric and passive movements*	
	Range of motion	May increase or decrease depending on swelling	
	Swelling	Major	
	Weakness	Major	
	Disability	Major	

* *When you completely tear a muscle, tendon, or ligament, the ability to feel pain in those structures is completely lost.*

Artificial Turf Versus Natural Turf

There is much debate about whether artificial playing surfaces are more dangerous than natural playing surfaces. Artificial surfaces provide greater friction, enabling athletes to run faster and change directions more quickly. However, these conditions also increase the loads placed on muscles, tendons, and ligaments, increasing the likelihood of sustaining a strain or sprain. Therefore, a trade-off exists between performance and potential for injury on artificial surfaces.

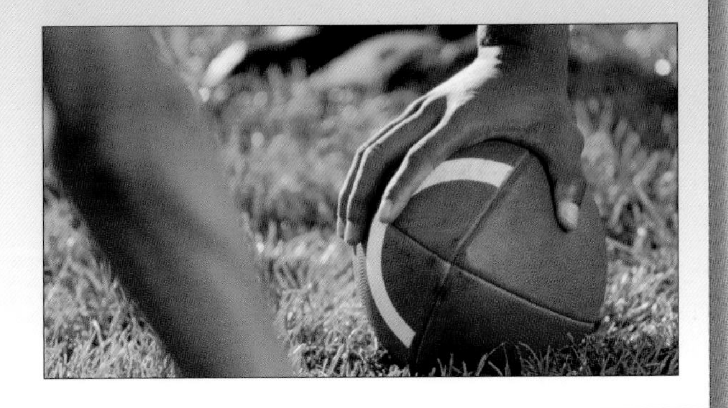

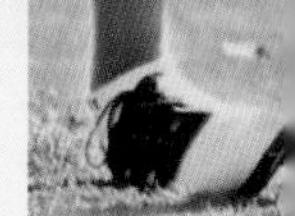

Management of an ACL Injury

Phase 1

- PRICE
- Range-of-motion exercises within pain-free limits
- Isometric exercises for quads, hamstrings, and hip adductors
- Cardiovascular exercise

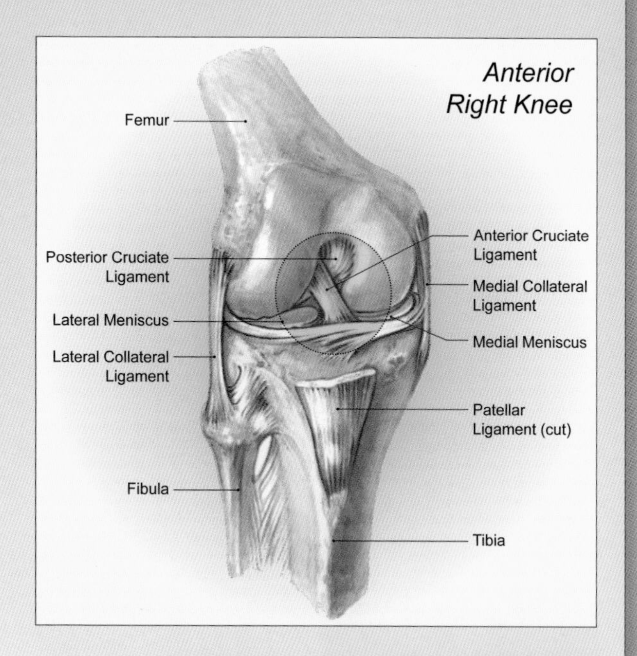

Phase 2

- Continued range-of-motion exercises
- Unilateral balance activities
- Slow, controlled balance activities (using a wobble board)
- Slow, controlled calf raises and straight leg raises
- Cardiovascular exercise

Phase 3

- Maintain range of motion
- Functional strengthening exercises (squats, leg presses, lunges)
- Cardiovascular exercise
- Continued balance activities

Phase 4

- All the activities of Phase 3, with increased sport-specific activities, such as running (circles, cross-over steps) and jumping drills (hopping, bounding, skipping)

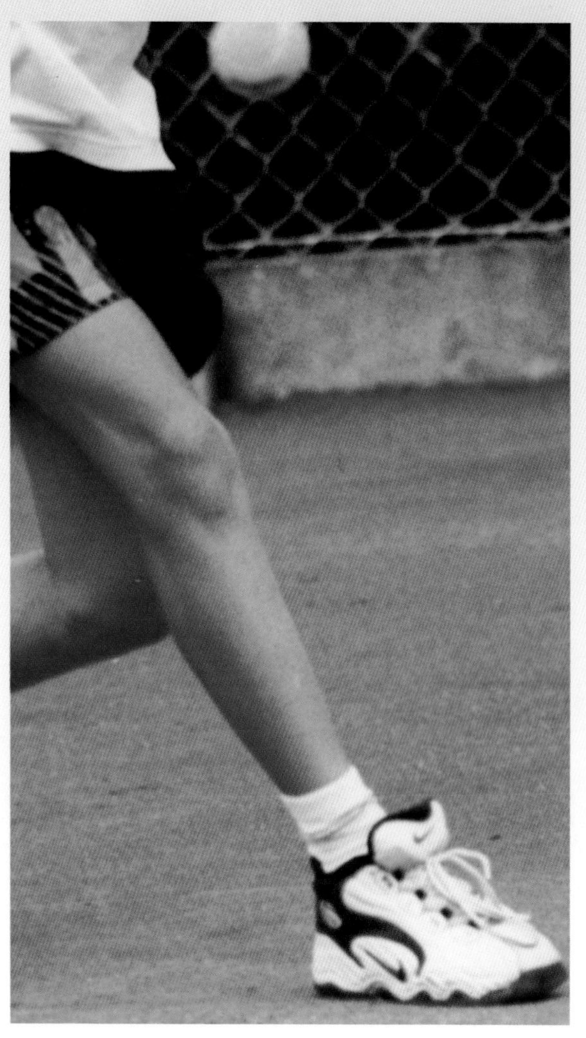

Surgery is often needed to repair a torn ACL. Your doctor replaces the damaged ACL with strong, healthy tissue usually taken from another area near your knee. Most commonly, a portion of the patellar ligament or hamstring is used. Your doctor threads the tissue through the inside of your knee joint and secures the ends to your femur and tibia.

After ACL surgery, rehabilitation exercises will gradually return your knee to maximal flexibility and stability. Building strength in the muscles around the knee joint (hamstrings, quadriceps, and calf) is important to stabilize the joint. Initially, a brace is usually required to protect the joint after surgery, but with successful rehabilitation, knee braces are slowly weaned off.

These are only general guidelines. Please consult a licensed health care practitioner for further details and individual situations.

Avoiding Hamstring Strains

Below is an example of a balanced leg workout designed to avoid strength imbalances in the muscles of the thigh.

Exercise	Reps x Sets
Squats	10 x 3
Lunges	10 x 3
Hamstring curls	10 x 3

Posterior Right Thigh

Ilium
Femur
Biceps Femoris (long head)
Semitendinosus
Biceps Femoris (short head)
Semimembranosus
Biceps Femoris (short head)
Tibia
Fibula

SQUATS

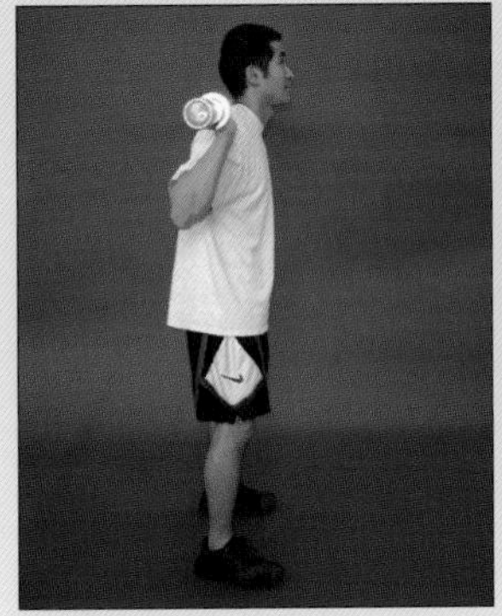

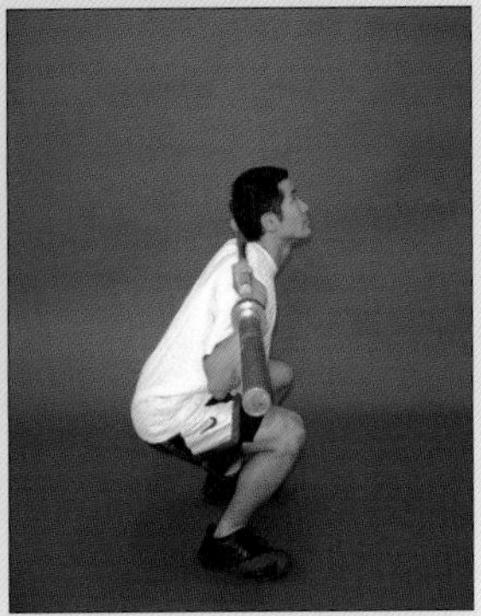

(1) Place the bar on your shoulders. Stand with feet shoulder-width apart. Point your feet slightly outward.

(2) Slowly bend your knees and hips in unison. The bar should descend in a straight line.

(3) Continue until your thighs are just above parallel to the ground.

(4) Using your legs, push back up to the starting position. You should feel most of the weight on your heels.

HAMSTRING CURLS

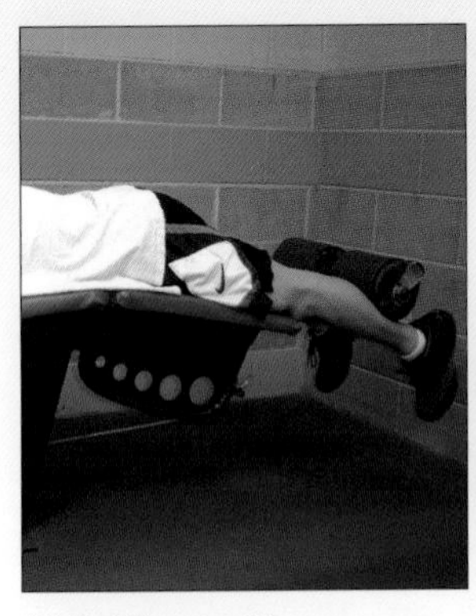

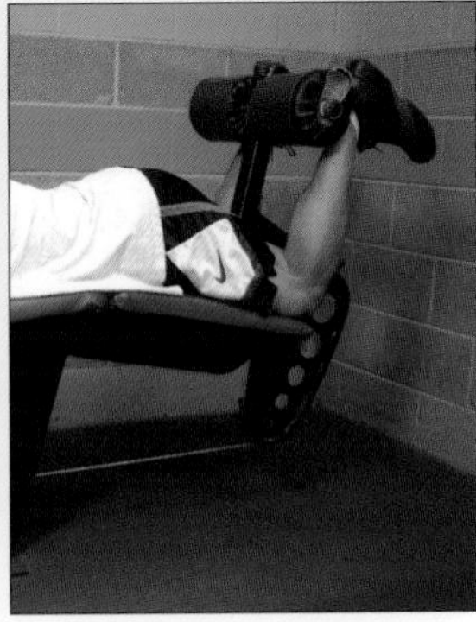

(1) Set the machine so your knees line up with its center of rotation.

(2) Lie on the padded surface.

(3) Slowly curl your feet toward your buttocks.

(4) Slowly lower your legs back to the starting position.

LUNGES

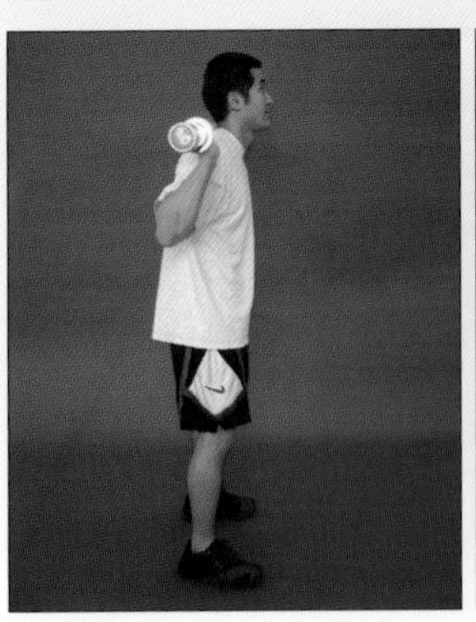

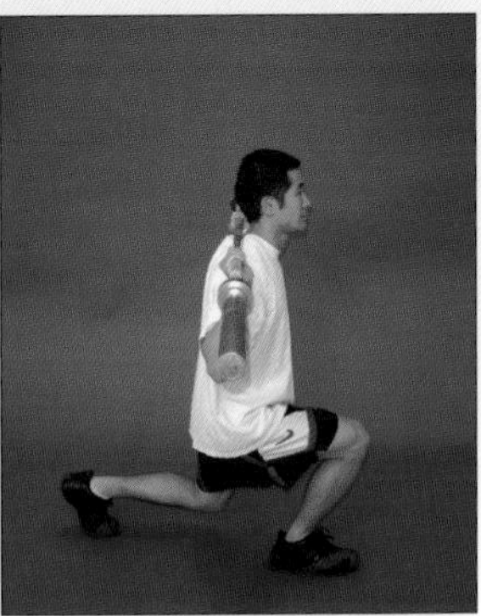

(1) Begin standing with legs together.

(2) Slowly take a step forward with one foot.

(3) Bend your knee, making sure you maintain your balance and your knee is in line with your toes.

(4) Return to starting position.

These are only general guidelines. Please consult a licensed health care practitioner for further details and individual situations.

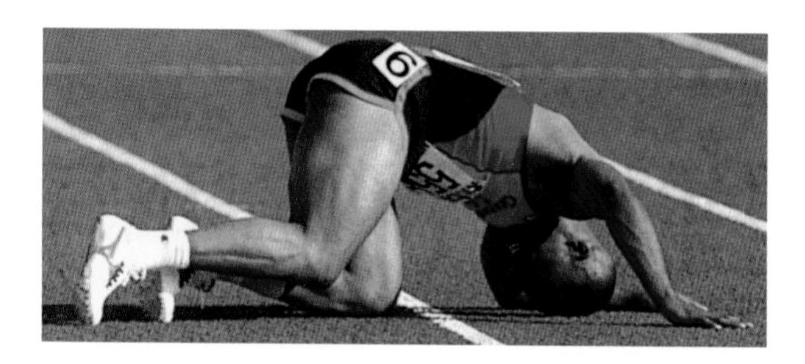

Figure 3.5 Hamstring strains are very common among sprinters and are often caused by muscle imbalances.

strong quadriceps are a main reason why hamstring strains occur so frequently. To reduce strength imbalances, rehabilitative exercises and strength and conditioning programs should emphasize the quadriceps and hamstrings equally. An example of a balanced workout program can be found in the box *Avoiding Hamstring Strains.*

Common Sprains

Ankle Sprains Ankle sprains are among the most common athletic injuries. You can sprain your ankle running, walking, dancing, or just stepping off a curb. Most common is the **lateral ankle sprain**. Lateral ankle sprains, or inversion sprains, occur when stress is applied (see box *Prevention of an Ankle Sprain*).

A "pop" or tearing noise is usually heard at the time of injury. The joint will swell rapidly, and the person is usually unable to walk. Point tenderness will be localized over the anterior talofibular ligament and may extend over the calcaneofibular ligament.

Proper rehabilitation is important to prevent reinjury. Research indicates that a main reason why ankle sprains reoccur is decreased proprioception following the initial sprain. **Proprioception** is the ability to sense the position of a joint in space. Balance exercises, such as wobble board exercises, help improve proprioception. This component of rehabilitation is often neglected because people tend to think they are healed once the pain is gone. Unfortunately their proprioceptive abilities are not healed, and they are more likely to suffer another injury.

Dislocations

If the forces acting on a joint are great enough to push the joint beyond its normal anatomical limits, a dislocation may occur. In a dislocation, the joint surfaces come apart. When the ligaments and other supporting structures of the joint are stretched and torn enough to allow the bony surfaces to partially separate, a **subluxation** has occurred. The joints of the fingers are the most commonly dislocated, followed by the shoulder. Dislocations may become chronic depending on the amount of damage to the ligaments and other supporting structures and on the treatment and rehabilitation of the original injury.

Dislocation of the Shoulder

The shoulder joint is the most mobile joint in our bodies, but by virtue of this mobility it is also the most unstable. There are two basic categories of dislocations: partial and complete. A **partial dislocation**, or subluxation, indicates that the head of the humerus (ball) is partially out of the glenoid fossa (socket). A **complete dislocation** occurs when the head of the humerus is completely out of the socket. Of course, the greater degree of joint dislocation indicates greater injury. A

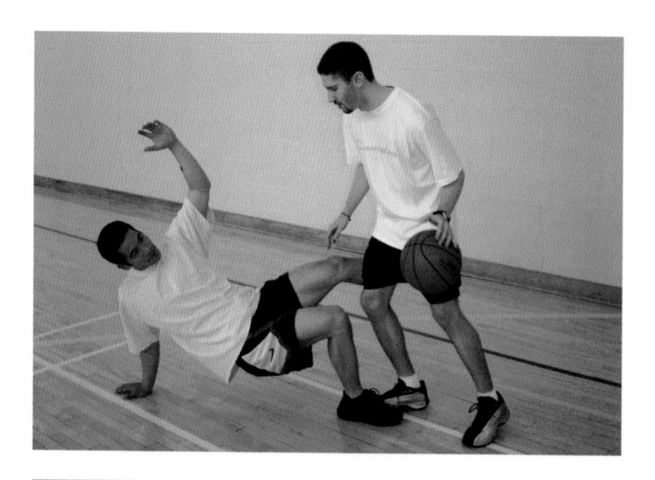

Figure 3.6 Falling and landing on an extended outstretched arm is one way to dislocate your shoulder joint.

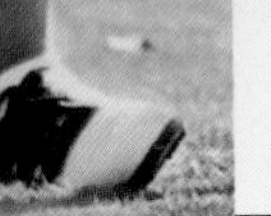

Prevention of an Ankle Sprain

Prevention

- **Limit running on uneven surfaces.** Uneven surfaces increase the chance of ankle sprains.
- **Improve balance.** Even if you don't have an ankle problem, balance exercises can help prevent possible future injuries.
- **Wear proper well-cushioned shoes.** Shoes that are worn or that don't fit properly should be replaced. Wear shoes that provide stability, especially if you play a sport that requires a lot of changes of direction, such as basketball.
- **Monitor fatigue.** If you are feeling unusually tired, stop and rest.
- **Stay hydrated.** Water is a key lubricant that permits bones, muscles, and connective tissues to slide against each other.
- **Strengthen the ankle stabilizers.** An excellent way to strengthen the muscles, tendons, and ligaments around the ankle joint is to run along the shores of a sandy beach.

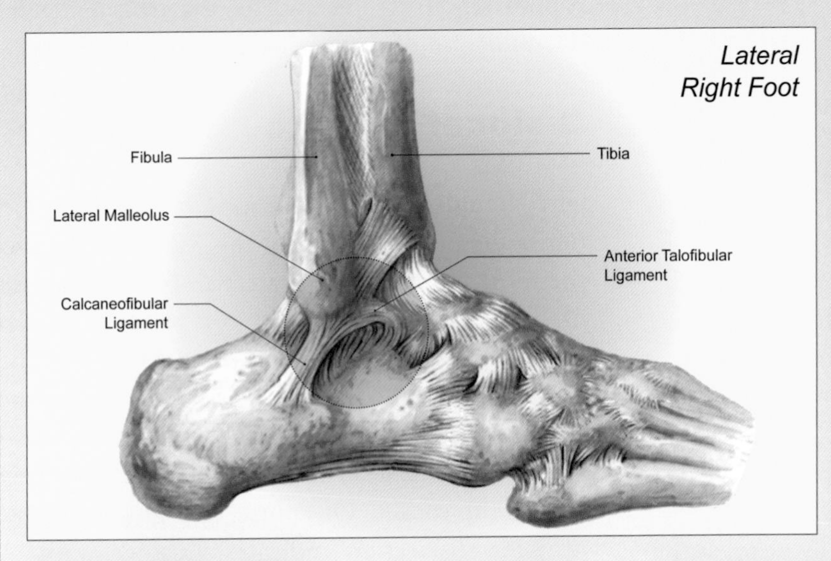

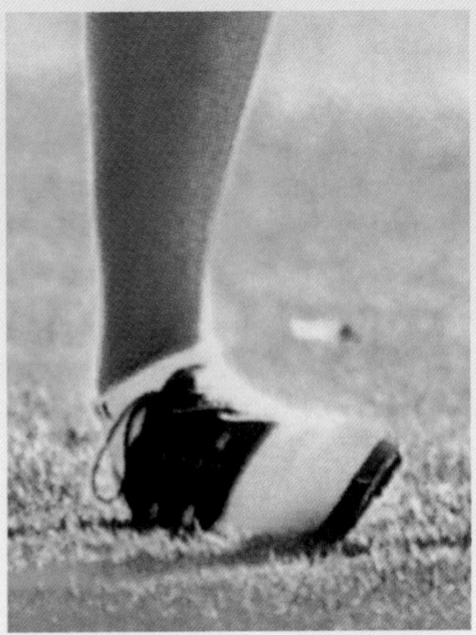

ONE-LEGGED BALANCE

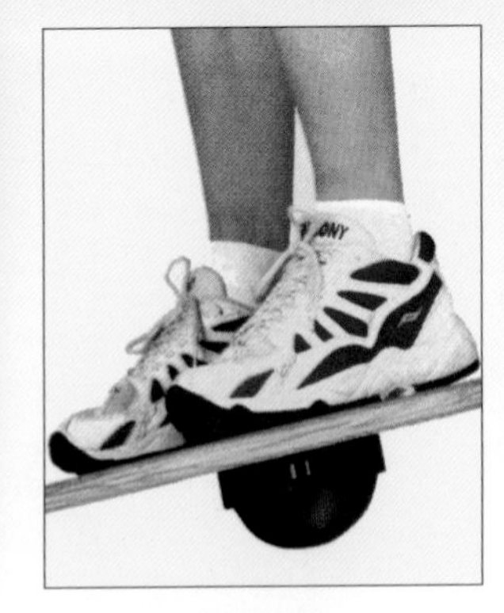

(1) Stand on one foot while performing simple movements of the arms and non-weight-bearing leg.

* Try writing letters or numbers with your arms or free leg.

WOBBLE BOARD

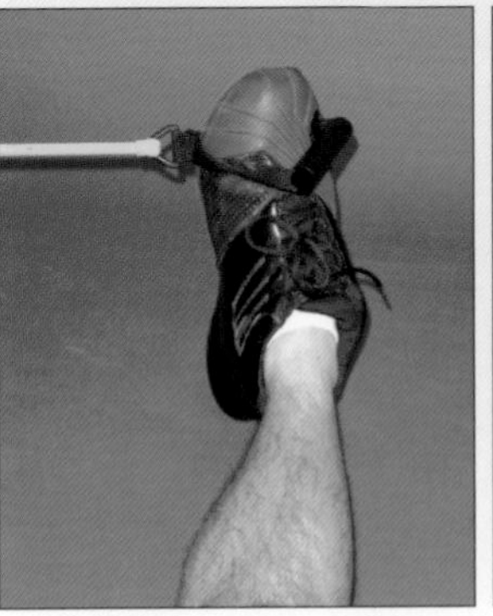

(1) Stand with your feet spread just inside shoulder-width on the wobble board.

(2) Balance.

* Try closing your eyes to challenge yourself.

ANKLE STRENGTHENING EXERCISES

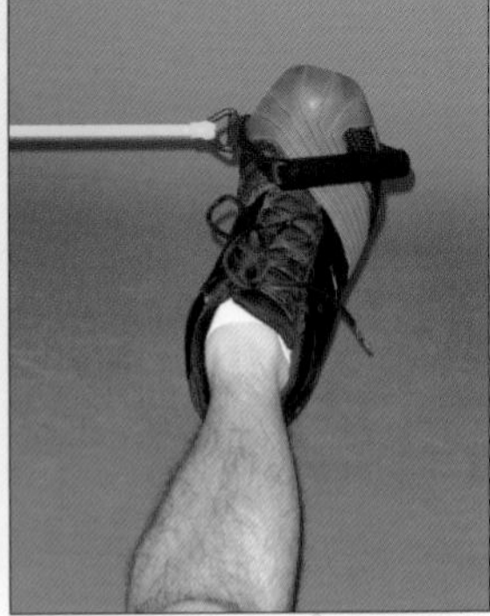

(1) Tie some exercise tubing around the outside of your foot.

(2) Attach the tubing to something solid.

(3) Begin exercises with foot inverted.

(4) Slowly evert your foot. You should feel the muscles on the outside of your leg (peroneals) contracting.

* Perform 15-20 reps x 3 sets, three times a week.

These are only general guidelines. Please consult a licensed health care practitioner for further details and individual situations.

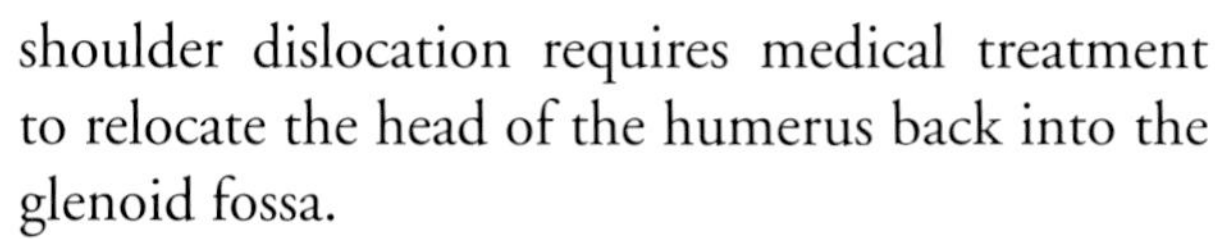

shoulder dislocation requires medical treatment to relocate the head of the humerus back into the glenoid fossa.

The most common type of shoulder dislocation occurs when the head of the humerus slips anteriorly. This can happen when you're falling backward and you land on an extended outstretched arm (Figure 3.6). Because your arm is locked, all the forces get transmitted to the front of the shoulder, causing the dislocation. The rotator cuff muscles help stabilize the joint, so a great deal of force is required for dislocations to occur.

Symptoms that occur with shoulder dislocations include swelling, numbness, pain, weakness, and bruising. In severe dislocations, the capsule that surrounds the shoulder joint can tear, along with muscles of the rotator cuff. An infrequent but serious complication of shoulder dislocations is injury to the brachial plexus. This is a group of nerves that exit from your neck and travel underneath the clavicle anterior to the head of the humerus. The brachial plexus innervates all the muscles of your chest, shoulder, arm, forearm, and hand. When the shoulder is dislocated forward, the brachial plexus may be injured.

Fractures

Bone fractures may be simple or compound. A **simple fracture** stays within the surrounding soft tissue, whereas a **compound fracture** protrudes from the skin. A **stress fracture** results from repeated low-magnitude training loads. Another type of fracture is an **avulsion fracture**, which involves a tendon or ligament pulling a small chip of bone away from the rest of the bone. Typically this occurs in children and involves explosive throwing and jumping movements.

Concussions

A **concussion** is an injury to the brain that usually develops from a violent shaking or jarring action of the head. The force of impact causes the brain to bounce against the inside of the skull. This results in confusion and a temporary loss of normal brain function, such as memory, judgment, reflexes, speech, muscle coordination, and balance.

Approximately 20 percent of concussions occur in organized sports. They are common in hockey, football, boxing, and many other contact sports. Athletes with a previous concussion are three to six times more likely to suffer another one.

For years, coaches would urge an injured player to "shake it off" and return after a brief rest. This casual attitude has changed in recent

Did You Know?

Helmets are a good idea for activities such as bicycling, in-line skating, and scooter riding. Skateboarders need special helmets that provide more coverage for the back of the head (especially for beginners, who tend to fall backward more often).

Research has shown that a properly fitted bicycle helmet offers up to 88 percent protection from brain injury (Figure 3.7).

Always replace helmets that have sustained a significant impact. Helmets are effective for one fall – one time use only! Also, avoid buying "used" helmets to ensure maximum protection.

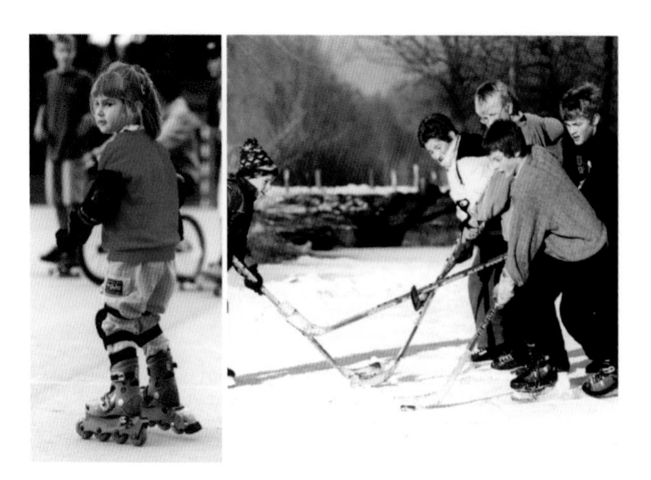

Figure 3.7 These kids are forgetting the most important piece of safety equipment – the helmet.

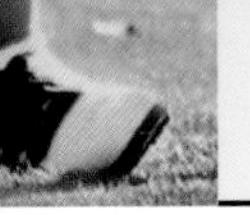

Concussion Awareness

Always assess airway, breathing and circulation.

All players who experience a concussion must be seen by a physician before the player can return to play.

Definition: Change in mental state (confusion) as a result of a trauma. May involve loss of consciousness.
Mechanism: Blow to the head, face or jaw. May result from a whiplash effect to the neck.

Types of Concussion

First Degree: Player experiences brief period of confusion. There is no loss of consciousness. Symptoms are completely gone in less than fifteen minutes.

Second Degree: Player experiences a loss of consciousness (however brief) or player experiences symptoms beyond fifteen minutes. ***Player should see a physician immediately.***

Common Symptoms and Signs

Vacant Stare	Dizziness
Poor coordination	Ringing in the ears
Delayed responses to questions	Seeing stars
Nausea, vomiting	Sensitivity to light
Inability to focus	Sensitivity to noise
	Headache

Please note that some symptoms/signs may appear later so player should be observed even after symptoms/signs seem normal.

Mental Status Testing

For information only. Do not attempt to treat a concussion. Always have the player consult a physician.

Orientation: Does the player know what the exact time and place is? Does the player know the circumstances of the injury?

Concentration: Can the player spell "world" backwards?

Memory: Does the player know the score of the game?

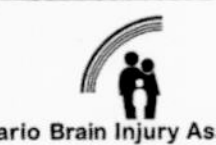

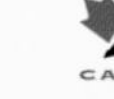

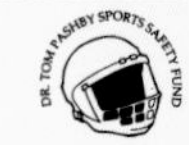

Ontario Brain Injury Association

CANADA

Concussion Management

Any Loss of Consciousness – Initiate Emergency Action Plan and Call an Ambulance

- **Rule out possible neck injury**
- **Remove the player from further play**
- **Do not administer medication**
- **Notify the parent or guardian about the injury**
- **The player does not return to play unless permitted to do so by a physician**

Return To Play

The return to play process only begins after a physician has given the player clearance to return to activity. If any symptoms/signs return during this process, the player must be re-evaluated by a physician.

1. No activity, complete rest. Proceed to step 2 only when symptoms are gone and a physician has given the player clearance.
2. Light aerobic exercise such as walking or stationary cycling. Monitor for symptoms.
3. Sport specific training (e.g. skating).
4. Non-contact drills.
5. Full contact practices.
6. Game play.

Note: Player should proceed through the steps only when it has been demonstrated that there are no return of symptoms. This includes long term symptoms such as, fatigue, irritable behaviour or sleep disturbance. If any symptoms return the player should drop down to the previous level and **must be re-evaluated by a physician.**

Prevention

Players
- Make sure your helmet fits snugly
- Get a custom fitted mouth guard
- Respect other players

Safety Person/ Trainer
- Discourage checks to the head
- Recognize signs and symptoms of concussion

These are only general guidelines. Please consult a licensed health care practitioner for further details and individual situations.

Figure 3.8 Hockey Canada Safety Program: Concussion Card.

years after the concussion-related retirements of Brett Lindros from hockey and Steve Young from football. Neurosurgeons and other brain injury experts emphasize that although some concussions are less serious than others, there is no such thing as a "minor concussion." The Canadian Hockey Association has developed a safety program using the "Concussion Card" to increase awareness of concussions (Figure 3.8).

Overuse Injuries

Overuse injuries are often the result of repeated microtrauma to the tissues, which do not have sufficient recovery time to heal. This accumulated microtrauma can result from poor technique, equipment that puts unusual stresses on the tissues, and the amount or type of training an athlete is

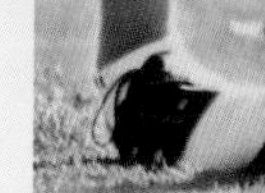

Preventing Lateral Epicondylitis

Lateral epicondylitis, commonly known as *tennis elbow*, tends to occur in people who play tennis or other racket sports. The most common cause of this condition is improper technique or overuse. Below are a few things you can do to prevent it.

Prevention

- **Analyze your arm motions.** This is very important to reduce unnecessary stress on the lateral epicondyle. Always seek professional guidance whenever starting a new activity.
- **Exercise to strengthen your forearm extensors/supinators.** Use either exercise tubing or free weights.
- **Stretch after exercise.** Stretching keeps your muscles flexible and better able to tolerate eccentric loads.
- **Use compression straps.** Straps reduce the tensile load at the lateral epicondyle.
- **Apply ice.** Even if you do not feel discomfort after the activity, it is important to ice.

Posterior Right Arm

Triceps Brachii

Lateral Epicondyle of Humerus

Forearm Extensors

FOREARM EXTENSOR EXERCISE

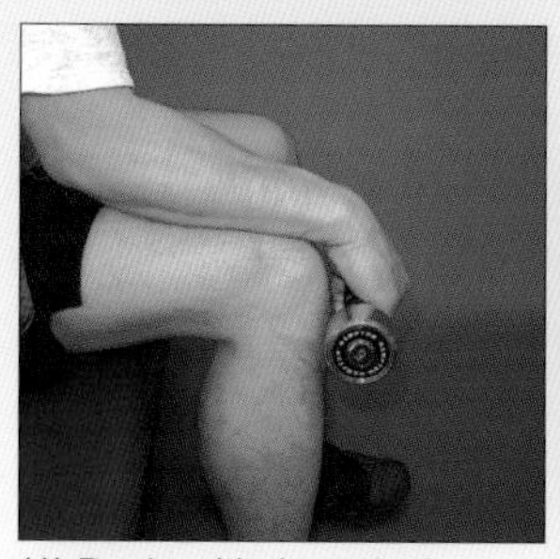

(1) Begin with the wrist in maximum flexion.

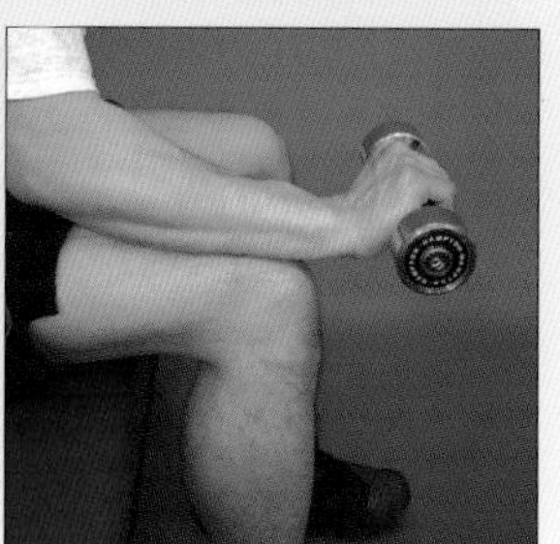

(2) Extend the wrist.

* Perform 15-20 reps x 3 sets, three times a week.

SUPINATOR EXERCISE

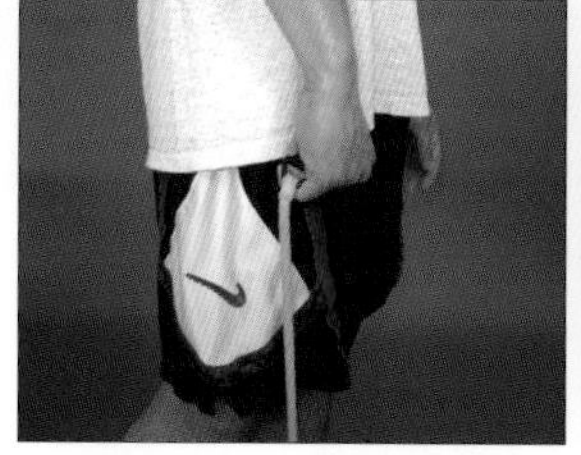

(1) Begin with the forearm in maximum pronation.

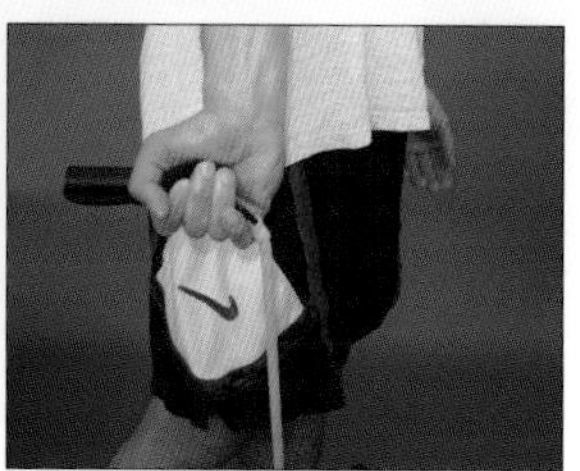

(2) Supinate the forearm.

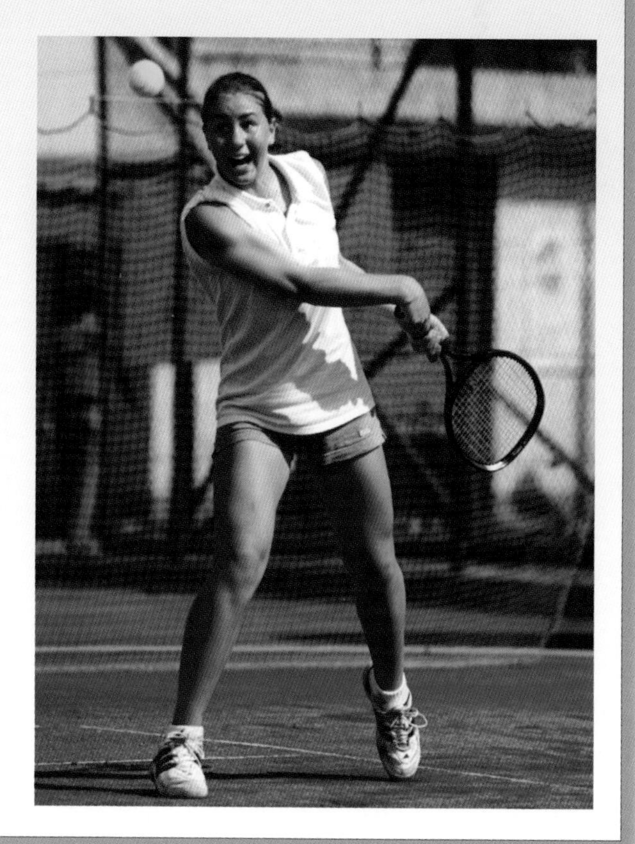

These are only general guidelines. Please consult a licensed health care practitioner for further details and individual situations.

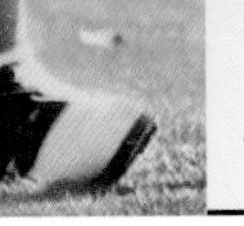

doing. Common types of overuse injuries include tendonitis, bursitis, shoulder impingement, and stress fractures.

Tendonitis

A tendon is a type of connective tissue that connects your muscles to your bones. **Tendonitis** occurs when a tendon becomes inflamed initially, then weakened and degenerative, and it is usually the result of a "microtrauma" in the tendon caused by excessive repetitive motions. Age can also contribute to the incidence of tendonitis because muscles and tendons lose their elasticity with age. Tendonitis produces pain, tenderness, and stiffness near a joint and is aggravated by movement.

Your risk of developing tendonitis increases if you perform excessive repetitive motions. For example, soccer and basketball players, runners, and dancers are prone to tendonitis in their legs and feet. Baseball players, swimmers, tennis players, and golfers are susceptible to tendonitis in their shoulders and elbows. The risk of developing tendonitis increases further if you use improper technique.

Tennis Elbow

Lateral epicondylitis, commonly known as **tennis elbow**, affects tendons of your forearm extensor/supinator muscles. These muscles attach to the lateral epicondyle of the humerus and are responsible for extending your wrist and fingers (see box *Preventing Lateral Epicondylitis*).

People who play tennis or other racket sports may develop this problem. Contributing factors include excessive forearm pronation and wrist flexion during forehand strokes, gripping the racket too tightly, improper size grip, excessive string tension, excessive racket weight or stiffness, faulty backhand technique, putting topspin on backhand strokes, or hitting the ball off-center.

Golfer's Elbow and Little League Elbow

Medial epicondylitis, commonly known as **golfer's elbow**, is similar to tennis elbow, but it occurs on the inner side. This condition affects the tendons of the forearm flexors/pronators, which attach to the medial epicondyle of the humerus. These muscles are responsible for flexing your wrist and fingers and pronating your forearm.

In severe injuries the ulnar collateral ligament and ulnar nerve can be injured. If the ulnar nerve is involved, tingling and numbness may radiate into the forearm and hand, particularly affecting the fourth and fifth fingers. Other activities that can irritate the medial epicondyle include racket sports and using a computer mouse.

Medial epicondylitis affecting the medial humeral growth plate in young children or adolescents is called **little league elbow.** This occurs primarily when young baseball players, usually around the age of 12 to 14, begin to throw curveballs. The excessive forces required to throw a curveball exceed the tissue tolerance of the medial epicondyle. For this reason, teaching players under the age of 16 how to throw a curveball is discouraged.

Jumper's Knee

Pain affecting the infrapatellar ligament, known as **patellar tendonitis** or **jumper's knee**, is caused by repetitive eccentric knee actions, such as jumping in volleyball, basketball, and track and field events. The eccentric load affects the quadriceps during jump preparation, when the forces experienced are several times larger than the athlete's body weight.

Bursitis

Bursitis describes inflammation of the bursae. Like tendonitis, it results from overuse and stress. Your body contains more than 150 bursae – tiny fluid-filled sacs that lubricate and cushion pressure points between your bones and tendons (Figure 3.9). When they become inflamed, movement and direct pressure cause pain.

Bursitis is most common in the shoulder, elbow, and hip joints. Again, the mechanism of injury is excessive repetitive movements. For

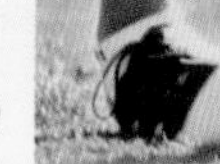

Preventing Medial Epicondylitis

Medial epicondylitis, also known as *golfer's elbow*, occurs commonly in people who play golf or racket sports. It also occurs frequently among people who use a computer mouse. Medial epicondylitis affecting the humeral growth plate in children or adolescents is called *little league elbow*. Listed below are a few things you can do to prevent this condition.

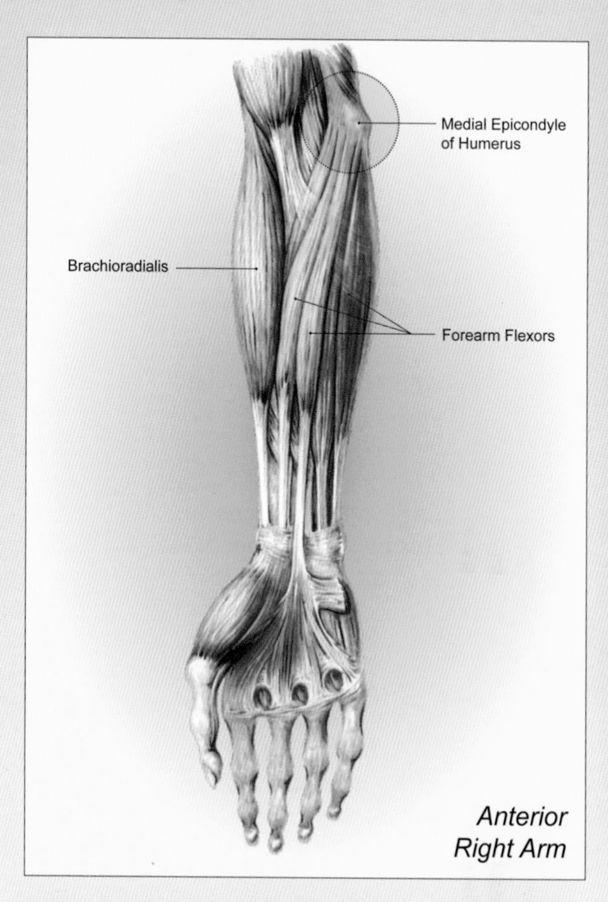

Anterior Right Arm

Prevention

- **Analyze your arm motions.** This is important to reduce unnecessary stress on the medial epicondyle. Always seek professional guidance whenever starting a new activity.
- **Exercise to strengthen your forearm flexors/ pronators.** Use either exercise tubing or free weights.
- **Stretch after exercise.** Stretching keeps your muscles flexible and better able to tolerate eccentric loads.
- **Apply ice.** Even if you do not feel discomfort after the activity, it is important to ice.

FOREARM FLEXOR EXERCISE

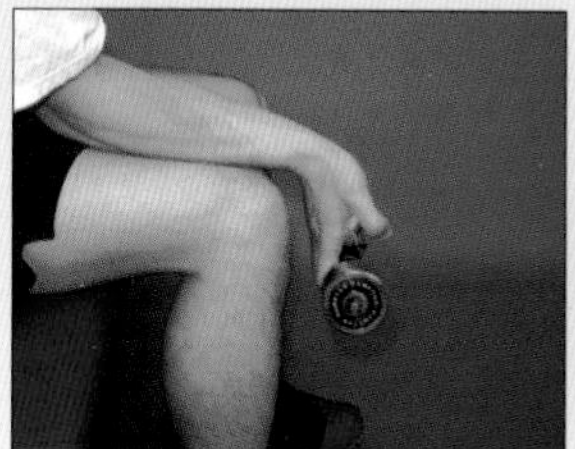

(1) Begin with the wrist in maximum extension.

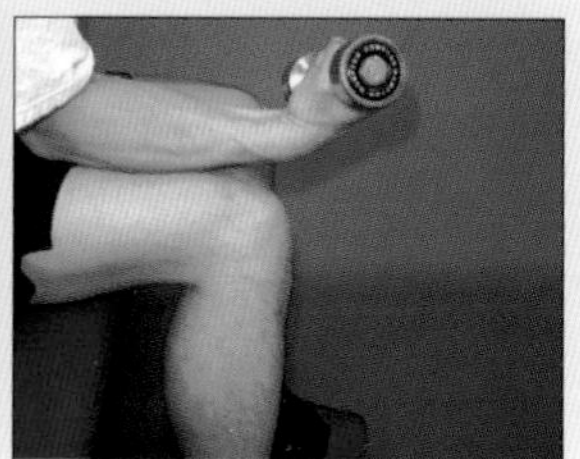

(2) Flex the wrist.

* Perform 15-20 reps x 3 sets, three times a week.

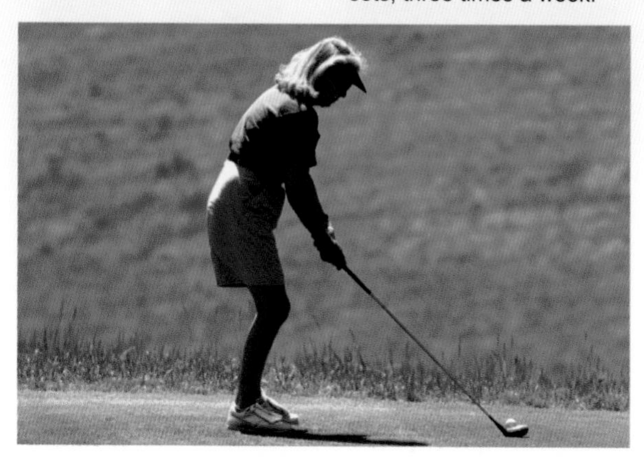

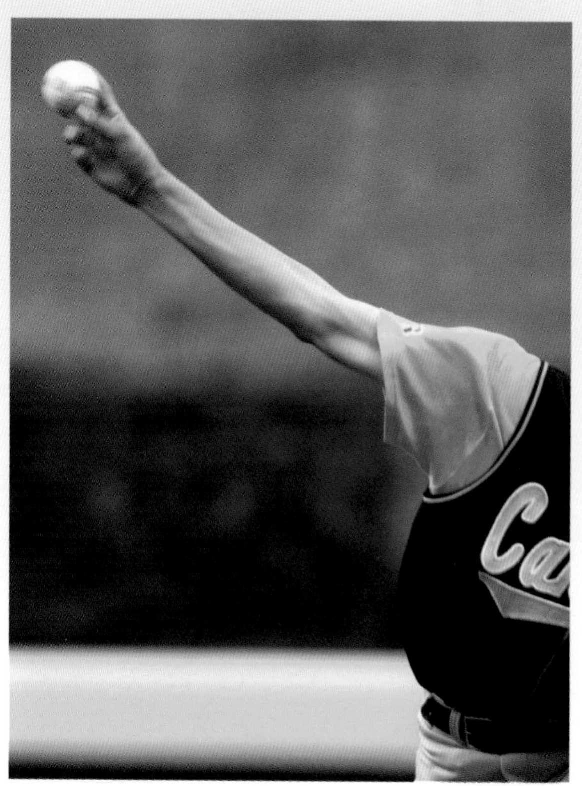

These are only general guidelines. Please consult a licensed health care practitioner for further details and individual situations.

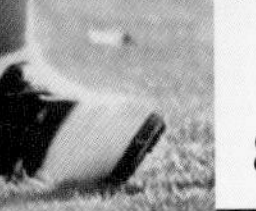

Prevention of Jumper's Knee

Prevention

- **Maximize quadriceps and hamstring strength.** A balanced workout program is important to prevent injury.
- **Perform repetitive eccentric quadriceps exercises.** Gradually increase load to prepare the body to withstand repetitive loading.
- **Stretch after exercise.** Stretching keeps your muscles flexible and better able to tolerate eccentric loads.
- **Train on cushioned surfaces and wear well-cushioned footwear.** This decreases the forces acting on the knee.
- **Apply ice.** Even if you do not feel discomfort after the activity, it is important to ice.
- **Seek medical treatment.** If you experience symptoms, seek medical attention to prevent future problems.

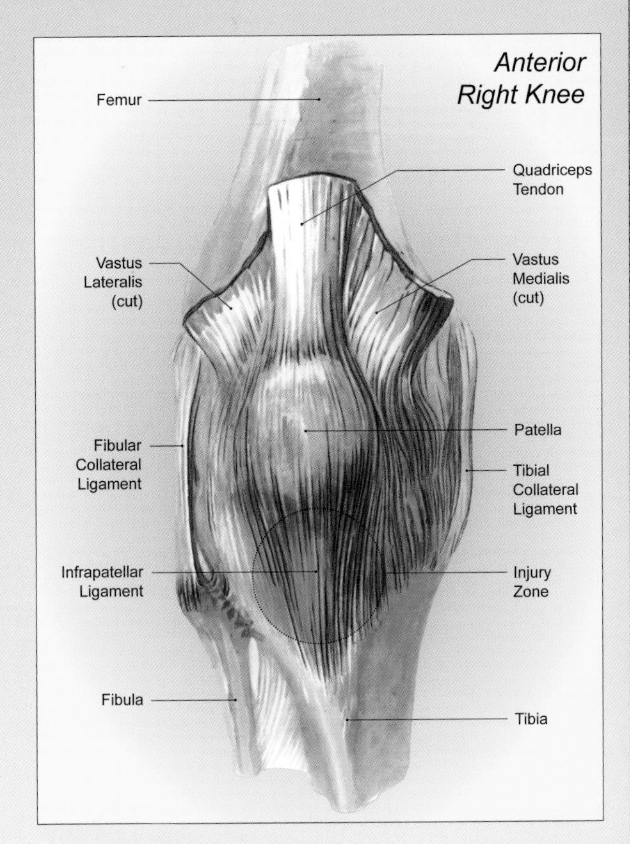

SINGLE LEG SQUATS

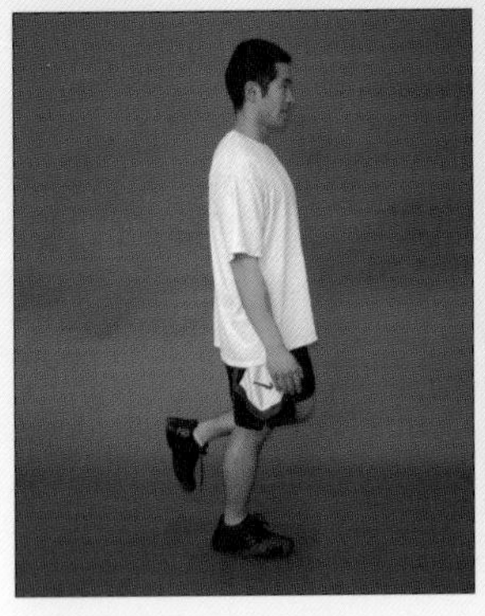

(1) Balance on one leg.

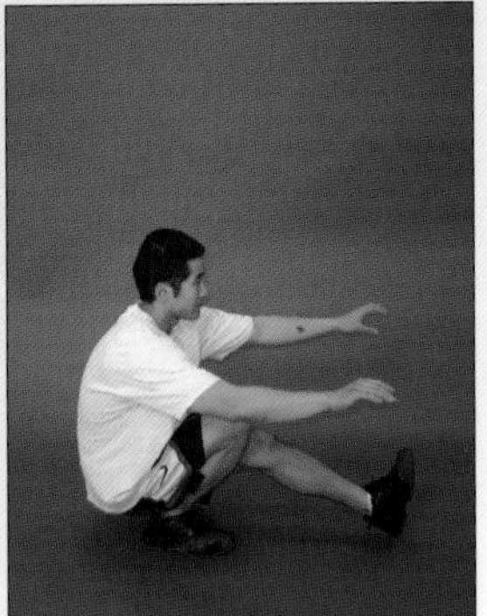

(2) Slowly lower yourself, making sure your knee and pelvis are in good alignment throughout the exercise.

(3) Only go as deep as you are able to maintain form.

* Perform 10 reps x 3 sets, three times a week.

QUAD STRETCH

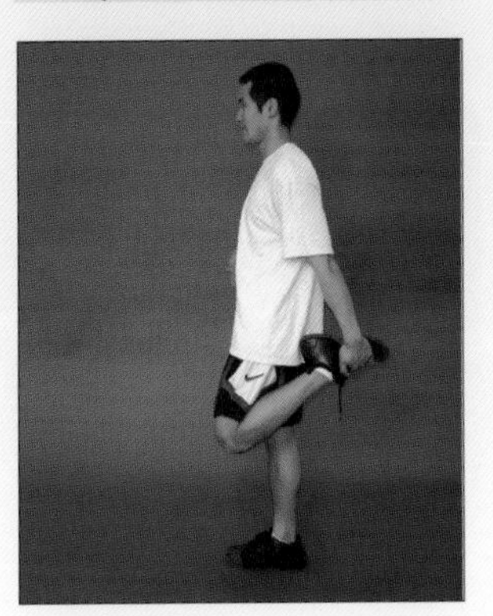

(1) Grasp your ankle.

(2) Slowly bring your foot to your buttocks.

* You may find it difficult on one foot, so try touching your belly button with your free hand.

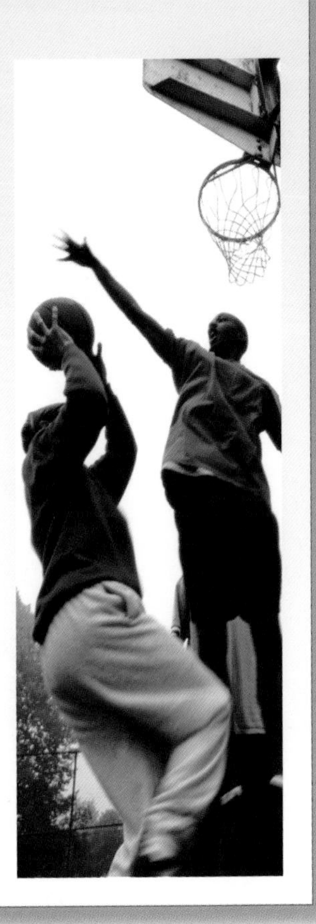

These are only general guidelines. Please consult a licensed health care practitioner for further details and individual situations.

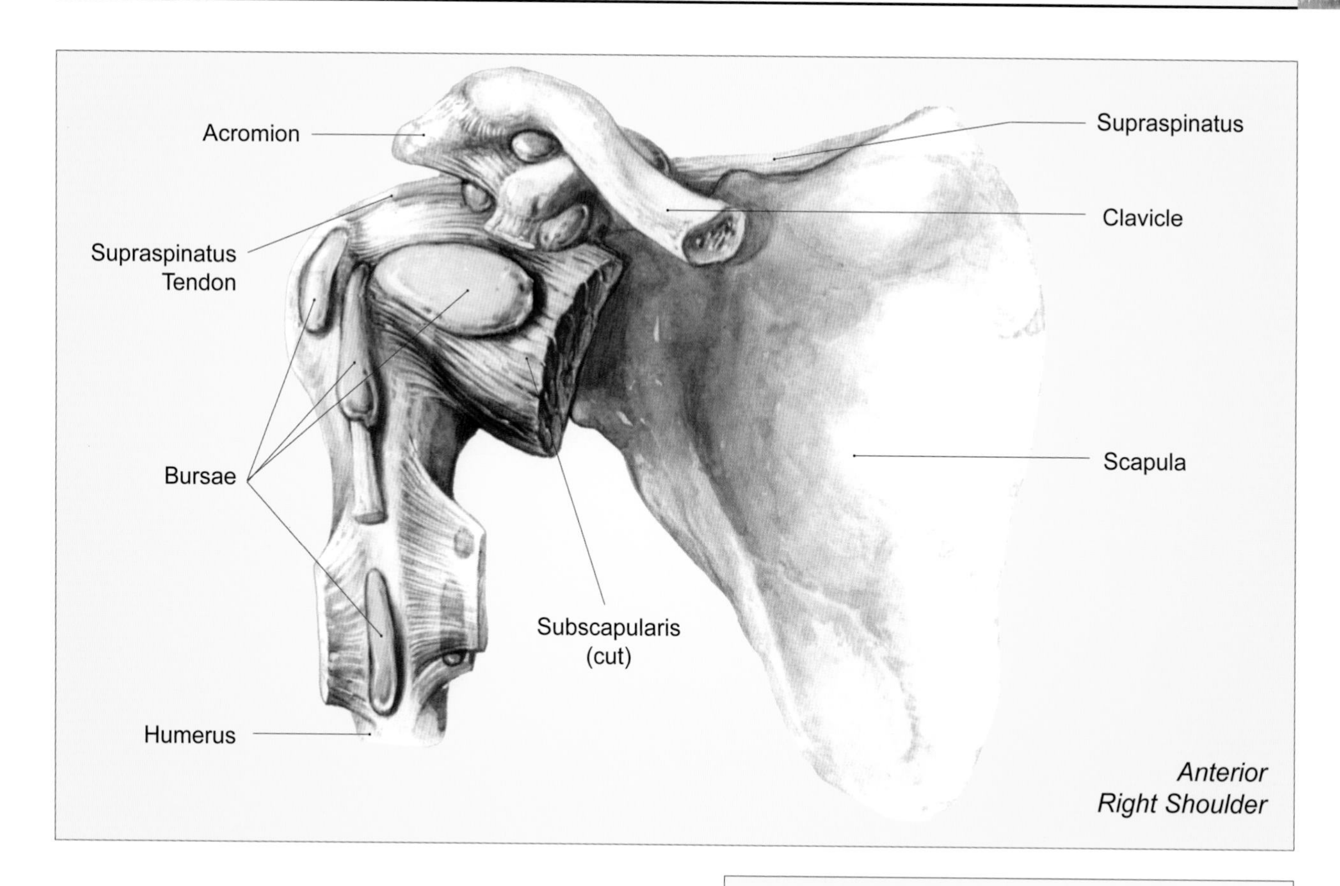

Figure 3.9 Bursae around the shoulder joint.

example, frequent extension of the arm at high speeds, such as in baseball pitching, can cause bursitis. Medical research indicates that you are more likely to develop bursitis with increasing age.

Shoulder Impingement

Shoulder impingement is a very common problem with athletes, industrial workers, and anyone who uses their shoulders repeatedly. Excess movement of the humeral head combined with a lack of space between the humeral head and the acromion causes inflammation in the bursae or rotator cuff tendons in the shoulder.

Muscle imbalances in the shoulder are largely responsible for development of shoulder impingement. The main culprit is weak shoulder depressors (lower fibers of the trapezius and serratus anterior) compared with the shoulder elevators (upper fibers of the trapezius). Likewise, a tight pectoralis major muscle may cause the humeral head to rotate anteriorly, increasing the potential for shoulder impingement.

Stress Fractures

A **stress fracture** is a special type of fracture that results from repeated low-magnitude forces. It begins as a small disruption in the continuity of the outer layers of cortical bone. With continued stress to the weakened bone, complete cortical bone fracture can occur. Stress fractures of the metatarsals, femoral neck, and pubis are common in runners who overtrain.

It is important to note the distinction between a stress fracture and shin splints, because the two terms are often used interchangeably. **Shin splints** describe pain that occurs along the inner surface of the tibia. Common causes include vigorous high-impact activity, training on hard surfaces, improper training protocols, poorly cushioned footwear, and having flat feet. Shin splints involve pain and inflammation without a disruption of

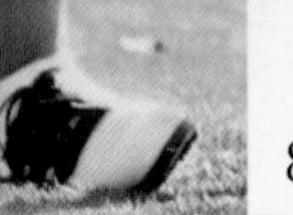

Avoiding Shoulder Impingement

Prevention

- **Make sure your shoulders are depressed when doing any exercises.** Elevating your shoulders while doing an activity decreases the space between the humerus and acromion, making impingement more likely.
- **Reduce activity.** If your shoulders become painful, reduce your activity levels.
- **Apply ice.** Even if you do not feel discomfort after the activity, it is important to ice.
- **Stretch the pectoralis major muscle.** A tight pectoralis major muscle may cause the humeral head to rotate anteriorly, thereby increasing the risk of shoulder impingement.
- **Strengthen the supporting muscles surrounding the shoulder joint.** These muscles help prevent anterior rotation of the humerus, thereby reducing the risk of shoulder impingement.

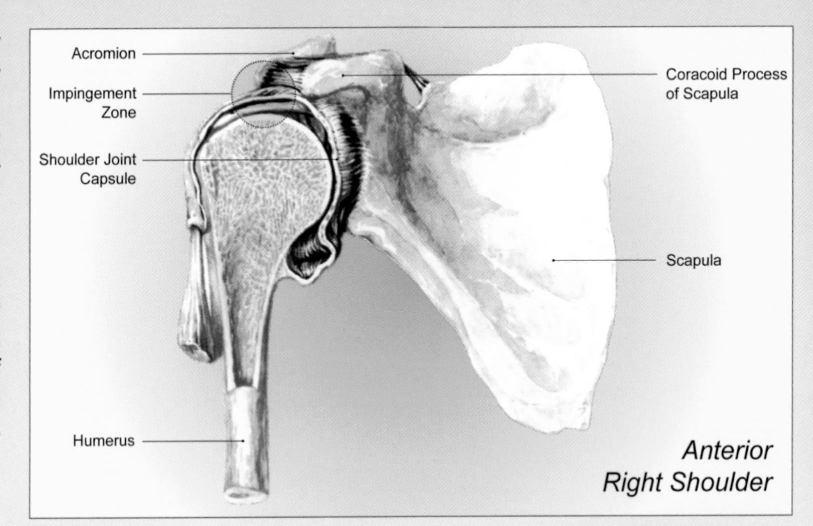

Anterior Right Shoulder

EXTERNAL ROTATORS EXERCISE

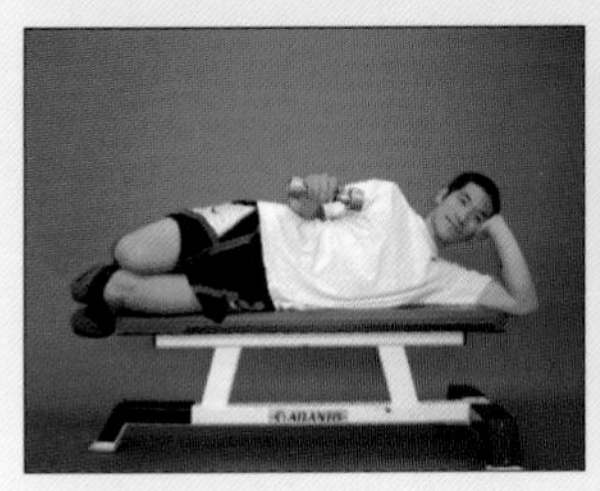

(1) Begin with your arm flexed at your side, with your shoulder internally rotated.

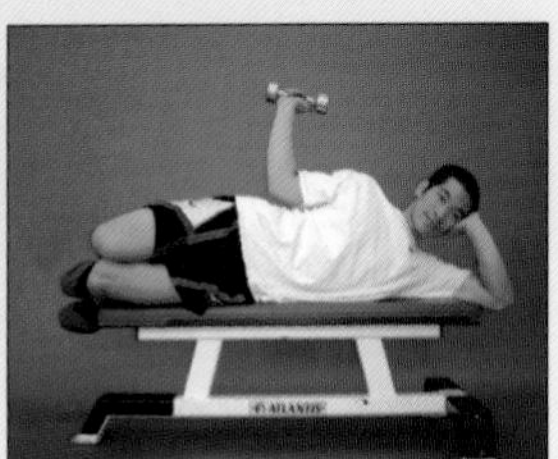

(2) Rotate your arm out to the side as if you are opening a door, making sure your shoulder is always depressed.

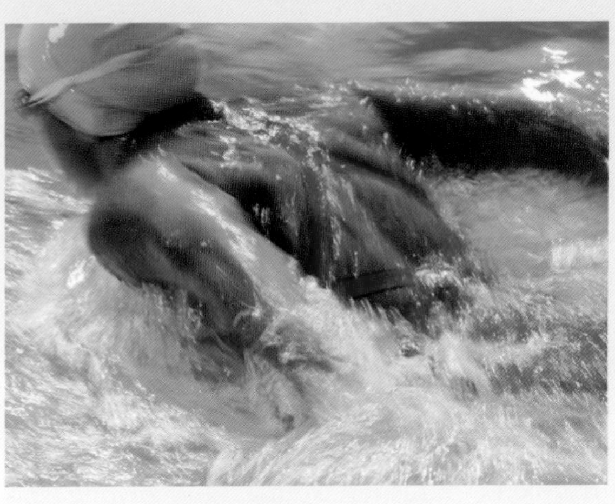

EMPTY CAN EXERCISE

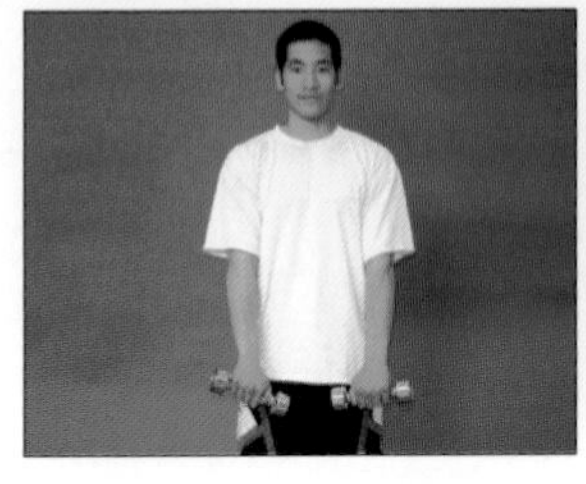

(1) Begin with your arm straight at your side, making sure your thumb is pointing down to the floor.

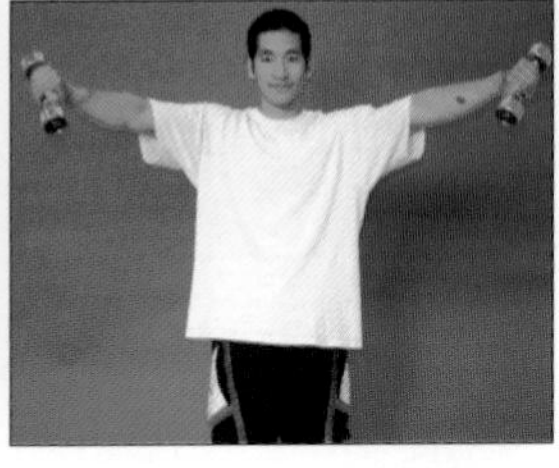

(2) Abduct your arm slowly, making sure there is about 30 degrees of horizontal abduction and your shoulders are depressed.

LOWER TRAPEZIUS EXERCISE

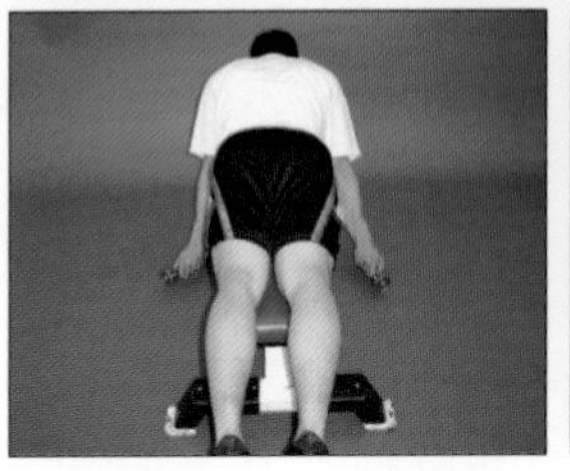

(1) Lie on the ground or on a bench with your arms abducted to 90 degrees. Your palms should face the ceiling.

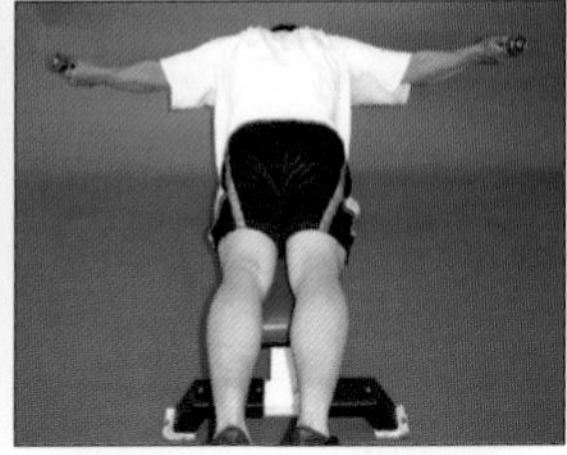

(2) Squeeze your shoulder blades together, making sure they are depressed and your palms are facing the ceiling.

These are only general guidelines. Please consult a licensed health care practitioner for further details and individual situations.

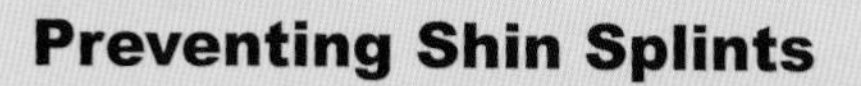

Preventing Shin Splints

Prevention

- **Limit running on hard surfaces.** Running on a variety of surfaces will force your supporting leg muscles to strengthen.
- **Join a running club.** Increasing mileage too quickly places excessive stress on the tibia. Proper training programs and technique are important. Guidance on this matter can be gained by joining a running club.
- **Seek medical treatment.** If you experience symptoms, seek medical attention to prevent future problems.
- **Address muscle imbalances.** Tight calf muscles and weak tibialis anterior muscles can decrease your ability to absorb forces.
- **Avoid biomechanical misalignment.** Anything from your toes to your head can affect the way you run.
- **Wear proper well-cushioned shoes.** Shoes that are worn or that don't fit properly should be replaced. Running shoes should be used for running, not basketball or tennis shoes.
- **Stay hydrated.** Water is a key lubricant that permits bones, muscles, and connective tissues to slide against each other.
- **Apply ice.** Even if you do not feel discomfort after the activity, it is important to ice.

TIBIALIS ANTERIOR EXERCISE

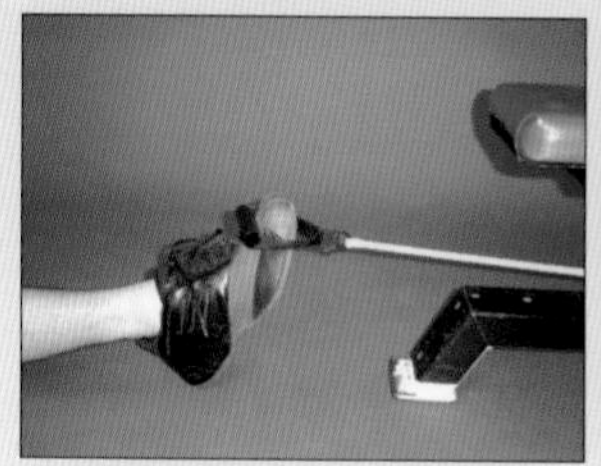

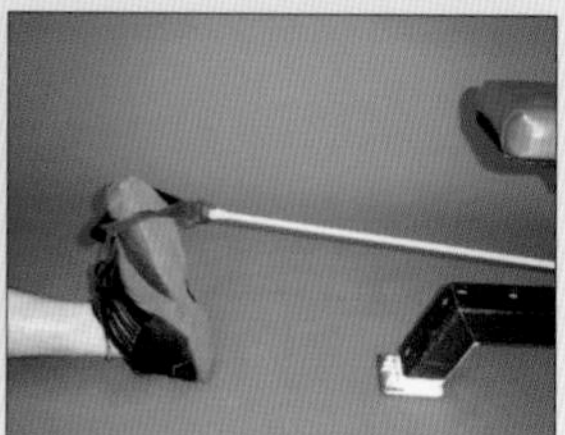

(1) Use a weight or exercise tubing.

(2) Begin the exercise with your foot pointed away.

(3) Begin with the ankle in plantar flexion (point toes down).

(4) Slowly dorsiflex your ankle (point toes up).

* You should feel the muscle in front of your shin contracting.
* Perform 15-20 reps x 3 sets, three times a week.

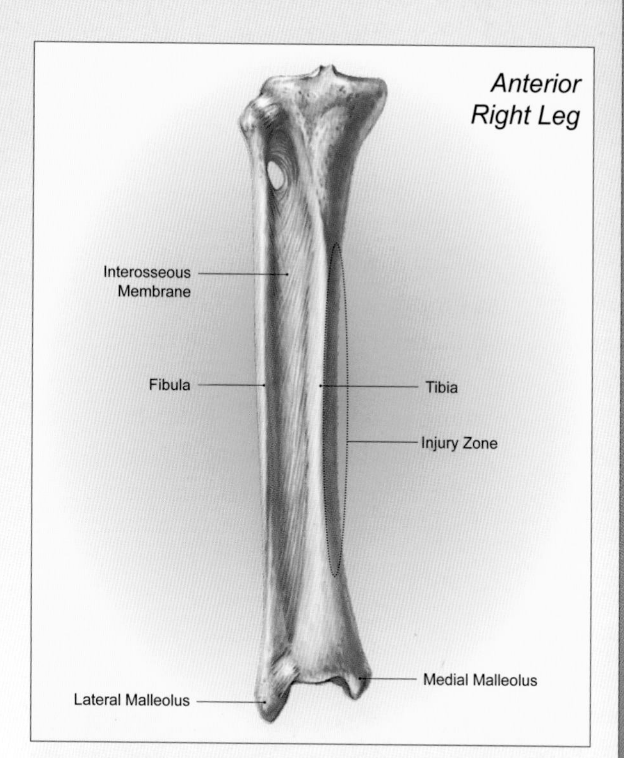

CALF MUSCLE STRETCHES

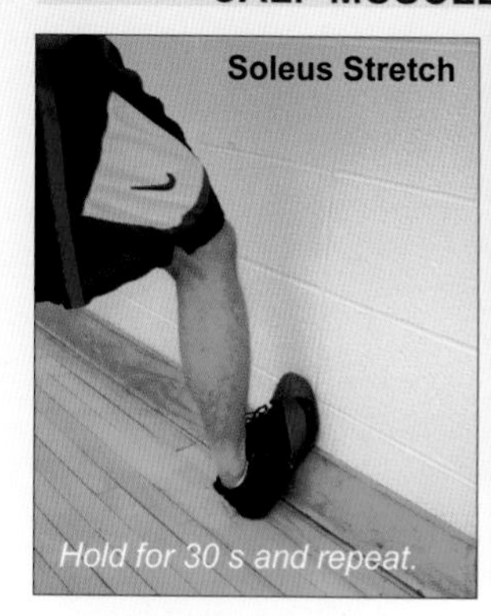

(1) Begin with your knee bent while standing.

(2) Maximally dorsiflex your ankle until you feel a stretch.

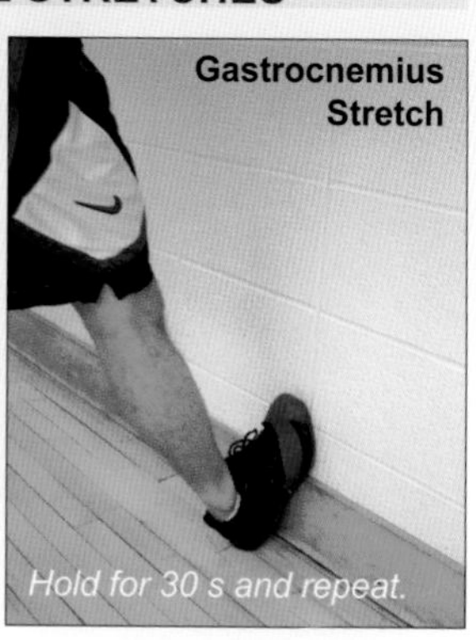

(1) Begin with your knee straight while standing.

(2) Maximally dorsiflex your ankle until you feel a stretch.

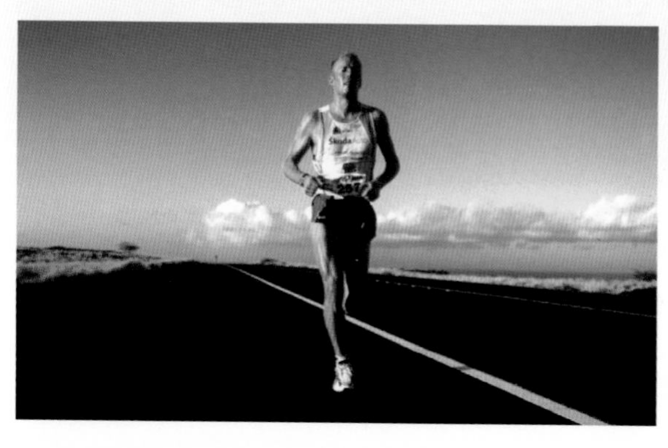

These are only general guidelines. Please consult a licensed health care practitioner for further details and individual situations.

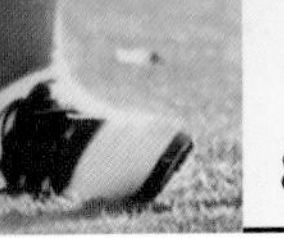

the cortical bone. X-rays and possibly bone scans are therefore needed to properly diagnose a stress fracture.

Injury Prevention

Not every injury can be avoided, but if you take the necessary precautions and make note of preventative factors, it is possible to develop a viable plan for injury prevention.

Protective Equipment

It sometimes takes a serious injury or a mountain of clinical evidence to wake people up to the risks associated with certain activities. For example, professional hockey players (including goalies) used to play the game without protective head gear. Today, helmets and face masks are mandatory. The use of helmets in many sports such as in-line skating and cycling has also received greater attention in recent years, and rightfully so. The consequences of participating in such activities without the proper head gear can be debilitating and even fatal. Injury prevention, however, goes far beyond knowing the risks and preventative factors; knowing is not doing. It is up to you to take advantage of whatever safety equipment is available for the activity in which you participate (Figure 3.10).

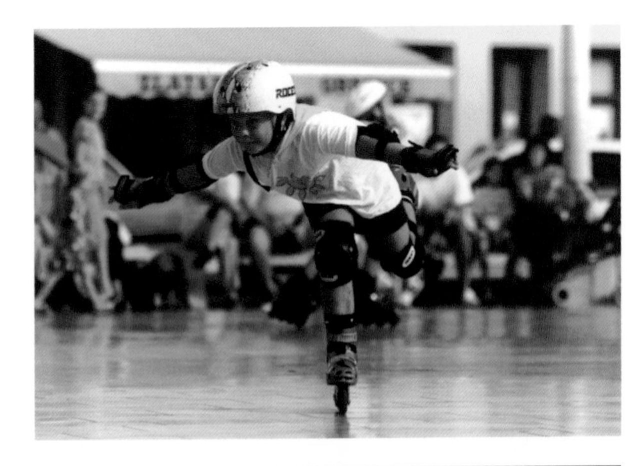

Figure 3.10 Here is someone who is properly protected and ready to have fun.

Warming Up and Cooling Down

Most athletes perform some type of warm-up before training or in preparation for an event, including stretching, light jogging or other aerobic activities, and sport- or activity-specific motions. Warming up helps an athlete prepare optimally (physically and mentally) for a competition or workout (Figure 3.11). Most research advocates a thorough and well-planned warm-up not only to improve performance but also to help prevent injury.

The issue of cooling down is overlooked by many athletes. After completing a long and tiring workout, many people are content to sit down and rest to allow their bodies to recover. This may lead to muscle stiffness, a condition that may make you

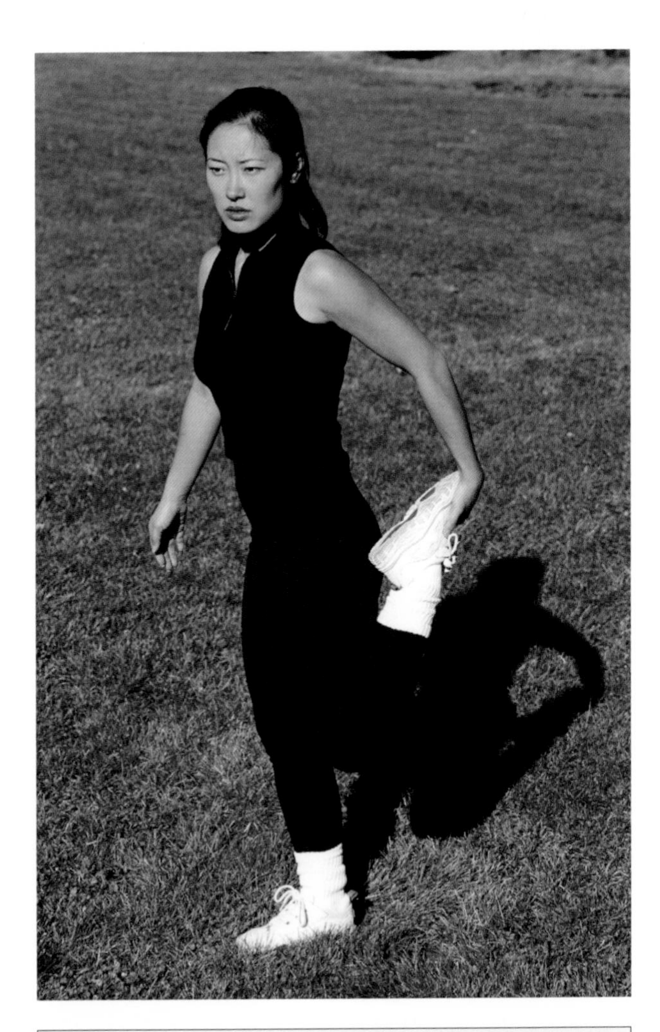

Figure 3.11 Stretching prepares not only your body but also your mind for physical activity.

more prone to injury the next time you take to the field or court. A short cool-down period removes lactic acid and other products of metabolism from the muscles and tissues, further reducing some of the stiffness and tightness that is often felt the next day. The cardiovascular system may also benefit from a gradual cool-down period since the abrupt lowering of an elevated heart rate is not ideal. So the next time you finish a long workout, don't just hit the showers; instead, walk a few laps and do some light stretching.

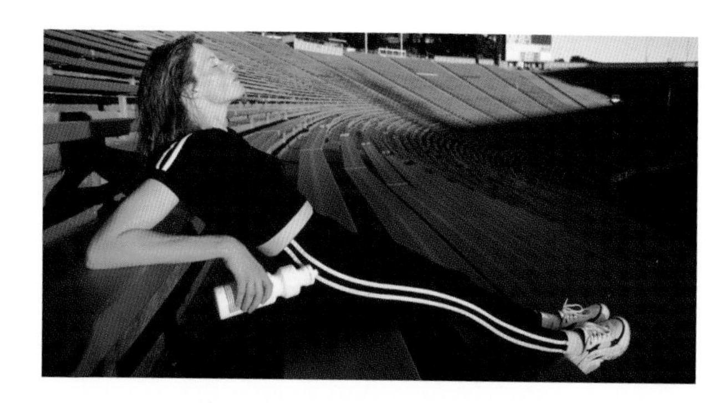

Figure 3.12 Resting and feeling a sense of accomplishment after a hard workout.

Keeping Fit and Flexible

As the saying goes, "use it or lose it." Seasonal athletes are well aware that training doesn't really end with the end of a competitive season. Sometimes the most important gains are made in the off-season. A fit athlete obviously has fewer adjustments to make at the beginning of a season than an athlete who is out of shape. The off-season is a time not only to develop and refine technical skills but also to maintain physical fitness (including strength, flexibility, and endurance). Most athletic injuries occur as a result of placing demands on a muscle or other tissue that is simply not prepared to withstand these demands.

The preseason claims many injury victims because many athletes do not stay in shape all year round. Some studies have shown that strength can be maintained with as little as one or two workouts a week at 90 percent of capacity. Fewer workouts are required to maintain aerobic capacity, so no excuses should be made for losing too much in the off-season.

Eating and Resting to Avoid Injury

Most athletes will agree that diet and rest play a major role, not only in enhancing performance but also in keeping the body well tuned for injury prevention. In order to function most effectively, the body must be fed the proper nutrients and must receive adequate rest. Not meeting these conditions inevitably opens the door to potential problems. Adhering to nutritional guidelines can prepare you for the stresses of physical exertion and lower your risk of sustaining an injury (see Chapter 14 for details on nutrients, hydration, and pre-event meals).

Because training and competition involve putting forth great physical effort, muscles need rest from these physical demands to recuperate for the next training or competitive session (Figure 3.12). Muscles forced to endure heavy demands when inadequately rested may snap (literally) under pressure. Overtraining can be just as detrimental to your performance as not training enough (see Chapter 12).

Inadequate sleep may lead to mishaps that could have been avoided with proper rest and alertness. It is up to each person to discover what amount of sleep is best for him or her – there is no set number of hours that applies to everyone.

Summary

With more people participating in sports and physical activity for health, fitness, and fun, avoiding injury is a notable concern. Injuries occur based on the biomechanical properties of tissue and where they are subjected to loads that exceed their elastic region.

Strains and sprains are common injuries. A strain occurs when muscle or tendon tissue is stretched or torn, and a sprain results when a ligament or the joint capsule is stretched or torn.

Another frequent sports injury is a contusion, or bruise, which occurs when a compression force crushes tissue. In a dislocation, either complete or partial (a subluxation), the joint surfaces come apart.

Bone fractures may be simple or compound. A simple fracture stays within the surrounding soft tissue, whereas a compound fracture protrudes from the skin. Overuse injuries are often the result of repeated microtrauma to the tissues. Examples include stress fractures, tendonitis, and bursitis. One potentially dangerous sports injury is a concussion, an injury to the brain that usually develops from a violent shaking or jarring action of the head.

Fortunately, we can train our bodies to make our tissues stronger and more resistant to deformation. We can also wear protective equipment, warm up and cool down before and after our activities, and make sure we perform the skill with good form in order to reduce our likelihood of injury.

No matter how hard we try to prevent them, injuries will always occur. The healing process begins immediately after injury and consists of three overlapping phases: the inflammatory response phase, the fibroblastic repair phase, and the maturation–remodeling phase. Many health care professionals have dedicated their lives to help us deal with problems resulting from injury. Doctors and various therapists can take us through treatment and rehabilitation programs that will help us return to our previous activities, if not beyond.

Key Terms

anterior cruciate tear
bending
bursitis
complete dislocation
compound fracture
compression
concussion
contusion
cryotherapy
deformation
elastic region
fibroblastic repair phase
inflammatory response phase
lateral ankle sprain
lateral epicondylitis
load
maturation–remodeling phase
medial epicondylitis
partial dislocation
patellar tendonitis
plastic region
positive training effect
PRICE
proprioception
rehabilitation
shear
shin splints
shoulder impingement
simple fracture
sprain
strain
stress
stress fracture
subluxation
tendonitis
tension
torsion
treatment
ultimate failure
yield-level point

Discussion Questions

1. Define the load–deformation curve and use it to describe any injury.
2. What is the role of training with respect to injury prevention?
3. Describe the complications associated with pain medication.
4. What is the difference between a sprain and a strain?
5. What should you do immediately after an injury?
6. Compare and contrast a dislocation and a fracture.
7. Name and describe three overuse injuries.
8. What is the difference between bursitis and tendonitis?
9. How do you distinguish between a stress fracture and shin splints?
10. What are the benefits of warming up and cooling down?

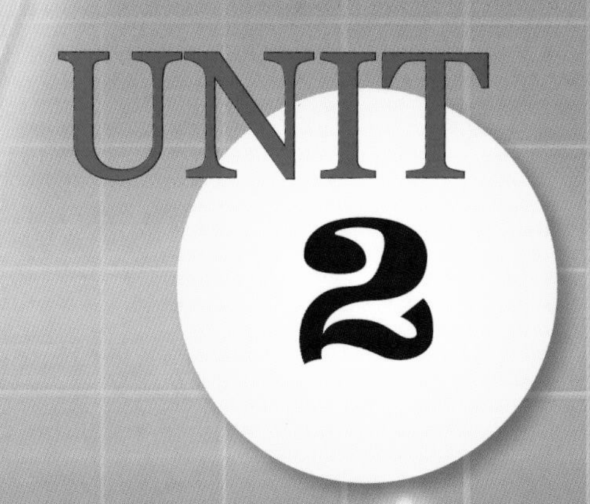

Physiology of Movement

- Muscle Structure and Function
- Muscles at Work
- Energy for Muscular Activity
- The Heart and Lungs at Work

In This Chapter:

CHAPTER 4

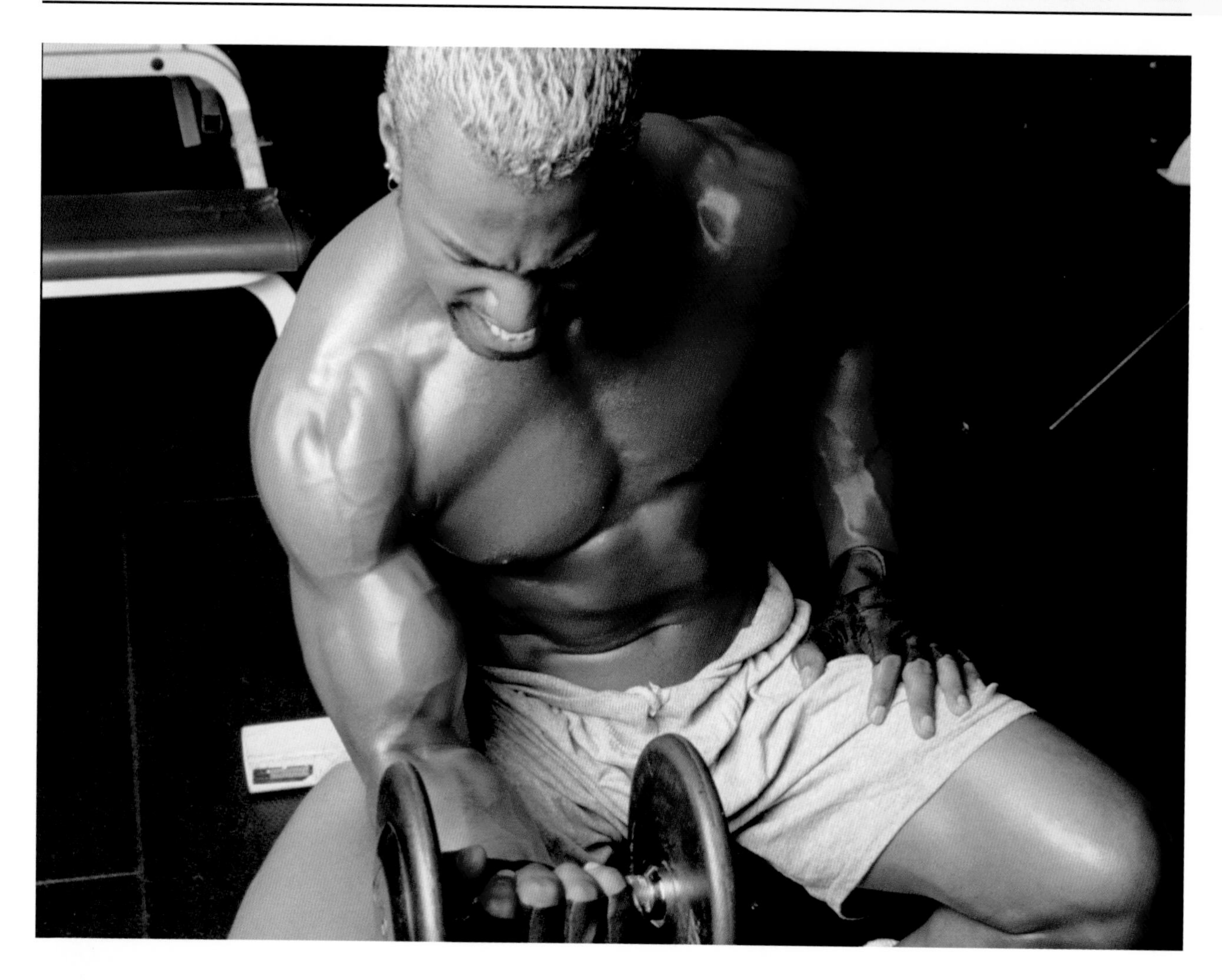

Muscle Structure and Function

After completing this chapter you should be able to:

- describe the macro and micro structures of skeletal muscle;
- describe muscle contraction and explain the sliding filament theory;
- demonstrate an understanding of nerve–muscle interaction;
- differentiate among types of muscle fibers;
- describe group action of muscles;
- discuss muscle's adaptation to strength training.

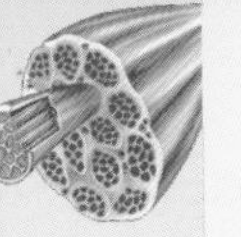

Structure determines function. This is a statement that defines the essence of human anatomy and physiology. Muscle tissue – the contraction specialist – provides a prime example of how the structure of a tissue is well adapted to perform a specific function. With approximately 660 muscles in the adult human body, making up nearly half of our body weight, the importance of muscular activity is obvious. The various structures and types of muscle tissue support numerous life functions, such as ventilation, physical activity and exercise, digestion, and of course, pumping life-sustaining blood throughout the body via specialized cardiac muscle. The focus in this chapter will be on skeletal muscle, which permits voluntary movement and is unique among other types of muscle in other important ways.

We often look at muscle as a single entity, but in so doing, fail to recognize the molecular complexity and hierarchical structure of this tissue. This specialized structure enables muscle to shorten and develop tension, allowing a myriad of human movements to occur. From movements as simple as waving good-bye or picking up a book, to more complex actions such as those required in athletics, the muscular system is vital to our daily functioning. But how does muscle activity integrate with the nervous system to produce movement? And what are the fundamental contractile properties of muscle?

Types of Human Muscle

On the basis of their structures, contractile properties, and control mechanisms, there are three types of muscle in the human body: (1) skeletal muscle; (2) smooth muscle; and (3) cardiac muscle.

Most **skeletal muscle** is attached to bone, and its contraction is responsible for supporting and moving the skeleton. The contraction of skeletal muscle is initiated by impulses in the motor neurons to the muscle and is usually under **voluntary** control.

Smooth muscle is under the control of the autonomic nervous system and is called **involuntary**. Smooth muscle forms the walls of blood vessels and body organs, such as the respiratory tract, the iris of the eye, and the gastrointestinal tract. The contractions of smooth muscle are slow and uniform and are very fatigue resistant. Smooth muscle functions to alter the activity of various body parts to meet the needs of the body at the time.

Cardiac muscle, the muscle of the heart, has characteristics of both skeletal and smooth muscle. Cardiac muscle functions to provide the contractile activity of the heart and has its own intrinsic beat. Like skeletal muscle, the contractile activity of cardiac muscle can be graduated; however, cardiac muscle is very fatigue resistant. Like smooth muscle, the activation of cardiac muscle is involuntary.

Although fitness training can benefit all three types of muscle systems, this chapter will deal primarily with the skeletal muscle.

Skeletal Muscle

Properties

Skeletal muscle refers to a number of muscle fibers bound together by connective tissue and is usually linked to bone by bundles of collagen fibers, known as **tendons**. Tendons are located at each end of the muscle (Figure 4.1 A). During muscle contraction, skeletal muscle shortens, and as a result of the tendinous attachments to bone, functions to move the various parts of the skeleton with respect to one another (joints) to allow changes in position of one skeletal segment in relation to another. Positioning several muscles on each "side" of a joint allows movement in several planes, and through graded activation the speed and smoothness of the movement can be graduated.

Skeletal muscles are capable of rapid contraction and relaxation. Intensive activity causes them to show early signs of fatigue. The assessment of the movement and the sequential pattern of muscle activation acting through joints to move

Origin–Insertion

In order for muscles to contract, they must be attached to bones to create movement. This is accomplished by tendons, strong fibrous tissues at the ends of each muscle. The end of the muscle attached to the bone that does not move is called the **origin**, while the point of attachment of the muscle on the bone that moves is the **insertion** (Figure 4.1 A). The origin tends to be the more proximal attachment (closer to the body), while the insertion is the more distal attachment (further from the body).

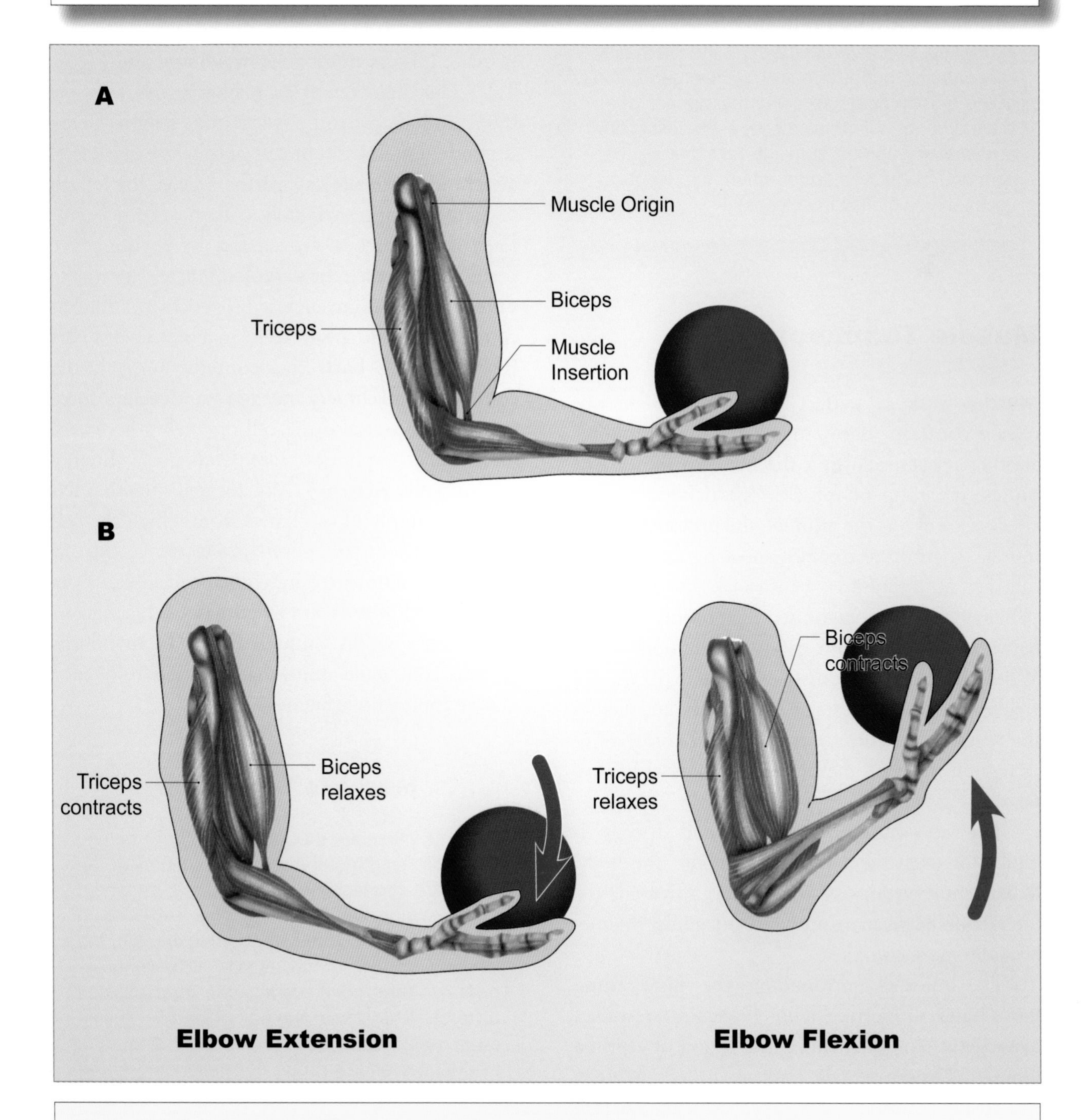

Figure 4.1 Bending or straightening the elbow requires the coordinated interplay of the biceps and triceps muscles.

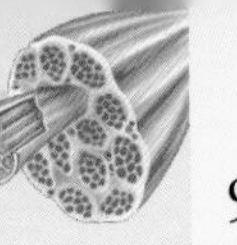

body segments is termed **biomechanics of human movement** (see Chapter 8).

> **Striated or Voluntary Muscle**
>
> Muscle attached to the skeleton to make it move is known as **skeletal muscle.** It is also known as voluntary or **striated muscle**. Skeletal muscle is considered *striated* because of the alternating light and dark bands (created by the organization of the muscle fibers, or cells) that appear when viewed under a light microscope. Its description as *voluntary* comes from the fact that we can contract skeletal muscle when we want to, voluntarily (e.g., flex the biceps).

Muscle Teamwork

Muscles work in perfect synchrony. When one muscle contracts (draws together) to move a bone, another relaxes, allowing the bone to move. The muscle or group of muscles producing a desired effect is known as the **agonist**, the **prime mover**. A muscle or group of muscles opposing the action is called an **antagonist.**

An agonist–antagonist relationship occurs between the biceps and triceps of the upper arm. When the biceps (agonist) contracts to bend the elbow, the triceps (antagonist) relaxes and allows the bend. When the triceps (agonist) contracts to straighten the arm, the biceps (antagonist) in turn relaxes (Figure 4.1 B).

The cooperation of biceps and triceps is typical of what takes place throughout the body. When entire groups of muscles get involved, the interaction between agonist and antagonist muscles becomes more complex.

The muscles surrounding the joint being moved and supporting it in the action are called **synergists** (complementing the action of a prime mover). Other muscle groups called **fixators** will steady joints closer to the body axis so that the desired action can occur. For example, if you want to climb a rope hand over hand, the muscles holding your shoulder girdle tightly to your rib cage are fixators, enabling you to use the muscles acting over the shoulder, elbow, wrist, and finger joints to perform their job and pull you up the rope.

Structure

Skeletal muscle is made up of numerous cylinder-shaped cells called **muscle fibers**, and each fiber is made up of a number of **myofilaments** (Figure 4.2). The diameter of each fiber varies between 0.05 and 0.10 mm, with the length being dependent mainly on the distance between skeletal attachments (in the case of the biceps, the length of a fiber is approximately 6 inches, or 15 cm). Each cell (fiber) is surrounded by a connective tissue sheath called the **sarcolemma**, and a variable number of fibers are enclosed together by a thicker connective tissue sheath to form a bundle of fibers (Figure 4.2 B). Each fiber contains not only the contractile machinery needed to develop force (Figure 4.3) but also the cell organelles necessary for cellular respiration (see Chapter 6, Energy for Muscular Activity). Also located outside each fiber is a supply of capillaries from which the cell obtains nutrients and eliminates waste.

A large number of individual threadlike fibers known as **myofibrils** run lengthwise and parallel to one another within a muscle fiber. The myofibrils contain contractile units that are responsible for muscle contraction (Figure 4.2 D).

> **Muscle's Tug of War**
>
> In some muscles, the individual fibers extend the entire length of the muscle, but in most the fibers are shorter. The shorter fibers, anchored to the connective-tissue network surrounding the muscle fibers, are placed at an angle to the longitudinal axis of the muscle. When muscle pulls on the bone during the transmission of force, it is like a number of people pulling on a rope, each person corresponding to a single fiber and the rope corresponding to the connective tissue and tendons.

Muscle: The Contractile Machinery

Within each myofibril, a number of contractile units, called **sarcomeres** (Figure 4.3 A), are organized in series (i.e., attached end to end). Each sarcomere consists of two types of protein myofilaments: **myosin**, the so-called thick filament, and **actin**, termed the thin filament. Looking at the filaments in a cross-section (i.e., looking at the myofilaments end-on), we see that each myosin filament is surrounded by actin filaments (Figure 4.3 A). Examining the sarcomere longitudinally (i.e., lengthwise), we see the distinctive banding pattern (striations) characteristic of skeletal, or striated, muscle (Figure 4.4). Projecting out from each of the myosin filaments at an angle of approximately 45 degrees are tiny contractile elements called **myosin bridges**; from this view, these elements look similar to the projections of oars from a rowing shell (Figure 4.3).

The Sliding Filament Theory During the contraction of a muscle, it is the sliding of the thin actin filaments over the thick myosin filaments that causes shortening of the muscle to create movement. This phenomenon is called the **sliding filament theory.** It is far more complex than described here, but you should still be able to appreciate all the intricate anatomical structures involved with every move we make.

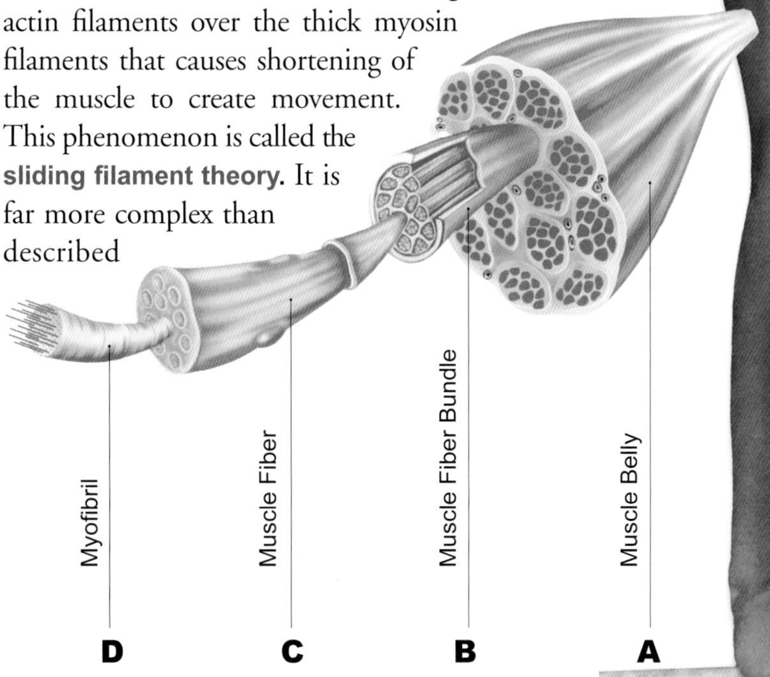

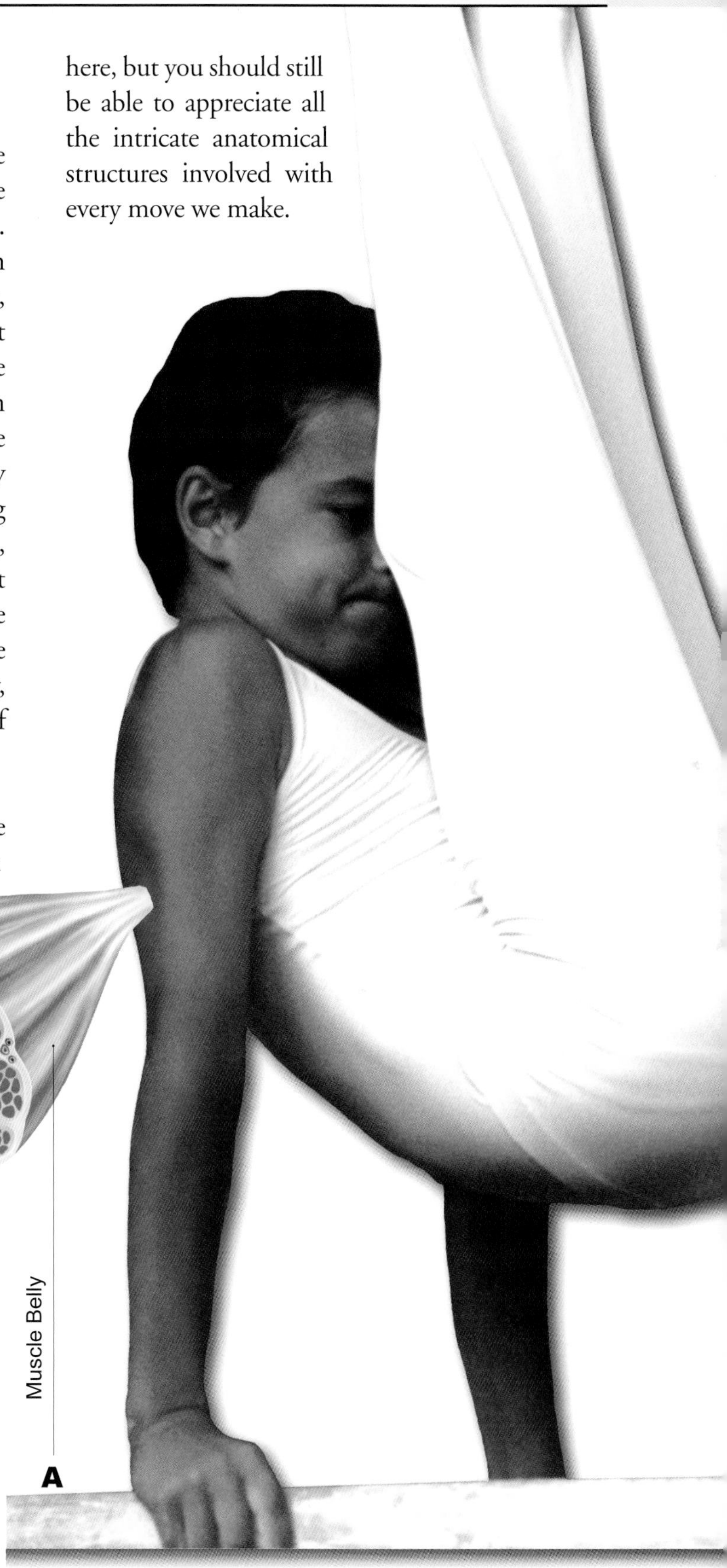

Figure 4.2 Components of skeletal muscle. **A.** Muscle belly (2 inches, or 50 mm, in diameter). **B.** Muscle fiber bundle (0.5 mm). **C.** Muscle fiber (0.05-0.1 mm). **D.** Myofibril (0.001-0.002 mm).

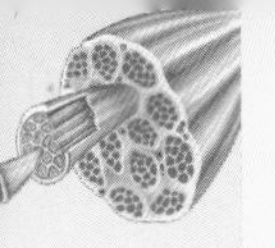

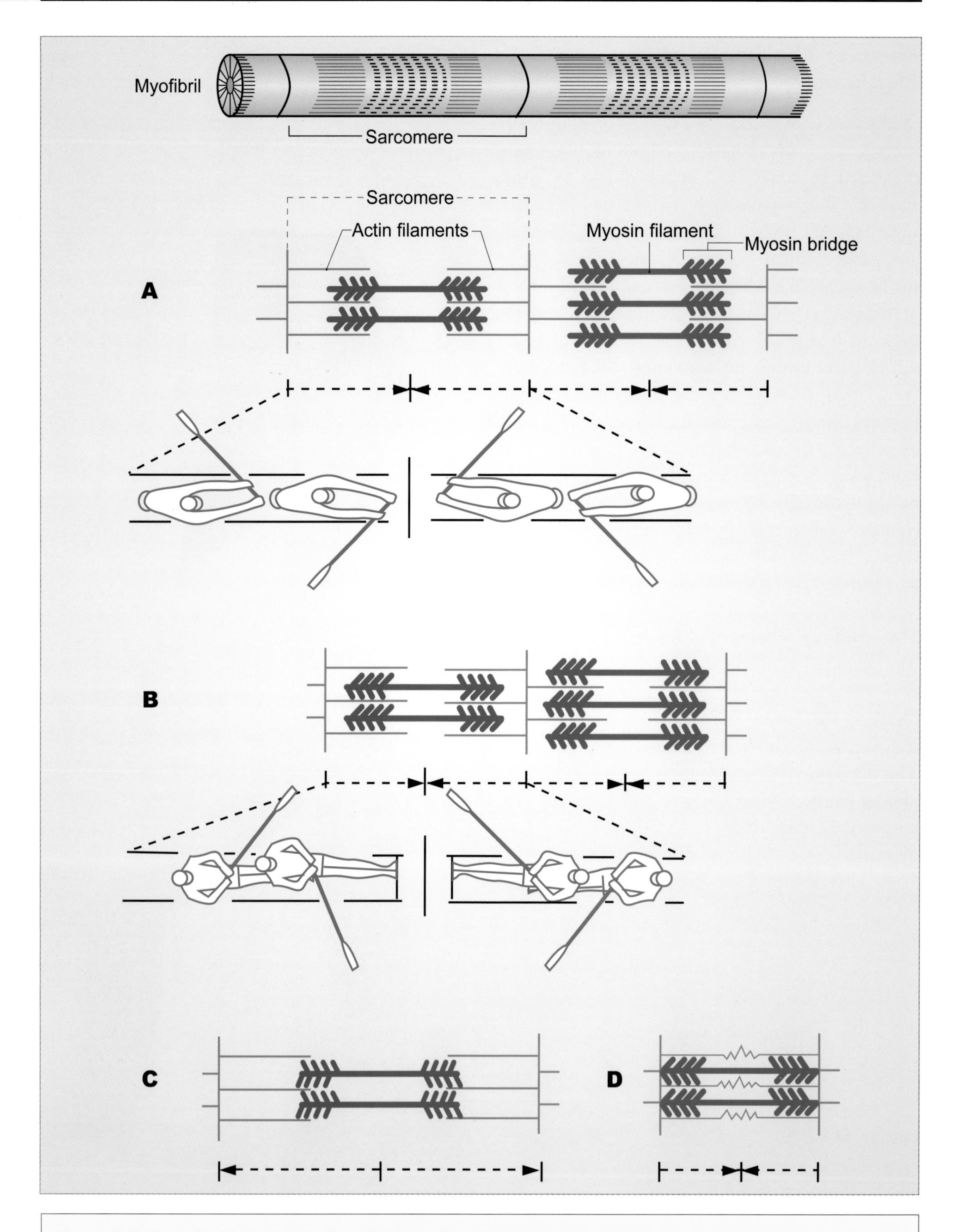

Figure 4.3 Longitudinal section of a myofibril and simplified representation of muscular contraction: **A.** At rest. **B.** Contraction. **C.** Powerful stretching. **D.** Powerful contraction.

Rowing Simulation When a signal comes from the motor nerve activating the fiber, the heads of the myosin filaments temporarily attach themselves to the actin filaments (Figure 4.3 D), a process termed **cross bridge formation**. In a manner similar to the stroking of the oars and the subsequent movement of a rowing shell, the movement of the cross bridges causes a movement of the actin filaments in relation to the myosin filaments, leading to shortening of the sarcomere. A single "stroke" shortens the sarcomere by approximately 1 percent of its length, and the nervous system is capable of activating cross bridge formation at a rate of 7 to 50 per second. Since the sarcomeres are attached to one another in series, the shortening of each sarcomere is additive. The total amount of fiber shortening amounts to some 25 to 40 percent of myofibril length.

To produce an efficient rowing stroke, the oars must be optimally placed (i.e., reaching far enough, but not too far); similarly, for optimal cross bridge formation, the sarcomeres should be an optimal distance apart. For muscle contraction, this optimal distance is 0.0019 to 0.0022 mm. When the sarcomeres are separated by this distance, an optimal number of cross bridges can be formed per unit time. If the sarcomeres are farther apart, or closer together, than this optimal distance, then fewer cross bridges can be formed, resulting in less force development. If the sarcomeres are stretched further apart, as occurs when the muscle is in a lengthened (i.e., extended or stretched) position (Figure 4.3 C), fewer cross bridges can form because the myosin projections have difficulty reaching the actin filaments; this results in a decreased ability to produce force. When the sarcomeres are too close together, as would occur when the muscle is shortened (flexed), the cross bridges in fact interfere with one another as they try to form, resulting in a smaller number of effective cross bridges being formed and, again, a decreased ability to develop force (Figure 4.3 D).

The distance between sarcomeres depends on the state of muscle stretch, which in turn is a product of the position of the joint. What this means to the development of muscle force is that maximal force is developed when an optimal number of cross bridges are formed, which occurs at an optimal joint angle. Thus, because muscle force depends on muscle length, maximal muscle force occurs at optimal muscle length. As a joint moves through its range of motion, the muscle(s) connecting the two segments of the joint will move from a stretched position to a compressed position, and therefore, at some point in the movement, will pass through a position, termed the optimal joint angle, at which the muscle is at optimal length for maximal force development (Figure 4.5). This means that there will be an optimal joint angle for maximal force development for each movement

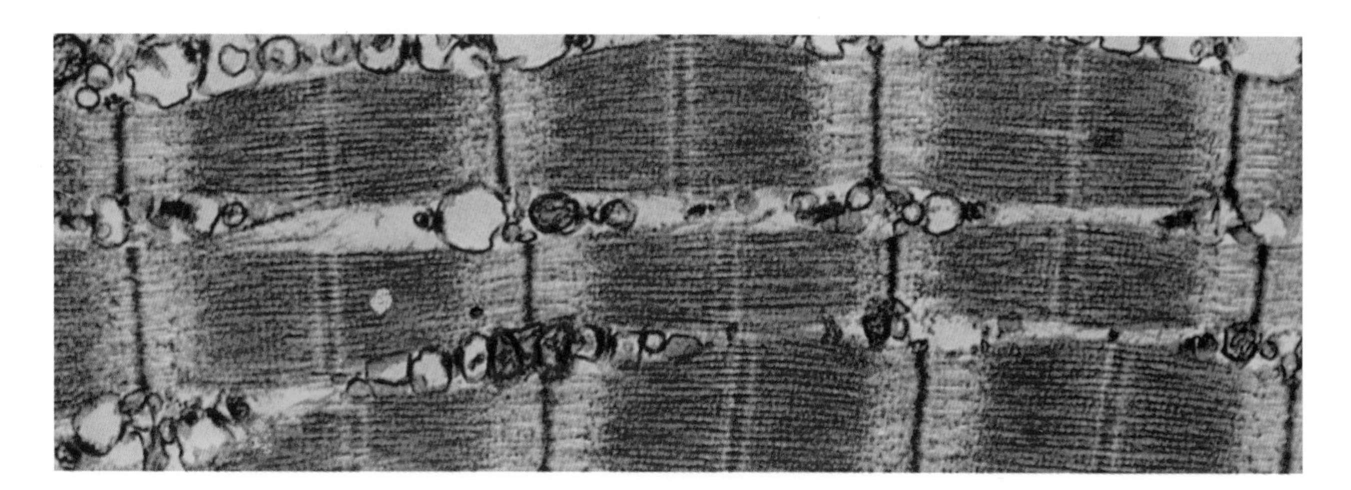

Figure 4.4 Microscopic view of several sarcomeres within a myofibril. The overlap arrangement of the actin and myosin strands results in the characteristic "striped" appearance of skeletal muscle.

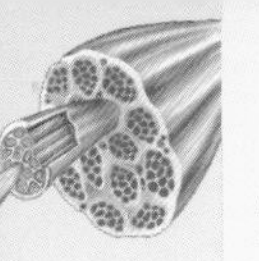

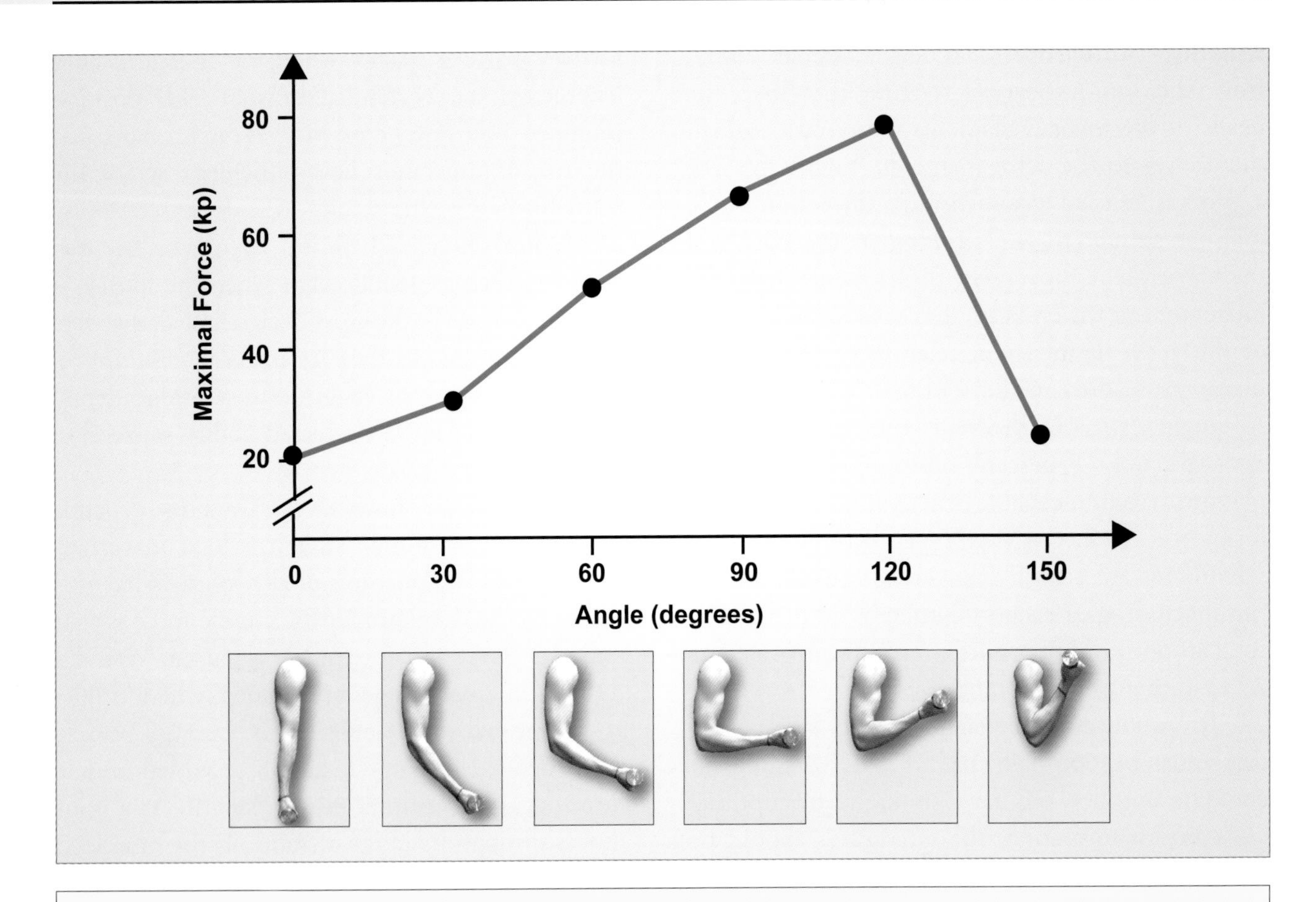

Figure 4.5 Maximal muscle force changes continuously throughout elbow flexion according to the joint angle.

Table 4.1 Relative involvement of muscle fiber types in sport events.

Event	Slow Twitch – Type I	Fast Twitch – Type II
100-m sprint	Low	High
800-m run	High	High
Marathon	High	Low
Olympic weightlifting	Low	High
Barbell squat	Low	High
Soccer	High	High
Field hockey	High	High
Football wide receiver	Low	High
Football lineman	High	High
Basketball	Low	High
Distance cycling	High	Low

of a joint. Knowledge of the joint angle at which maximal force can be developed is important in the development of optimal biomechanics of the movement.

Muscle Fiber Types

There are also different types of skeletal muscle fibers. Some fibers can reach maximum tension more quickly than others. Based on this distinction, muscle fibers can be divided into the categories of **fast twitch** (FT or type II) (also called white fibers based on their microscopic appearance) and **slow twitch** (ST or type I) (also called red fibers based on their microscopic appearance). FT fibers are more anaerobic, larger, fatigue faster, and have a faster contraction speed than ST fibers. This makes these fibers ideal for actions that are short and require quick bursts of power and energy, such as sprinting or jumping. On the other hand, events that require endurance, such as long-distance running, swimming, or cycling, depend on the smaller, slower contracting, fatigue-resistant ST fibers that rely on oxygen (Table 4.1). There are also fiber types that fall in between these extremes, with characteristics of both fiber types. Thus, type II is further divided into type IIa and type IIb fibers. The distinction between the two is mainly in their contractile strength and their capacity for aerobic-oxidative energy supply. The type IIa fibers have greater capacity for aerobic metabolism and more capillaries surrounding them than type IIb and therefore show greater resistance to fatigue.

The muscle fiber composition of an individual is dictated through heredity. The fiber composition of an individual cannot be *altered* by training (i.e., the transformation of a fiber from one type to another as a result of the training stimulus does not occur).

Most skeletal muscles, however, contain both FT

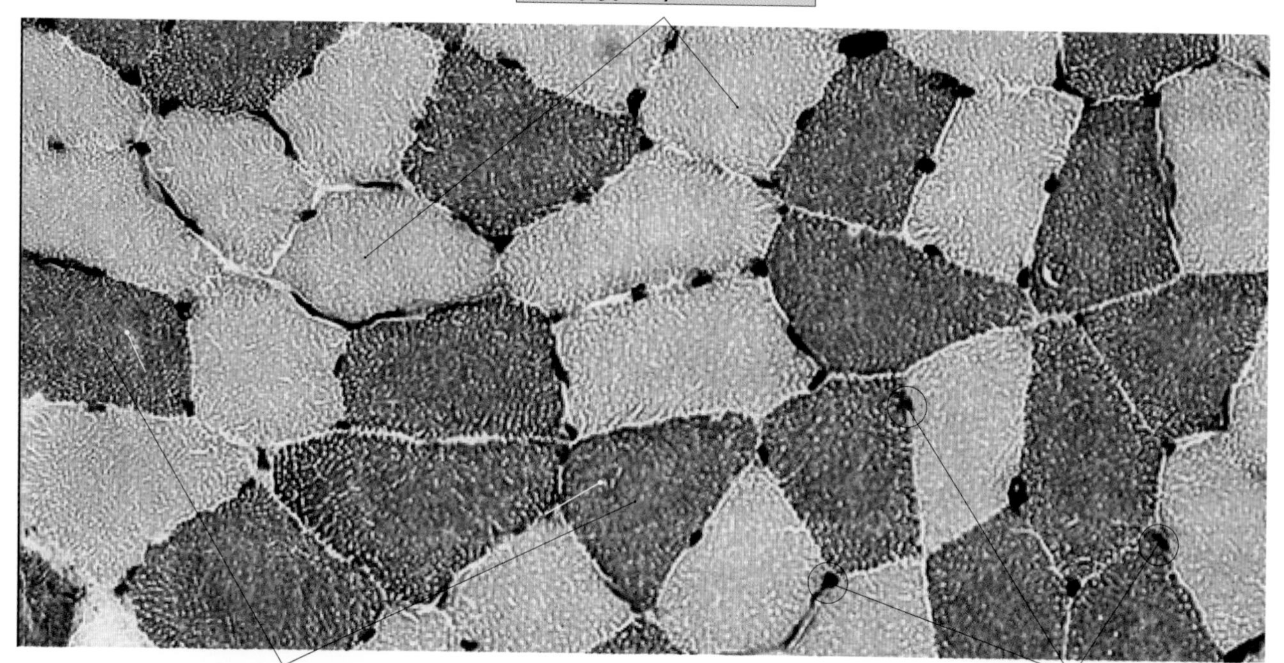

Figure 4.6 Muscle biopsy.

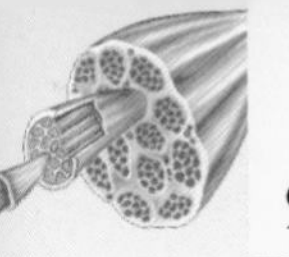

and ST fibers, with the amount of each varying from one muscle to another, as well as among different individuals. Therefore, individual performance differences occur as a result of varying percentages of the muscle fiber types, making some individuals suited to some activities more than others (that is not to say that training will not *improve* what fibers you do have).

Muscle Biopsy

Muscle fiber type is determined from a **muscle biopsy**. In this procedure, a small incision (about 5 to 7 mm) is made in the skin and fascia of the muscle following injection of a local anesthetic into the muscle. A tiny piece of tissue is cut and removed from the muscle and then analyzed under a microscope (Figure 4.6). In addition to determining muscle fiber type, it is possible to study the metabolic characteristics of the muscle and to assess changes in metabolic capability following various types of training programs.

Biopsy = *bio* (life) + *opsis* (sight)

Nerve–Muscle Interaction

As with bone, muscle is a living tissue, and as such, is richly supplied with blood vessels and nerves. Skeletal muscle activation is initiated through neural activation (Figure 4.7), and therefore it is under conscious control. The nervous system is organized at two levels – the **central (CNS)** and **peripheral (PNS) nervous systems**, with the central system being composed of the brain and spinal cord (Figure 4.7 A) and the peripheral system being made up of numerous nerves of various sizes (Figure 4.7 C).

The nervous system can also be divided in terms of function, namely motor and sensory activity. The sensory section (Figure 4.7 E) collects information from the various sensors located throughout the body and transmits the information to the brain, where it is processed and acted upon. This sensory information is also stored away so that future responses to similar input can be acted upon more quickly. The motor section (Figure 4.7 D) is involved directly in conducting the signals from the CNS to activate muscle contraction (see Chapter 10, Information Processing in Human Movement).

Motor Unit

Motor nerves extend from the spinal cord to the muscle fibers. Each fiber is activated through impulses delivered via its **motor end plate**. A group of fibers activated via the same nerve is termed a **motor unit**, the basic functional entity of muscular activity. A muscle can be composed of a different number of motor units, and each motor unit can in turn consist of a different number of muscle fibers.

All muscle fibers of one particular motor unit, however, are always of the same fiber type (FT or ST fibers). Muscles that need to perform delicate and precise movements (the eye and finger muscles) generally consist of a large number of motor units (1,500 to 3,000), each containing only a few muscle fibers (8 to 50). Relatively unrefined movement, however, is carried out by muscles composed of fewer motor units with many fibers (approximately 600 to 2,000), each of which innervates up to 1,500 muscle fibers. In the tibialis anterior muscle, approximately 650 muscle fibers are innervated by each motor unit; in the gastrocnemius muscle, the number is approximately 1,600, and in the extensors of the back, it is about 2,000.

The specific number of fibers in a motor unit of any given muscle can vary. The biceps may be composed of motor units that innervate 1,000, 1,200, 1,400, or 1,600 fibers. Furthermore, each muscle fiber can be innervated by only one motor unit. This cannot be altered through exercise.

All-or-none Principle

Muscle movement is controlled by the motor nerve

impulses transmitted from the CNS and spinal cord out to the motor unit, which when activated causes the muscle fibers to contract. Whether or not a motor unit activates upon the arrival of an impulse depends upon the so-called **all-or-none principle.** This principle, discussed in more detail in Chapter 10, requires an impulse of a certain magnitude (or strength) to cause the innervated fibers to contract. The principle is analogous to firing a gun. Once a sufficient amount of pressure is placed on the trigger, the gun fires; pulling on the trigger harder will not cause the bullet to go faster or farther.

Activation Threshold Every motor unit has a specific threshold that must be reached for such activation to occur. For the biceps muscle, for example, all of the 1,500 fibers that may make up a single motor unit will contract maximally providing the nerve impulse has reached a certain magnitude. However, if the nerve impulse does not reach the required magnitude, then none of the fibers will contract.

A weak nerve impulse activates only those motor units that have a low threshold of activation. A stronger nerve impulse will additionally activate motor units with higher thresholds. As the resistance increases, more motor units must be activated by stronger, more intensive impulses. An athlete needs increasingly more willpower to exceed the excitatory thresholds of the motor units. This process is extremely fatiguing as a result of lactic acid accumulation in the muscle tissue and blood, the depletion of high-energy compounds, and the fatigue of the nervous system processes.

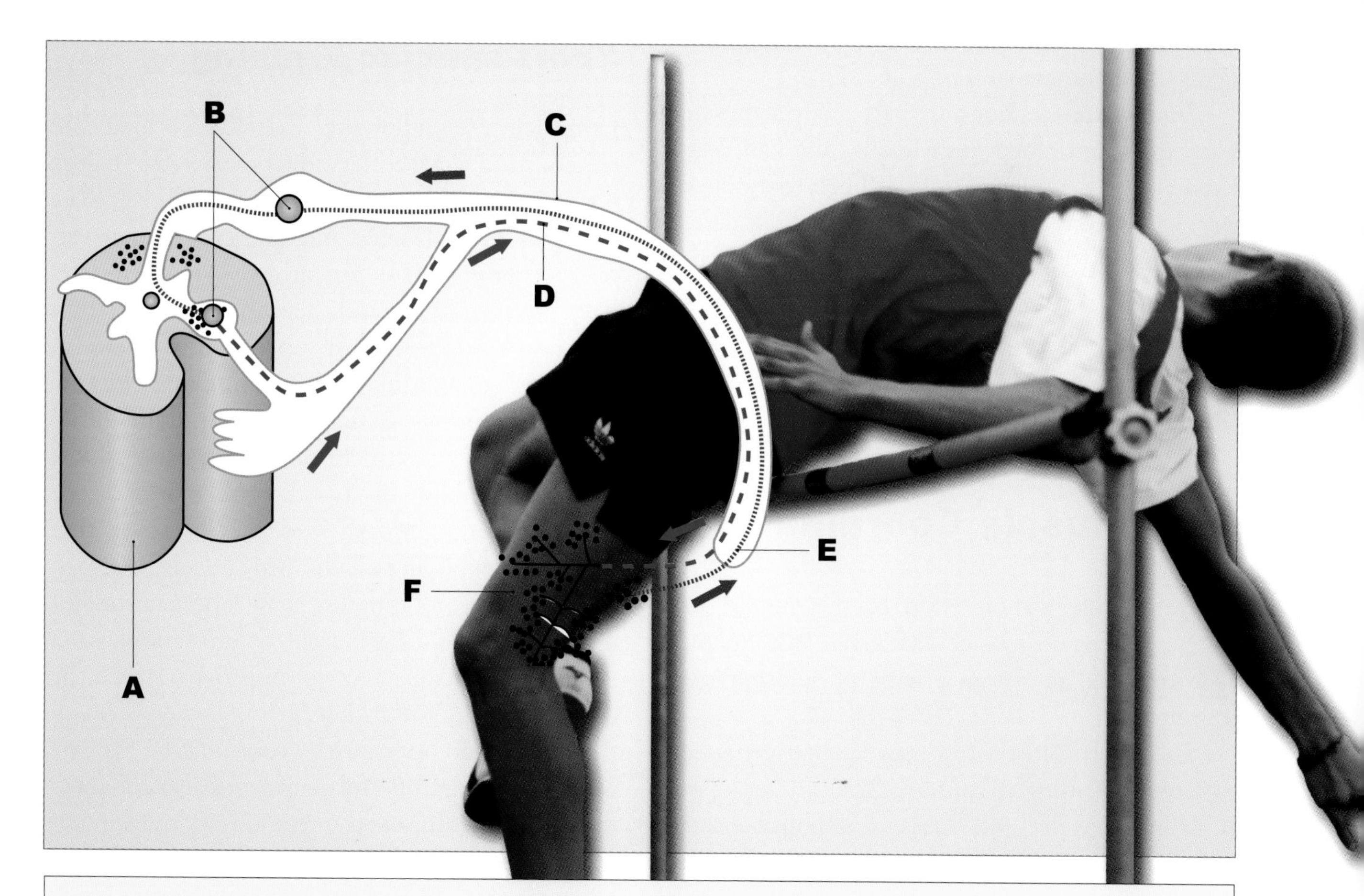

Figure 4.7 Sensory neurons transfer messages to the central nervous system, where they are analyzed and responded to by motor neurons. Activation of a motor unit and its innervation systems: **A.** Spinal cord. **B.** Cytosomes. **C.** Spinal nerve. **D.** Motor nerve. **E.** Sensory nerve. **F.** Muscle with muscle fibers.

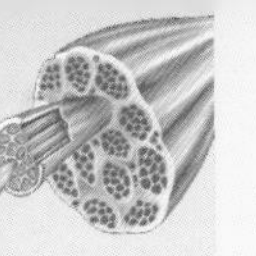

Intramuscle Coordination

The capacity to activate motor units simultaneously is known as **intramuscle coordination**. Although it is impossible to use all the motor units of a muscle at the same time, many highly trained power athletes, such as weightlifters, wrestlers, and shot-putters, are able to activate up to 85 percent of their available muscle fibers simultaneously, thus generating great strength. Untrained individuals, on the other hand, can normally activate only up to 60 percent of their fibers.

Research has shown that under hypnosis a trained athlete can elevate the maximal force application for a given muscle by approximately 10 percent. The difference between assisted and voluntarily generated maximal force is regarded as the **muscle force deficit** of the muscle contraction. For untrained individuals, this deficit is much larger (approximately 20 to 35 percent).

Trained athletes not only have a larger muscle mass than untrained individuals but can also exploit a larger number of muscle fibers to produce force. However, for this reason, such athletes are more restricted than untrained individuals in further developing strength by improving intramuscle coordination. For this same reason, trained individuals can further increase strength only by increasing muscle diameter.

Intermuscle Coordination

It requires considerable effort by the muscles or muscle groups to master any given movement. This requires an optimal level of **intermuscle coordination**.

The interplay between muscles that generate movement through contraction, the agonists or prime movers, and muscles responsible for opposing movement, the antagonists, is of particular importance to the quality of intermuscle coordination. The cooperation between agonist and antagonist muscles during the bench press, for example, provides a useful illustration. From a supine position, an athlete explosively stretches his or her arms against a high resistance. During the movement, a considerable number of motor units in the triceps and in cooperating muscles are synchronously activated, while the motor units of the antagonist muscles relax.

The greater the participation of muscles and muscle groups, the higher the importance of intermuscle coordination for strength capacity. To benefit from strength training, technically demanding sport-specific movements are often broken down into partial movements so that the individual muscle groups responsible for these movements can be trained in relative isolation. The exercises used closely resemble the movement structure of the sport-specific movement, such that the training allows for the key muscle groups to be loaded relatively heavily.

Sport-specific Training

Consider the following exercises, which are beneficial to weightlifters: the bench press (Figure 4.8 A), lateral trunk curl (Figure 4.8 B), knee bend, or squat (Figure 4.8 C), and heel or calf raise (Figure 4.8 D). An athlete whose muscles have been trained and developed in isolation using such exercises must subsequently engage in training that coordinates these muscles within the complete, sport-specific movement. Difficulties may occur if the athlete fails to develop all the relevant muscles in a balanced manner. For instance, a weightlifter who uses exercises that increase strength in only the arm and leg extensors, but not the trunk muscles, may experience major disturbances of intermuscle coordination. As a result, performance may not improve or reach the level desired by the athlete.

High-level intermuscle coordination greatly improves strength performance and also enhances the flow, rhythm, and precision of movement. Unlike an ordinary individual, a highly trained athlete is able to translate strength potential more effectively into strength performance through enhanced intermuscle coordination.

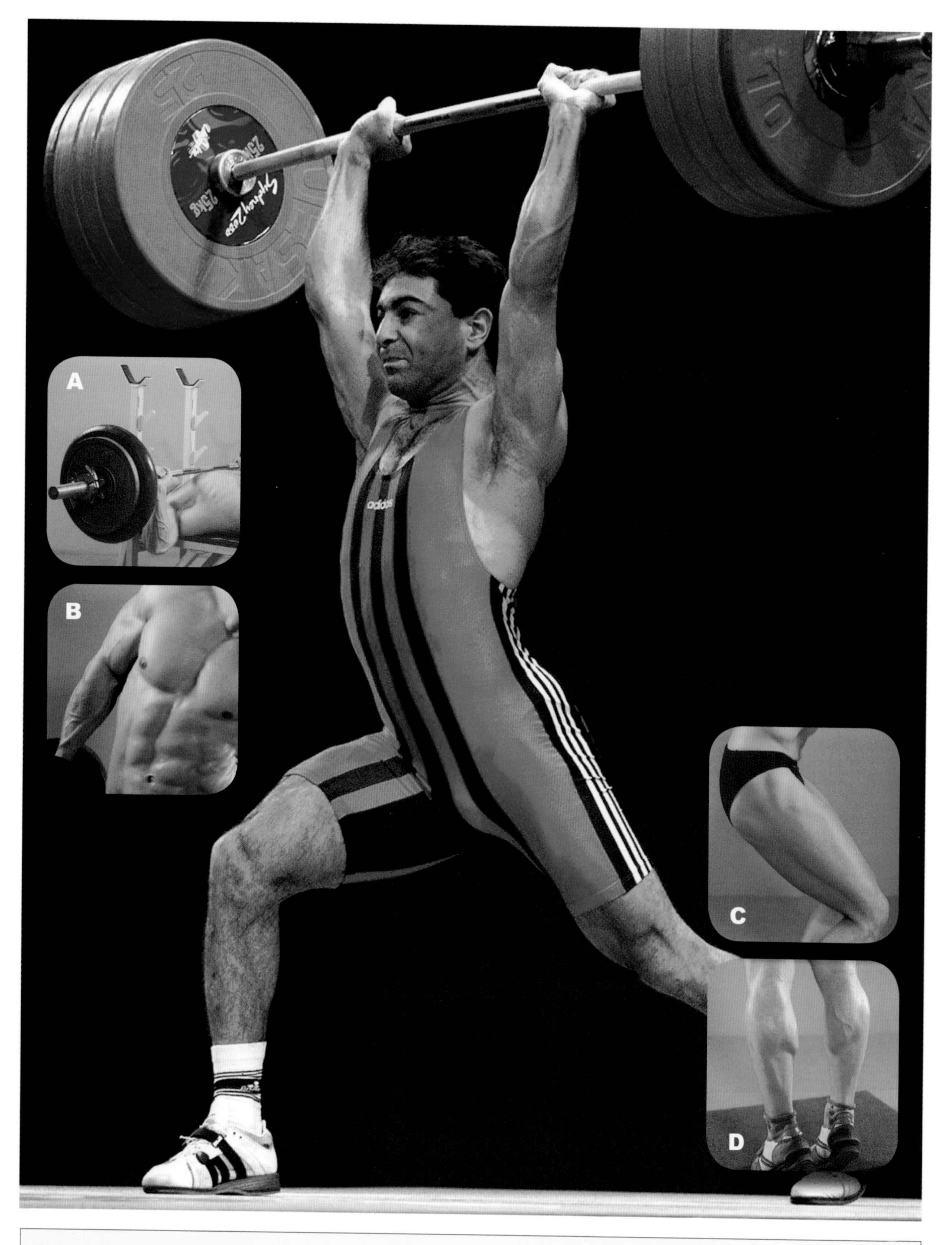

Figure 4.8 A weightlifter's training includes exercises that work several prime movers in isolation. **A.** Bench press. **B.** Lateral trunk curl. **C.** Knee bend, or squat. **D.** Heel or calf raise.

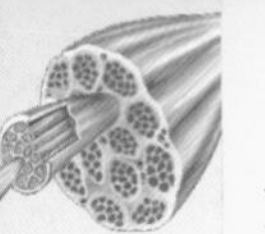

Trainable Versus Nontrainable Factors

The performance capacity of muscle is determined by several trainable and nontrainable factors.

Trainable factors:

- fiber diameter
- intramuscle coordination
- nerve impulse frequency
- intermuscle coordination
- elasticity of muscle and its tendons
- energy stores of muscle and liver
- capillary density of muscle

Nontrainable factors:

- number of fibers
- fiber structure (ST or FT fibers)

Muscle's Adaptation to Strength Training

In strength training, an individual's performance improvements occur through a process of **biological adaptation**, which is reflected in the body's increased strength. Similar types of adaptation may occur in any form of training. Indeed, they are the building blocks for improved performance in any athletic activity.

In strength training, the adaptation process proceeds at different time rates for different functional systems and physiological processes. The adaptation depends on a variety of factors, in particular on intensity levels used in training and on an athlete's unique biological makeup. Specific substances of the metabolism, such as enzymes, adapt within hours; the energy supply in the liver and muscle increases at a more moderate pace, within 10 to 14 days, by which time the first adaptations in the cardiovascular circulation also occur (see Chapter 7). The muscle mass increases slowly, within four to six weeks, its growth caused by an increase in the structural proteins in the skeletal muscle fibers.

Recruitment of Muscle Fibers

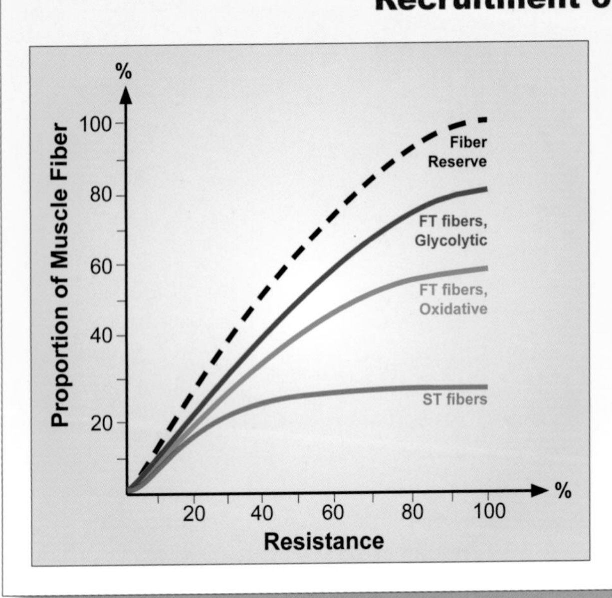

Recruitment of muscle fibers during resistance work depends on the level of muscle tension. As the tension rises, more and more of the various fiber types are recruited into the movement, as shown by the curves. Muscle tension below 25 percent of one's maximal resistance recruits mostly ST fibers. At higher resistance, FT fibers also become active. Furthermore, which fiber is involved depends upon the muscle force that needs to be mobilized as well as the rate of acceleration of the mass to be moved. High accelerations of small loads and low accelerations of high loads require the intensive involvement of the FT fibers. Also, it is primarily the FT fibers that generate the explosive-type movements requiring a lot of strength.

Summary

Muscles attached to skeletal bones work together and with tendons to enable body movement. Thin fibers called myofibrils constitute muscle, and end-to-end units called sarcomeres within each myofibril enable muscles to contract, causing movement in response to motor nerve stimulation.

Motor nerves extend from the spinal cord to muscles throughout the body, and each motor unit is specific to either fast twitch or slow twitch muscle types. FT fibers, which are anaerobic in nature and fatigue faster than ST fibers, are best suited for activities requiring short bursts of power and energy. Endurance events such as long-distance running, swimming, or cycling make use of the fatigue-resistant ST fibers, which rely on oxygen. Motor units require threshold levels of nerve impulses before they can react – and some motor units have higher resistance thresholds than companion units in the same muscle.

Movement requires precise coordination of muscles and the muscle fibers themselves. Intramuscle coordination is the ability to activate motor units simultaneously, while intermuscle coordination refers to the synchronization of different muscles and muscle groups. Cooperation of the agonists and antagonists is necessary for smooth, controlled motion.

Key Terms

actin
agonist
all-or-none principle
antagonist
biological adaptation
cardiac muscle
cross bridge formation
fast twitch (FT) fiber
fixator
insertion
intermuscle coordination
intramuscle coordination
involuntary muscle
motor end plate
motor unit
muscle biopsy
muscle fiber
muscle force deficit
myofibril
myofilament
myosin
origin
prime mover
sarcolemma
sarcomere
skeletal muscle
sliding filament theory
slow twitch (ST) fiber
smooth muscle
striated muscle
synergist
tendon
voluntary muscle

Discussion Questions

1. What are the three types of muscle found in the human body?
2. Describe the structure of a muscle from the largest structural unit to the smallest.
3. Explain how the sarcomere contracts, resulting in muscle shortening.
4. What are the three types of muscle fibers? Give two characteristics of each type of fiber.
5. Explain nerve–muscle interaction.
6. Discuss the differences between inter- and intramuscle coordination.

In This Chapter:

CHAPTER 5

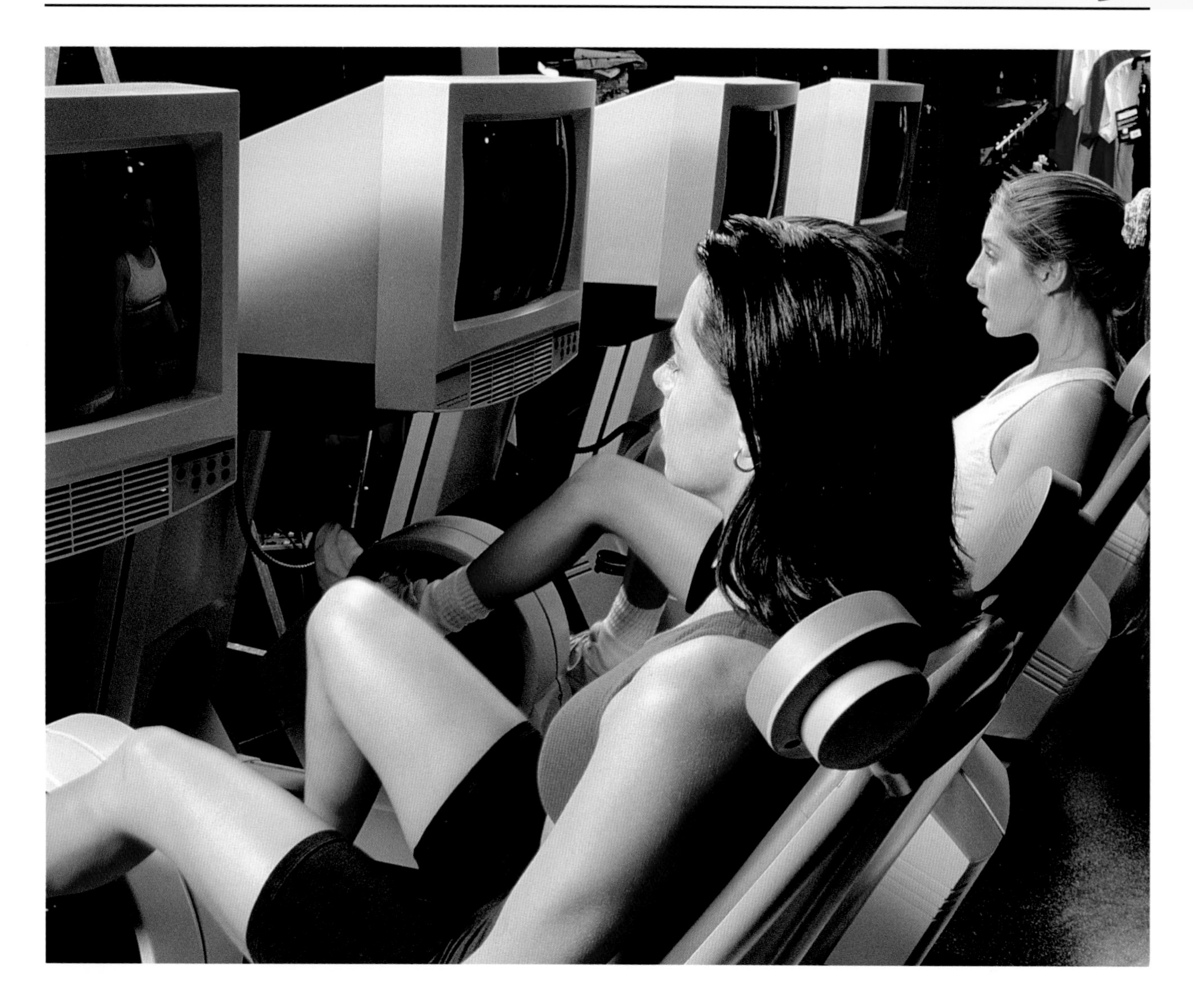

Muscles at Work

After completing this chapter you should be able to:

- differentiate between the various types of muscle contractions;
- describe the factors that influence strength development;
- identify the components of strength;
- discuss the relationships between the various components of strength.

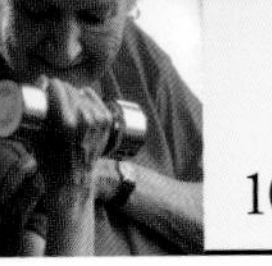

Muscle is an organ that creates movement. Its structure and function presented in the previous chapter can adapt according to some important training principles. These principles are designed to improve general and specific fitness, which is an important component of overall health. However, before we present the various principles of training in Chapter 12, you must become familiar with the various types of muscle contraction. You must also understand the concept of muscular strength, its components, and the interrelationships between these components, which provide the basis of training for fitness and athletic performance.

Types of Muscle Contraction

Several types of muscle contraction are relevant to a fitness and strength training program. The first distinction is made between static and dynamic contraction.

Static and dynamic work involves four types of muscle contraction: isometric, isotonic, isokinetic, and plyocentric. Each of these types of contractions is further divided into two forms of movement: concentric and eccentric.

> **Did You Know?**
>
> It is interesting to note that the terminology for major muscle contractions has been developed from the Greek language (Figure 5.1).

Static Contraction

Static contraction refers to a contraction in which the muscle tension or force exerted against an external load is equal or weaker, so no visible movement of the load occurs. Consider an athlete who attempts to flex an arm against the resistance of a fixed bar. Even if all energy and strength are mobilized, the athlete will not succeed in moving the arm or the bar. Nonetheless, the exerted muscle force is substantial.

In most sports, maximal static tension is rare. It may occur, however, in gymnastics (in the iron cross and hanging scale) or in wrestling and judo (in floor grips, holding techniques, and bridges). In general, most sport activities require low to **submaximal static contraction**. Sailing in close contact with the wind, shooting, and alpine downhill events often require static work over extended periods (Figure 5.2).

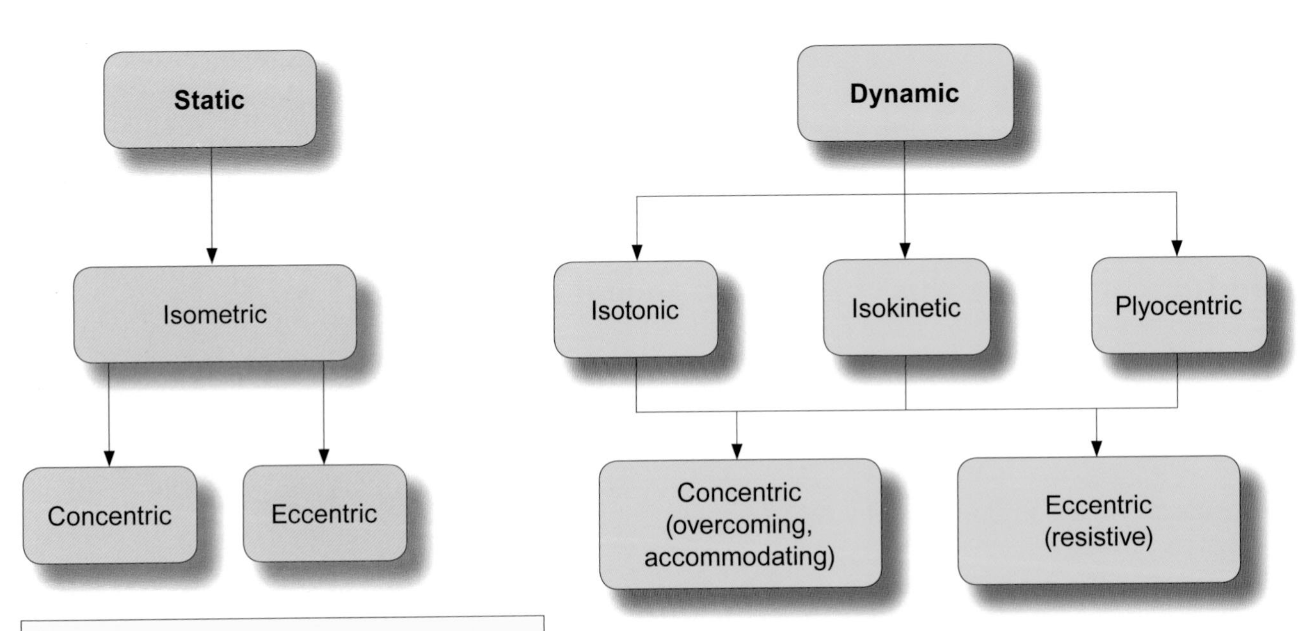

Figure 5.1 Types of muscle contractions.

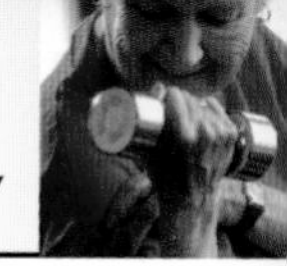

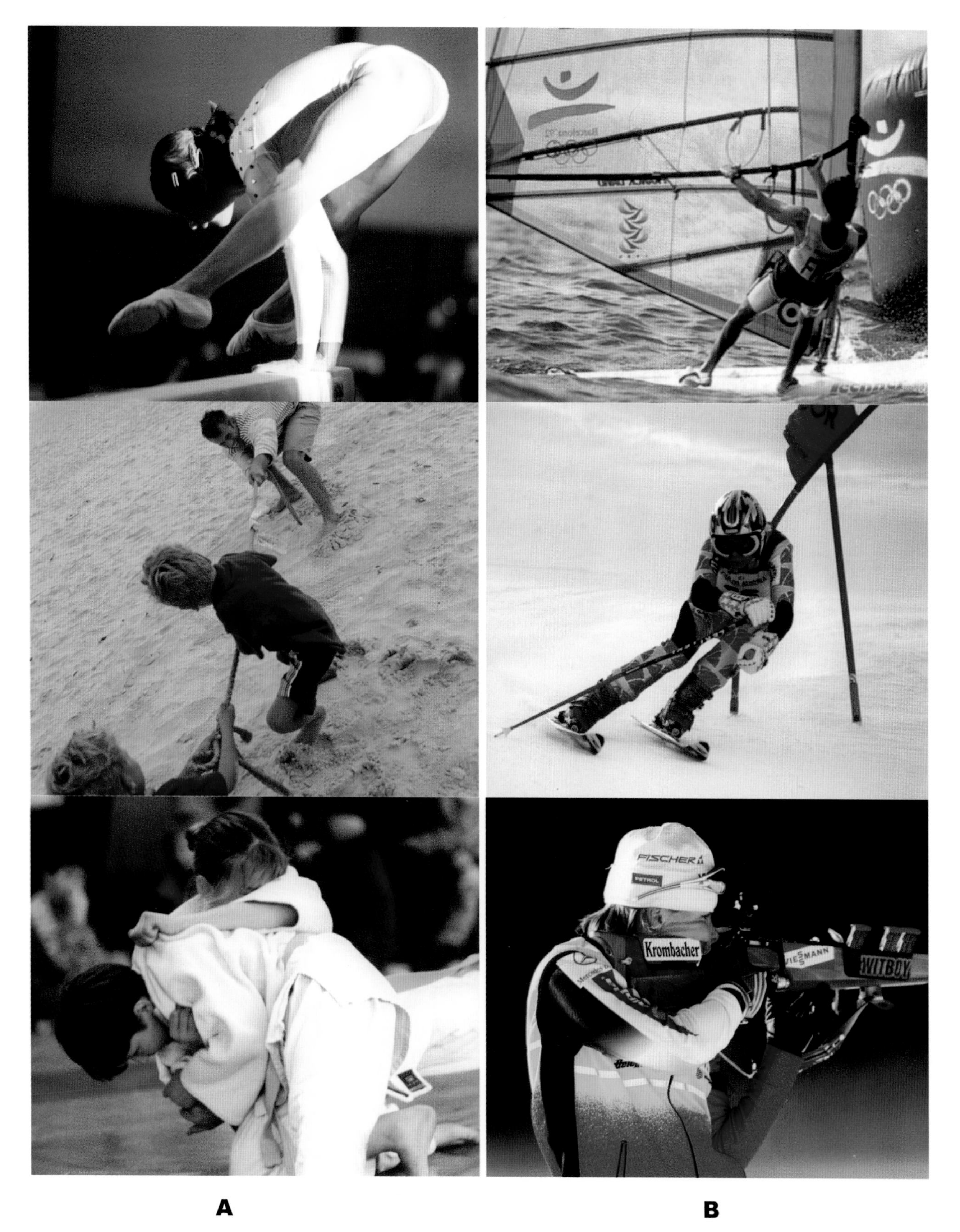

A B

Figure 5.2 Static or isometric contractions. **A.** Activities requiring maximal static muscle tension. **B.** Activities requiring submaximal static muscle tension.

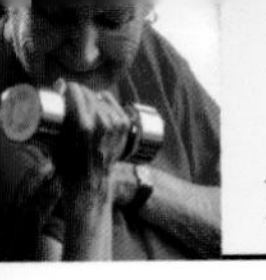

Isometric Contraction

An **isometric contraction** (*iso* = same, *metric* = length) is one in which there is no visible change in muscle length, even though the muscle has undergone muscle contraction. In this case, the contraction is against a load that is beyond the capability of the muscle(s) to move, and therefore, no movement of the load occurs. We also know that considerable force has been produced by the tiredness that one feels. The issue here is that no external movement is registered. Isometric contraction is a static contraction.

Strictly speaking, no work is performed during an isometric contraction (work = force x distance); nonetheless, a relatively high amount of tension is developed and energy is used. Therefore, an isometric contraction is not defined by the work performed but by the rate of tension developed and by the duration over which the tension lasts.

When two individuals of equal strength compete in arm wrestling, an isometric contraction occurs. There will be no movement of the hands until one individual fatigues (loses some of the cross bridges) and therefore can no longer maintain the status quo. For more on cross bridge formation, see Chapter 4.

Can you name other activities that are based on isometric contraction?

Dynamic Contraction

The neuromuscular system is said to work dynamically if internal and external forces are unbalanced. For instance, an athlete may be able to exert enough force to lift a weight through the full range of an exercise. When the external force (gravity of a weight or object) is smaller than the internal force generated by the athlete, the latter will be able to resist, and the result will be movement. Thus, a **dynamic contraction** involves movement.

Isotonic Contraction

Under normal circumstances, dynamic work is based on **isotonic contraction** (*iso* = same or constant, *tonos* = tension). Because of the continual change in joint angle and speed that occurs during dynamic work, the muscle needs to contract at either increasing or decreasing tension. The constant addition or subtraction of motor units recruited causes the muscle to adapt to constantly changing tension requirements. Isotonic contraction is a dynamic contraction.

When an athlete bends the arms while holding a barbell, the mass of the barbell obviously remains the same or constant during the entire range of movement. The strength needed to perform this movement is not, however, constant, but depends upon the physique of the athlete, the athlete's leverage, the angle position of the limbs, and the speed of movement (Figure 5.3). Also see Figure 4.5 in Chapter 4.

Lateral arm raises, too, require greater strength initially, reaching a maximum at 90 degrees and then dropping constantly. When lifting the trunk from a horizontal position, an athlete needs to mobilize maximal strength at the beginning of the movement, gradually reach peak values, and then decline continuously toward zero.

The issue of changing muscle force or tension throughout a movement also poses a problem to those using free weights to train. What often happens is one of two scenarios. If the chosen load can be lifted throughout the complete range of motion, it provides adequate stress for training in the initial and final stages of the movement but does not stress the muscle as much in the area of movement corresponding to optimal cross bridge formation. It is often in this area that the athlete wants to train, whether it is for the development of additional strength or the building of muscle bulk.

If the load is chosen to provide training stress to the muscle in that part of the range of movement corresponding to optimal cross bridge formation, then the load is often too great for the individual to be able to move at either end of the complete range of movement. In this case, the individual often gets the bar moving by "bumping" it with his thighs, and, at the end of the curl, lets it fall onto the shoulders. When lowering the bar, the

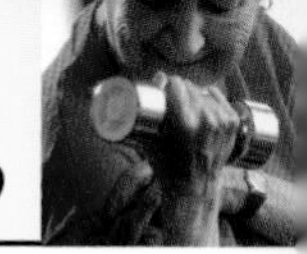

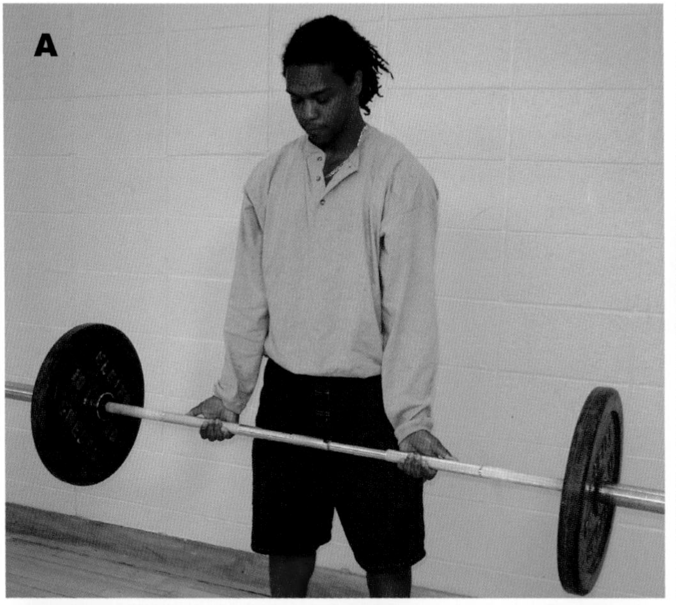

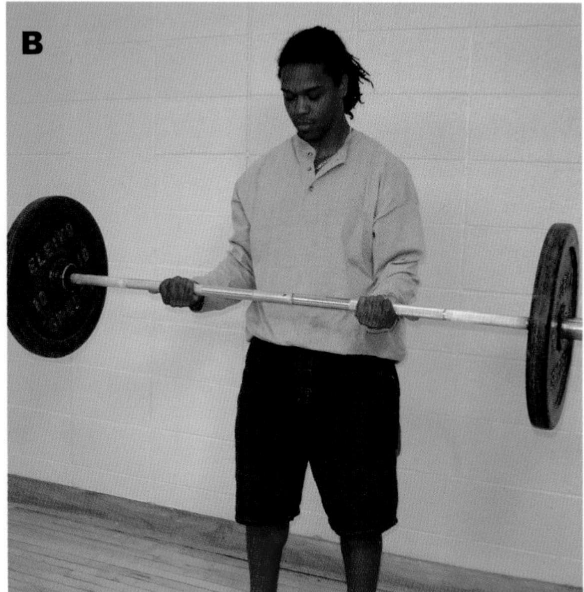

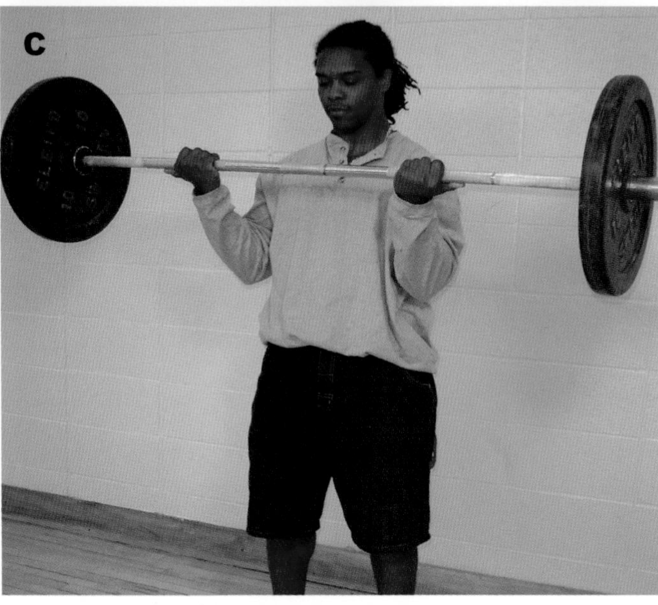

Figure 5.3 Muscle tension during elbow flexion varies according to the joint angle.

first movement is to drop the bar until sufficient cross bridges can form to stop its falling, and the movement ends with the bar falling onto the thighs.

Most often, the latter course of action is taken, and the result is that the individual does not train throughout the full range of motion, often resulting in the appearance that the arms can't be straightened! What you would like to do is optimally stress the muscle throughout the range of motion. To do this, the load must be increased as the lift is made and then decreased as you pass the region where optimal cross bridge formation occurs, a difficult task to say the least when training with free weights.

Isokinetic Contraction

In **isokinetic contraction** (*iso* = same or constant and *kinetic* = motion), the neuromuscular system can work at a constant speed during each phase of movement (despite the constantly changing leverage or torque) against a preset high resistance. This allows the working muscles and muscle groups to release high tension over each section of the movement range. This type of contraction is effective for strengthening the musculature

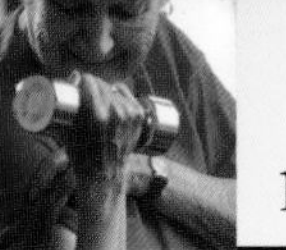

uniformly at all angles of motion.

As in the auxotonic contraction, however, the precise amount of muscle tension release is always dependent upon the corresponding joint angle and the velocity of movement. This is accomplished, with varying degrees of success, by a number of expensive dynamometers, including the Cybex, the Kin-Com, and the Lido, which keep the speed of movement constant electronically, and the HydraGym and Nautilus, which use mechanical means to produce movements that are "isokinetic" in nature (Figure 5.4).

The relatively constant speeds involved in swimming and rowing are similar to those produced in isokinetic exercise forms. For this reason, these sports use isokinetic training to increase performance levels. However, the majority of sports contain few pure isokinetic movements as they continuously require changes in velocity and force application throughout movements.

Isokinetic contractions are classified as dynamic contractions.

Plyocentric Contraction

The last type of muscle contraction, a **plyocentric contraction**, is a hybrid contraction in that the muscle performs an isotonic concentric contraction

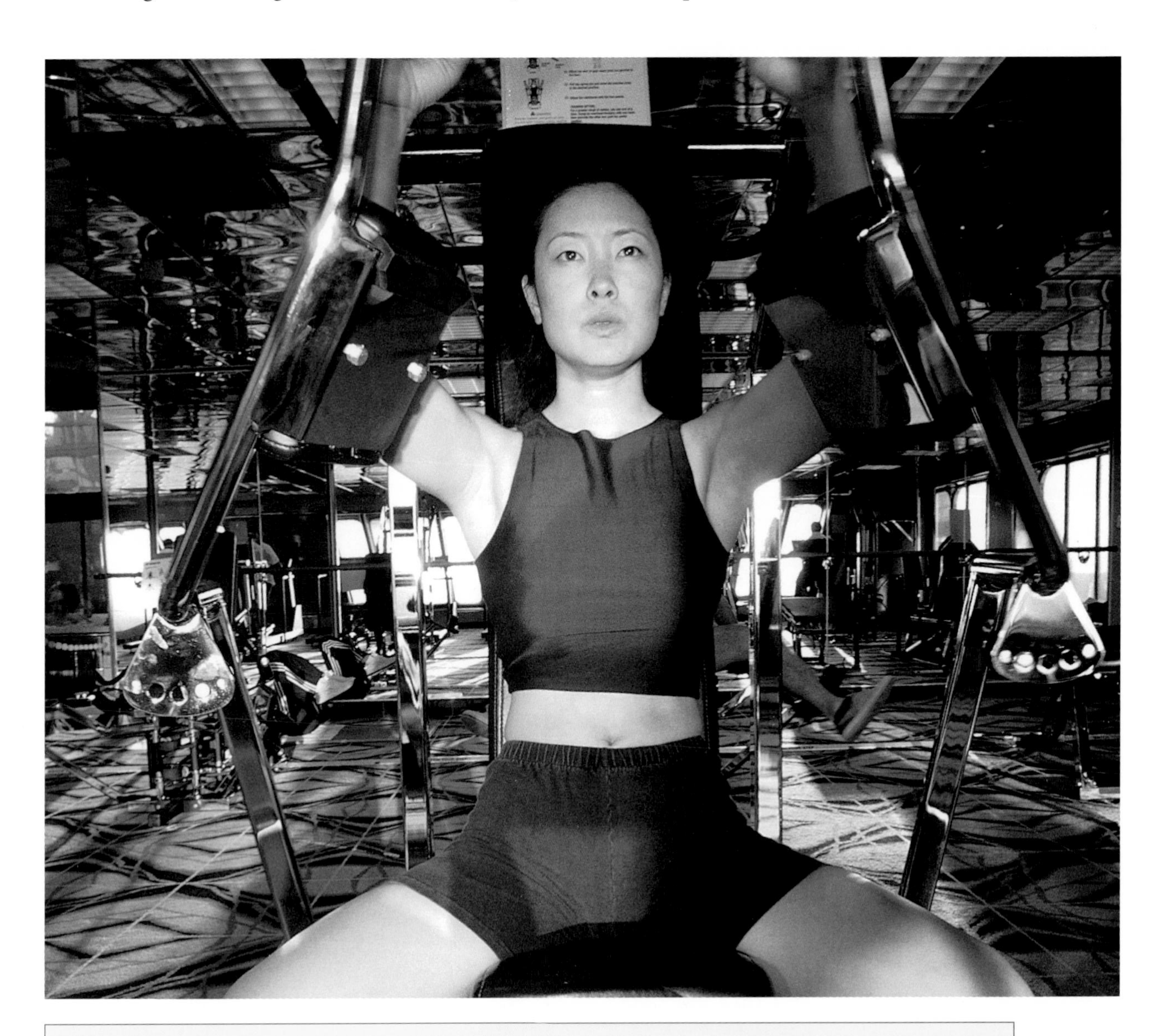

Figure 5.4 Isokinetic contractions are generated by a variety of very expensive dynamometers.

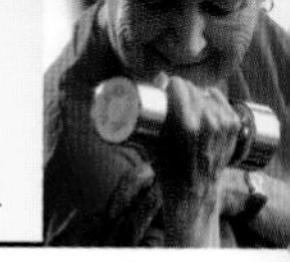

> **Which Is Best?**
>
> Isotonic muscle contractions involving dumbbells and barbells are considered to be the most effective method for developing overall strength.

from a stretched position. The "prestretching" of the muscle is achieved by jumping off an object (box) from a height of 10 to 15 inches, or 25 to 40 cm (depth jumping).

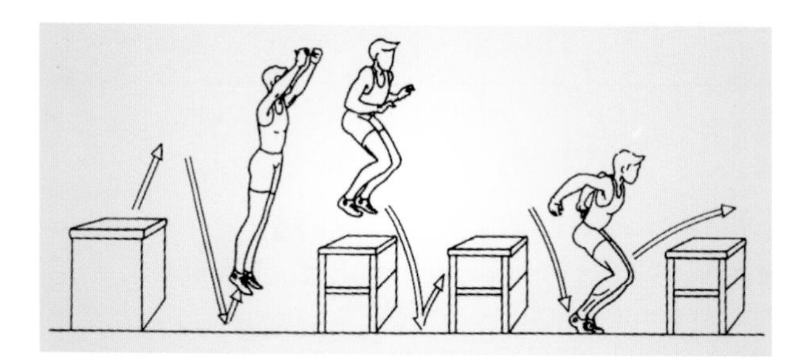

This not only prestretches the muscles but also sets off the **Golgi tendon organ** reflex, which functions to protect the muscle from too much stretch. The reflex causes the muscles to contract. Activities that utilize this type of contraction to train jumping ability include leaping and bounding, such as in plyometric training.

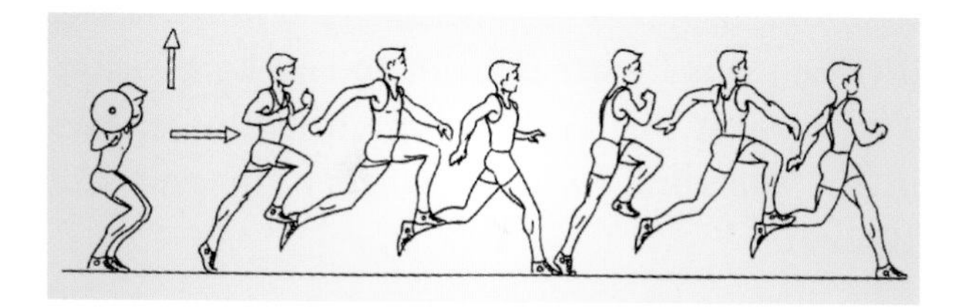

Research has shown that this type of strength and power training leads to a greater increase in jump height than that developed by strength training alone.

Concentric and Eccentric Contractions

A **concentric contraction** is one in which the muscle shortens as it goes through the range of motion; this is usually termed **flexion**. An **eccentric contraction** is one in which the muscle lengthens during the movement, usually termed **extension**. Again, let's use the arm curl with free weights as an example (Figure 5.3). The movement of the bar from the thighs to the shoulder region (i.e., flexion of the biceps brachii) is an auxotonic concentric contraction. The movement from the shoulder area back to the thighs (i.e., extension of biceps brachii) is an isotonic eccentric contraction.

Factors Influencing Muscle Contraction

There are numerous factors that can affect the force and power output of a muscle, including the individual's **state of health** and **training status**. Other factors that affect force and power output include: (1) joint angle; (2) muscle cross-sectional area; (3) speed of movement; (4) muscle fiber type; (5) age; and (6) sex.

Joint Angle

Let us again consider the example of elbow flexion during a barbell lift (Figure 5.3). Contraction of the elbow flexors is initially isometric (static). The muscle does not visibly shorten until after the internal forces generated by muscle flexing exceed the external forces of the barbell. As the arms flex at the elbow joints, the barbell is moved toward the shoulders. The barbell accelerates in proportion to the degree that the internal forces exceed the load of the barbell. A short phase of static work, often lasting only a few hundredths of a second, occurs between the dynamic work of concentric contraction and the lowering of the barbell.

On lowering the barbell into its initial position, external forces exceed internal ones. The same muscles that previously were involved in lifting the barbell are now being stretched, and with the arms extended at the elbow joint, the barbell is lowered. Elbow flexors, which on lifting the load performed dynamic concentric contractions, are now involved in lowering the load by performing dynamic eccentric contractions. The greater the

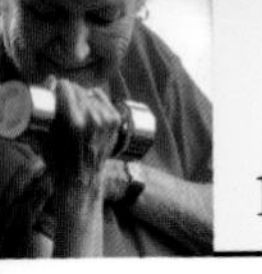

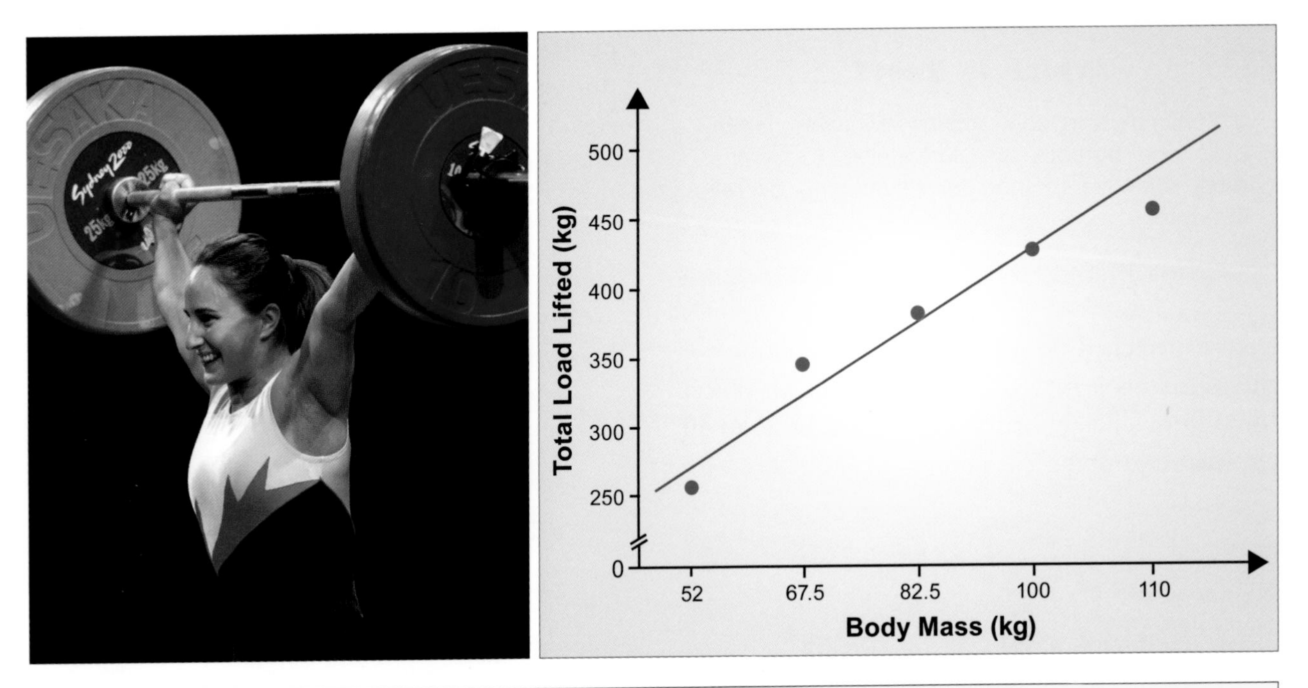

Figure 5.5 Relationship between body weight and maximal load lifted for the combined clean and jerk and snatch events (data from the Seoul Olympics weightlifting competition).

external force, the higher the speed at which the load is lowered. "Muscle teamwork" (agonist versus antagonist) was discussed in Chapter 4.

An athlete doing knee bends performs an eccentric contraction during the flexing phase and a concentric contraction during the ensuing extension phase.

Athletic activities involving only one muscle or muscle group are rare. During each phase of movement, some muscles contract in a dynamic concentric mode, others in a dynamic eccentric mode, and some contract statically. For example, an athlete doing knee bends activates over 75 percent of the body's skeletal musculature to generate the total movement.

Muscle Cross-sectional Area

Human beings have always recognized the close connection between body mass and strength. The relationship between body mass and strength is indeed valid. The greater one's stature, the greater one's strength – provided body mass is composed mainly of muscle and not fat. In other words, strength is determined by the volume of active body matter (i.e., the entire body mass minus body fat). This mass is also referred to as the fat-free or lean body mass (see discussion on this topic in Chapter 15). This fact has been emphasized by the performances of weightlifters across various weight categories (Figure 5.5). The world record in the 62-kg division is greater than that in the 52-kg division; and in the 85-kg division, it is higher than in the 62-kg division. The heaviest weights of all are lifted by athletes in the superheavyweight category (in excess of 105 kg).

Maximal or Absolute Strength

From the above discussion we can conclude that the greater the active body mass, the greater the maximal or **absolute strength**. This general rule is based on the notion that strength depends to a high degree on the size of the muscle cross-section (Figure 5.6). However, this statement requires qualification. Because intra- and intermuscle coordination, anatomical structure, and the elasticity of muscle also play an important part in the performance capacity of the muscle, it is

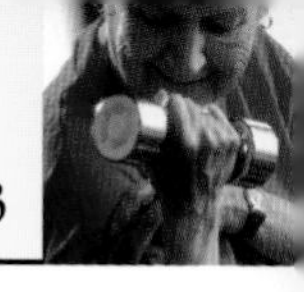

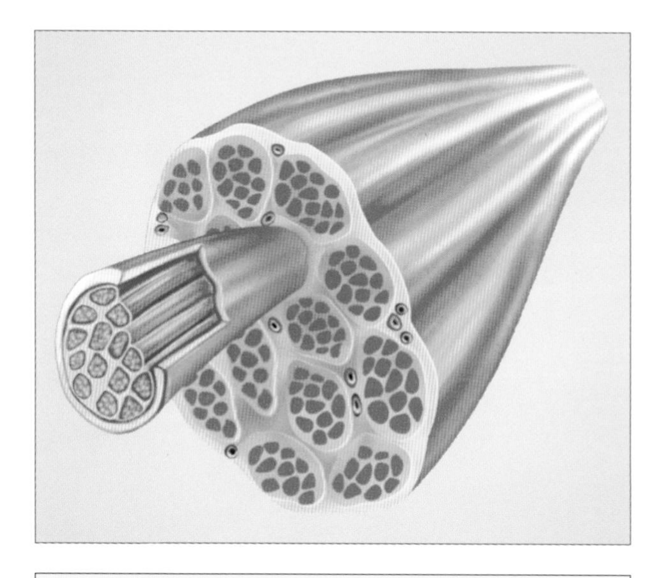

Figure 5.6 The larger the muscle cross-sectional area, the more force it can generate.

possible for individuals of a small and lighter physique to possess a relatively high strength potential. For discussion on inter- and intramuscle coordination, refer to Chapter 4.

Strength is also of critical importance to athletes who are not classified by weight but whose prime aim, nevertheless, is to overcome the resistance of a partner or equipment. Thus, wrestlers, judokas, and weightlifters competing in the highest weight category, as well as shot-putters, javelin throwers, and hammer throwers, may all want to increase their strength by increasing muscle mass (and therefore total body mass). Weightlifters may also strive to increase their overall strength through an extreme thickening of the muscle fibers.

Relative Strength

The performance of athletes classified by weight (such as weightlifters) and athletes who must overcome their own body mass (such as jumpers, runners, and gymnasts) depends less on maximal strength than on the proportion of maximal strength to body mass. A gymnast, for instance, will be unable to perform an iron cross unless his neuromuscular system can generate approximately 10 Newtons of force per kilogram of body mass.

From Greek Mythology

The alertness and great strength of Hercules, the hero of Greek mythology, allowed him to perform extraordinary deeds. Even today, the name Hercules itself suggests a human being of giant stature and great physical strength.

The relationship between maximal strength and body mass is also referred to as **relative strength**.

$$\text{Relative Strength} = \frac{\text{Maximal Strength}}{\text{Body Mass}}$$

Consider the following example. Two athletes performing bench presses can lift a maximal barbell load with full arm extension. Suppose both are able to lift 200 lb (i.e., each develops equal maximal strength for the movement), but athlete A weighs 165 lb, athlete B 200 lb. Using the formula above, athlete B's relative strength is 1.0 (200 / 200 = 1.0), whereas athlete A's is 1.2 (200 / 165 = 1.2). It follows that the lighter athlete's (A) relative strength is higher than the heavier athlete's (B) (Figure 5.7).

Recreational athletes are usually interested in increasing their active strength by stabilizing their maximal strength and reducing body mass. Overweight athletes who want to lose superfluous fat also follow this method. It is of little use to competitive athletes, however, because a reduction of body mass is often linked with loss of muscle mass and therefore with a decrease in maximal and relative strength.

Another way to increase relative strength is to increase strength and stabilize body mass. Because maximal strength is dependent not only upon muscle diameter but also upon intramuscle coordination, this variation is often quite promising, provided that the correct and relevant training methods are chosen.

For young recreational athletes, the more favorable training programs are those that hold out the prospect of strength development in

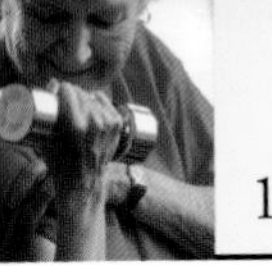

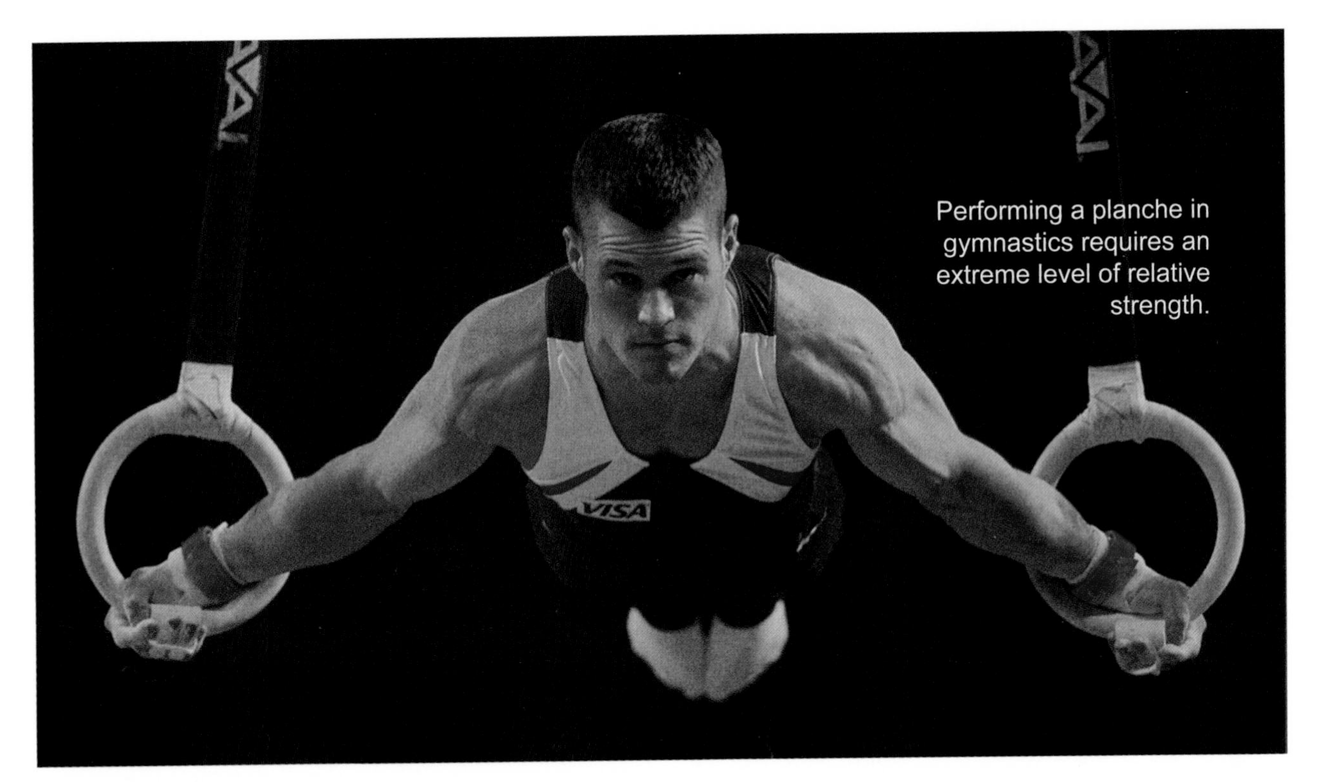

conjunction with a sensible and adequate increase in active body mass.

Speed of Movement

For movements occurring at fast velocities, the cross bridges cannot couple and uncouple fast enough to establish and maintain a large number of cross bridges. This results in a decreased ability to develop force at fast velocities. This means that as the speed of movement is increased, the force that the muscle can develop is decreased.

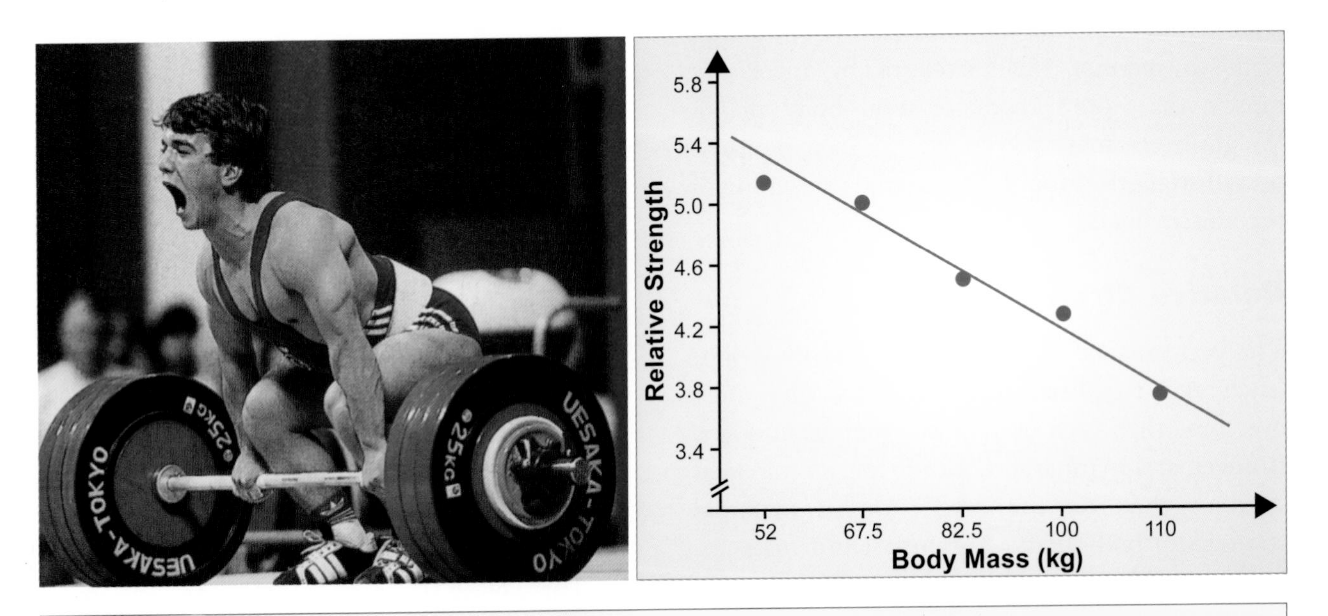

Figure 5.7 Relationship between relative strength and body weight based on the combined clean and jerk and snatch events (data from the Seoul Olympics weightlifting competition).

Speed of movement is closely linked to the main components of strength: maximal strength, power, and muscle endurance. The relationships between these components also interact to affect speed of movement.

Maximal Strength

Maximal strength is the ability of the athlete to perform maximal voluntary muscular contractions in order to overcome powerful external resistances. It is the greatest force an athlete can exert for a given contraction of muscles. In other words, it is the highest load the athlete can lift in one attempt, or **one repetition maximum (1RM)**. A higher absolute strength is necessary for such activities as weightlifting and field events in track and field (shot put, hammer, discus, and javelin throws). Its importance for an athletic performance diminishes as the resistance that must be overcome in competition is reduced and as the period of competition increases.

Power

Power, often referred to as **speed–strength**, is the ability of an athlete to overcome external resistance by developing a high rate of muscular contraction. The ability to develop power is decisive in the speed of execution of individual movements performed in activities such as the high jump and long jump in track and field. It is also important for the achievement of high push-offs, for throw or takeoff velocity in ball games, for mastering quick movement in individual activities, and for starting and acceleration of sprinters and skaters, as well as for fast starts and accelerations in rowing and similar events.

Muscular Endurance

Muscular endurance, or **strength endurance**, is the ability of an athlete to resist fatigue in strength performance of longer duration. It determines performances in those endurance activities where exceptional resistance must be overcome over relatively longer periods of time, such as in rowing, swimming, and cross-country skiing.

Muscular endurance is also important in predominantly acyclic (nonrepetitive) activities where high demands are placed on strength and endurance, such as gymnastics, wrestling, boxing, downhill skiing, and most games.

The Relationship Between Maximal Strength and Power

It is a well-known fact that top-class heavyweight weightlifters achieve outstanding results in tests measuring power, such as standing high jump and long jump, in 40-yard sprints, and in other events that require speed and strength performance. This contradicts the deep-rooted notion that strength training and increases in maximal strength lead to slowed muscle performance (Figure 5.8).

Much research has been conducted to investigate this area in greater depth. The following is a summary of the results:

- The more internal force an athlete can generate to overcome external resistance, the more movement acceleration increases. If an athlete must mobilize as much as 90 percent of maximal strength to merely lift a barbell off the ground (i.e., to resist gravity), little strength reserve is left to accelerate the barbell lift. This means the movement must be performed at a relatively slow speed. If, however, the athlete needs to apply only 30 percent of maximal strength to lift the barbell off the ground, a high volume of strength is reserved for acceleration of the barbell. Indeed, the movement can then be performed explosively.
- The higher the external resistance to be overcome, the more important the maximal strength for power performance.

In general, high power output sports, such as 100-meter and 200-meter track events, high jump and triple jump, speedskating, and rowing, require the application of more than 25 to 30 percent of one's maximal strength, which in turn depends upon the use of ST and FT fibers (see discussion on muscle fibers in Chapter 4). FT fibers respond very effectively to high-resistance training, which

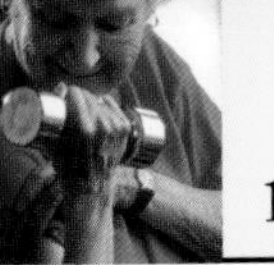

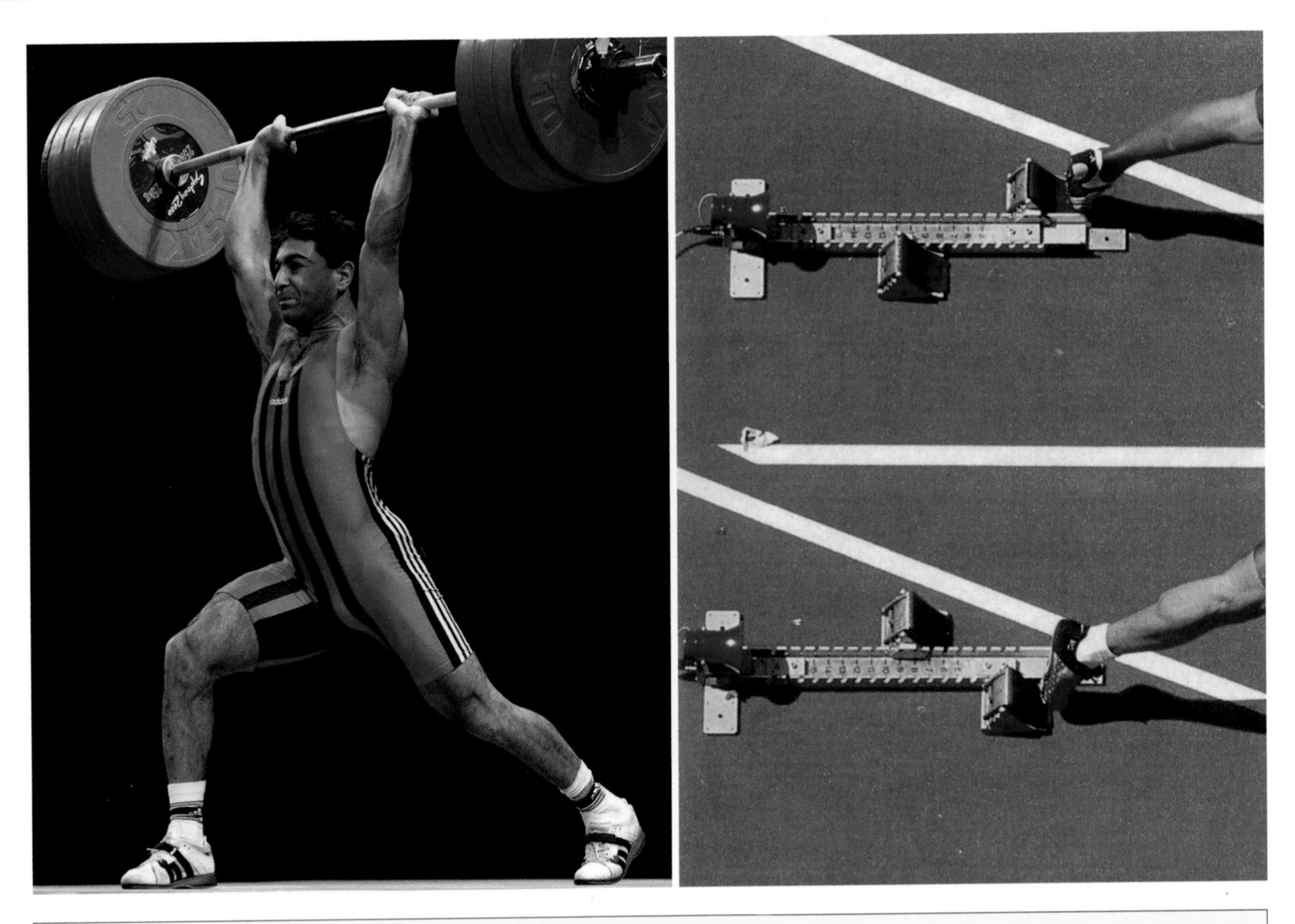

Figure 5.8 Heavy weightlifters and field event specialists in track and field are among the quickest athletes off the starting block. They also hold the world record in the standing long jump.

generates an increase in diameter of the contractile elements (myofibrils) of the fibers. Furthermore, this type of training results in a progressive increase in the number of fast motor units that can be mobilized. This results in improved intramuscle coordination (Figure 5.9).

Enlarged diameter of the FT fibers and improved intramuscle coordination are beneficial to power performances, providing that the capacity of the FT fibers for fast contraction does not deteriorate following high-resistance training. This implies that, despite relatively slow movements during maximal resistance training, the myosin and actin filaments must be able to retain their capacity for swiftly establishing cross bridge formation and, after completion of the contraction, removing the bridging formation. Coaching experience has shown that the high contraction speed of FT fibers can be maintained and even considerably increased if maximal strength training is carried out explosively at all times. It follows that a high level of maximal strength is an invariable prerequisite for fast movements in medium- to high-resistance training. Maximal strength training can thus be beneficial to the development of power.

The Relationship Between Maximal Strength and Muscular Endurance

The relationship between maximal strength and muscular endurance can be illustrated best with the following example. Athlete A is able to lift a 220-lb (100-kg) barbell, but partner B masters only 200 lb (91 kg). If both athletes are challenged to clean and press a barbell of 185 lb (84 kg) as often as possible, athlete A will perform 7 to 8 repetitions and B only 2 to 3 repetitions. Using a 175-lb (79-kg) barbell, athlete A can do 10 to 12 repetitions and athlete B

Table 5.1 Maximum number of repetitions as a function of resistance.

Resistance Level	100%	95%	90%	85%	80%	75%
Repetition Maximum	1	2-3	5-6	7-8	approx. 10-12	approx. 12-16

only 5 to 6. The comparison shows that the number of repetitions against high resistance is dependent on the maximal strength of the athlete. Table 5.1 shows the maximal number of repetitions possible for load levels of different resistance.

The maximal feasible number of repetitions of a particular load is referred to as the **repetition maximum (RM)**. If the RM of an exercise is 2 to 3, it can be deduced that an athlete can resist a force corresponding to approximately 95 percent of maximal strength capacity. If the athlete is able to perform maximally 7 to 8 repetitions with a particular weight, then this weight approximates 85 percent of maximal strength capacity.

Therefore, it is not always necessary that you work against maximal resistance (which may be very dangerous in most cases) in order to calculate your maximal strength capacity for a given exercise. Determining an athlete's maximal number of repetitions against submaximal resistance will produce an accurate assessment of maximal strength. However, as the number of repetitions increases (or as the level of resistance decreases), the RM becomes a less accurate criterion of maximal strength.

Issues Related to the Relationship Between Strength and Endurance It is a commonly held belief that the development of strength hinders and even impairs the development of endurance, and vice versa. The validity of this notion depends upon the type of training and event in question. Vigorous training for running long distances leads to an increase in cardiorespiratory fitness (increased aerobic power). However, the simultaneous decrease in the diameter of the fast twitch muscle fibers causes a corresponding decrease in muscle volume. These processes, then, result in increased endurance and decreased muscle strength.

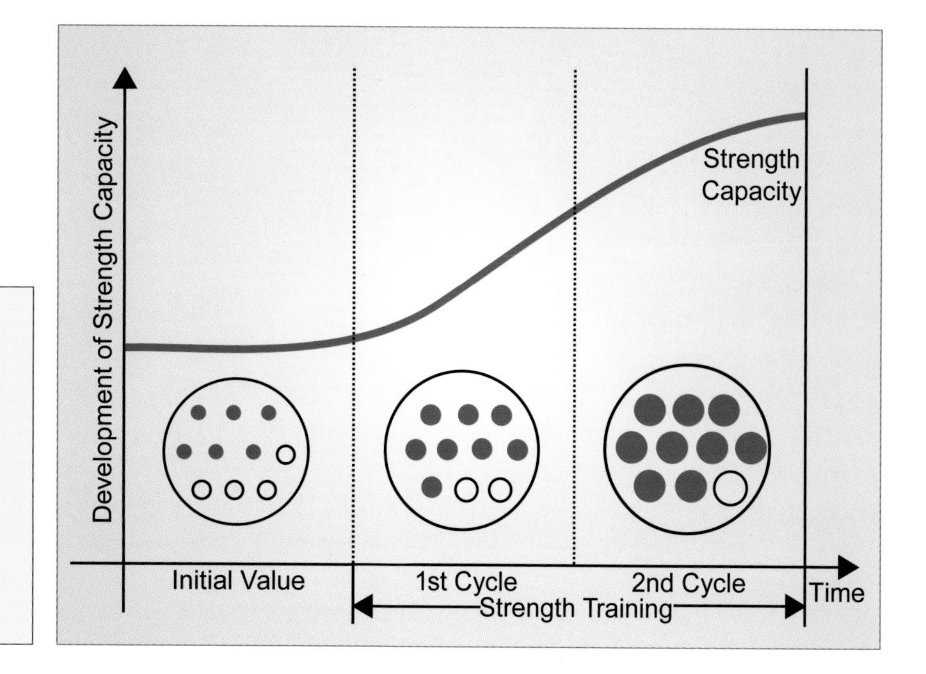

Figure 5.9 Development of maximal strength through muscle hypertrophy and increased intramuscular coordination using a training method that combines repetition training at submaximal loads and short-term maximal resistance training.

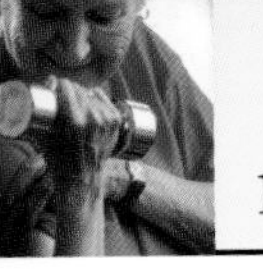

Conversely, repetitive maximal strength training decreases endurance but increases strength. Thus, the training of a weightlifter or shot-putter is geared toward the development of maximal strength and power; endurance is hardly improved. However, unless a specific sports event requires the possession of a maximal level of endurance or strength, training should achieve a balance between strength and endurance (Figure 5.10).

Competitive athletes should be capable of coping with high-intensity, short-term anaerobic loads and at the same time be able to master long-term, low-intensity aerobic loads. The proof that such training is possible has been demonstrated in sports requiring both strength and endurance, such as Nordic events that combine cross-country skiing and ski jumping. A Nordic skier, however, will not normally achieve the distances of a skier specializing in jumping or approximate the times of a cross-country skier (Figure 5.11).

Thus, relatively high levels of both strength and endurance can be achieved either by training for strength and endurance in separate training sessions or by developing both in combination. Both methods can be used effectively. Using one method, an athlete doing four training sessions a week might devote two sessions to track exercises and two sessions to strength exercises. Using the other method, an athlete may develop a program that trains both strength and endurance within each session.

Muscle Fiber Type

Fiber type is another factor that will greatly affect muscle force output. In general, the greater the fast twitch fiber content of a muscle, the greater will be the force output, the overall speed of contraction, and the fatigability, when the muscle has been maximally activated. On the other hand, a muscle dominated by a slow twitch fiber population will produce less force and will contract slower, but it will have far superior endurance characteristics. Submaximal responses are much more difficult to predict, as we need to keep in mind the order of fiber recruitment (discussed in Chapter 4) when examining submaximal activities.

Age

Aging has a significant influence on muscle force output. Research indicates that there is a selective loss of fast twitch fibers, mainly fast twitch

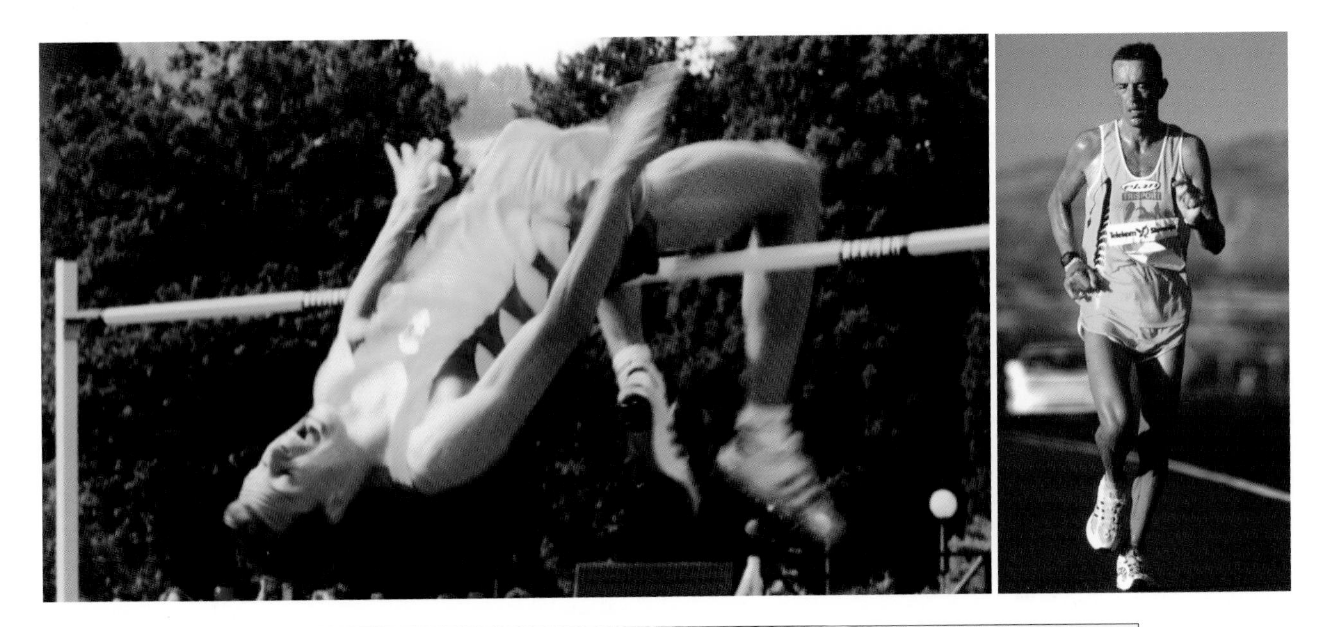

Figure 5.10 Training for explosive power is significantly different from training for endurance.

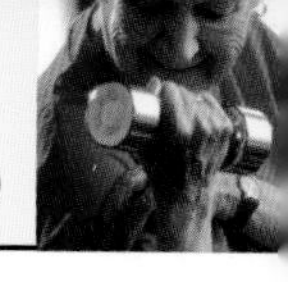

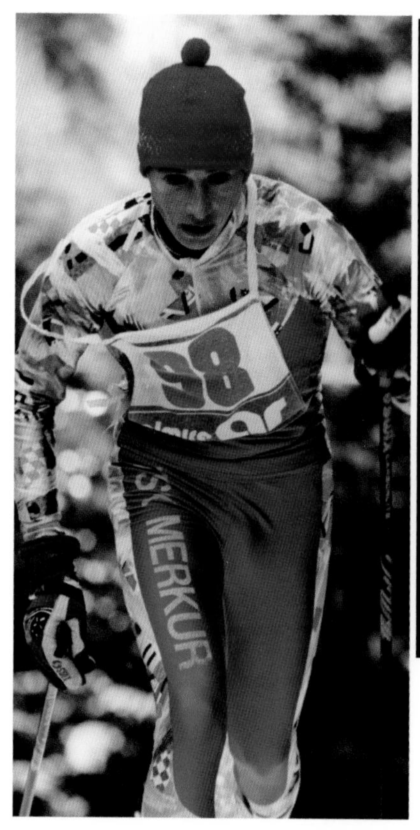

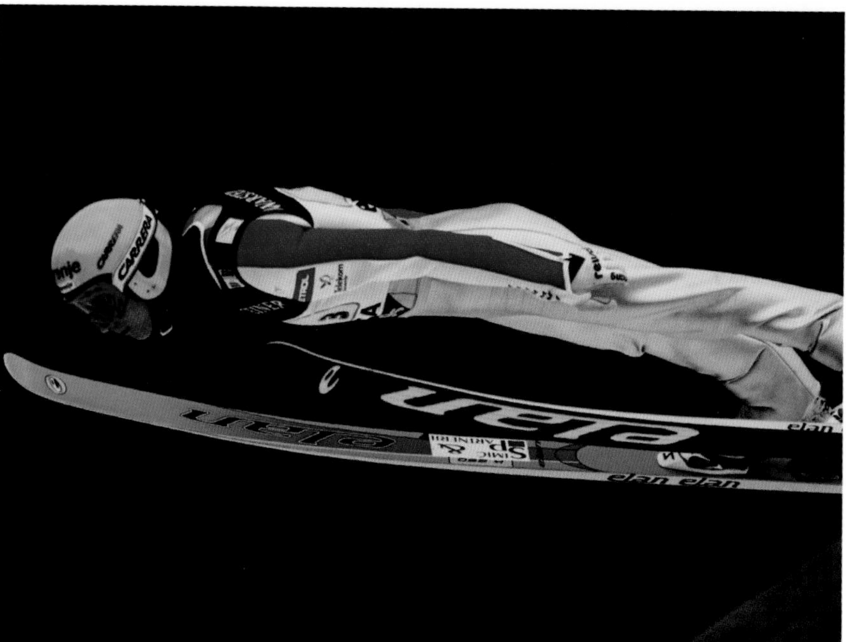

Figure 5.11 A Nordic event skier competing in ski jumping and cross-country skiing events must successfully combine training for maximal strength and muscular endurance.

glycolytic, with aging. Obviously, this loss will significantly affect the force-generating potential of a muscle. What remains unknown at this time is why this loss takes place. It is possible that it is preprogrammed to occur with aging (i.e., **apoptosis**). Alternatively, the loss may represent a "use it or lose it" phenomenon. As people age they become less active, which results in muscle atrophy (Figure 5.12).

Muscle loss has become a very real medical condition known as **sarcopenia** (Greek for "vanishing flesh"). Research shows that by age 70, sedentary individuals have lost 30 percent or more of the muscle they had at 30, the age at which muscle mass peaks. Muscle loss inevitably means diminished strength and balance. These developments may lead to falls and fractures, a major cause of age-related disabilities.

Sex

From a physiological standpoint, men and women are more similar than they are dissimilar. Aside from the obvious distinctions between men and women, the average woman is approximately 70 percent as strong as a man of the same size. However, differences between the sexes may not be as great as is commonly thought. In fact, in some cases, the differences may not be at all what is typically assumed.

Strength-to-Weight Ratio

One of the major factors accounting for the physical performance differences between men and women is the ratio of strength to weight – where women are clearly at a disadvantage. Women do not have the physiological or structural capacity to develop the same strength and muscular bulk that men do, due to the ratio of muscle to adipose tissue. In general, women have less muscle tissue and considerably more adipose tissue. However, recent research has shown that a single fiber of the same diameter from a man and a woman produces similar amounts of force when activated by electrical stimulation. It follows that when adipose tissue is factored out of the equation and strength

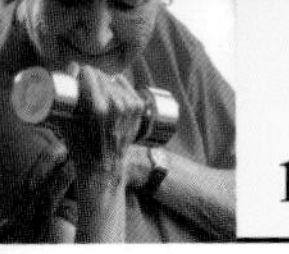

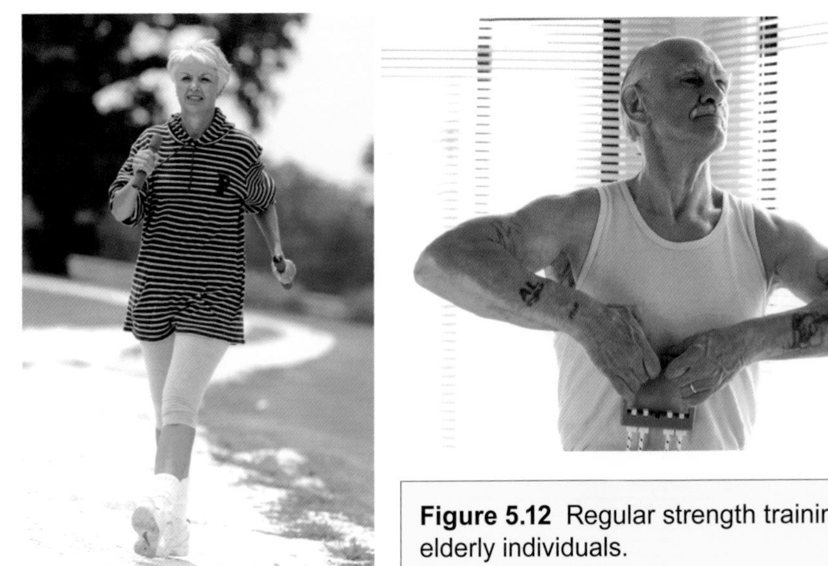

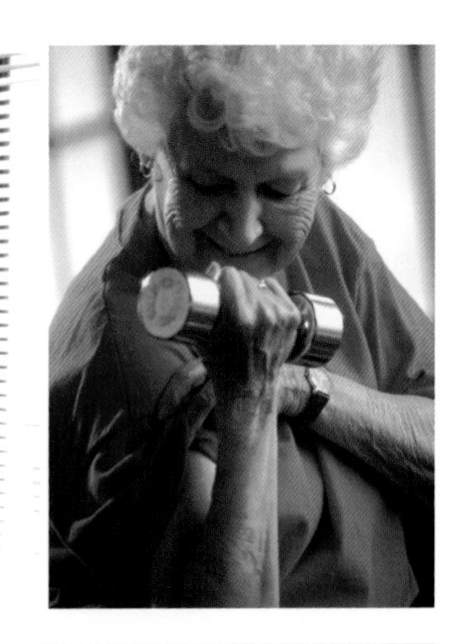

Figure 5.12 Regular strength training can slow down muscle atrophy in elderly individuals.

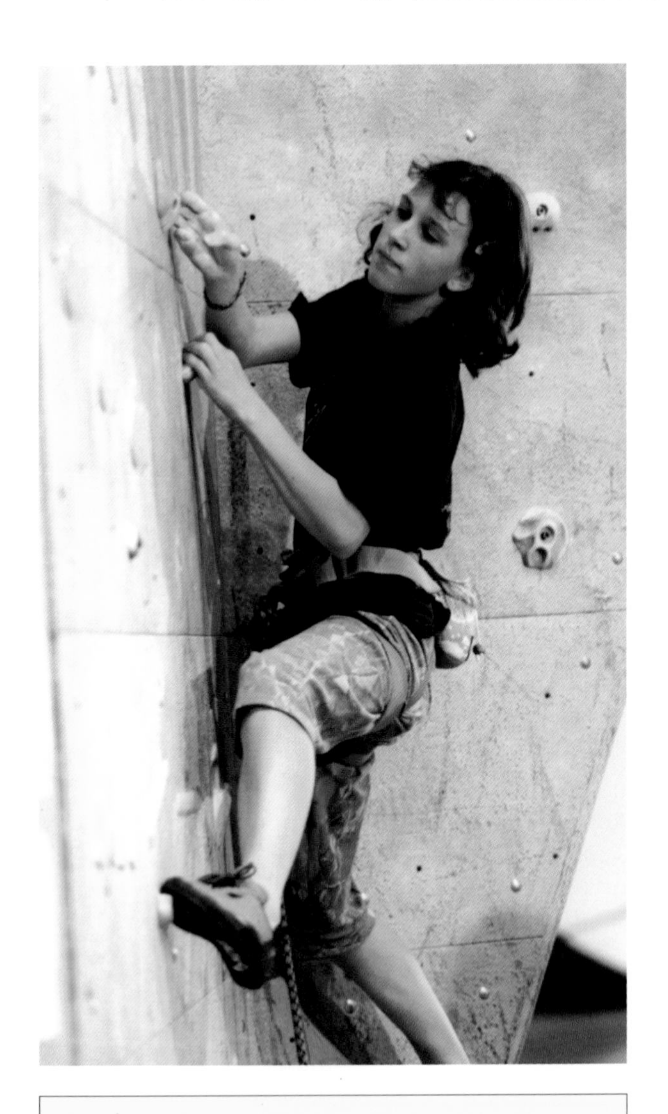

Figure 5.13 Females are able to perform challenging tasks requiring maximal strength.

is looked at in terms of lean body mass, women are just as strong as men in total body strength (Figure 5.13).

Muscle Cross-sectional Area

The cross-sectional area of a muscle fiber is smaller in women largely because they have proportionally more type I (slow twitch) fibers, while men have proportionally more type II (fast twitch) fibers. Type II fibers are considered to be more conducive to increasing muscle size and strength, whereas type I fibers are responsible more for muscular endurance.

Variation in Testosterone Level

A difference in testosterone levels is another significant reason accounting for the difference between men and women in the development of muscle size and strength. Men produce 20 to 30 times more testosterone – the anabolic hormone responsible for muscle growth – than do women.

Summary

When discussing exercise prescription for the development of general fitness among recreational individuals or the design of training programs for athletes, it is important to distinguish between the various forms of muscle contractions. In static contractions, tension develops in the muscle, but it is insufficient to move the intended load. Dynamic contractions, on the other hand, involve movement.

Muscle contractions can be characterized further as either concentric or eccentric. A concentric contraction is one in which the muscle shortens as it goes through its range of motion (flexion); an eccentric contraction is one in which the muscle lengthens during the movement (extension). When there is no visible change in muscle length, even though the muscle has undergone muscle contraction, an isometric contraction is said to have occurred. It is important to know the functional value of training equipment that is designed to enhance specific muscle contractions.

Maximal strength is the highest load an athlete can lift in one repetition. This value is known as the athlete's one repetition maximum (1RM). Power refers to the ability of an athlete to overcome external resistance by developing a high rate of muscular contraction. Finally, muscular endurance is the ability of an athlete to resist fatigue in strength performance of longer duration. Many factors affect the force and power output of muscle contraction. Some of these factors, including joint angle, muscle cross-sectional area, speed of movement, muscle fiber type, age, and sex, were discussed in detail in this chapter.

Key Terms

absolute strength
apoptosis
concentric contraction
dynamic contraction
eccentric contraction
isokinetic contraction
isometric contraction
isotonic contraction
maximal strength
muscular endurance
one repetition maximum (1RM)
plyocentric contraction
power
relative strength
repetition maximum (RM)
sarcopenia
speed–strength
static contraction
strength endurance
submaximal static contraction

Discussion Questions

1. Identify the major types of muscle contraction and give two examples of each.
2. Discuss the major differences between static and dynamic muscle contractions.
3. Muscle cross-section influences the amount of force a muscle can generate. Explain.
4. List the factors that influence muscle contraction. Provide an example of each.
5. Differentiate between absolute and relative strength and give examples of each.
6. Discuss the differences between strength, power, and endurance sporting activities.
7. Briefly discuss the relationship between maximal strength and power. Present two examples.
8. Briefly discuss the relationship between maximal strength and muscular endurance. Present two examples.
9. What happens to muscular strength as one ages? Why?

In This Chapter:

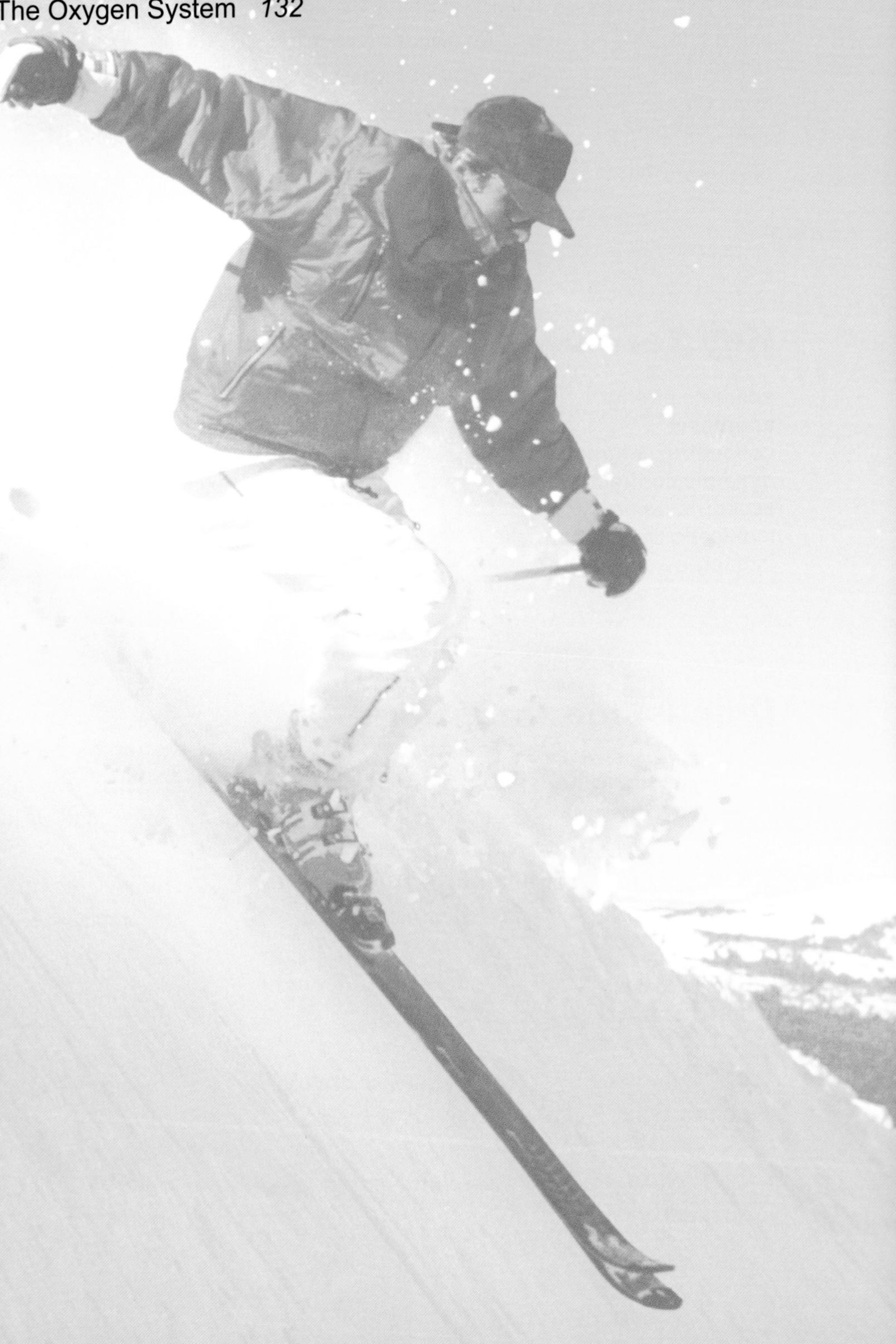

CHAPTER 6

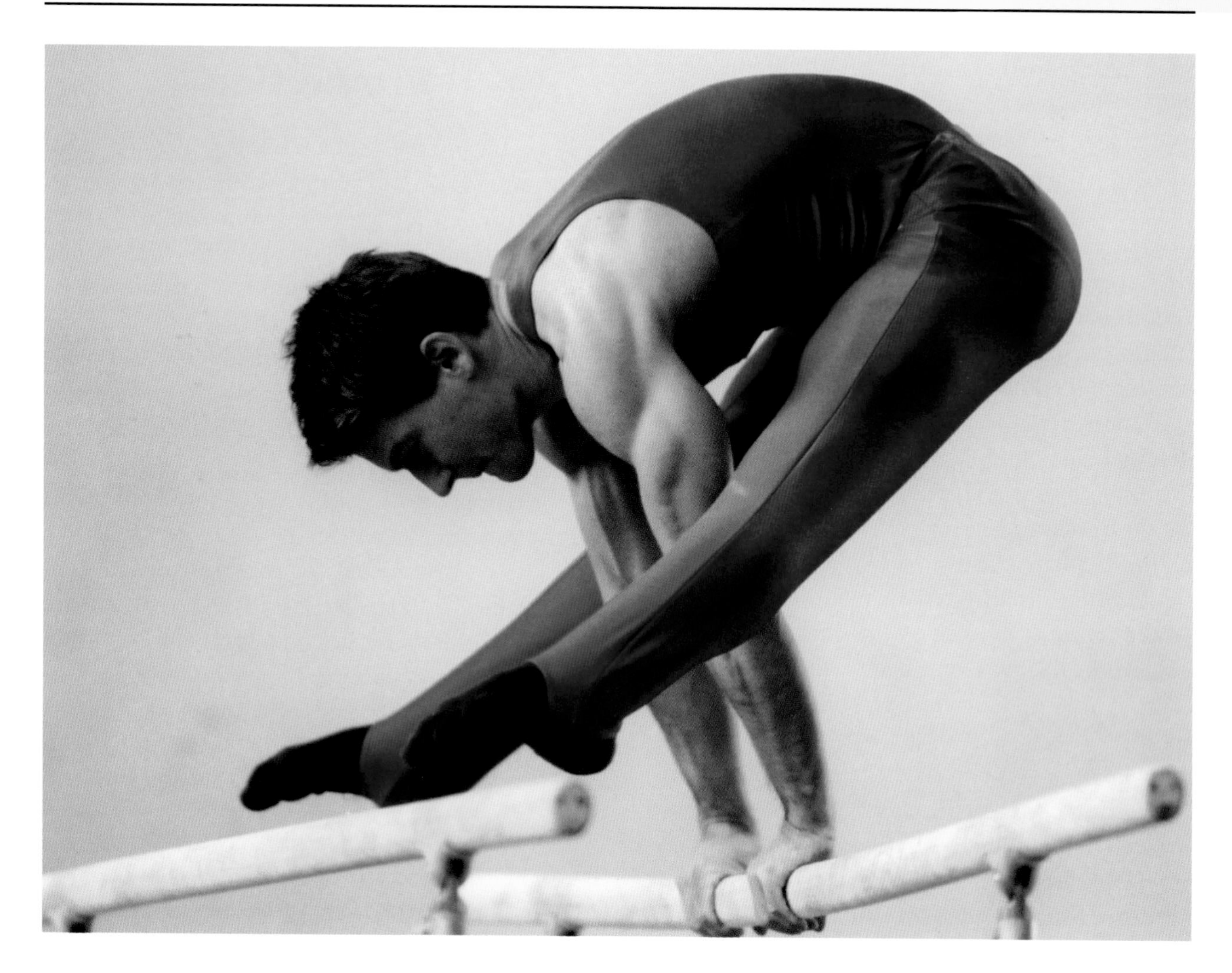

Energy for Muscular Activity

After completing this chapter you should be able to:

- use and understand the basic terminology of human metabolism related to exercise;
- describe the basic chemical processes the body uses to produce energy in the muscles;
- demonstrate an understanding of the body's three energy systems and their contribution to muscular contraction and activity;
- discuss the effects of training and exercise on the energy systems.

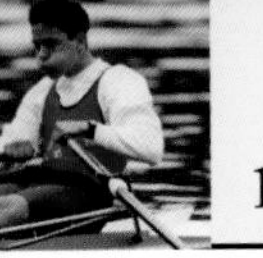

Humans are capable of performing amazing physical feats. Sprinters run down the track with astonishing speed and power; power lifters hoist hundreds of pounds of weight, making it look effortless; swimmers traverse an entire lake or channel against the elements; hurdlers gracefully clear all obstacles in their way; and basketball players seem to defy the laws of gravity in their flight to the basket. While various combinations of physical ability, skill, and training are required to accomplish these feats, the common denominators in each case are the muscle activation patterns described previously and the development of energy at rates, and in sufficient quantity, to meet the needs of the activity.

The energy needs for endurance events performed at relatively low intensity levels significantly differ from those requiring immediate power output performed at highest intensity levels. For effective planning of training programs, coaches need to know the energy demands of their sport.

The production of a movement during contraction occurs as the muscle pulls on the bones through the tendinous attachments to the bones. Even a single contraction requires a significant input of energy. Just as a car requires the appropriate fuel to run efficiently, so too do our muscles require energy for maximal performance. However, depending on the activity in which you are engaged, the body will make use of different energy systems that have been adapted for supplying energy at the required rate and in the necessary amount for that particular activity (i.e., the body will produce energy at a higher rate – but for a shorter duration – during an activity demanding power than one requiring endurance, where energy is required in greater quantities but at a lower rate).

What are the body's primary sources of energy? What other fuels do we use? Why do our muscles produce energy differently under varying circumstances? These are some of the many questions that will be answered in this chapter. We will also explore some methods of testing and assessing energy production as well as the way the body adapts to exercise.

The Chemistry of Energy Production

All energy in the human body is derived from the breakdown of three complex nutrients: carbohydrates, fats, and proteins. The end result of the breakdown of these substances is the production of various amounts of the molecule **adenosine triphosphate (ATP)**, the energy currency of the body. ATP provides the energy for fueling all biochemical processes of the body such as muscular work or digesting food. The capacity to perform muscular work depends on sufficient energy supply at the required rate for the duration of the activity.

Energy is liberated for muscular work when the chemical bond between ATP and its phosphate subgroup is broken through **hydrolysis** according to the following biochemical reaction:

$$\text{ATP} \longrightarrow \text{ADP} + P_i + \text{Energy}$$

The breakdown of ATP into **adenosine diphosphate (ADP)** and a **free phosphate group (Pi)** is the fuel for contractile activity (i.e., the formation of cross bridges in working muscles) (see Chapter 4, Muscle Structure and Function). The amount of energy released is about 38 to 42 kilojoules (kJ) or 9 to 10 kilocalories (kcal) per mole of ATP (Note: a **kilocalorie** is the amount of heat energy needed to raise 1,000 grams of water by 1 degree Celsius).

When the body performs physical work, it needs a continuous supply of ATP. The muscle has a small supply of ATP stored within it, satisfying initial requirements of the body, but the initial stores of ATP in the muscles are used up very quickly. Therefore, if activity is to continue, ATP must be regenerated. ATP is a renewable resource that can be regenerated by the recombination of ADP with a free phosphate. The metabolic process that results in the recombination of ADP and P_i to form ATP is termed **ATP resynthesis**.

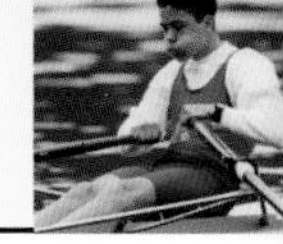

This reaction can occur at a very fast pace in the body. The resynthesis of ATP is described by the following reaction:

$$ADP + P_i + \text{Energy} \longrightarrow ATP$$

The regeneration of ATP, however, requires the addition of energy, which is supplied through the breakdown of complex food molecules, such as carbohydrates and fats.

The Three Energy Systems

The production of ATP involves three energy systems, each of which produces ATP at a distinct

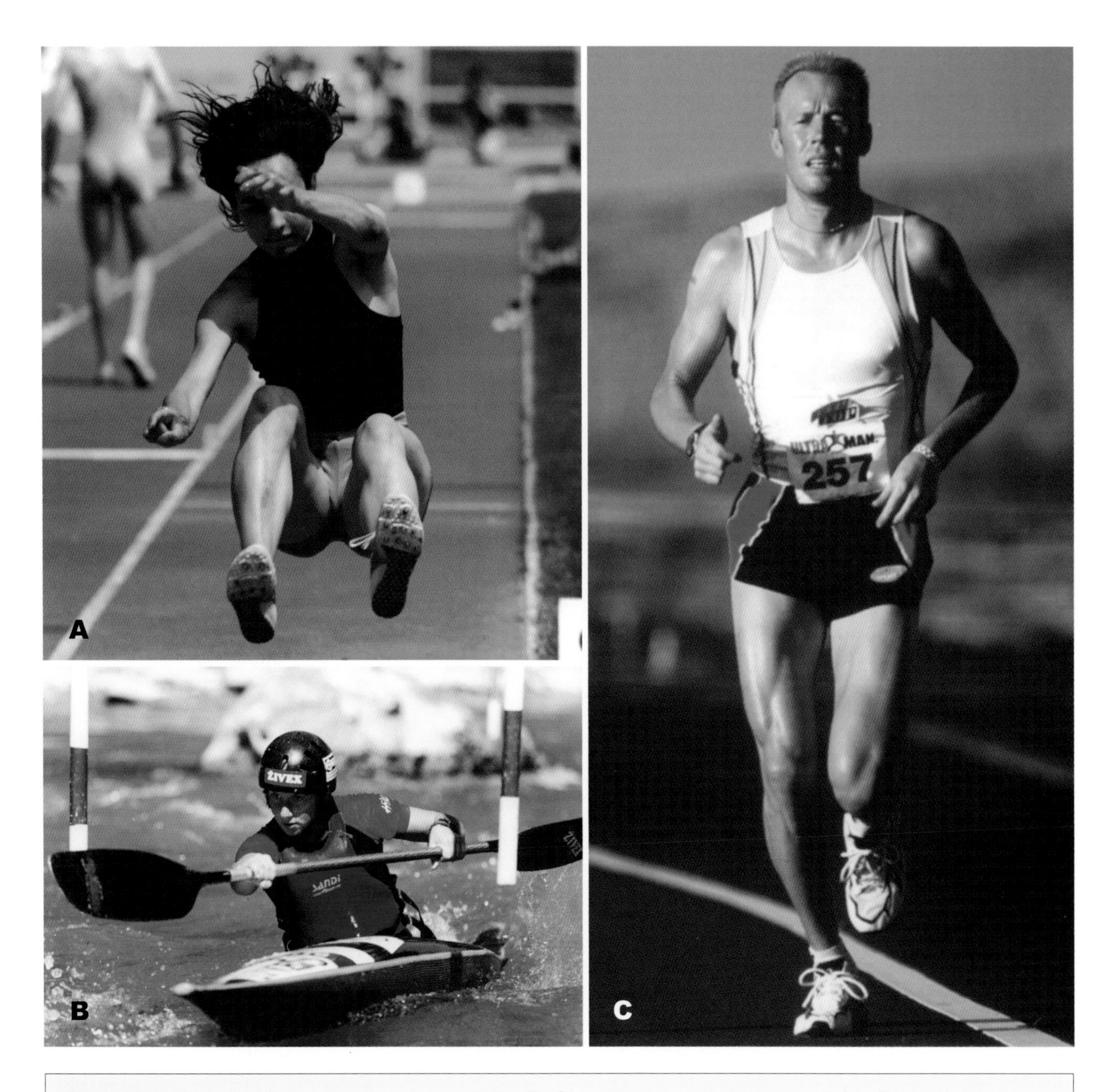

Figure 6.1 **A.** Immediate energy system activity. **B.** Short-term energy system activity. **C.** Long-term energy system activity.

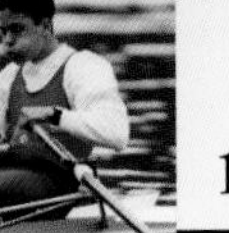

Table 6.1 The roles of the three energy systems in competitive sport.

Energy Pathways	Anaerobic Pathways			Aerobic Pathway	
Primary Energy Source	ATP produced without the presence of O_2			ATP produced with the presence of O_2	
Energy System	Immediate Alactic	Short-term Lactic		Long-term Oxygen	
Fuel	ATP, CP	Glycogen, glucose		Glycogen, glucose, fat, protein	
Duration	0 s 10 s	40 s	70 s 2 min	6 min 25 min	1 hr 2 hr 3 hr
Sport Event	Sprinting 100-m dash Throwing Jumping Weightlifting Ski jumping Diving Vaulting in gymnastics	Track 200-400 m 500-m speed-skating Most gym events Cycling, track 50-m swimming	100-m swimming 800-m track Floor exercise gymnastics Alpine skiing Cycling, track: 1,000 m and pursuit	Middle-distance track, swimming, speedskating 1,000-m canoeing Boxing Wrestling Rowing Figure skating Synchronized swimming Cycling, pursuit	Long-distance track, swimming, speedskating, canoeing Cycling, road racing Triathlon
	Most team sports/racket sports/sailing				

rate and for a given maximal duration: (1) the immediate or high energy phosphate system (anaerobic alactic system); (2) the short-term or glycolytic system (anaerobic lactic system); and (3) the long-term or oxygen system (aerobic system) (Figure 6.1). The main roles of the three energy systems in competitive sport are summarized in Table 6.1.

The three energy systems are designated as **aerobic** or **anaerobic**, depending on whether oxygen is needed by the system in the production of the energy. While oxygen is not needed by either the **high energy phosphate** or **glycolytic** systems, the **oxidative phosphorylation** system depends on oxygen to produce energy. Similarly, the two anaerobic systems can be separated on the basis of whether or not lactic acid is produced during the energy production. With the glycolytic system, lactic acid is produced as part of energy production (hence **anaerobic lactic**), but no lactic acid is produced during energy production by the high energy phosphate system (hence **anaerobic alactic**).

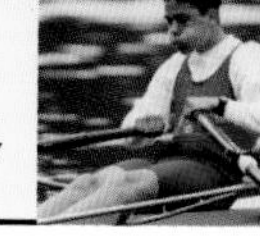

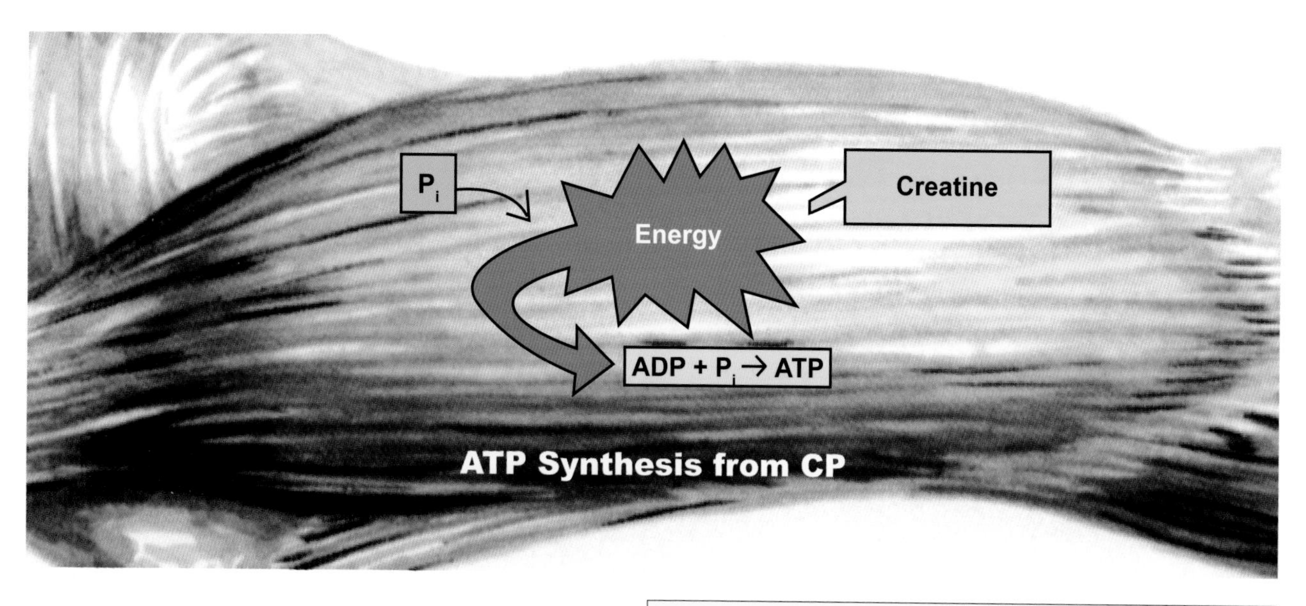

Figure 6.2 The immediate (alactic) energy system.

Immediate Energy: The High Energy Phosphate System

Many sporting activities, such as weightlifting, high jump, long jump, 100-meter run, or 25-meter swim, sometimes described as **high power output activities**, require an immediate high rate of energy production as intensive muscle activity is done over a short time interval. The primary fuel source for these activities is the **immediate** or high energy phosphate system. Under these conditions, creatine phosphate (CP), another high-energy compound in the muscle cell, can be broken down to produce phosphate and creatine. The free phosphate then bonds with ADP to reform ATP (Figure 6.2). As there is only a small amount of ATP and CP stored within each muscle fiber, and because this system produces energy at a very high rate, this system can only provide immediate energy for muscles in the initial 7 to 12 seconds of high-intensity activity.

This system is also known as the alactic energy source or the ATP-CP system.

Characteristics of the High Energy Phosphate System

The utility of the high energy phosphate system is that (1) it can produce very large amounts of energy in a short amount of time and (2) its rate of recovery is relatively rapid. The system can supply energy only until the intramuscular stores of ATP are exhausted, and thereafter, for as long as there is a sufficient local supply of creatine phosphate to resynthesize ATP from ADP. However, the total muscle stores of ATP are very small and are depleted after only a few seconds of high-intensity work. Because the store of creatine phosphate in muscle is also small, it too is depleted rapidly during high-intensity work.

The initial concentrations of high energy phosphates in the muscle are limiting factors in an individual's ability to perform short-term high-intensity work. If the athlete must continue the activity for a period longer than 7 to 12 seconds of very highly vigorous work, or for 15 to 30 seconds of moderately intensive work, the high energy phosphate supply cannot provide all the energy for the activity. It is for this reason that a 100-meter runner often loses speed after only 80 meters as the store of high energy phosphates is exhausted and the body begins using another energy source, the short-term or glycogen energy source (Table 6.1 and Figure 6.3).

Similarly, in weight training, short-term sets (three of 30-second duration) during maximal

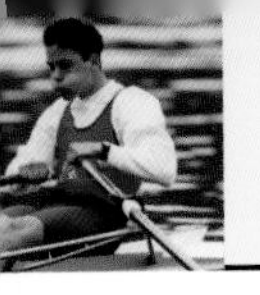

strength and power training are dependent on stored ATP and CP as the primary energy source.

Short-term Energy: The Lactic Acid System

A second energy system results in the production of ATP at the expense of producing lactic acid, an unwanted by-product. This process is called **anaerobic glycolysis**. It involves the breakdown of glycogen (stored carbohydrate in the muscle) into pyruvic acid and ATP (Figure 6.3).

The **lactic acid system** uses a complex biochemical process called anaerobic glycolysis to release energy in the form of ATP by a stepwise breakdown of the carbohydrate fuels glycogen and glucose. During glycolysis, each step in the sequential breakdown (a total of 10 steps; Figure 6.4) involves a specific **enzyme** breaking down the chemical bonds of glycogen or blood glucose in the absence of oxygen (hence the term *anaerobic*). The last product in the series of breakdowns is termed **pyruvate**. When the rate of work is high, the pyruvate is converted into **lactic acid**. The exercise intensity at which lactic acid begins to accumulate within the blood is known as the **anaerobic threshold**. The anaerobic threshold can be thought of as the point during exercise when you begin to feel discomfort and a burning sensation in the muscles.

The source of substrates for the anaerobic energy system is carbohydrate. Glycogen (stored form of carbohydrate in the muscles and the liver) and blood glucose (circulating form of carbohydrate) are derived from the carbohydrates that make up one's diet. Carbohydrates (pasta, rice, bread, potatoes, starchy foods, sweets; Figure 6.5) are the primary dietary sources of glucose and serve as the primary energy fuels for the brain, muscles, heart, liver, and various other organs. Once ingested, these foods are broken down into glucose by the digestive system. Glucose then enters the bloodstream and is circulated around the body. Some glucose stays in the blood, but most is stored in the liver and the muscles as glycogen. Glycogen consists of hundreds of glucose molecules linked together to form a chain. The process of forming glycogen from glucose is termed **glycogenesis**.

Characteristics of the Lactic Acid System

Lactic acid is the substance that makes your muscles "burn" when you exercise intensely

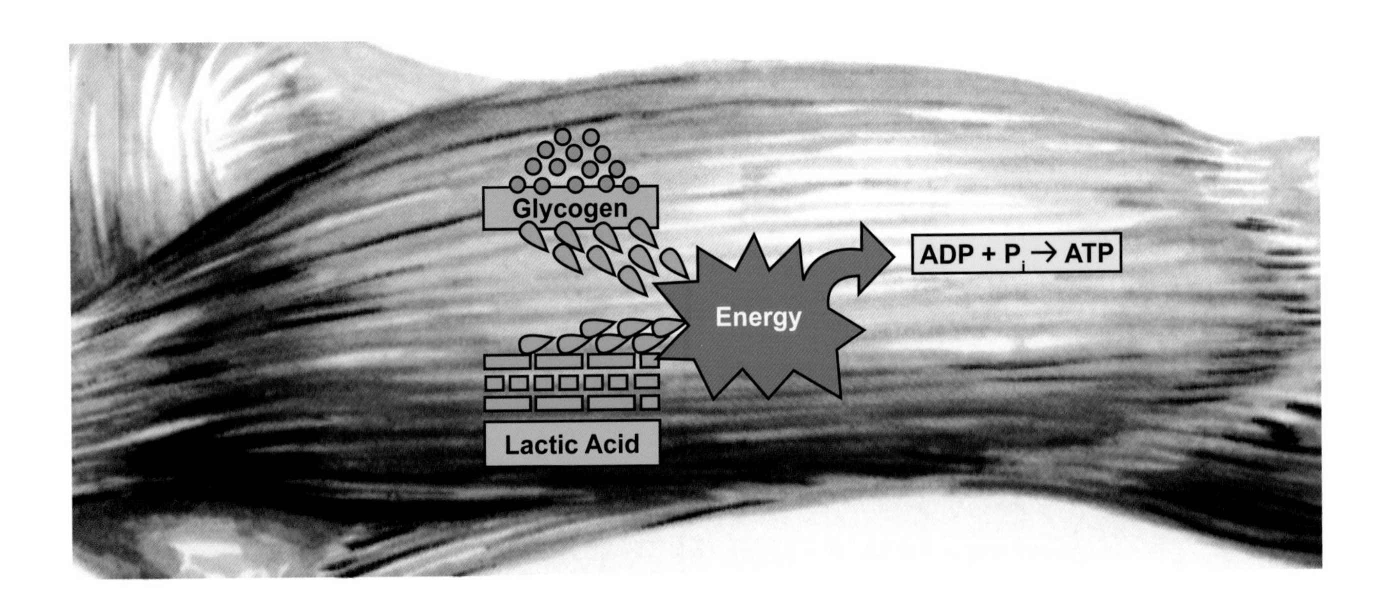

Figure 6.3 The short-term (lactic acid) energy system.

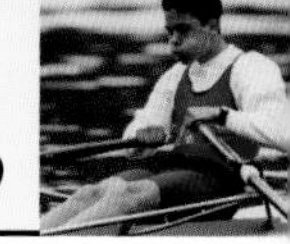

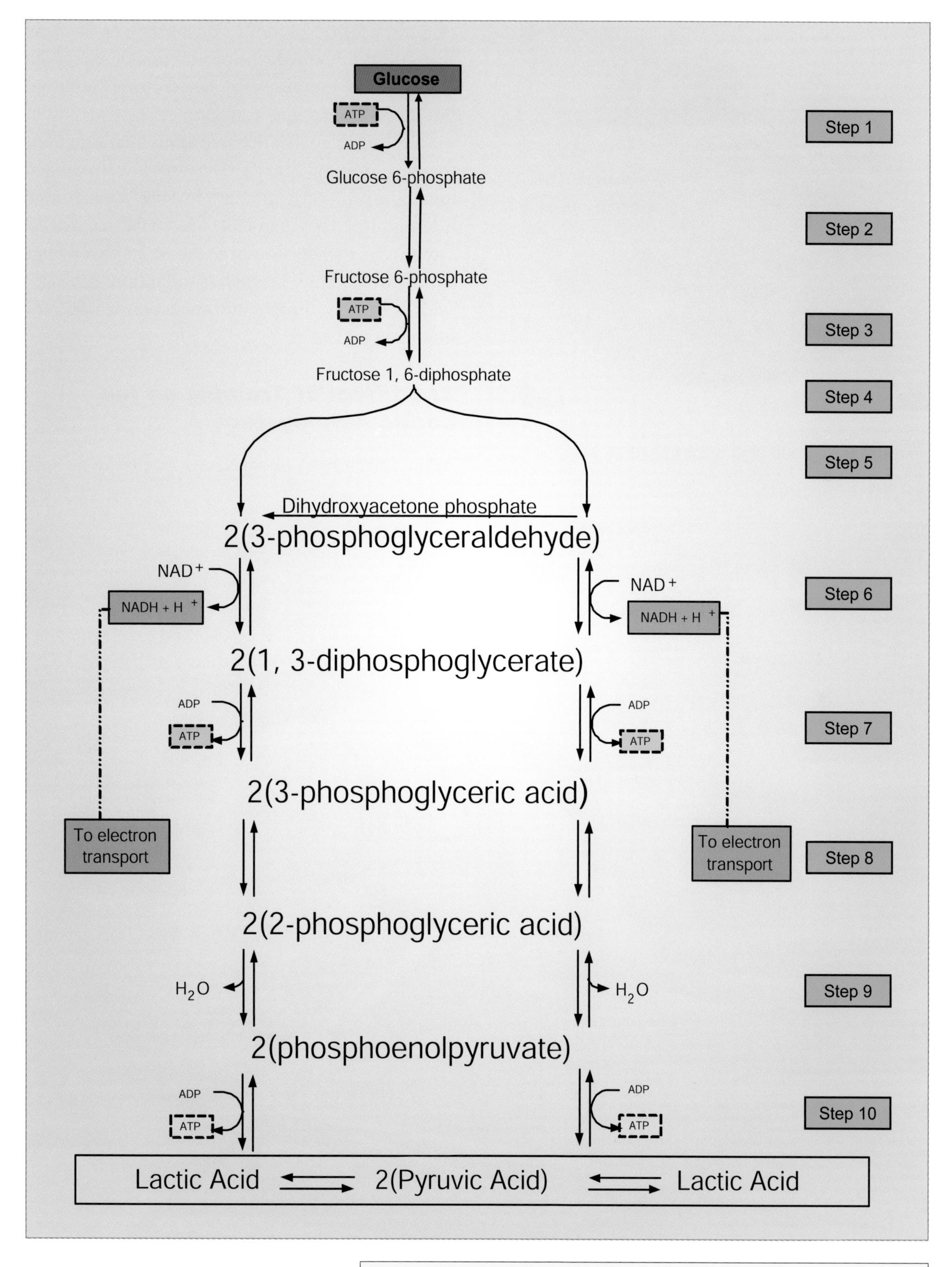

Figure 6.4 The highly complex metabolic pathways of glycolysis.

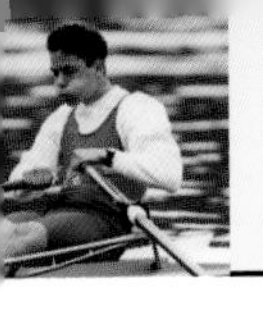

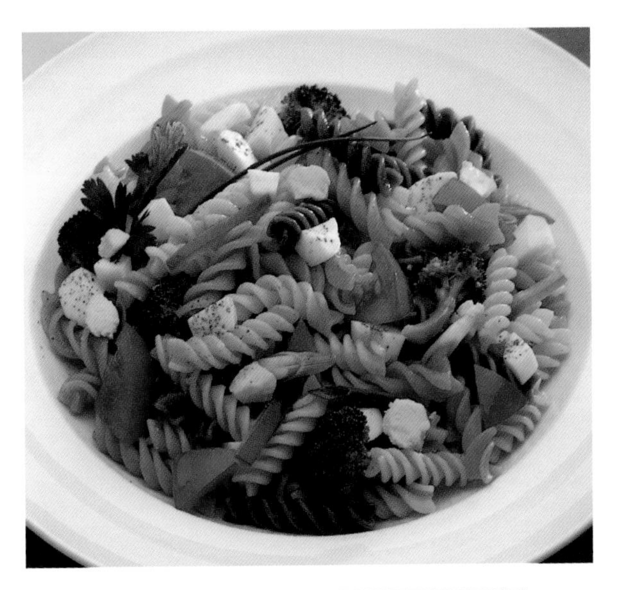

Figure 6.5 Food high in carbohydrates.

(Figure 6.6). Not only does the lactic acid concentration impede the production of energy via glycolysis by inhibiting proper enzyme function, but the hydrogen ions also hamper transmission of the electrical signal at the neuromuscular junction, thereby limiting fiber activation. The hydrogen ions compete with calcium for the cross bridge binding sites (see Chapter 4, Muscle Structure and Function), thereby limiting the strength of fiber contraction. Thus, a high production of lactic acid ultimately limits continued performance of intense activities.

The Effect of Training on the Lactic Acid System

At any given level of work, the rate of lactic acid

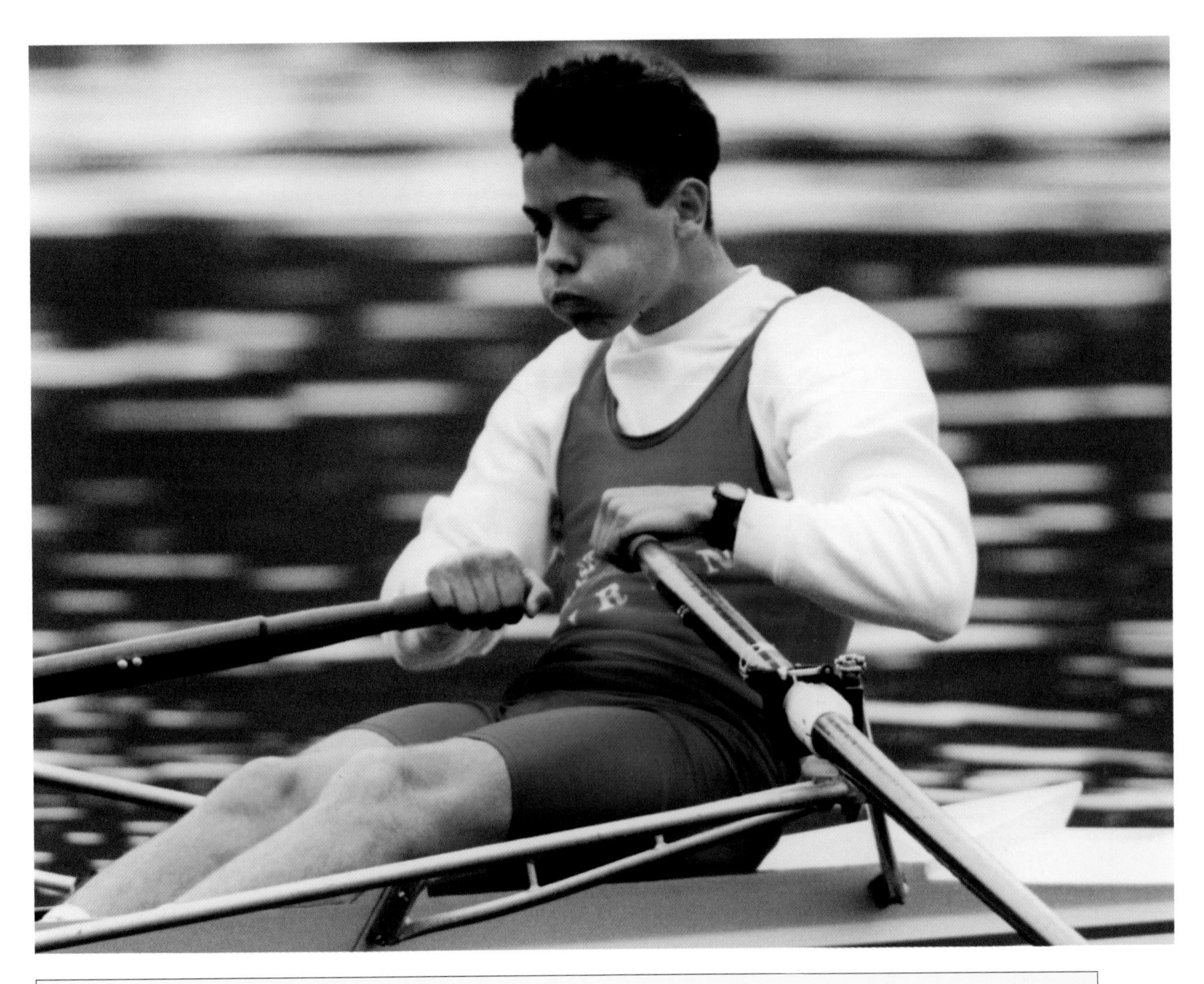

Figure 6.6 Extreme pain at the end of a rowing race is due to lactic acid concentration in muscles.

accumulation is decreased in the trained individual (i.e., the so-called anaerobic threshold is higher, meaning that the individual can work at a higher rate of activity before the accumulation of lactic acid begins).

During high-intensity exercise, the rate of lactic acid production can be decreased by decreasing the intensity of the activity or by increasing the ability to "handle" the lactic acid. Decreasing lactic acid production at any given rate of work can be achieved by increasing the effectiveness of the aerobic system (described in the next section of this chapter), thereby lessening the need for energy from anaerobic sources. Note, however, that this is not a strategy that will work for sprint- or power-oriented performances because the rate of energy demand for this purpose is always going to be higher than the ability of the aerobic system to provide ATP. For these types of performances, other adaptive responses are needed to manage the lactic acid production if higher or sustained levels of performance are to be achieved.

Endurance trained individuals are able to remove lactic acid faster from exercising muscle. Faster lactate removal will allow people to continue to exercise at higher intensities for longer periods of time. Major factors that can lead to an increased rate of lactate removal from the muscle following training are (a) an increased rate of lactic acid diffusion from active muscles (requires an increase in the capillary supply to the muscle in order that the lactic acid can be diffused into the circulatory

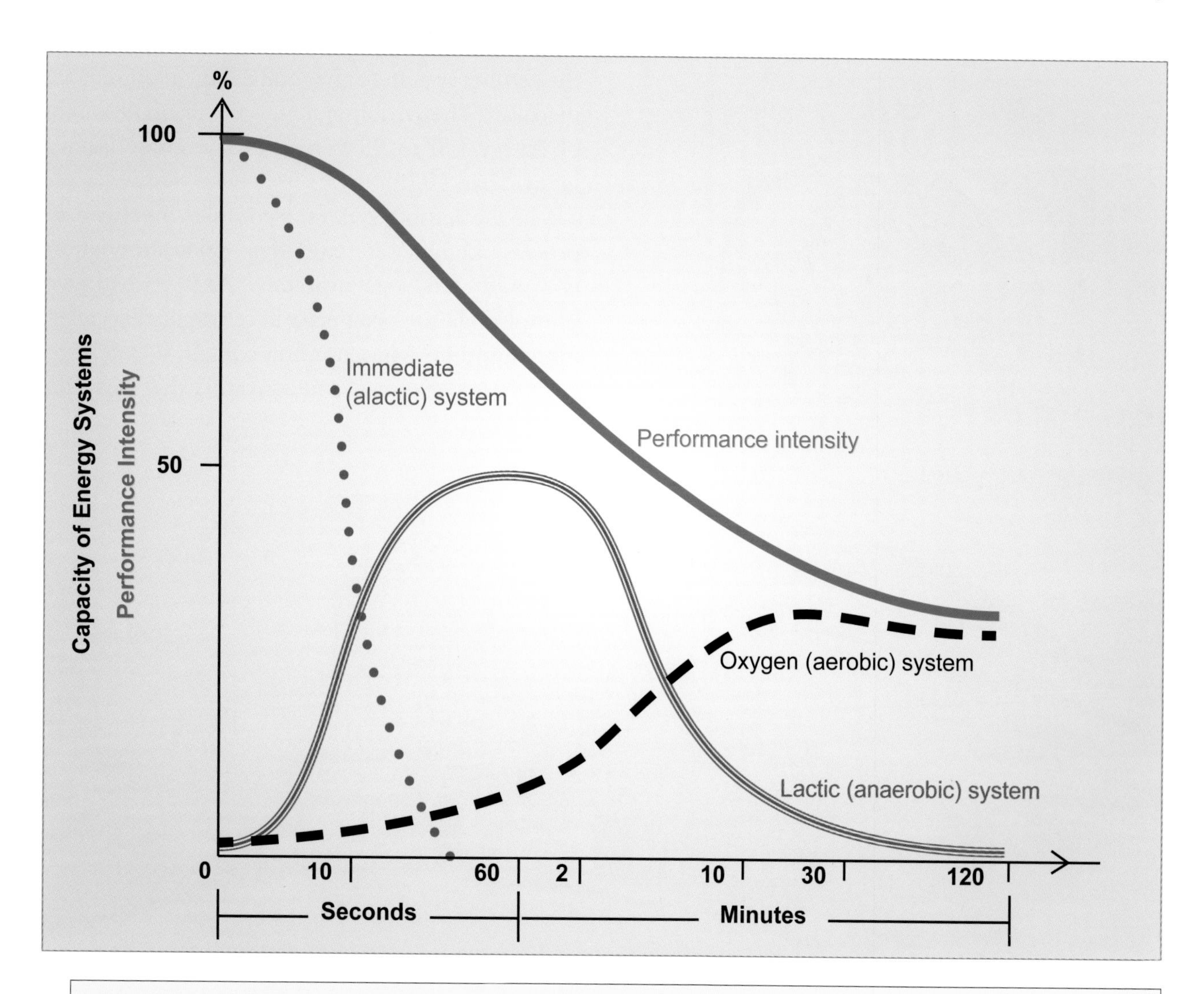

Figure 6.7 The role of the three energy systems during an all-out exercise activity of different duration.

system); (b) an increased muscle blood flow; and (c) an increased ability to metabolize lactate in the heart, liver, and nonworking muscle fibers. Key elements in this adaptation process are changes in the cardiovascular system – the development of more capillaries and the expansion of the body's ability to deliver an increased blood flow to the working muscle either through an increased cardiac output or by the redistribution of blood flow to the muscle. Blood flow is increased in trained individuals through an increase in the number of blood vessels in the muscle, more red blood cells, greater total blood volume, and greater efficiency of the heart (see Chapter 7, The Heart and Lungs at Work).

Long-term Energy: The Oxygen System

The **oxygen** or **long-term** energy system is the most important energy system in the human body, as it represents the primary source of energy for a broad range of activities. Most daily activities use energy provided by the aerobic system. Exercise performed at an intensity lower than that of the anaerobic threshold relies exclusively on the aerobic system for energy production. Thus, during aerobic activities, blood lactate levels remain relatively low.

For intensive work of 2 to 3 minutes' duration, approximately half the energy is supplied from **anaerobic metabolism** and the other half from **aerobic metabolism** (Figure 6.7). As the duration of the activity increases, the relative contribution of the aerobic system to the total energy requirement increases. The aerobic system is the primary source of energy (70 to 95 percent) for exercise lasting longer than 10 minutes.

In the aerobic system, a complex biochemical process known as **oxidative phosphorylation** is used to resynthesize ATP. Oxidative phosphorylation takes place in cell organelles called **mitochondria**. Mitochondria contain a system of enzymes, coenzymes, and activators that carry on

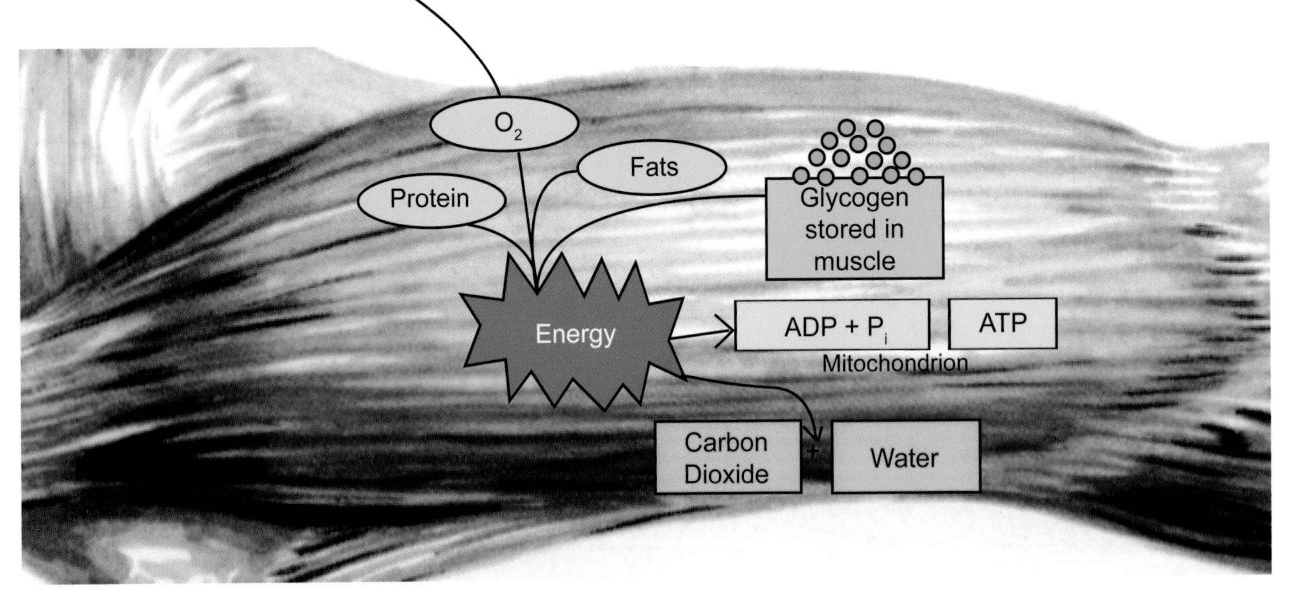

Figure 6.8 The long-term (oxygen) energy system.

an extensive breakdown of fuels, providing large quantities of ATP.

The aerobic energy system is the primary energy system used in exercise provided that (a) the working muscles have sufficient mitochondria to meet energy requirements; (b) sufficient oxygen is supplied to the mitochondria; and (c) enzymes or intermediate products do not limit the rate of energy flux through the aerobic energy production system, called the **Kreb's cycle**. The Kreb's cycle is a metabolic process where pyruvic acid is metabolized, as are other fuel sources including glucose, fat molecules, and protein.

Characteristics of the Oxygen System

The aerobic system is highly efficient. For example, the energy yield from the aerobic breakdown of a glycogen molecule is approximately 12 times more efficient than that of the anaerobic system breakdown of the same molecule of glycogen. Even more energy is derived from the utilization of fats. When fats are oxidized (note fats cannot be broken down anaerobically), the energy yield may be increased by more than 4.5 times the yield from carbohydrates. Thus, fats are an important energy source for athletic events that require large outputs of energy over a long period of time as they provide nearly limitless energy supplies to the human body. At the end of the aerobic breakdown of carbohydrates and fats, water and carbon dioxide are given off as the metabolic by-products (Figure 6.8).

Cori Cycle Another important feature of the oxygen system is its ability to remove lactic acid from the muscle. As indicated earlier, the removal of lactic acid from muscle tissue is important for the maintenance of skeletal muscle function. The removal of lactic acid allows the muscle to continue to contract and allows for exercise to continue. The aerobic system allows for removal of lactic acid through the conversion of lactic acid back into usable glucose. Lactic acid, once produced in the muscle fiber, passes out of that fiber and is taken to the liver to be metabolized back into pyruvic acid and then glucose. This process is called the **Cori cycle** (Figure 6.9).

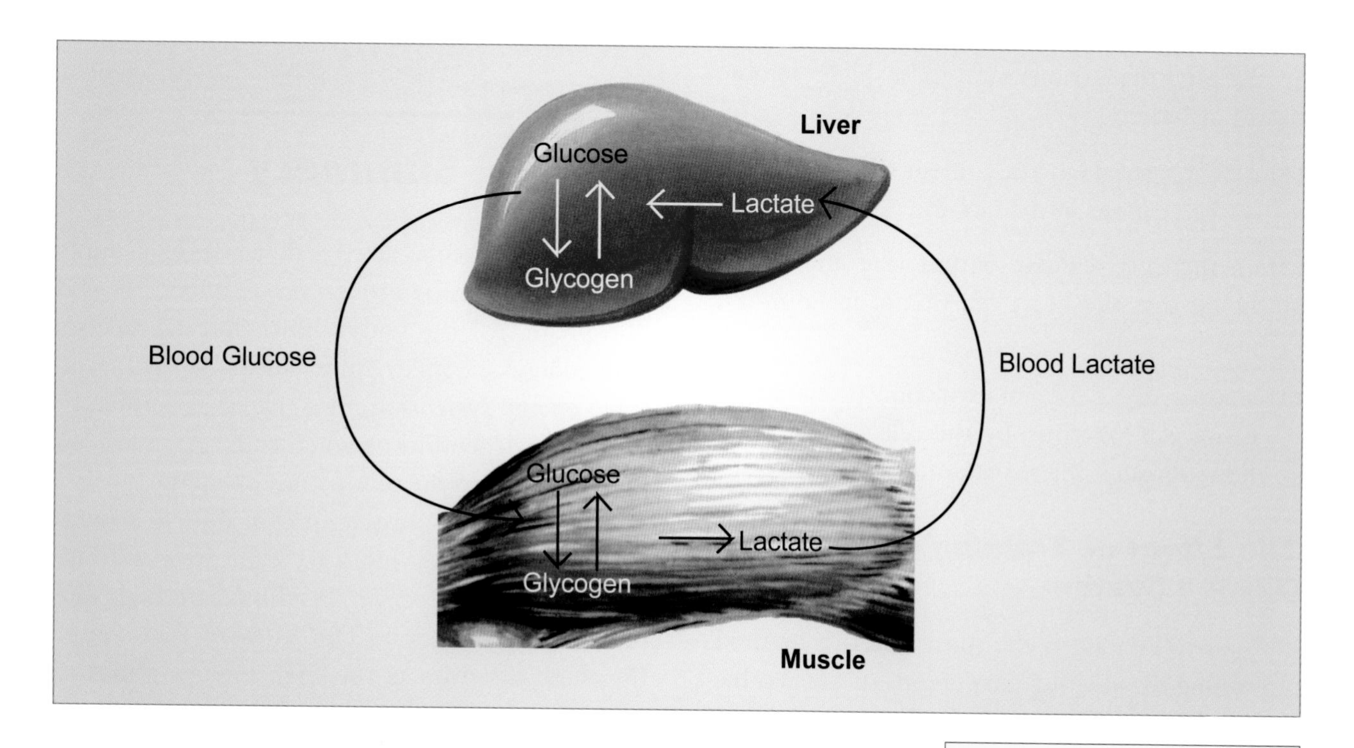

Figure 6.9 The Cori cycle.

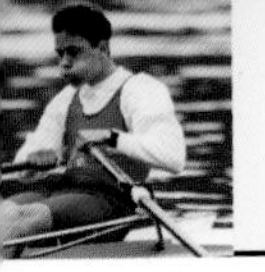

Limitations of the Oxygen System

There are, however, two limitations of the aerobic energy system. First, the system requires continuous and adequate supplies of oxygen and fuel sources that are necessary for aerobic metabolism. Second, the rate of ATP utilization must be relatively slow to allow the process to meet the energy demands. Therefore, the aerobic system is well suited for low- to moderate-intensity activities.

Aerobic Power

The power of the aerobic system is generally evaluated by measuring the maximal volume of oxygen that can be consumed in a given amount of time during maximal effort (units of L/min). This measure is called **maximal aerobic power**, or **$\dot{V}O_2$max**, and is most often expressed relative to body mass to yield a measure that describes the efficiency of the working body (units of ml/kg/min). The average sedentary, healthy 20-year-old male will have a $\dot{V}O_2$max of 40 to 44 ml/kg/min, and the average sedentary 20-year-old female has a value of 36 to 40 ml/kg/min. In comparison, the values of trained athletes will reach 80 to 90 ml/kg/min for males and 75 to 85 ml/kg/min for females.

Factors that contribute to a high aerobic power include:

(1) a high arterial oxygen content (the amount of oxygen carried in the blood);

(2) an increased cardiac output (the amount of blood that the heart can pump per minute); and

(3) a larger tissue oxygen extraction (the amount of oxygen taken up by the cells as the blood flows through the tissue).

The Effect of Training on the Oxygen System

Endurance exercise is the most effective method of training for eliciting adaptations in the aerobic oxidative energy system. Endurance training consists of repeated, sustained efforts of long duration several times per week. Examples of endurance exercise include running, swimming, or biking for 40 minutes or more at a heart rate of 130 to 140 beats per minute. Endurance training has four major effects on aerobic metabolism:

(1) it increases vascularization within the muscles so that there is an enhanced delivery of nutrients and oxygen to the muscle;

(2) it increases the number and size of mitochondria within the muscle fibers;

(3) it increases the activity of the enzymes involved in the aerobic metabolic pathways; and

(4) it results in the preferential use of fats over glycogen during exercise, which saves the muscles' rather limited store of glycogen.

Endurance training increases the maximal aerobic power of a sedentary individual by 15 to 25 percent regardless of age. Genetics plays a large role in determining the rate of adaptation, with some individuals adapting quickly and others more slowly. Age also plays a role in the training adaptation in that an older individual adapts more slowly than a younger person. Maximal aerobic power peaks between the ages of 18 and 25 and declines at a rate of 0.5 to 1.5 percent per year after that.

Summary

Energy for muscular activity depends on a supply of ATP that can be broken down into ADP and phosphate. All the body's biochemical processes and energy systems require adequate ATP. The three energy systems are designated as aerobic or anaerobic, depending on whether oxygen is needed by the system in the production of energy.

Activities that involve intense muscle activity over a short time interval (e.g., weightlifting, 100-meter dash) require an immediate high rate of energy production. The primary fuel source for these activities is the high energy phospate system, or ATP-CP system. This energy system can produce large amounts of energy in a short time, with a relatively rapid recovery rate.

A second energy system called anaerobic glycolysis results in the production of ATP at the expense of producing lactic acid – the substance that makes your muscles "burn" when you exercise intensely. Anaerobic glycolysis involves the breakdown of glycogen (stored carbohydrate in the muscle) into pyruvic acid and ATP. The point during exercise when lactic acid begins to accumulate in the blood is known as the anaerobic threshold.

The oxygen, or long-term, energy system is the most important energy system in the human body, as it represents the primary source of energy for a broad range of activities. Most daily activities use energy provided by this highly efficient aerobic system. In the aerobic system, a complex biochemical process known as oxidative phosphorylation is used to resynthesize ATP.

The body's energy production is one of the more complex factors affecting athletic capacity, especially with athletics involving high-endurance requirements such as running, swimming, cross-country skiing, and rowing. Trained individuals are able to utilize ATP and remove lactic acid more efficiently than untrained individuals, and endurance training can significantly improve the aerobic energy system.

Key Terms

adenosine diphosphate (ADP)
adenosine triphosphate (ATP)
aerobic metabolism
anaerobic alactic
anaerobic glycolysis
anaerobic lactic
anaerobic metabolism
anaerobic threshold
ATP resynthesis
Cori cycle
enzyme
glycogenesis
glycolytic system
high energy (immediate) phosphate system
Kreb's cycle
lactic acid
lactic acid system
maximal aerobic power ($\dot{V}O_2max$)
mitochondria
oxidative phosphorylation
oxygen system
pyruvate

Discussion Questions

1. What are the differences between the three energy systems?

2. List one advantage and one disadvantage of each of the three energy systems.

3. Give an example of three activities or sports that use each of (a) the high energy phosphate system; (b) the anaerobic glycolytic system; and (c) the aerobic glycolytic system as its primary source of energy (one sport for each energy system).

4. What is the most important source of fuel in the body for all types of energy production, a substance also known as the energy currency of the body?

5. Distinguish ATP turnover from ATP resynthesis.

6. Describe how each of the three energy systems could be trained most efficiently.

In This Chapter:

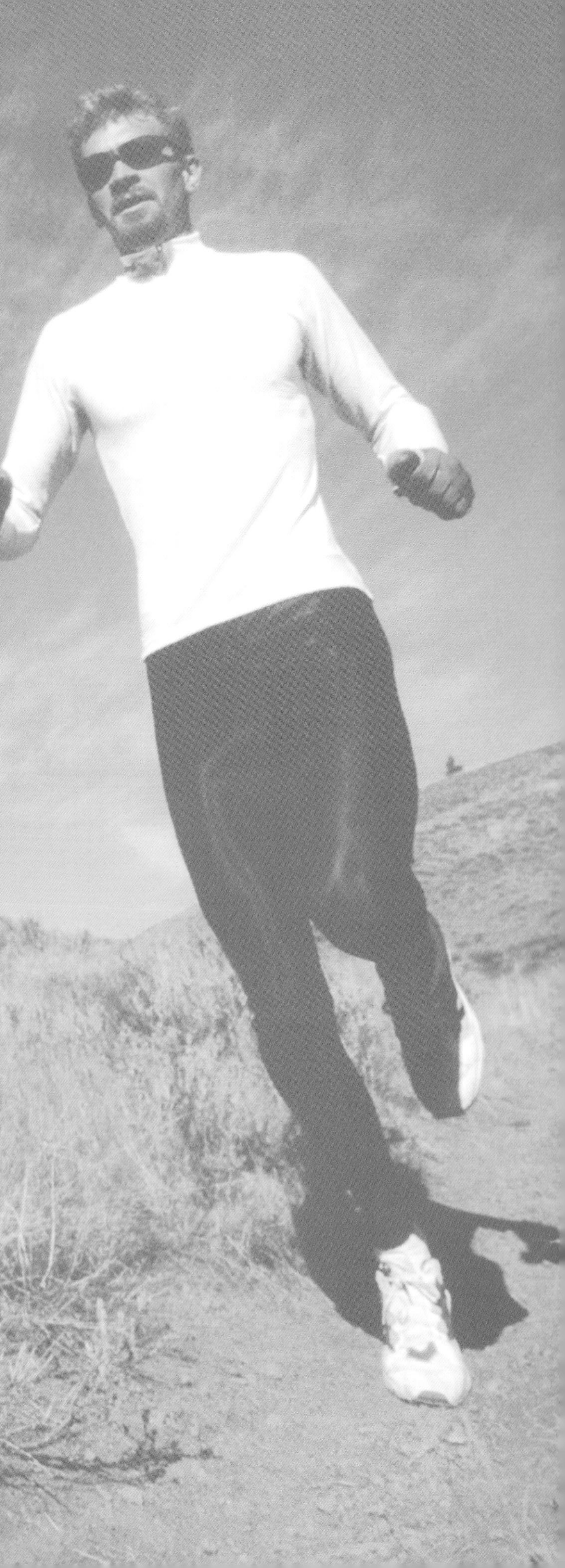

CHAPTER 7

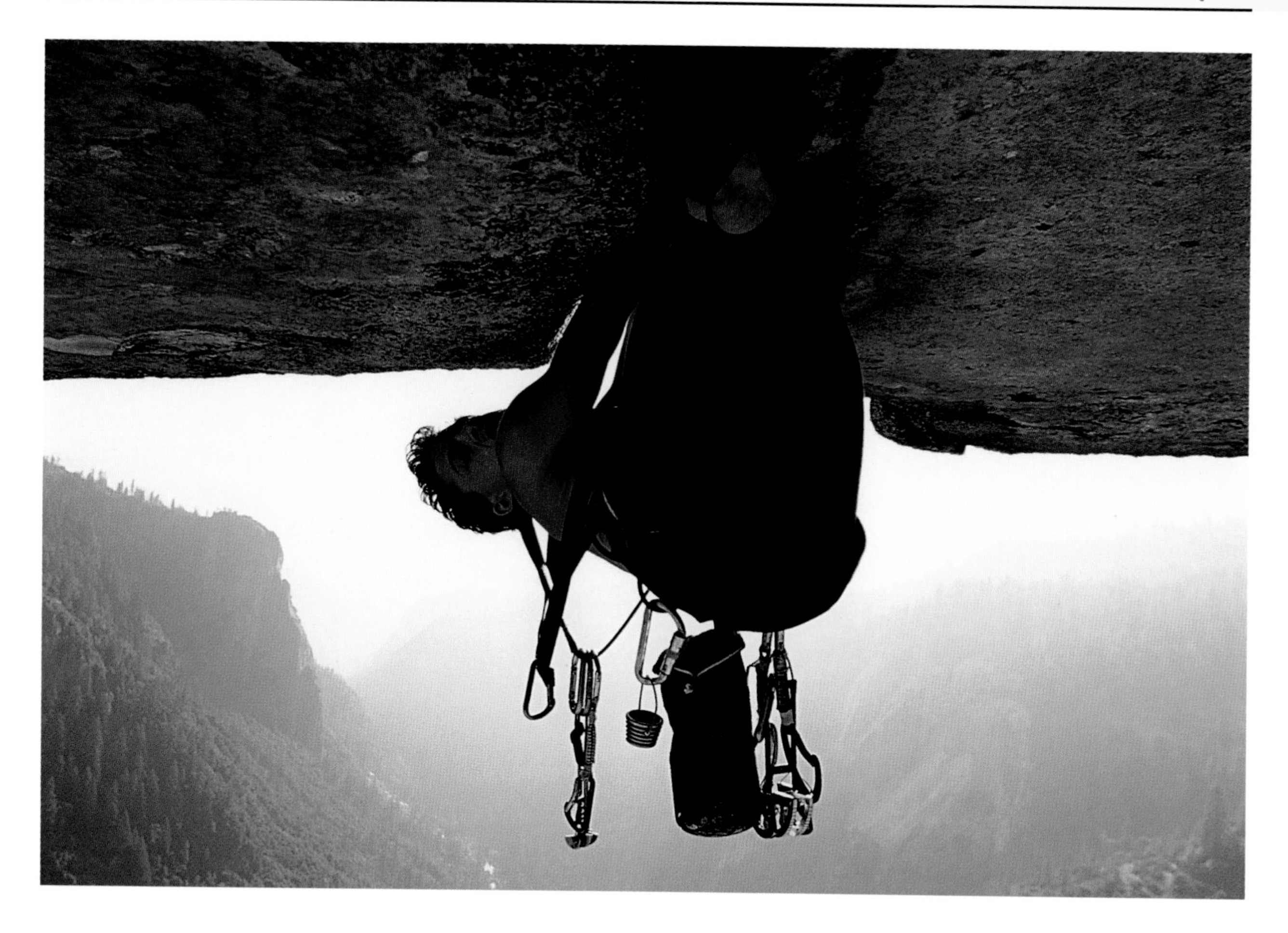

The Heart and Lungs at Work

After completing this chapter you should be able to:

- explain the function and control of the cardiovascular and respiratory systems;
- describe the relationship between the cardiorespiratory system and energy production;
- explain the measures that are used to evaluate and describe the various components of the cardiovascular and respiratory systems;
- describe the acute and chronic effects of physical activity on the body;
- analyze the effects of different environmental conditions on the body during physical activity.

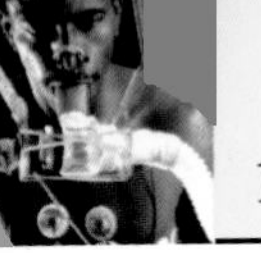

During an average human life the heart will beat about three billion times, beginning at conception and continuing until death. The heart is one of the first organs to begin functioning and is often associated with life and death. This life-sustaining organ that pumps blood throughout our bodies is only one part of our circulatory system. The others – blood vessels (the passageways) and blood (the transport medium) – complete the transport system that delivers supplies to the tissues that need them for survival and growth. Oxygen is perhaps the most important supply to be delivered at rest and during exercise.

The systems of the body, however, are by no means independent of one another. Pulmonary structure and function are closely linked with the cardiovascular system; without getting oxygen into the body through breathing (ventilation), diffusion, and gas exchange in the lungs, there is no oxygen to transport to the body's tissues. Thus, the body's systems must work together in order to function most efficiently.

Because cardiovascular function is so vital to our existence, it is important to be aware of the advantages that can result from training, and their implications for health. Exercise offers numerous benefits, and enhanced cardiovascular function is one of them. Understanding the changes that occur during exercise will enable you to train more effectively for performance and will improve your cardiovascular health. How are blood flow and blood volume controlled? What is actually involved in the transport of oxygen? And what role does hemoglobin play in oxygen transport? The answers to these and other questions will be presented in this chapter; this material will provide the foundation you will need to attain and maintain optimal cardiovascular health.

Cardiovascular Anatomy

The primary role of the cardiovascular system is supplying the muscles and organs with the oxygen and nutrients that they need to function properly and removing metabolic by-products from areas of activity. Optimal functioning of the cardiovascular system is critical for human performance. The anatomy and physiology of the heart and the blood vessels are described in this section.

The Heart

Structure

The heart is an organ made up of striated muscle that serves to pump blood through the human body. The heart pumps blood through the body by using two different pumps, called **ventricles** (Figure 7.1). The blood comes to the heart from the peripheral organs. The right ventricle receives deoxygenated blood from the body and pumps it to the lungs, and the left ventricle receives oxygenated blood from the lungs and pumps it to the rest of the body. Since the **left ventricle** has to pump blood through the entire body, it is larger and its muscle walls are stronger than that of the **right ventricle**, which has to pump blood only a short distance to the lungs. The heart has two smaller chambers called **atria** (singular = atrium). These smaller pumps receive blood from the body (**right atrium**) or the lungs (**left atrium**) and then pump the blood into the right and left ventricles, ensuring that the ventricles have a sufficient supply of blood for distribution to the lungs and other areas of the body, respectively.

Function

The heart contracts in a constant rhythm that may speed up or slow down depending on the need for blood (and oxygen) in the body. For example, if you start running, your leg muscles will need more oxygen to do the work of running. Therefore your heart will have to pump more oxygen-carrying blood to those working muscles and will have to beat more rapidly in order to supply that blood. The beating of the heart is governed by an automatic electrical impulse that is generated by the sinus node. The **sinus node** is a small bundle of nerve fibers that are found in the wall of the right atrium near the opening of the **superior vena**

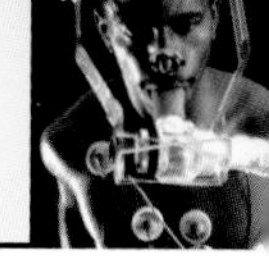

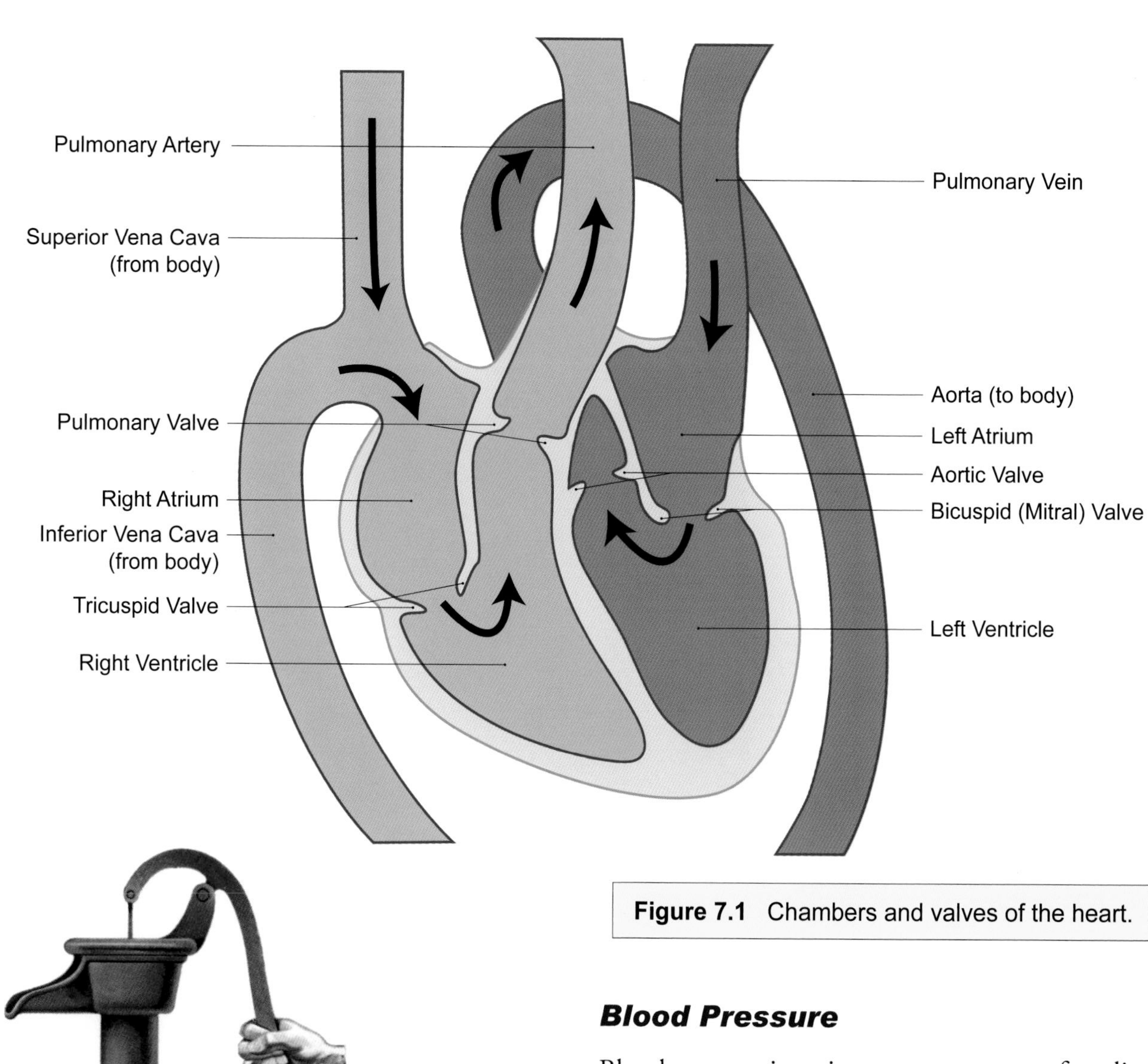

Figure 7.1 Chambers and valves of the heart.

The heart works like an efficient pump.

cava (see Figure 7.5). The sinus node generates an electrical charge called an **action potential** that causes the muscle walls of the heart to contract. The atria contract before the ventricles contract, which allows for the blood to be quickly pumped into the ventricles from the atria and then from the ventricles to the lungs and the body. The sinus node determines the rate of beating of the entire heart (Figure 7.2).

Blood Pressure

Blood pressure is an important measure of cardiac function (Figure 7.3). There are two components to the measure of blood pressure. The first component is the pressure in the ventricles when they are contracting and pushing blood out into the body. This is called **systole.** *Systolic pressure* provides an estimate of the heart's work and the strain against the arterial walls during the contraction. In healthy young adults, systolic pressure is normally around 120 mm Hg.

The second component of blood pressure, called **diastole**, describes the pressure in the heart when it is in the relaxation phase of the cardiac cycle (the ventricles are relaxed and being filled with blood). *Diastolic pressure* is used as an indicator of peripheral blood pressure (the blood pressure in the body outside the heart). It provides an indication of the ease with which the blood

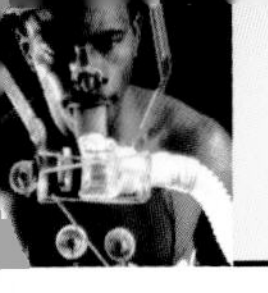

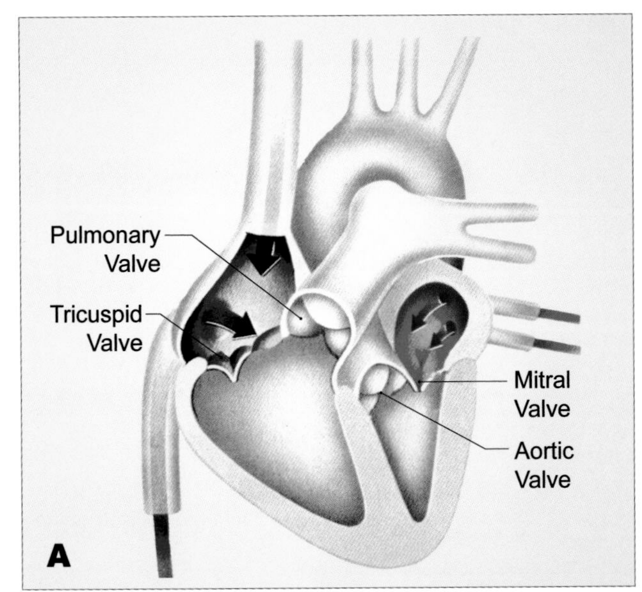

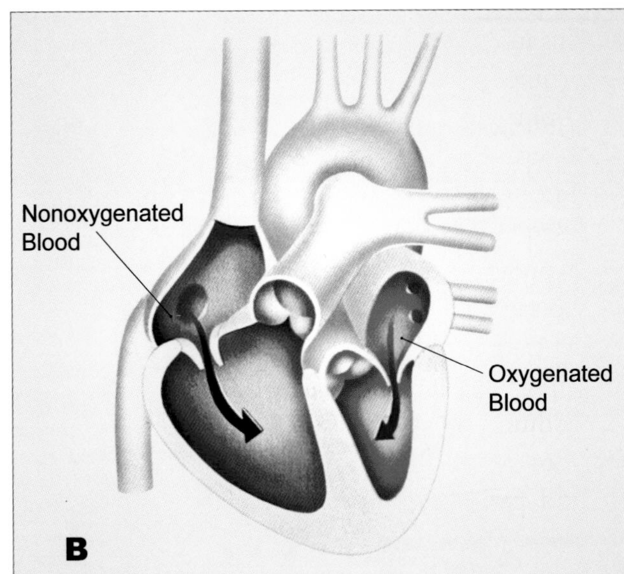

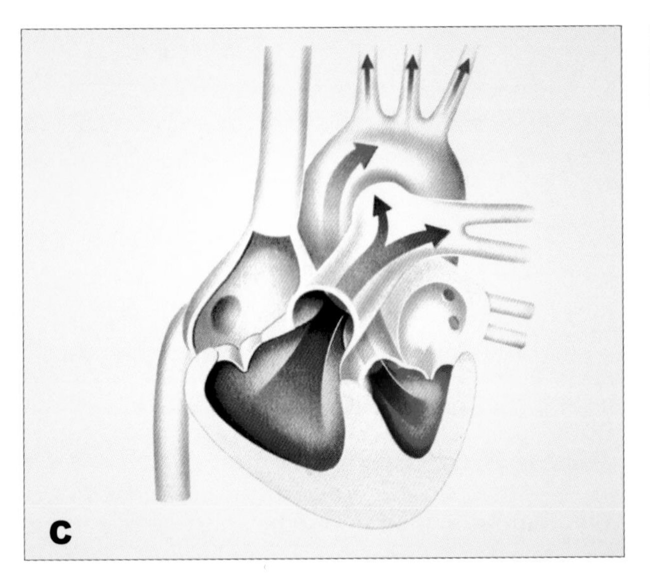

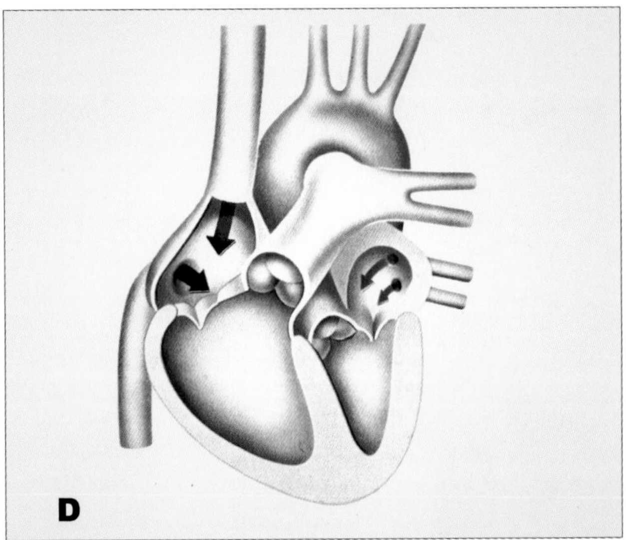

Figure 7.2 The finely tuned cardiac cycle. **A.** As the heart relaxes in diastole, both atria and ventricles simultaneously fill with blood. **B.** The atria, squeezing into systole, force blood into the ventricles. **C.** As the ventricle compartments fill with blood, they contract, thereby ejecting blood to the lungs and body. **D.** The atria and ventricles relax as the cycle begins anew.

flows from the arterioles into the capillaries. The normal diastolic pressure in healthy young adults is about 70 to 80 mm Hg.

Cardiac Output

The amount of blood that is pumped into the aorta each minute by the heart is known as the **cardiac output** (measured in liters per minute). Cardiac output is the product of stroke volume (measured in liters per minute) and heart rate (measured in beats per minute) and is therefore representative of the quantity of blood that flows to the peripheral circulation. Cardiac output can be described by the simple equation presented below:

Cardiac Output = Stroke Volume x Heart Rate

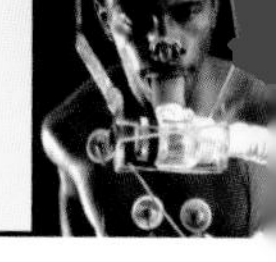

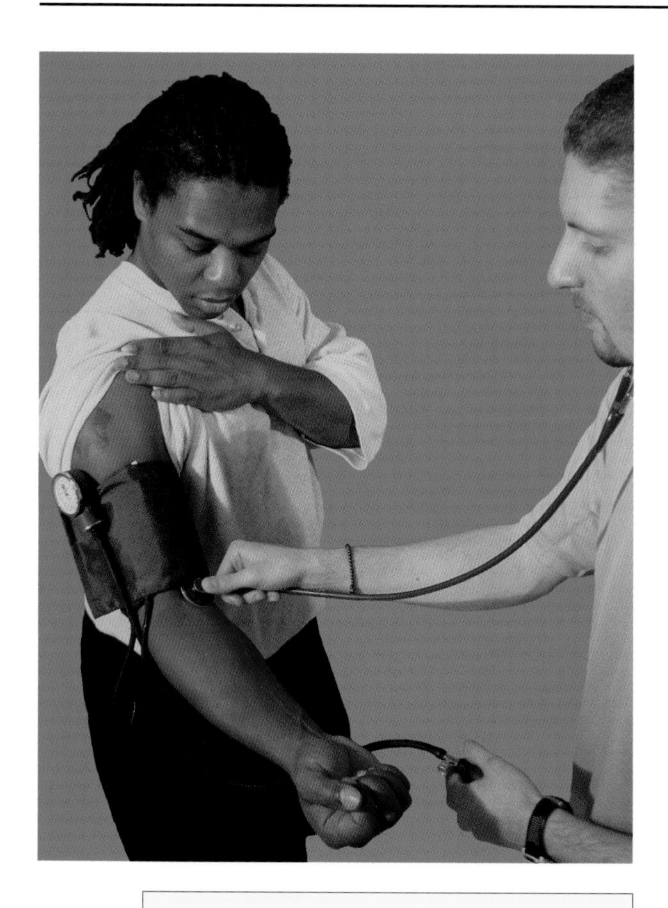

Figure 7.3 Measuring blood pressure.

Stroke Volume The amount of blood that is pumped out of the left ventricle with each heartbeat is the **stroke volume**. The stroke volume of the heart is measured in milliliters (1 liter = 1,000 ml). A typical stroke volume for a normal heart is about 70 ml of blood. Regular exercise and sports training can serve to increase stroke volume.

Heart Rate The rhythmical contraction of the walls of the heart is commonly known as a **heartbeat**. **Heart rate** is the number of times the heart beats in one minute and is measured in beats per minute (bpm). At rest the normal heart rate of an adult can range from 40 bpm in a highly trained athlete to 70 bpm in a normal, healthy person. During intense exercise, the heart rate may increase to up to 200 bpm and occasionally even higher. The maximum expected heart rate for most people can be estimated by using the following equation:

Maximum Heart Rate = 220 – Age (in years)

Intensity of Work The intensity of aerobic exercise can be estimated by measuring heart rate as the two are highly related. The higher the intensity of exercise, the higher the heart rate per minute. Since heart rate is a measure that is easily

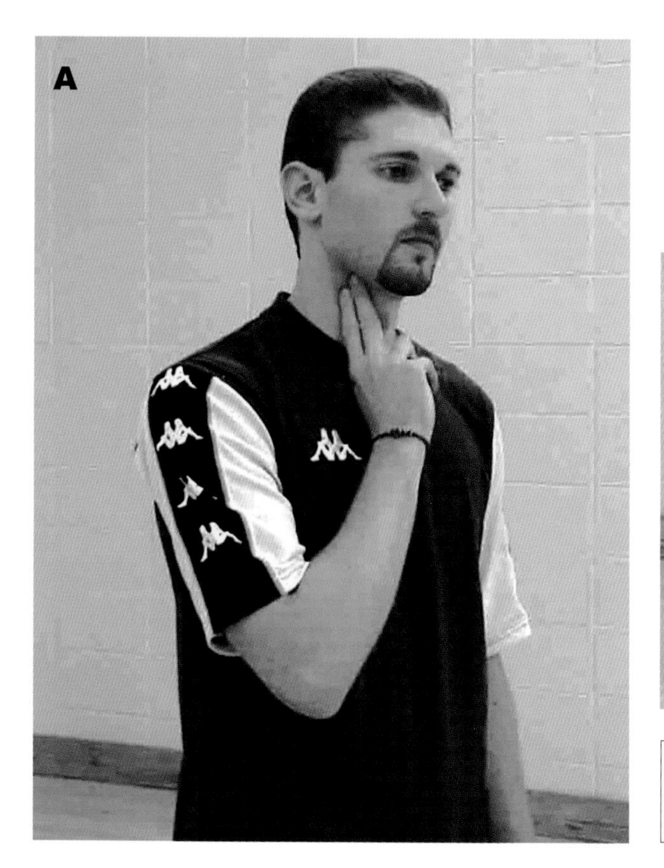

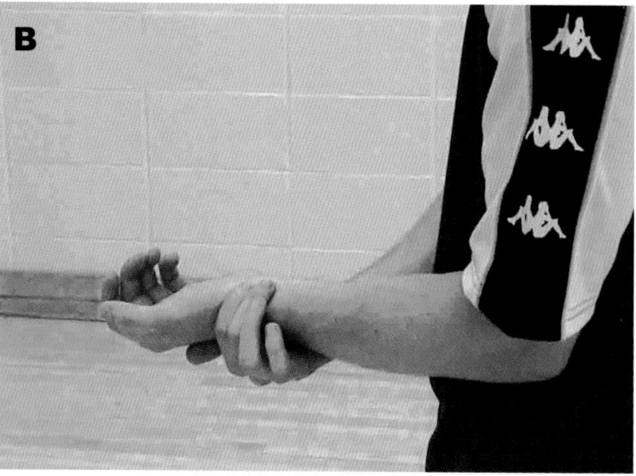

Figure 7.4 **A.** Measuring the carotid pulse. **B.** Measuring the radial pulse.

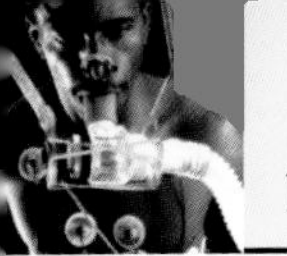

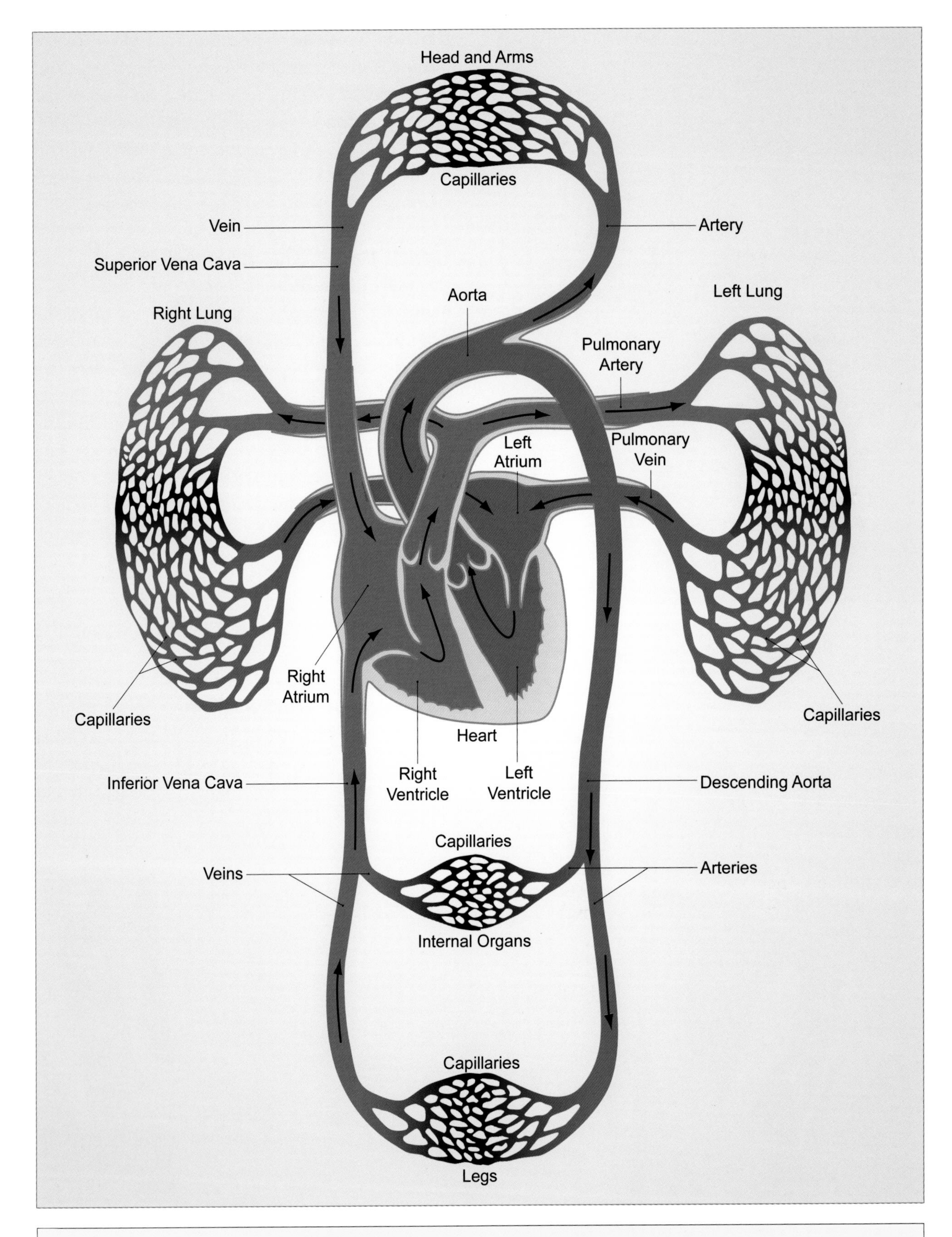

Figure 7.5 Circuitry of the heart and cardiovascular system. Oxygenated blood is shown in red, deoxygenated blood in blue.

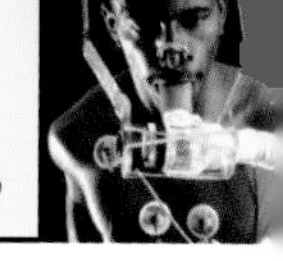

obtained, it becomes very practical for estimation of intensity of work and/or exercise. The heart rate can easily be measured by feeling the carotid or radial pulses with the middle three fingers as in Figure 7.4. By placing two or three fingers and applying light pressure between the trachea and the sternocleidomastoid muscle in the neck, you can feel the carotid pulse. Then count the number of beats in 10 seconds and multiply the figure by 6 to get the number of beats per minute.

For example, a count of 17 beats in 10 seconds multiplied by 6 would result in a heart rate of 102 beats per minute. This elementary procedure allows you to quickly determine how hard you are working without any specialized equipment.

The Peripheral Circulatory System

All of the larger blood vessels of the body are made up of tubes composed of layers of tissue. Smooth muscle cells that allow them to contract or relax also surround the fibrous tubes of the arteries, arterioles, venules, and veins. This enables the vessels of the peripheral circulatory system to regulate blood flow and alter the pattern of circulation throughout the body.

The peripheral circulatory system is made up of the vessels that carry blood away from the heart to the muscles and organs (lungs, brain, stomach, intestines) and then return the blood to the heart. The vessels that carry blood away from the heart are called arteries, and the vessels that return blood to the heart are called veins (Figure 7.5).

Arteries

As the **arteries** carry blood away from the heart, they branch into smaller and smaller vessels called **arterioles**. The arterioles also branch into smaller and smaller vessels until they are composed of vessels that are about the width of one red blood cell. At this point, they are called **capillaries** (Figures 7.5 and 7.11). The capillaries are small vessels composed of only endothelial cells that allow for the exchange of oxygen and nutrients from the blood to muscles and organs and also allow blood to pick up the waste products and carbon dioxide from metabolism.

Veins

As the blood begins to return to the heart, the capillaries connect to form larger and larger vessels called **venules**. The venules then merge into even larger vessels called **veins**. Veins have an additional feature that facilitates the return of blood to the heart, sometimes against the pull of gravity. In comparison to arteries, veins have **valves** that open with the flow of blood in the direction of return to the heart (e.g., from the

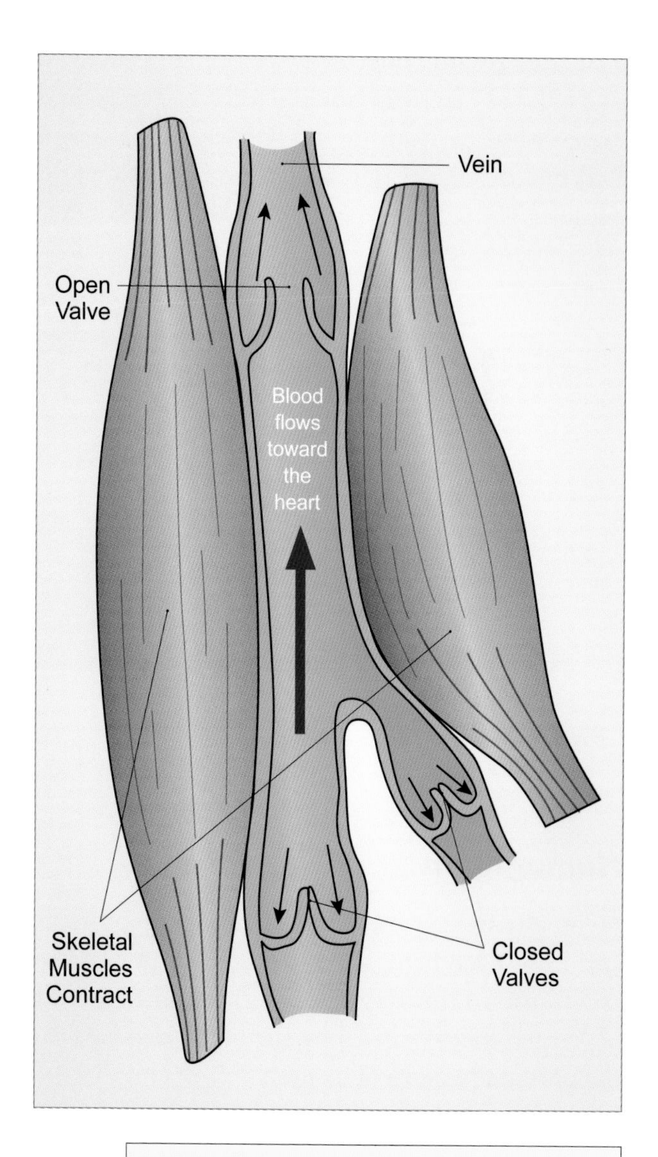

Figure 7.6 The skeletal muscle pump.

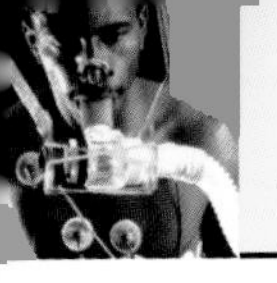

knee to the hip) and close to prevent blood flow in the opposite direction (Figure 7.6). Blood can be pushed through veins by smooth muscle that surrounds the veins, by contraction of the various skeletal muscles (or muscle groups), or to a minor extent by the pumping action of the heart.

Red Blood Cells

Red blood cells, or **erythrocytes** (Figure 7.7), are specialized cells (approximately 8 µm in diameter) that are present in the blood. Other components of blood include **white blood cells** and a clear fluid called **plasma**. The percentage of the blood that is made up of red blood cells is called the **hematocrit**, which normally is about 45 percent. The primary function of the red blood cells is to transport oxygen from the lungs to the tissues and carbon dioxide from the body back to the lungs. Red blood cells are able to perform this function because they contain an oxygen-binding substance called **hemoglobin**.

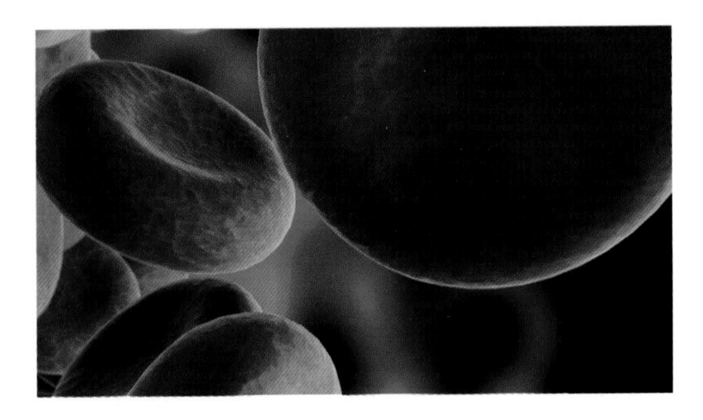

Figure 7.7 Red blood cells.

Hemoglobin

Hemoglobin is a molecule made up of proteins and iron. Each hemoglobin molecule can bond to and transport four oxygen molecules. The amount of oxygen that is carried by the blood depends on the **partial pressure of oxygen (PO_2)**. Thus, in the lungs where the partial pressure of oxygen is high because of the fresh air that is present, hemoglobin binds easily to oxygen, and the red blood cells become saturated with oxygen. However, once the blood has reached the tissues, the partial pressure of oxygen is usually much lower because the metabolism of the body uses up the oxygen that is present. When the partial pressure of oxygen is lower, oxygen unbinds (dissociates) from hemoglobin and is diffused to the tissues, where it is used to produce energy. The difference in the amount of oxygen that is present in the blood as it leaves the lungs and the amount of oxygen that is present in the blood when it returns to the lungs is called the **arterial–venous oxygen difference (a–v O_2 difference)** and is measured in milliliters of oxygen per deciliter of blood (i.e., ml O_2/100 ml blood). This is an important physiological measure of the amount of oxygen that is being used by the body. If the a–v O_2 difference increases, it means that the body is using more oxygen. A typical a–v O_2 difference at rest is about 4 to 5 ml O_2/dl of blood, while at exercise the a–v O_2 difference may increase to 15 ml O_2/dl of blood.

The total mass of red blood cells in the circulatory system is regulated within very narrow limits. New red blood cells (**reticulocytes**) are produced in the bone marrow. The principal factor that stimulates red blood cell formation is the circulating hormone **erythropoietin (EPO)**. EPO is secreted in response to low oxygen levels (when one is at high altitude; Figure 7.8) and also in response to exercise. Thus, exercise can increase the percentage of new red blood cells in the body. New red blood cells contain more hemoglobin than older red blood cells and thus can carry greater amounts of oxygen.

Cardiovascular Physiology

The Transport of Carbon Dioxide

Carbon dioxide (CO_2) is produced in the body as a by-product of metabolism. Once formed, carbon dioxide diffuses from the cells to the blood where it is transported to the lungs via one of three mechanisms: (1) a small percentage of the

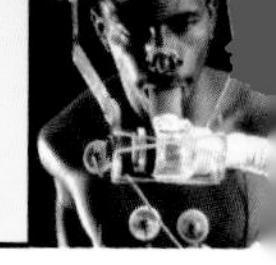

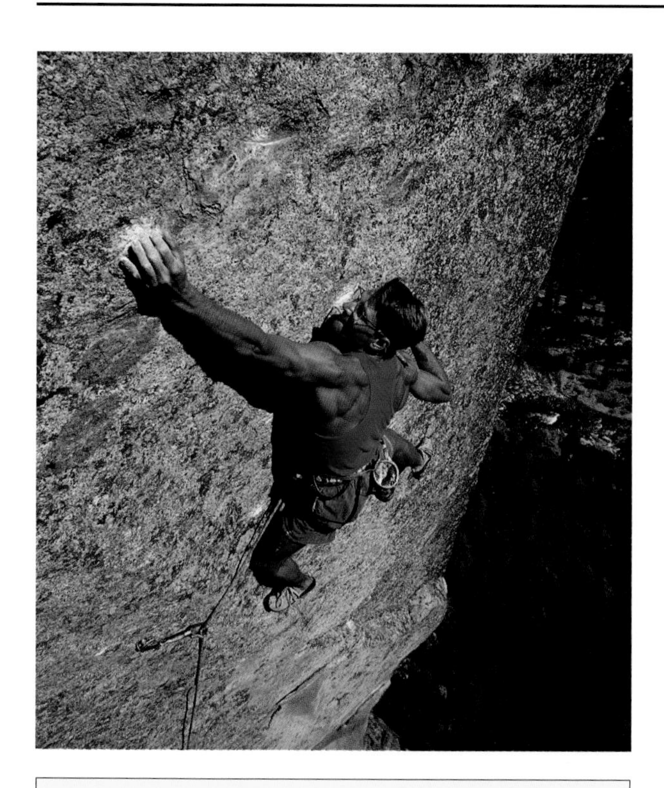

Figure 7.8 High altitude has an effect on EPO production which in turn generates a high production of red blood cells.

produced CO_2 is dissolved in the blood plasma; (2) CO_2 also bonds to the hemoglobin molecule (remember that hemoglobin has unloaded its oxygen at the tissues so is capable of carrying CO_2 from the tissues to the lungs); and (3) CO_2 combines with water (primary mechanism) to form bicarbonate molecules (H_2CO_3), which are then transported through the body. This happens according to the following reversible reaction:

$$CO_2 + H_2O \longleftrightarrow H_2CO_3 \xleftrightarrow[\text{Anhydrase}]{\text{Carbonic}} H^+ + HCO_3^-$$

This reaction is also critical for the body's defense against changes in acidity.

Oxygen Uptake

Oxygen uptake is the amount of oxygen that is consumed by the body due to aerobic metabolism. It is measured as the volume of oxygen (in liters) that is consumed ($\dot{V}O_2$) in a given amount of time, usually a minute. Oxygen uptake increases in relation to the amount of energy that is required to perform an activity; however, there is a limit to the amount of oxygen that the body can consume. One measure that is commonly used to evaluate the maximal volume of oxygen that can be supplied to and consumed by the body is **maximal aerobic power ($\dot{V}O_2$max)** (Figure 7.9).

The cardiovascular system can have an impact upon the amount of oxygen that is consumed by the body. For example, since the cardiac output determines the amount of blood that is delivered to the body, and blood is what carries oxygen to the tissues, any changes in cardiac output will alter the $\dot{V}O_2$. Changes in hematocrit (concentration of red blood cells) can also alter the oxygen uptake by increasing or decreasing the amount of oxygen that is supplied to working tissues. The ability of the tissues to extract oxygen (a–v O_2 difference) directly affects the oxygen uptake. Increases in a–v O_2 difference may arise from an increased

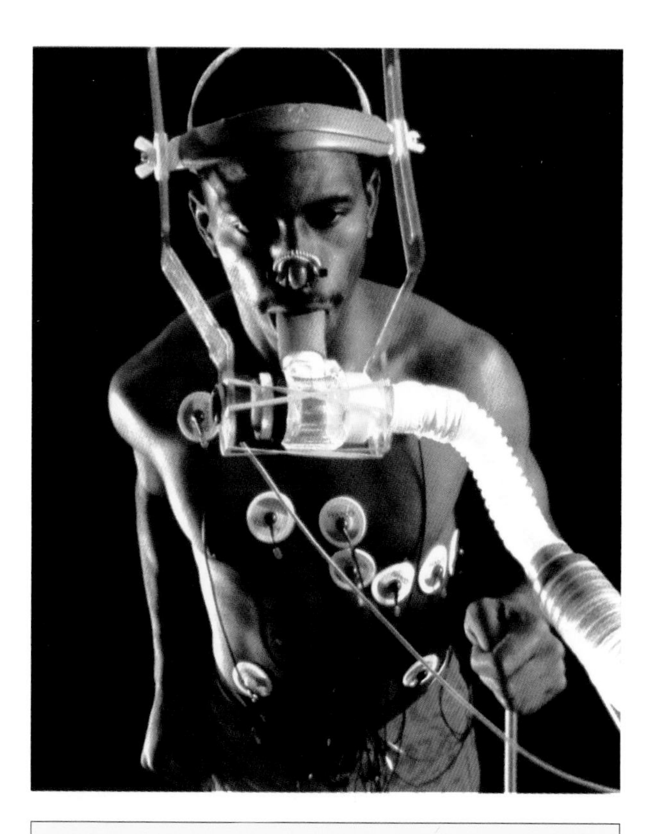

Figure 7.9 Testing for maximal oxygen uptake or aerobic power.

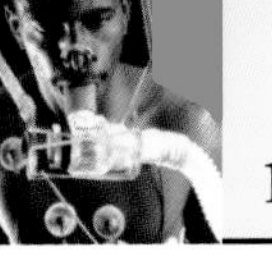

number of mitochondria in muscles, increased enzyme efficiency in working tissues resulting in increased processing of oxygen, or for other reasons. Increased **capillarization** (number of capillaries in tissue) can affect the ability of the circulatory system to place red blood cells close to the tissues that are using the oxygen, thus increasing the ability of those tissues to extract the required oxygen because of a shorter diffusion distance.

> **Terminology Alert!**
>
> In most literature, the following terms are used synonymously with $\dot{V}O_2$max:
>
> - aerobic power;
> - maximal aerobic power;
> - maximal oxygen uptake; and
> - maximal oxygen consumption.

Cardiovascular limits ($\dot{V}O_2$max) can be described by multiplying the central component, cardiac output, by the effectiveness of peripheral factors (a–v O_2 difference). The central component primarily concerns the effectiveness of the heart and the ability of the lungs to oxygenate the blood. The peripheral factors include the ability of the body to extract that oxygen. Training can increase the maximal oxygen consumption of the human body by improving both the central and peripheral components. How this is accomplished will be presented in the next section.

Respiratory Anatomy and Physiology

One can survive without food for as much as several weeks and without water for several days, but if one stops breathing for only three to six minutes, death is likely. The respiratory system is closely integrated with the cardiovascular system. Both these systems have similar functions in that they deliver oxygen and nutrients to the body and remove carbon dioxide and waste products. The primary role of the respiratory system is to deliver oxygenated air to the blood and remove carbon dioxide, a by-product of metabolism, and to aid in acid–base balance.

Structure

The respiratory system includes the lungs, the several passageways leading from outside to the lungs, and the muscles that are responsible for the mechanical movements that move air into and out of the lungs. The two lungs are located within the thoracic cavity (the chest). Unlike most organs in the human body, the lungs are asymmetrical. The right lung is larger than the left lung because the heart takes up more space on the left side.

The air passages of the respiratory system are divided into two functional areas, the conduction zone and respiratory zone. The **conduction zone** consists of the anatomical structures through which air passes before reaching the respiratory zone. Air enters through the **nose** and/or **mouth**, where it is filtered, humidified, and adjusted to body temperature in the **trachea** (windpipe). The trachea branches into the **right** and **left bronchi**, which enter the lungs and continue to branch into smaller and smaller tubes called **bronchioles**, and finally, the **terminal bronchioles**. The whole system inside the lungs looks so similar to an upside-down tree that it is commonly called the **"respiration tree"** (Figure 7.10).

The bronchioles continue to branch into the **respiratory zone**, the region where gas exchange occurs. The functional units of the lungs are tiny air sacs, known as **alveoli**. It is in these 300 million alveoli where gas exchange occurs. A single alveolus looks like a bubble. Alveoli are clustered in bunches like grapes, with a common opening into an alveolar duct, and each cluster is called an alveolar sac (Figures 7.10 and 7.12).

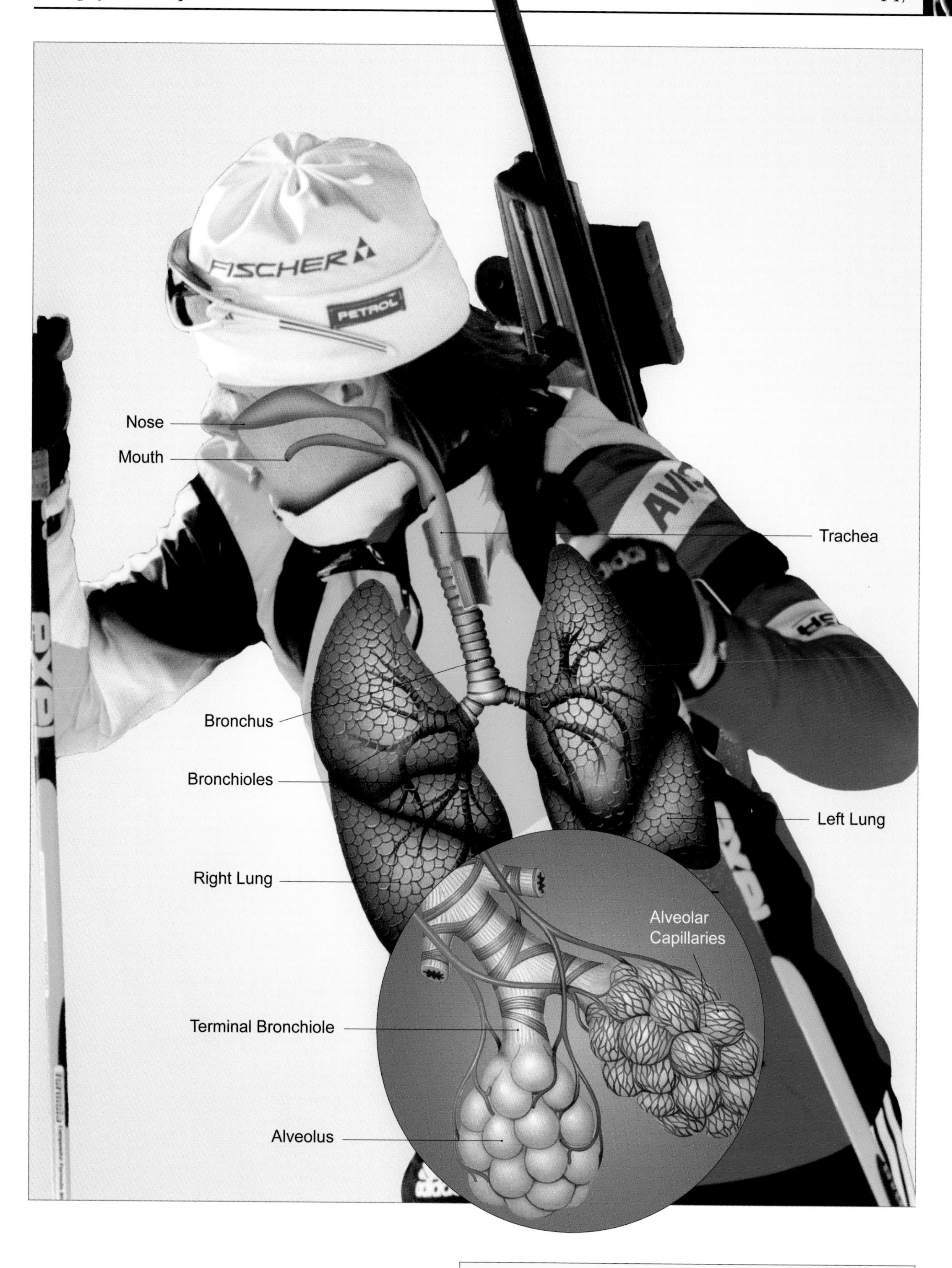

Figure 7.10 The structure of the respiratory system.

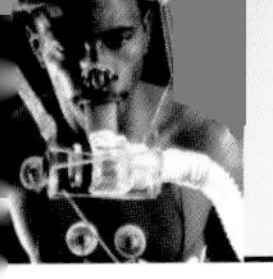

Function

Ventilation

Several phases are involved in human respiration:

(1) **ventilation** or **breathing**, which includes two phases, inspiration and expiration;

(2) **gas exchange**, which occurs between the air and blood in the lungs and between the blood and other tissues of the body; and

(3) **oxygen utilization** by the tissues for **cellular respiration.**

Atmospheric air is composed mainly of oxygen and nitrogen, with a small amount of carbon dioxide. The gases of interest in respiration are oxygen and carbon dioxide. Ventilation involves the movement of air into (**inspiration**) and out of (**expiration**) the lungs.

Changes in the size of the thoracic cavity, and thus of the lungs, allow us to inhale and exhale air. Lungs are normally light, soft, and spongy to allow for expansion in the thoracic cavity. It is the continual work of the muscles surrounding the thoracic cavity that results in the change in the thoracic cavity. These muscles include the **diaphragm** (Figure 7.12) and the **intercostal muscles.** During inspiration, the thoracic cavity expands via muscle contractions, causing the air pressure inside to be lowered, forcing a flow of air into the lungs. When the thoracic cavity shrinks during expiration via muscle relaxation, the increased pressure inside causes air contained in the lungs to flow out.

Gas Exchange in the Lungs

Gas exchange between the air and blood in the lungs occurs at the alveoli. Alveoli are only a single cell layer thick, thus facilitating gas diffusion. Each bubble-like alveolus is surrounded by a vast network of pulmonary capillaries (Figure

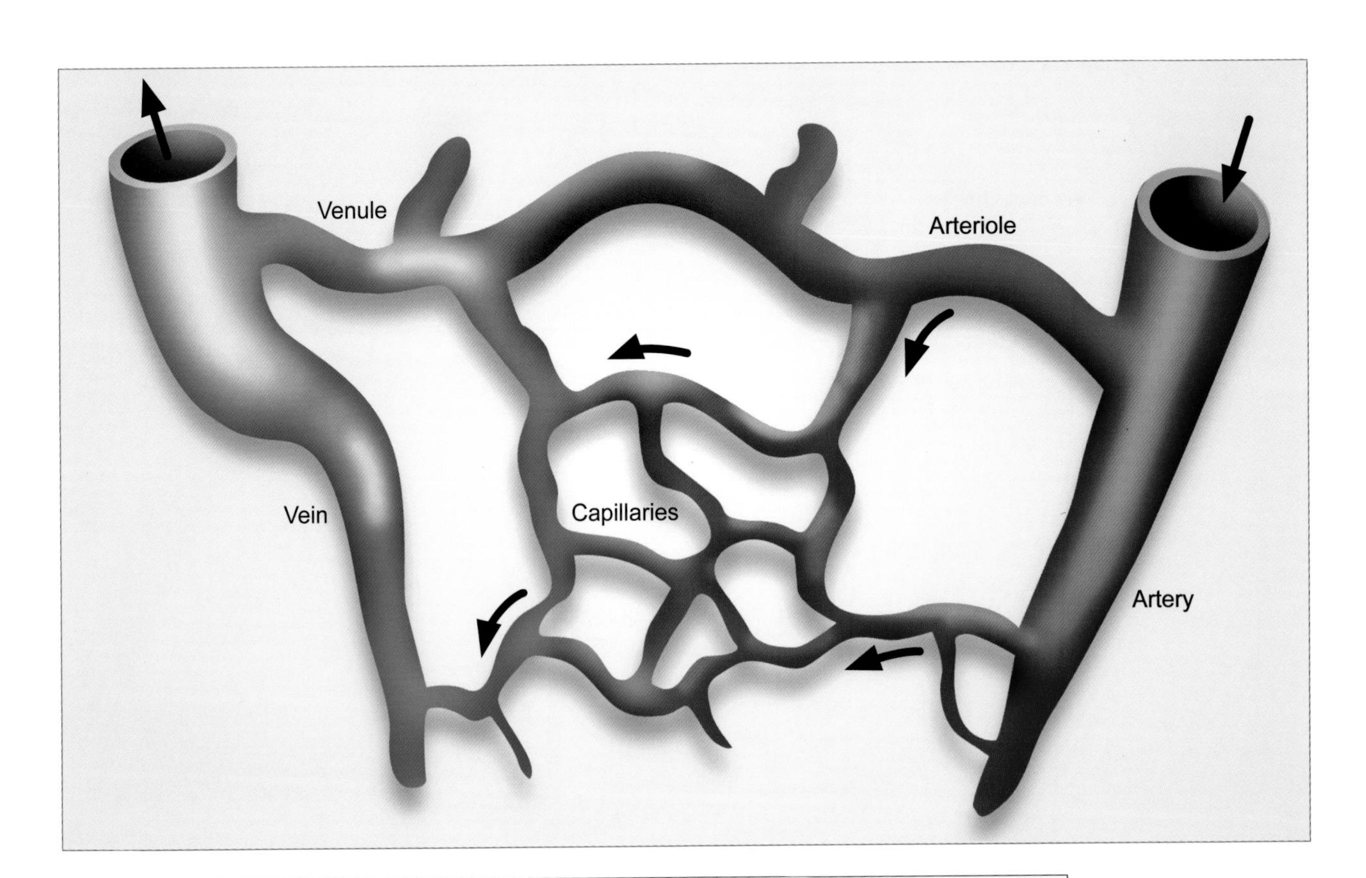

Figure 7.11 The network of pulmonary capillaries where gas exchange takes place.

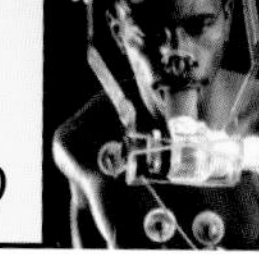

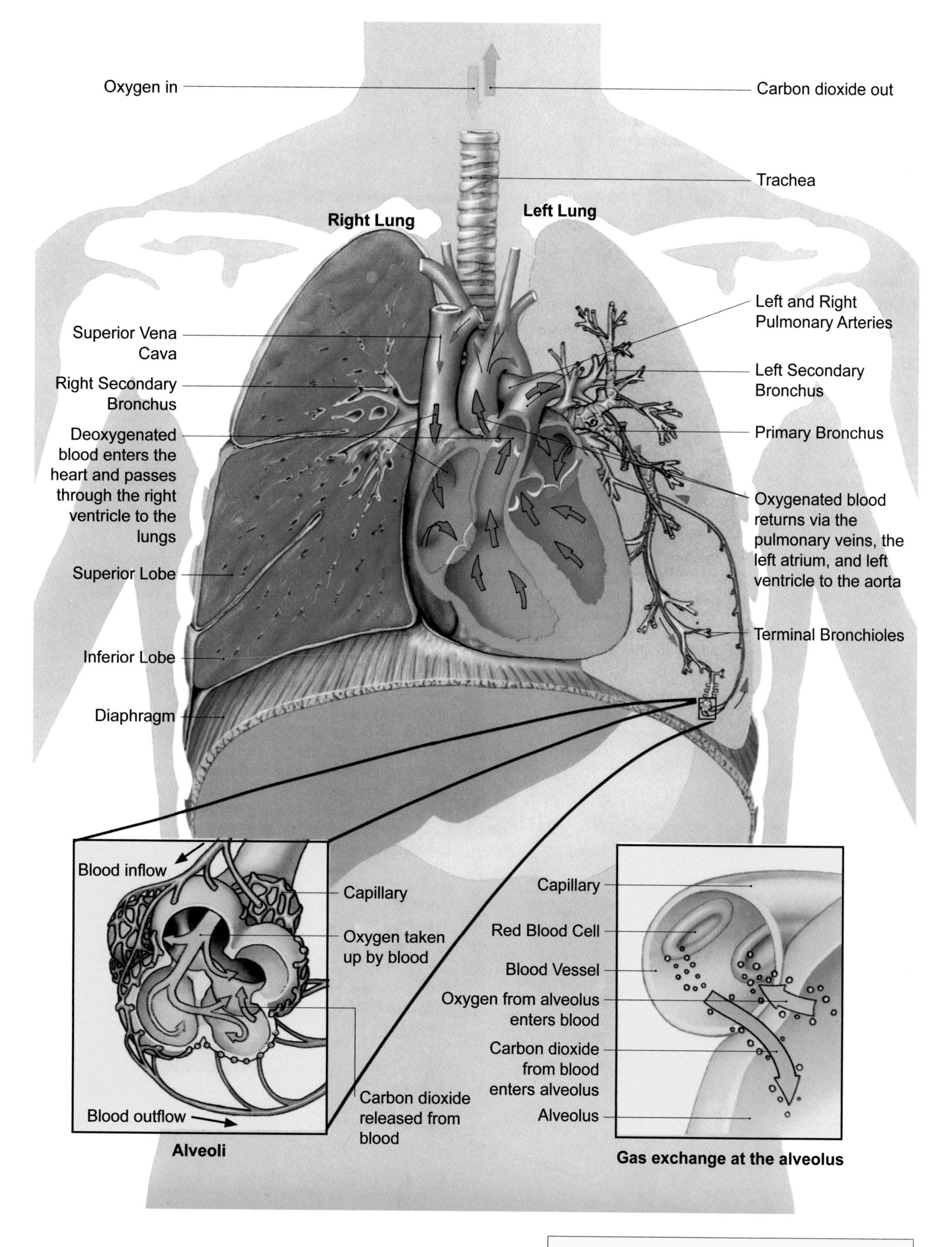

Figure 7.12 Gas exchange in the alveoli.

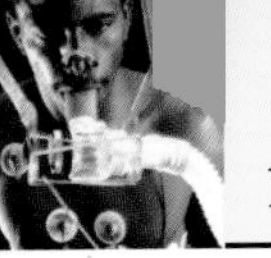

7.11). The atmospheric air, which has made its way into each alveolus, is rich in oxygen. The blood in the pulmonary capillaries is loaded with the waste product of carbon dioxide. This difference in concentration in these gases sets up ideal conditions for **gas diffusion**. Diffusion is the movement of molecules (gases) from a higher concentration to a lower concentration. Therefore, the oxygen from the atmospheric air diffuses through the alveolar membrane into deoxygenated pulmonary capillaries (Figure 7.12). Carbon dioxide diffuses in the opposite direction, from the carbon dioxide–rich pulmonary blood into the alveoli, where the concentration of carbon dioxide is lower. The carbon dioxide is exhaled. The oxygenated blood follows the pulmonary circulation to reach the heart's left ventricle, where it is distributed throughout the body via the systemic circulation.

Exercise Effects on the Cardiovascular and Respiratory Systems

Exercise can have many beneficial effects on the cardiovascular and respiratory systems. The cardiovascular system adjusts to meet the demands of exercise. These adjustments ensure an adequate blood supply to working muscles, the brain, and the heart and ensure that heat and waste products generated by muscles are dissipated and removed. The benefits are important as they can lead to an improvement in quality of life by allowing people to do more with less effort, as well as by reducing disease and improving overall health and vitality. These benefits, known as exercise training effects, are presented in Figure 7.13 and discussed in this section.

Cardiac Output

The first effect of training on the cardiovascular system concerns changes in the heart (Figure 7.13 A). Endurance training has been shown to increase the size of the heart. The increase in heart size may arise from an increase in the size of the heart cavities (ventricles and atria) as well as an increase in the thickness of the walls of the heart. The benefits to the cardiovascular system realized by an increase in heart size include: the larger atria and ventricles allow for a greater volume of blood to be pumped each time the heart beats; and the increased thickness of the walls of the heart (the walls of the heart are made up of cardiac muscle) allows for an increased contractility (rate of contraction) and also a greater emptying of the ventricles each time the heart beats. The end result is a greater cardiac output (heart rate x stroke volume) during each heartbeat and thus an increase in the efficiency of the heart.

Capillary Supply

Increased capillarization (number of capillaries in a given space) is another benefit that may arise as a result of endurance training (Figure 7.13 B). An increased capillarization allows for a greater surface area and reduced distance between the blood and the surrounding tissues, thus increasing diffusion capacity of oxygen and carbon dioxide, as well as easing the transport of nutrients to cells. An increased capillarization also occurs in cardiac muscle, reducing the possibility of cardiac disease and heart attacks. The a–v O_2 difference of the body can be improved by endurance training. Essentially this means that the body can be trained to extract more oxygen from the blood. This can be achieved because endurance training increases circulation (blood flow) to the capillaries that are next to muscle fibers, as discussed. This provides a greater surface area for the exchange of nutrients, oxygen, and carbon dioxide. Another factor that increases the ability of the body to extract oxygen is the ability of muscle cells to process oxygen through aerobic metabolism that occurs in mitochondria (see Chapter 6, Energy for Muscular Activity). Endurance training increases both the number and activity levels of mitochondria in muscle fibers.

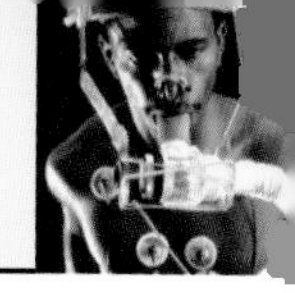

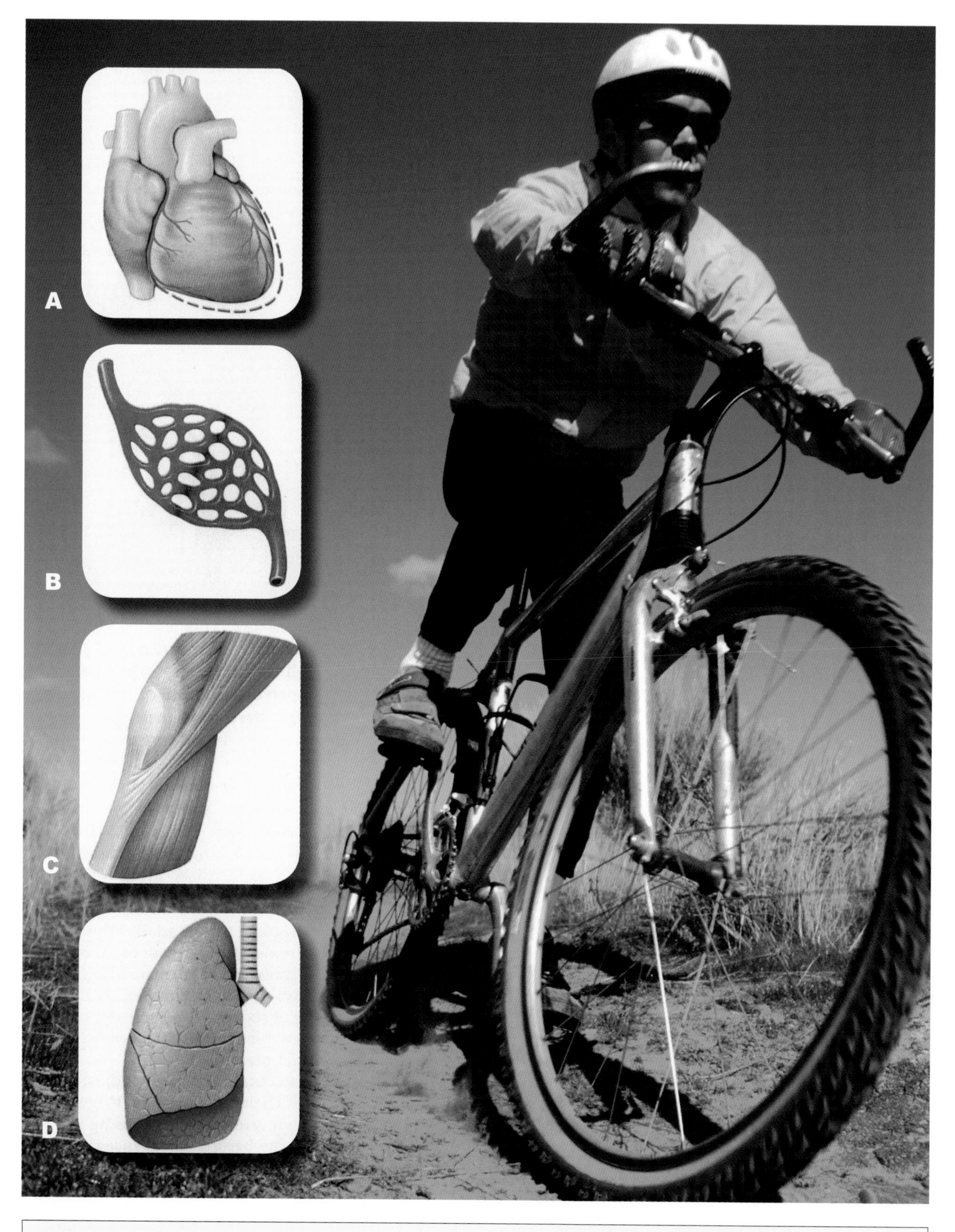

Figure 7.13 The dynamic exercise (aerobic) training effect on the cardiovascular and respiratory systems. **A.** Increase in the size of the heart. **B.** Increased capillarization. **C.** Increase in the amount of extracted oxygen from circulating blood in working muscles. **D.** Increased efficiency in gas exchange.

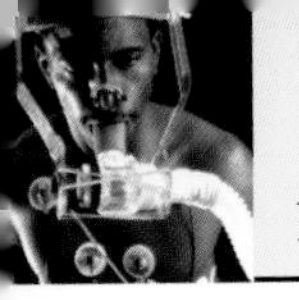

Blood Volume

Total blood volume has been shown to increase with training as the number and total volume of red blood cells are increased through stimulation of erythropoiesis (formation of new red blood cells) in the bone marrow. Both of these factors can have positive effects on the efficiency of the cardiovascular system, primarily by increasing the ability of the blood to carry a greater amount of oxygen and by decreasing the thickness (viscosity) of the blood. The amount of extracted oxygen from the circulated blood is significantly increased in the working muscles, thereby increasing their efficiency (Figure 7.13 C).

Ventilation

During dynamic exercise, breathing becomes deeper and more rapid. Ventilation increases with exercise in order to meet the increased demand of gas exchange. During exercise, ventilation can increase from 6 L/min at rest to over 150 L/min during maximal exercise. The increased air flow allows for more gas exchange to occur. With continuous dynamic activity such as running, swimming, cross-country skiing, and bicycling, the lungs become more efficient in gas exchange (Figure 7.13 D).

The Bohr Effect

During exercise, body temperature increases. An increased body temperature, in turn, promotes oxygen extraction. This phenomenon is known as the **Bohr effect**. It describes the reduced effectiveness of hemoglobin to hold oxygen. This phenomenon, accompanied by an increase in metabolic heat, carbon dioxide production, and lactic acid concentration, is important in vigorous exercise because even more oxygen is released to the working muscle tissue. However, in the alveoli the Bohr effect is negligible, thus allowing hemoglobin to maximally load with oxygen.

The Bohr effect is another example of an exercise training effect that occurs in the human body.

Exercise and Environments

In general, the environmental conditions under which exercise takes place do not change much. If the environment does change, it creates additional stresses on the various physiological systems of the body.

Two common examples of environmental changes are altitude and temperature.

Altitude

The air we breathe is primarily made up of 79.04 percent nitrogen, 20.93 percent oxygen, and 0.03 percent carbon dioxide. At **altitude**, the percentages of these molecules remain the same but the density of molecules changes. The term **thin air** is often used to describe the condition of air at altitude. Since the body requires a certain amount or volume of oxygen (obtained during each breath), a lower density of oxygen molecules per unit volume of air means a person at altitude must breathe more frequently or more deeply to obtain the necessary amount of oxygen. This **hyperventilation** is a hallmark of altitude exposure.

Although hyperventilation provides the necessary amount of oxygen to the body, it has

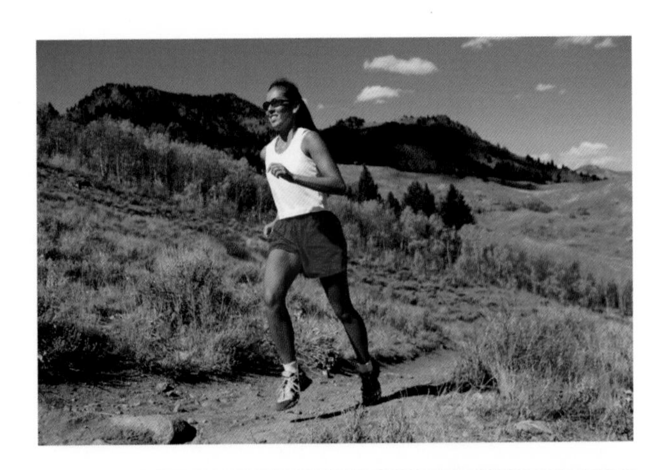

Figure 7.14 Exercising at altitude results in various positive physiological adaptations.

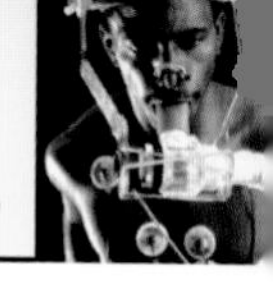

the negative consequence of "blowing off" a greater than normal amount of carbon dioxide, which changes the acid–base (pH) balance and thus influences other physiological systems and processes. With sudden or large changes in altitude, the body cannot always adequately adapt, and **acute mountain sickness (AMS)** can occur. The symptoms and severity of AMS vary from a headache to cerebral or pulmonary edema, which can cause death.

One consequence of exercising at altitude is that the heart must work harder to compensate for the reduced amount of available oxygen. This partially explains the higher heart rates observed upon initial altitude exposure. However, given enough time, the body offsets the increased cardiac work by improving the oxygen-carrying capacity of the blood. This is accomplished by increasing both the number of red blood cells (*hematocrit*) and the amount of hemoglobin (the protein that carries oxygen) in the red blood cells. After a few weeks, these adaptations ease the work of the heart, and homeostasis is restored (Figure 7.14). Athletes often train at altitude in hopes of acquiring these adaptations so that when they return to lower altitudes, they can derive the benefits of an increased oxygen-carrying capacity. Whether altitude training actually provides benefits is currently under investigation.

Temperature

While at rest, the body loses heat primarily through radiation. That is, heat warms the surrounding air and objects and is dissipated electromagnetically. During exercise, heat must be released to maintain a constant core temperature. About 80 percent of the energy released during exercise is released as heat.

As heat builds up in the body, sweat glands produce sweat on the skin surface. As the sweat evaporates, heat is removed from the body. In humid conditions, when the air already holds a great deal of water, it becomes more difficult for the sweat to evaporate, and heat tends to be stored in the body. Core temperature increases as a result, along with the possibility of developing the potentially fatal condition of **hyperthermia**, or **heat stroke**.

Heat generated by the muscles is transported to the skin by the blood. During exercise in the heat, the circulatory system performs the dual function of delivering oxygen to the tissues as well as transporting blood to the skin (*peripheral vasodilation*) to allow for heat dissipation. Since these two events are mutually exclusive, athletes exercising in the heat often exhibit an increased heart rate at submaximal workloads to accommodate for the reduced blood flow to the muscles. This means that the heart will have to work harder than normal and maximal heart rate will be reached sooner. In addition, fluid loss through sweat will eventually lead to a reduced stroke volume, which further compromises cardiac output. An athlete is therefore unable to work at the same absolute intensity under hot or humid conditions than when exercising in a normal environment.

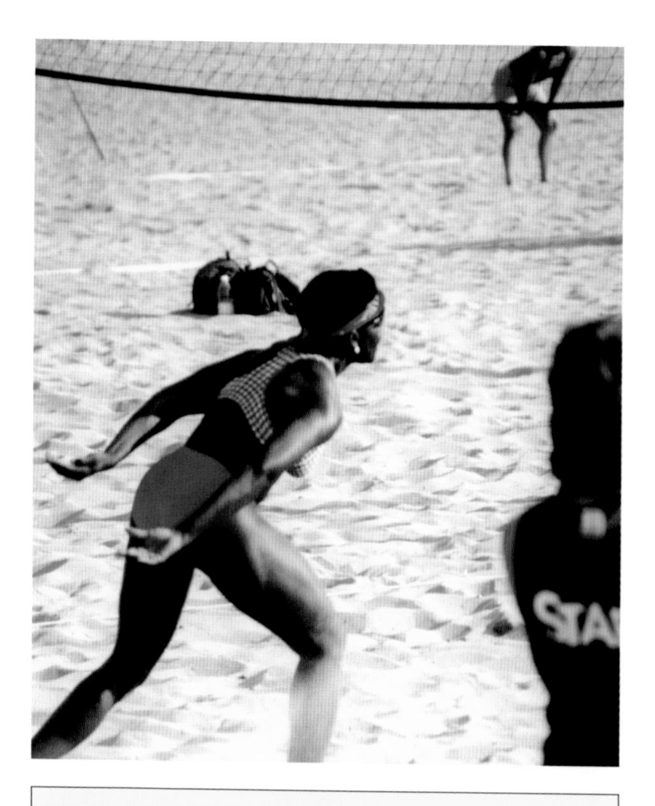

Figure 7.15 Fluid replenishment is vital to avoid the potentially dangerous effects of hyperthermia when exercising in the heat.

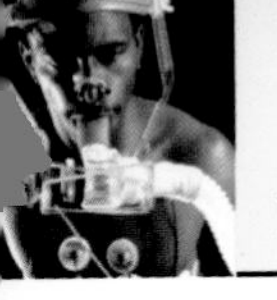

Since the body is sweating at a high rate, fluid replenishment is vital. If fluids are not replaced, core temperature will rise and hyperthermia may occur (Figure 7.15). Over time, the body can adapt to exercise in the heat by maintaining core temperature and minimizing increased heart rate, as well as by increasing the ability to sweat and therefore lose heat.

Summary

The cardiovascular and respiratory systems are made up of interconnected organs that include the heart, lungs, and blood vessels, as well as the blood itself. These systems' four primary functions are the transportation of (1) oxygen from the lungs to the tissues; (2) carbon dioxide from the tissues to the lungs; (3) nutrients from the digestive system to other areas in the body; and (4) waste products from sites of production to sites of excretion.

Several key aspects of the cardiovascular system can be measured and monitored. Blood pressure (systolic and diastolic) is an important gauge of cardiac function. Heart rate is the number of times the heart beats in one minute, and the amount of blood pumped by the left ventricle with each heartbeat is known as the stroke volume. Another factor, cardiac output, is the product of stroke volume and heart rate. Cardiac output represents the amount of blood that is pumped into the aorta each minute by the heart; it therefore indicates the quantity of blood that flows to the peripheral circulation.

Oxygen uptake is the amount of oxygen consumed by the body due to aerobic metabolism. One measure commonly used to evaluate the maximal volume of oxygen that can be supplied to, and consumed by, the body is maximal aerobic power, or $\dot{V}O_2max$, expressed in liters per minute. The difference in the amount of oxygen that is present in the blood as it leaves the lungs and the amount of oxygen that is present in the blood when it returns to the lungs is called the arterial–venous oxygen difference (a–v O_2 difference).

Key Terms

action potential
acute mountain sickness (AMS)
altitude
alveoli
arterial–venous oxygen (a–v O_2) difference
arteriole
artery
bohr effect
bronchiole
bronchus
capillary
cardiac output
conduction zone
diaphragm
diastole
erythropoietin (EPO)
expiration
gas diffusion
heart rate
hematocrit
hemoglobin
hyperthermia (heat stroke)
hyperventilation
inferior vena cava
inspiration
left atrium
left ventricle
maximal aerobic power ($\dot{V}O_2max$)
plasma
red blood cell (erythrocyte)
respiratory zone
reticulocytes
right atrium
right ventricle
sinus node
stroke volume
superior vena cava
systole
terminal bronchiole
trachea
valve
vein
ventilation
venule
white blood cell

Discussion Questions

1. Describe the path and all related steps that a molecule of oxygen would take from the air in the lungs to a muscle cell.

2. Describe the path and all related steps that a molecule of carbon dioxide could take from a muscle cell to the air in the lungs.

3. Define and provide the units for blood pressure, heart rate, cardiac output, stroke volume, and arterial–venous oxygen difference.

4. List the ways in which training improves the effectiveness of the cardiovascular and respiratory systems.

5. Describe the two components of blood pressure. What do they measure?

6. What is hemoglobin? Where is it found? What is its purpose?

7. What is hematocrit?

8. Describe the ways in which carbon dioxide can be transported through the blood.

9. What is $\dot{V}O_2max$? What factors influence this measure? How is it affected by training?

10. Discuss the many benefits of exercise on the cardiovascular and respiratory systems.

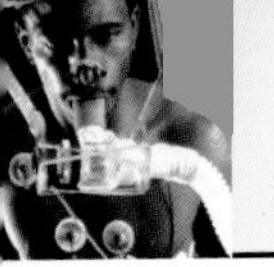

A Career in Fitness

NAME: Susan S. Lee
OCCUPATION: Personal Trainer-Manager
Executive Director, Canadian Personal Trainers Network
Program Manager, University of Toronto Athletic Centre
EDUCATION: Harbord Collegiate (Secondary School)
BPHE, University of Toronto (Bachelor of Physical and Health Education)
MPE, University of British Columbia (Master in Physical Education)

What do you do?

I work in the field of personal training as the executive director of the Canadian Personal Trainers Network (CPTN), an organization which specializes in education, certification, leadership, and advocacy for fitness professionals. Since 1993, I have provided leadership for the development of a national certification program for personal trainers, and specialty workshops (such as The Art and Science of Personal Training, Golf Conditioning Specialist, Post-Rehabilitation Functional Training, Nutrition 101, and Pilates Mat and Ballwork Specialist). At the University of Toronto Athletic Centre, I implemented and supervise the personal training program which services the students, staff, faculty, and community members.

What is unique about your roles?

I am often viewed as a resource person for the fitness and personal training industries. I have had the opportunity to develop curriculum for new workshops and technical manuals for the industry. I co-authored a book entitled *Business Strategies for Personal Training*. I am often quoted by the media as a result of interviews for magazines and newspapers. I speak on fitness and personal training at national and international conferences, allowing me to share my insights with international audiences in China, Australia, Canada, and the U.S.

How did studies in physical and health education benefit your career choice?

My university degrees provided me with a solid foundation in the theoretical frameworks and practical applications of physical and health education. The combination of a strong academic background and broad work experiences provided me with the confidence to pursue my professional career. My education has allowed me to develop new products and services for the fitness industry, and to become a leader and mentor for novice personal trainers.

What are the future prospects in the field?

Personal training is becoming a popular career choice for individuals who enjoy physical activity and want to share this enthusiasm with others. The demand for personal training is on the rise as a result of the aging population, as well as concerns about the rise in obesity among children, youth, and adults. Physical activity through personal training will be one career to address the health needs of the general population.

What career advice would you give to students interested in this field?

Students interested in personal training will need a solid background in physical and health education through university or college, or personal training workshops. Most trainers now become certified with a reputable organization to identify themselves as quality trainers. The public is looking for well-educated personal trainers. To succeed in the industry, learn about cardiorespiratory, strength training, and flexibility training techniques. Excellent communication skills are required as well. You can practice your communication skills through public speaking and develop your interpersonal skills by working on projects with peers or participating on a sports team. To be an entrepreneur in the industry, business courses will provide you with the skills to become successful in your own personal training business.

What do you enjoy most about your profession?

I enjoy meeting people and learning about their unique needs and interests, and then being able to provide them with an exercise program and the professional support to reach their goals. I often find myself training people for the sport of life. I am in the business of improving people's quality of life by helping them become stronger and more confident through physical activity. A sedentary client who can be transformed into an active one is one of my greatest rewards.

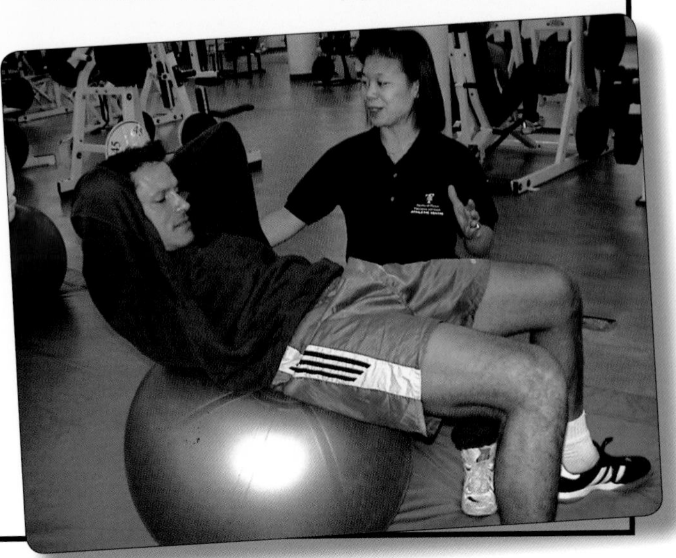

UNIT 3

Biomechanics and Motor Control

- How Do I Move? The Science of Biomechanics
- Technology and Sport
- Information Processing in Human Movement
- Movement Intelligence: A Vast Store of Motor Programs

In This Chapter:

CHAPTER 8

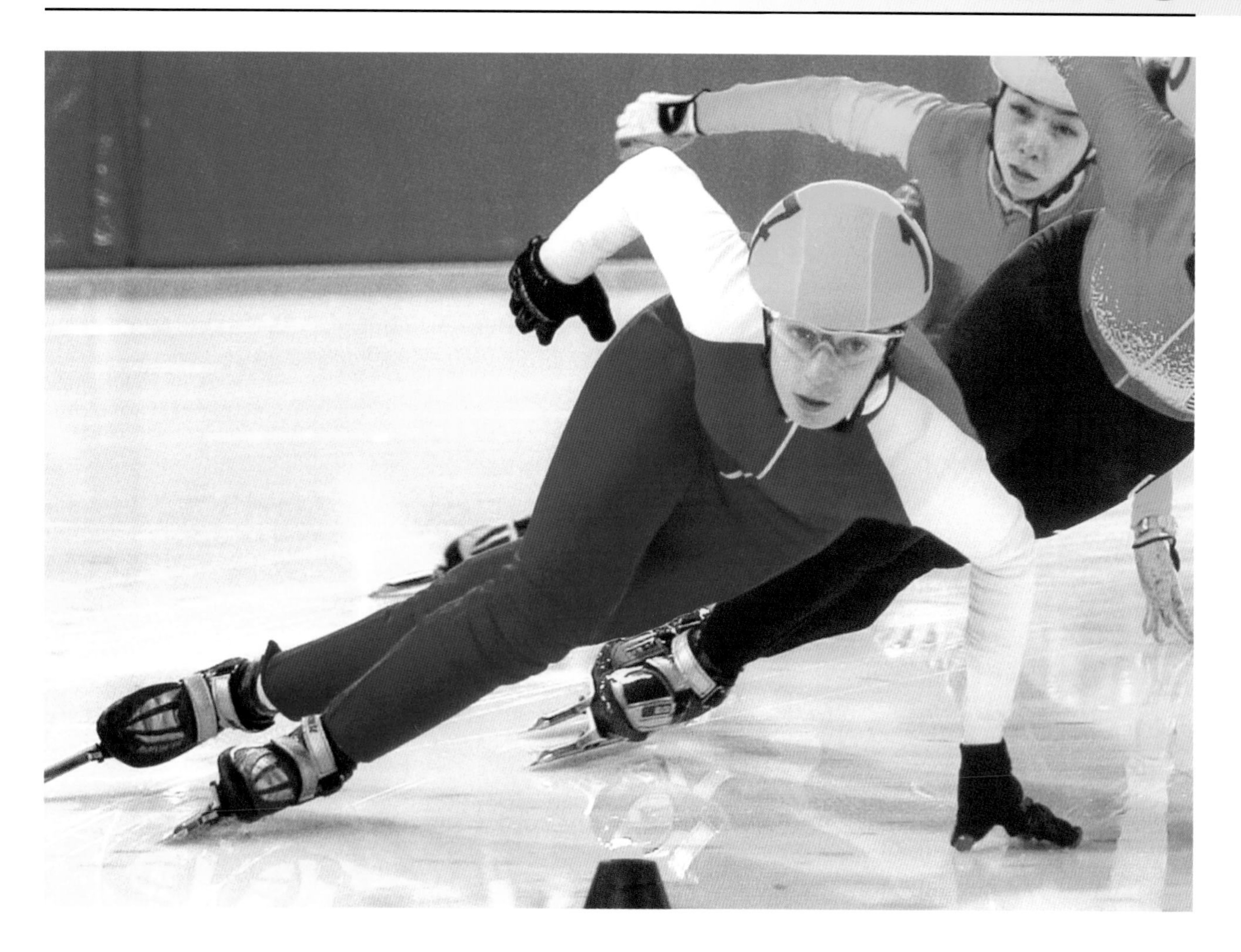

How Do I Move? The Science of Biomechanics

After completing this chapter you should be able to:

- distinguish between different types and causes of human motion;
- identify Newton's laws of motion and describe practical illustrations of the laws;
- describe the expected path and motion of a projectile;
- describe the conservation of momentum within the body, and explain why changes in the configuration of a rotating airborne body produce changes in its angular velocity;
- explain the role of friction in the context of fluid dynamics;
- evaluate qualitative analyses of human motion.

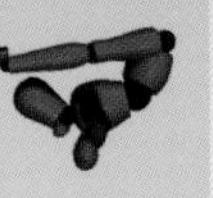

The capabilities of the human body seem endless. From a baby's first step, to an Olympic performance, we marvel at the wide range of human movements that are possible. We have all witnessed the powerful gymnast who explodes off the floor to perform three rotations in the air before landing on his or her feet, or the diver who twists and turns in the air before entering the water with delicate precision. But what causes these movements? How do we describe them? Are there limitations to what we can do? Biomechanics, one of the biophysical sciences that make up the field of physical and health education, tries to describe the causes and effects of how the body moves.

Biomechanics is a science that examines the internal and external forces acting on the human body and the effects produced by these forces. It is considered a relatively young field of scientific inquiry, but many other scientific disciplines and professional fields make use of biomechanical considerations. People in various walks of life, including physical and health education, use the principles of biomechanics. Academic backgrounds in fields such as sports medicine, physical therapy, kinesiology, biomechanical engineering, and even zoology can offer important knowledge to the biomechanical aspects of the structure and function of living things.

For example, biomechanics allows us to understand why humans walk the way we do, what effect gravity has on the human musculoskeletal system, how mobility impairment in the elderly can be improved, and how a prosthesis can aid individuals with below-knee amputations. These are real concerns that can have a significant impact on the lives of many people. Sport biomechanists and engineers have also contributed invaluably to improving performances in selected sports, such as wheel and helmet designs for cycling, optimal body positioning for ski jumping during the flight phase, and the most effective technique for throwing a discus. Have you ever wondered why some golfers tend to slice the ball, or why pole-vaulting records have continued to fall since the introduction of fiberglass poles?

From playing surfaces and equipment to shoes, biomechanics plays an important role in recognizing what practices are perhaps less effective and less dangerous and how athletes optimize performance. Research continues to be conducted in an attempt to highlight these concerns and provide more effective alternatives.

Obviously, research involving biomechanics is extremely diverse and multifaceted. From analyzing technique to developing innovative equipment designs, biomechanics has significantly added to our knowledge of human movement. Before the advent of fiberglass poles, clearing a height of 20 feet (6 meters) in pole vaulting would have seemed unreachable. Understanding the mechanical principles that underlie human movement can help answer questions related to human health and performance. This chapter will provide you with the foundation necessary to identify, analyze, and effectively answer questions related to the biomechanics of human movement.

Types of Study

Quantitative Versus Qualitative Analysis

Biomechanists spend a great deal of time devising techniques to measure those biomechanical variables that are believed to optimize performance. These scientists may investigate (1) the pattern of forces exerted by the foot onto the sprinter's starting block; (2) the sequence of muscle activity during running using electromyography; or (3) the three-dimensional movements of each body segment during a high jump using high-speed cinematography or an automated motion analyzing system. These studies are examples of **quantitative analyses** of performance. A quantitative analysis is intended for use by researchers and will be left for further study.

Coaches and teachers do not always have available to them the necessary equipment to perform these analyses and thus must rely on

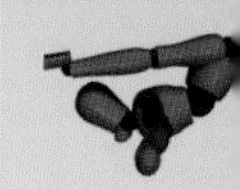

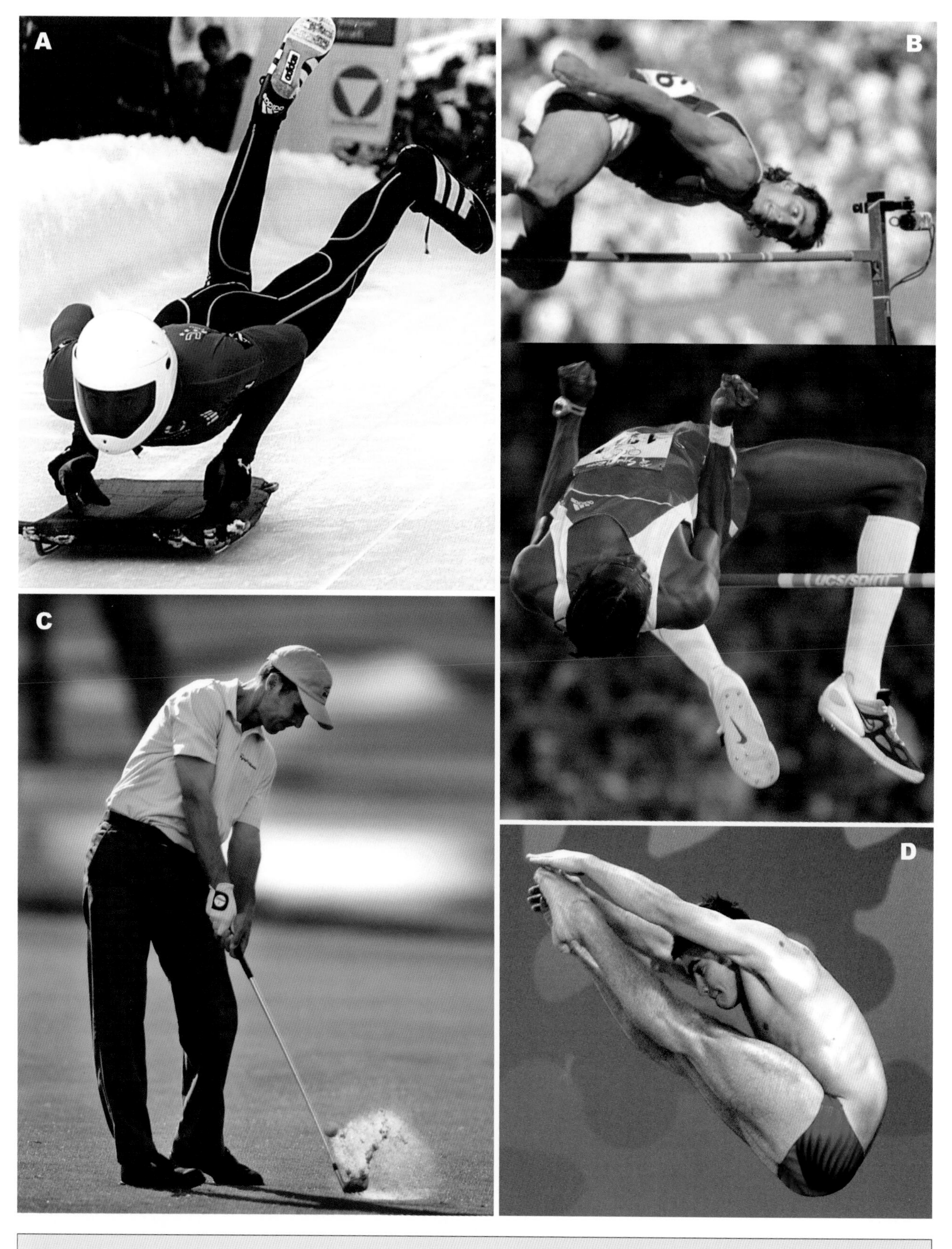

Figure 8.1 Biomechanics can help us understand sport performances by suggesting better teaching and coaching techniques (A), comparing different techniques for performing the same skill (B), and improving error detection and correction techniques (C, D).

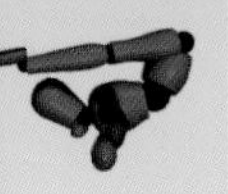

Kinematic Variables

Time

How long does it take to run a race, to swing a bat, to perform a karate chop, or to prepare to jump in volleyball? How long is a diver airborne before entering the water? *How long* refers to the temporal characteristics of a performance, either of the total skill or of its phases. It is a time interval calculated as the difference between the beginning and end of two instants of time.

Displacement

Displacement is the **length** and **direction** of the path an athlete traverses from the start to finish of a performance or portion thereof. Sprinters run 100 meters east. Volleyball players jump 0.8 meters up during a block.

Angular Displacement

Angular displacement measures the direction of and **smallest angular change** between the rotating body's initial and final position. In standing up from a chair, the knee joint and hip joint both rotate through approximately 90 degrees but in opposite directions (i.e., clockwise and counter-clockwise). A diver performing a front 1½ dive would have an angular displacement of 180 degrees clockwise or counterclockwise.

Velocity

Velocity is the measure of the displacement per unit time. Velocities can be calculated as instantaneous (i.e., occurring over a very small time interval) or as average, where the time interval is longer (i.e., the time it takes to run a complete race). The top sprinters in the world, such as Asafa Powell of Jamaica, have reached peak velocities over 12 m/s and average velocities over 10 m/s (e.g., 100 m / 9.77 s = 10.24 m/s) in competition.

Angular Velocity

Angular velocity is the measure of angular displacement per unit time, or how fast a body is rotating. The rotation of the arm about the shoulder joint during the delivery swing of a bowling ball has a lower angular velocity than the same movement in a fastball pitcher.

Acceleration

Acceleration is the rate of change of velocity. Success in many sports activities depends upon the athlete's ability to increase or decrease speed and/or direction rapidly, such as changes of direction in basketball or football, or stealing a base in baseball, or sprinting a 100-meter dash, or throwing a shot, or decreasing the velocity of a ball when catching in handball.

Angular Acceleration

Angular acceleration is the measure of change in angular velocity per unit time. During a giant swing, a gymnast begins from a handstand and swings once around the bar. The gymnast accelerates clockwise on the way down but experiences deceleration clockwise during the up phase.

any information they can readily obtain, visual or aural, to assess performance. This type of analysis is known as a **qualitative analysis**. A qualitative analysis requires a framework within which skilled performances can be observed, a set of principles within which movement can be analyzed, a checklist to use when identifying errors, and techniques to use to correct errors in performance. Good qualitative analyses lead to good quantitative analyses.

Whether they are working with developing or advanced athletes, biomechanists can provide coaches and instructors with (1) knowledge on how a skill is done; (2) a basis for the comparison of techniques; (3) better teaching and coaching techniques; and (4) improved ability to detect and correct errors in performance (Figure 8.1).

Kinematics Versus Kinetics

The study of **kinematics** describes spatial and timing characteristics of motion of the human body and its segments. These variables are used to describe both linear and angular motion (see box *Kinematic Variables*). They answer four questions: how long? how far? how fast? and how consistent was the motion?

Kinetics, on the other hand, focuses on the various forces that cause a movement: that is, the forces that produce the movement and the resulting motion. The forces, which act on the human body, can be **internal** or **external.** Internal forces refer to forces generated by muscles pulling on bones via their tendons and to bone-on-bone forces exerted across joint surfaces. External forces on the body refer to those forces acting from without, such as the force of **gravity,** or the force from any body contact with the ground, environment, sport equipment, or opponent. In general, internal forces *cause* individual body segment movements, while external forces *affect* total body movements.

Biomechanical Models of Human Motion

Biomechanics has been defined as the science that examines the internal and external forces acting on the human body and the effects produced by these forces. For example, a hockey player skating down the ice is generating internal forces in the leg muscles during each skating stroke. The net result of all of these internal muscle forces is a sequence of pushes against the ice with the skate blade. With each push against the ice, the ice pushes back upon the hockey player (note: the ice is an external force), and as a result the skater experiences forward movement. Other external forces also act upon the skater such as gravity, the weight of the hockey stick, or an opposing player who gives the skater a body check into the boards. Each of these external forces in turn has an effect upon the motion of the human body. A body check, for example, causes the hockey player to crash into the boards.

While we can visualize the hockey player crashing into the boards, the actual human body with all its bones, muscles, connective tissue, and internal organs is too complex for most biomechanical analyses. Anatomical differences exist between people due to race, age, sex, health, and lifestyle. Furthermore, all body tissues undergo shape deformations during sport movements. Moreover, the human body is multisegmented, such that the same total body or limb movement can be performed using different segment movement sequences. And finally, most sports skills occur in three dimensions, which adds a great deal of complexity to understanding and observing human movements.

To make the study of human movement possible, biomechanics has adopted three simplified models of human motion analysis: the particle, stick figure, and rigid segment body models.

The Particle Model

The **particle model** is a simple dot representing the center of mass (see box *Center of Mass*, page 173) of the body or object (Figure 8.2 A). Particle models are used when the human body or object is airborne and in flight. When the body is airborne it is already free from its surroundings. Most often, gravity (see box *Gravity*, page 174) is the only external force acting on the body through its center of mass. For objects that possess a relatively large velocity, such as baseballs, javelins, and discuses, the surrounding air will also apply a force to the object (see Figure 8.13, page 181). This external force, known as air resistance, will also affect the motion of the object.

Since particle models involve only the center of mass of an object, they are limited to bodies in flight. In sport, these include any ball or object that is thrown, struck, hit, or kicked, as well as the human body in flight such as during diving, high jumping, or tumbling. In all of these examples, the object or body is said to be a projectile.

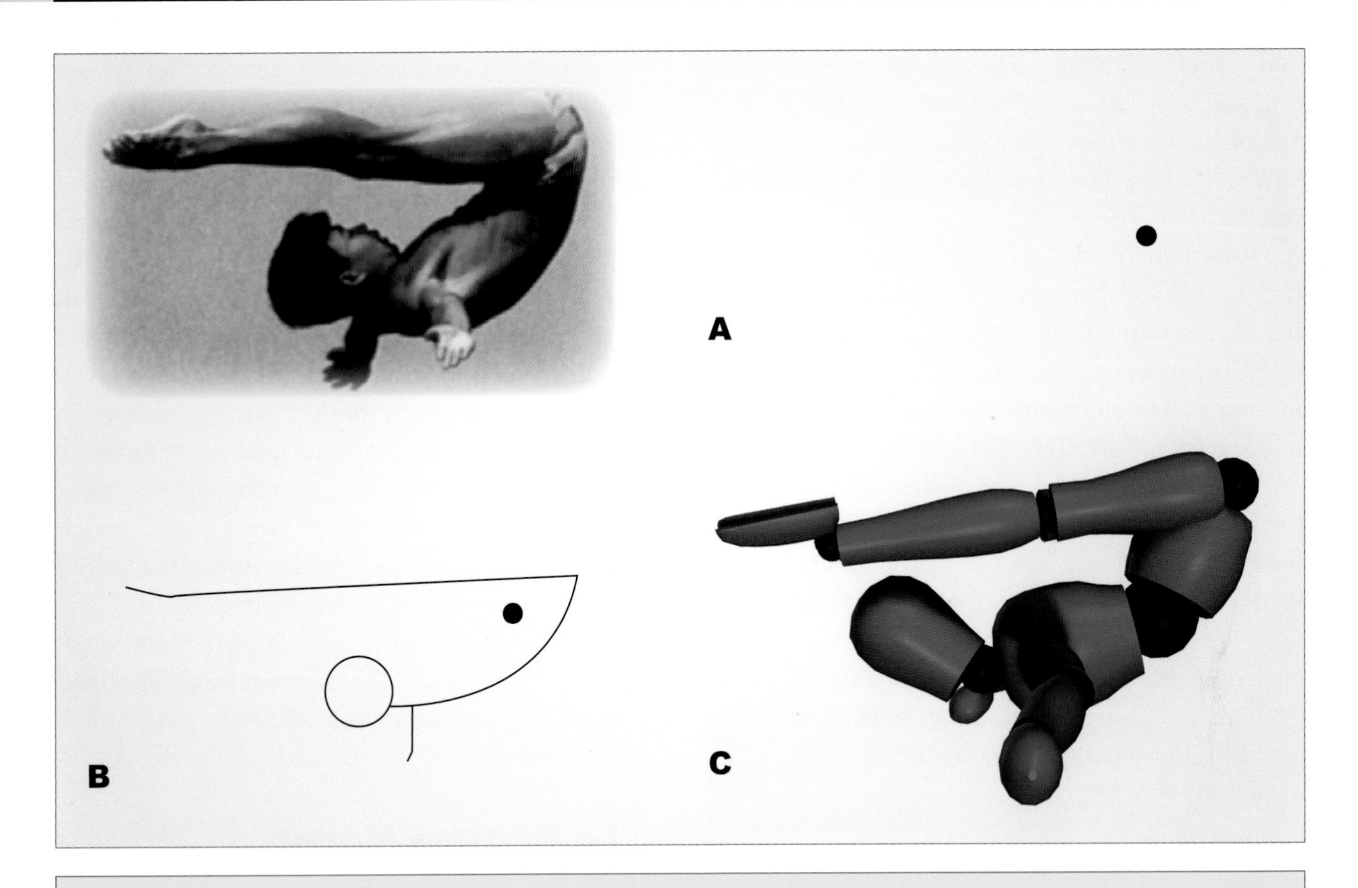

Figure 8.2 Three models used to represent the diver pictured above. **A.** Particle model. **B.** Stick figure model. **C.** Rigid segment body model. Choice of model is based on the type of biomechanical analysis to be made.

The Stick Figure Model

For athletes who are in contact with the ground or other earth-bound objects (e.g., diving board) a **stick figure model** is used to represent their bodies (Figure 8.2 B). Body segments are represented by rigid bars (sticks) linked together at the joints. Stick figures indicate approximate body segment positions, their connections, and size. External forces, represented by vectors, can be shown acting on the stick figure at the appropriate locations.

Stick figure models are used to represent the total body configuration for gross motor skills that occur in two dimensions. Sprint starts, running, and somersaults are good examples. They cannot easily represent small or fine local muscle movements, such as the grip on a baseball. Nor can they represent longitudinal rotations, either total body twisting movements or segment rotations such as pronations. Total body skills, which occur with many three-dimensional movements, are also difficult to draw.

A sequence of stick figures representing either the total body or portion thereof is known as a **composite diagram** (Figure 8.3). Composite diagrams give a quick picture of the body actions involved in a skill. To our mind's eye, they resemble our visual impression of a skill. However, because the stick figure links have no volume, the stick figure cannot be truly individualized to the athlete.

The advantage of the stick figure over the particle model is that multiple force vectors can be drawn on the free body diagram. These vectors can represent gravity or air resistance forces acting at the center of mass and reaction forces (described later in the chapter) acting on the body wherever contact is made with the environment. Some of these forces may create moments of force and thus indicate rotation of the body or its segment parts

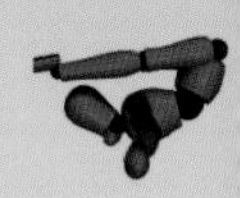

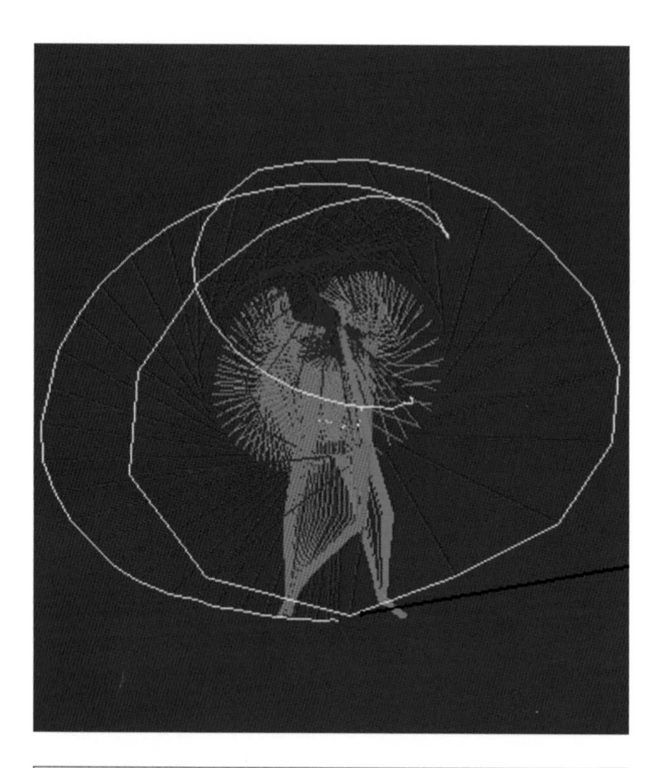

Figure 8.3 Composite diagrams provide a pictorial overview of the performance. However, if the motion does not occur in the two-dimensional plane of the diagram, then accurate measurements, such as angular velocity of the golf club, will be difficult.

(Figure 8.9, page 172).

The Rigid Segment Body Model

For sophisticated three-dimensional (3D) analyses, biomechanists employ a **rigid body segment model** in which each body segment is represented as an irregularly shaped 3D volume (Figure 8.2 C). The shape deformation of body segments during vigorous activity adds to the complexity of these analyses.

Steps of Analysis

There are three preliminary steps that must be completed before any human or object motion can be described using the three biomechanical models.

Step 1

Identify the system to be studied: in other words, isolate the object of analysis from its surroundings (e.g., arm, leg, tennis racket, or total body of a runner) (Figure 8.4).

Step 2

Identify the frame of reference (or coordinate system) in which the movement takes place (e.g., a runner changes his position relative to the ground and to some starting point; Figure 8.4). While many sport movements are usually described as occurring in two dimensions (running, somersaulting), most sport activities (or components) actually occur in three dimensions.

Step 3

Identify the type of motion that is occurring, the **body planes** in which movement takes place (sagittal, frontal, and transverse, see Chapter 2), and the **axes of rotation** about which rotational motion occurs (either through a joint or the total body).

Types of Motion

Human movement is composed of a number of fundamental types of motion. We differentiate between linear, angular, and general motion.

Linear Motion

Linear motion occurs when all parts of the body move the same distance, in the same direction, and at the same time, such as a toboggan run, a skater's glide, or a sprinter (Figure 8.5 A). Another term often used for linear motion is **translation**, which refers to movement of the body as a unit without individual segment parts of the body moving in relation to one another.

Rectilinear motion occurs when the movement follows a straight line (a 100-meter sprinter's movement); a **curvilinear motion** occurs when the

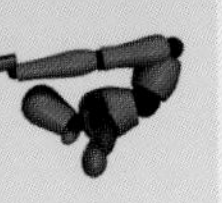

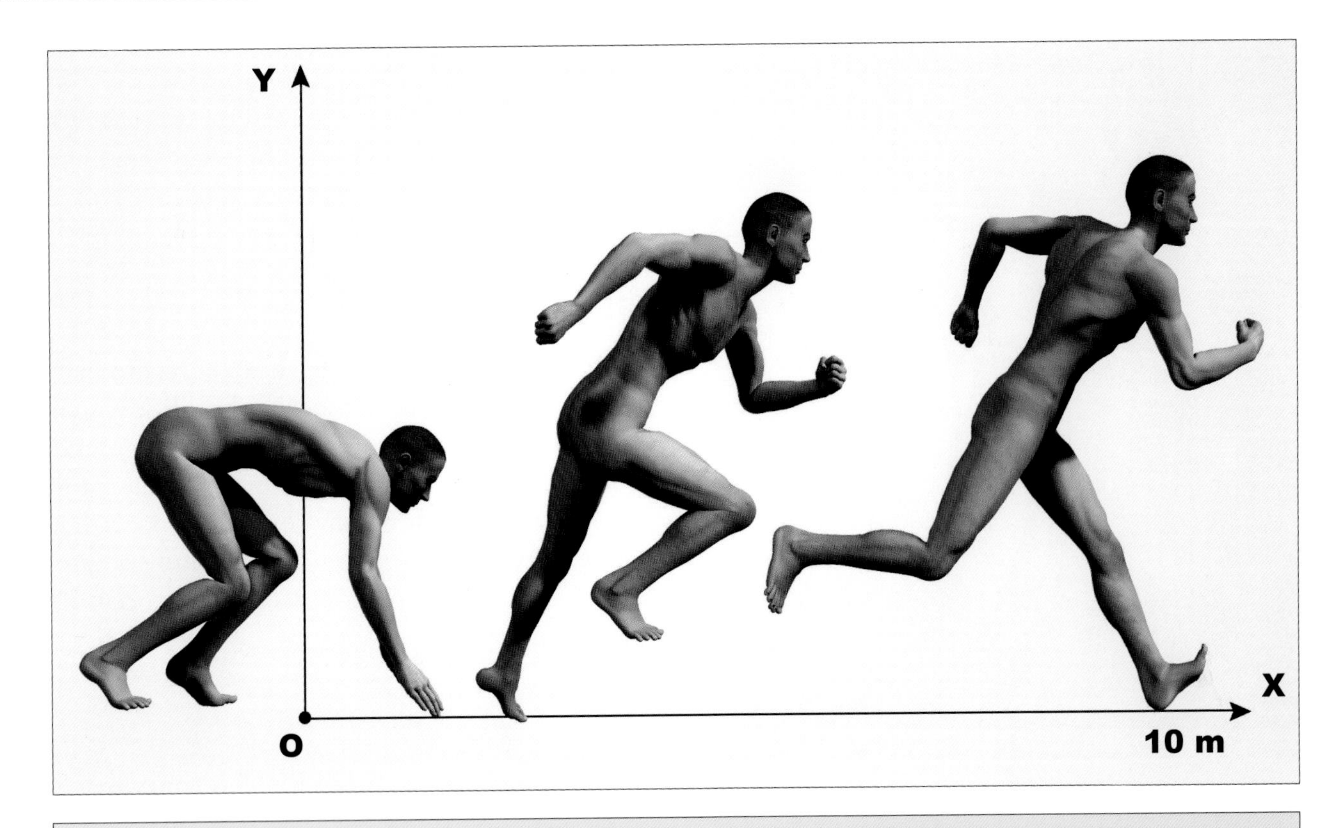

Figure 8.4 Identifying the system and reference frame. The system is the total body of a runner. The reference frame is the two-dimensional xy plane, with the origin at the start line.

movement path is curved (a ski jumper's flight).

Angular Motion

When a body moves on a circular path and in the same direction, then the body is experiencing **angular motion** or **rotation**. The line about which bodies rotate is called the axis of rotation. A good example of this type of motion is a gymnast executing giant swings on a high bar (Figure 8.5 B).

Body segments also experience angular motion about their joints as they flex, extend, and longitudinally rotate. Twisting somersault dives, the shot put, and an automobile's wheels turning around their axes are good examples of angular motion.

General Motion

A combination of linear and angular motion (i.e., body moving linearly and rotating simultaneously) is referred to as **general motion**. This is true for most athletic and many everyday activities (e.g., gymnastics floor routine, wrestling, a diver falling downward while simultaneously rotating in a somersault; Figure 8.5 C).

Causes of Motion

The cause of motion of the human body is the application of internal and external forces. A force is any action, a push or pull, that tends to cause an object to change its state of motion by experiencing acceleration. If an object is not accelerating, then it experiences a state of constant **velocity** (note: rest, or no motion, is just the state of constant "zero" velocity).

There are two types of motion resulting from the application of a force, linear motion and angular motion. Forces that act through a body's center of mass will cause linear motion, such as

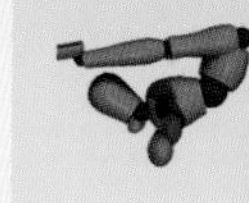

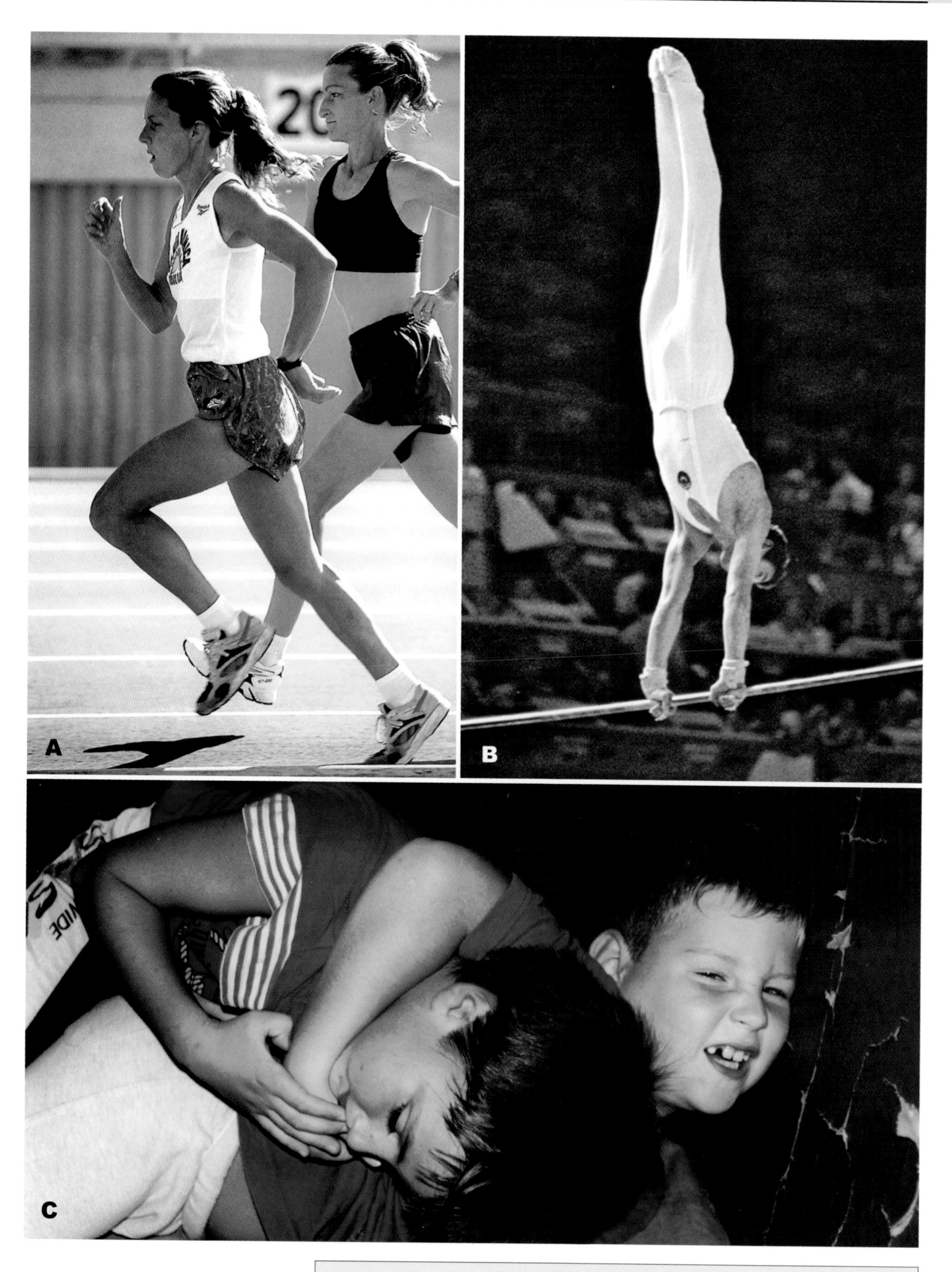

Figure 8.5 Types of human motion. **A.** Linear. **B.** Angular. **C.** General.

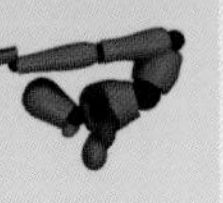

throwing a ball or pushing a cart (Figure 8.6 A).

Forces that do not go through the center of mass or pivot point of an object cause a rotation about an axis of rotation. These actions cause the object to change its state of angular motion by experiencing an angular acceleration. When a force causes angular motion, the effect is known as a **moment of force**, or **torque**. Moments of force are generated to open a door, flex a joint, or move an opponent (Figure 8.6 B).

Calculating Moment of Force

Consider a balanced teeter-totter (Figure 8.7 A). If each person was to sit alone on the teeter-totter, this would cause the teeter-totter to rotate about its axis, the **fulcrum** of the teeter-totter. Each person creates a moment of force by applying his or her

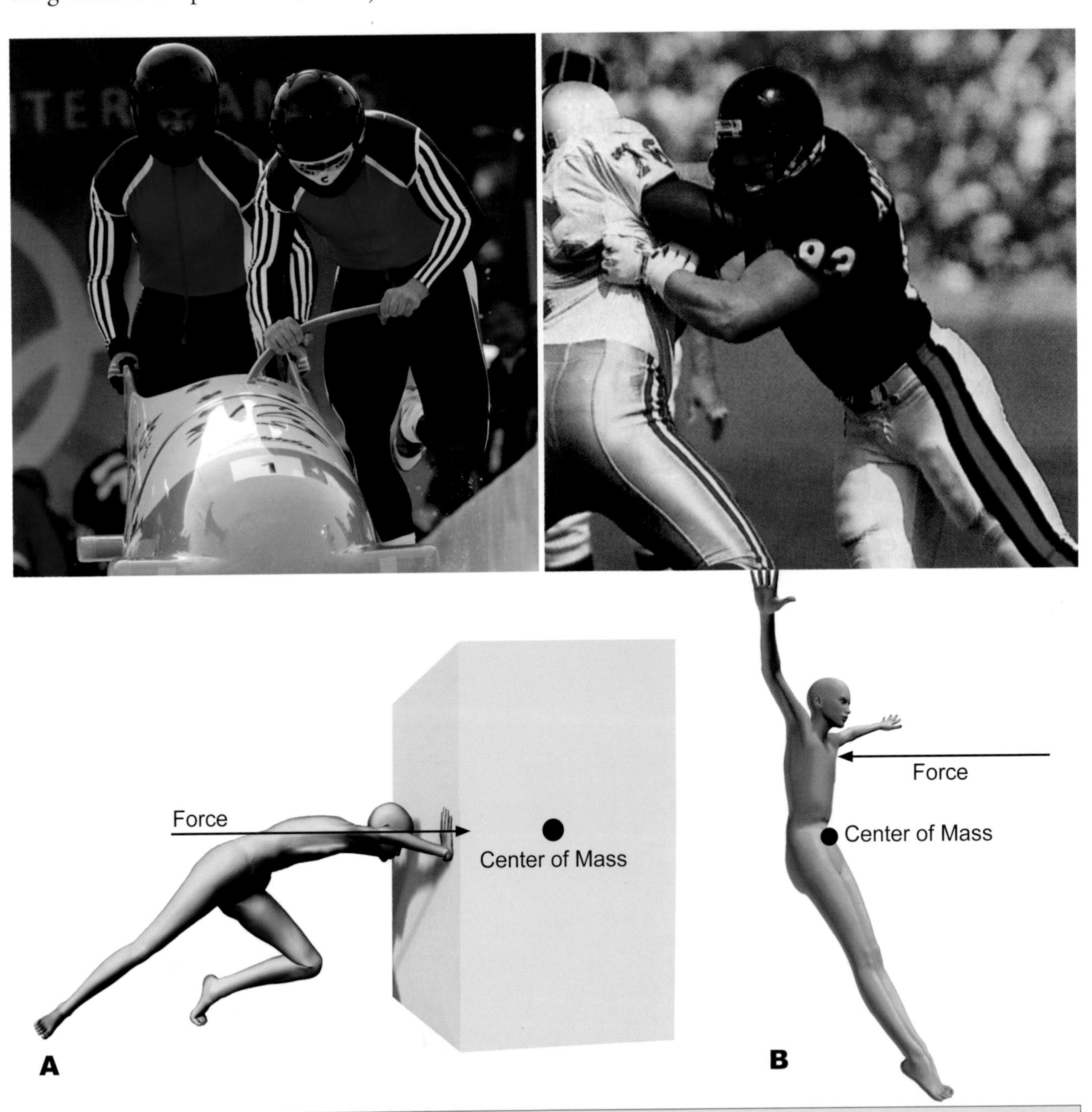

Figure 8.6 Causes of linear and angular motions. **A.** Linear motion results when the forces are applied through the center of mass. **B.** Angular motion results when forces are applied away from the center of mass.

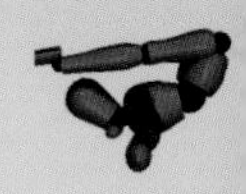

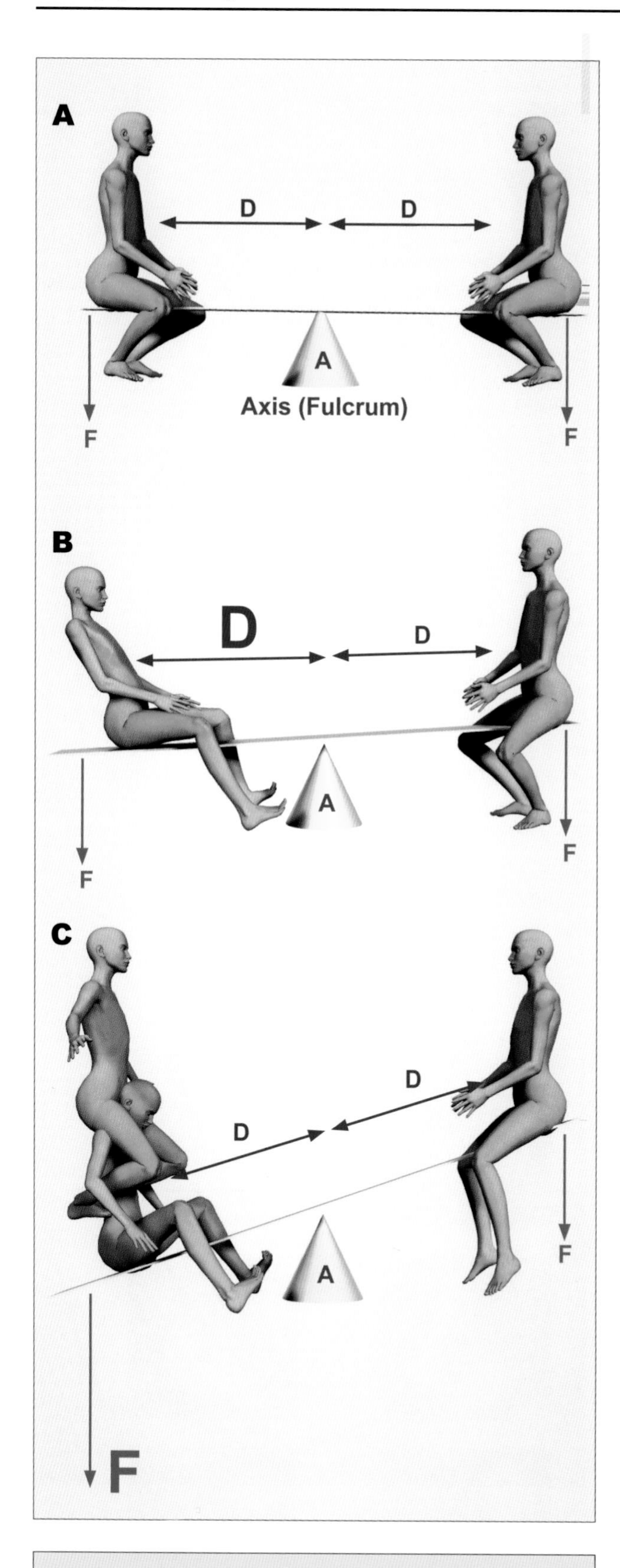

Figure 8.7 Factors affecting the moment of force. **A.** Balanced teeter-totter. **B.** Increasing the moment arm by leaning back. **C.** Increasing the applied force by adding a friend.

weight away from the axis of rotation. However, if the moments of force created are equal, then the teeter-totter will be balanced (Figure 8.7 A).

What could you do to unbalance the teeter-totter? One method is to lean back, away from the fulcrum, increasing the distance from the fulcrum to the point of application of your weight vector (Figure 8.7 B). The shortest (perpendicular) distance from the axis of rotation to the line of action of the force is known as the **moment arm (D)**. Therefore, by increasing the moment arm, you can create more moment of force and rotate the teeter-totter in your direction.

Another method to unbalance the teeter-totter would be to ask a friend to join you on your side of the teeter-totter (Figure 8.7 C). In this case, you have increased the applied force acting on the teeter-totter and thus have increased the moment of force your side creates.

Thus two factors, moment arm and magnitude of force, influence the magnitude of the moment of force that can be generated. The magnitude of the moment of force is calculated by using the equation:

Moment of Force = Moment Arm x Force

Levers

Levers are simple mechanical devices that augment the amount of work done by an applied force. A lever is a rigid body (e.g., long bone) that rotates about a fixed point (e.g., joint) called an axis (A) or fulcrum. Acting on the lever is a resistive force (R, e.g., weight of a limb segment) and an applied force (F, e.g., muscle contraction). There are three classes of levers, first, second, and third, which differ by placing the fulcrum, resistive force, and applied force respectively between the other two. They are presented in the box *Lever Systems and Muscle Actions*.

The teeter-totter is just one example of a lever. There are many levers found in the human body and in sports skills. Can you think of examples for each type of lever?

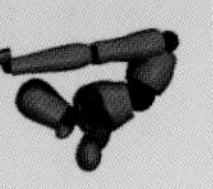

Lever Systems and Muscle Actions

Functions of Levers

Levers perform different functions. Some levers help to balance forces and resistive loads. In other levers, the application of a relatively small amount of force can overcome a relatively large resistive force (e.g., crowbar). Finally in some levers, the application of a force results in the lever (and resistive force) moving quickly through a large range of motion (e.g., forearm flexion).

First Class Levers When the applied force and the resistance are located on opposite sides we speak of **first class levers**. The applied force and resistance may be at equal distances from the axis, or one may be farther away from the axis than the other.

In everyday life, the teeter-totter in Figure 8.7 is an example of a first class lever. In the human body, flexion and extension of the head about C1 is an example of a first class lever. The simultaneous action of agonist and antagonist muscle groups (see Chapter 4) on opposite sides of a joint axis is another. During contraction, the agonists provide the applied force and the antagonists supply a resistance force.

Second Class Levers The applied force and the resistance are on the same side of the axis in a **second class lever**, and the resistance is closer to the axis. In everyday life, a wheelbarrow or a nutcracker may serve as examples of second class levers. In the human body, second class levers are hard to find. Contraction of the calf muscles to raise the body onto the toes – the fulcrum is at the distal end of the metatarsals – serves as an example.

Third Class Levers A **third class lever** exists when the applied force and the resistance are on the same side of the axis, but the applied force is closer to the axis. In everyday life, a screen door with a spring closing or snow shoveling can serve as third class levers. Most muscle–bone lever systems of the human body are examples of third class levers during concentric contractions. Forearm flexion may serve as an example: the biceps, attaching to the bone at a short distance from the joint center, supplies the applied force; the weight, at much greater distance from the joint center, supplies the resistance.

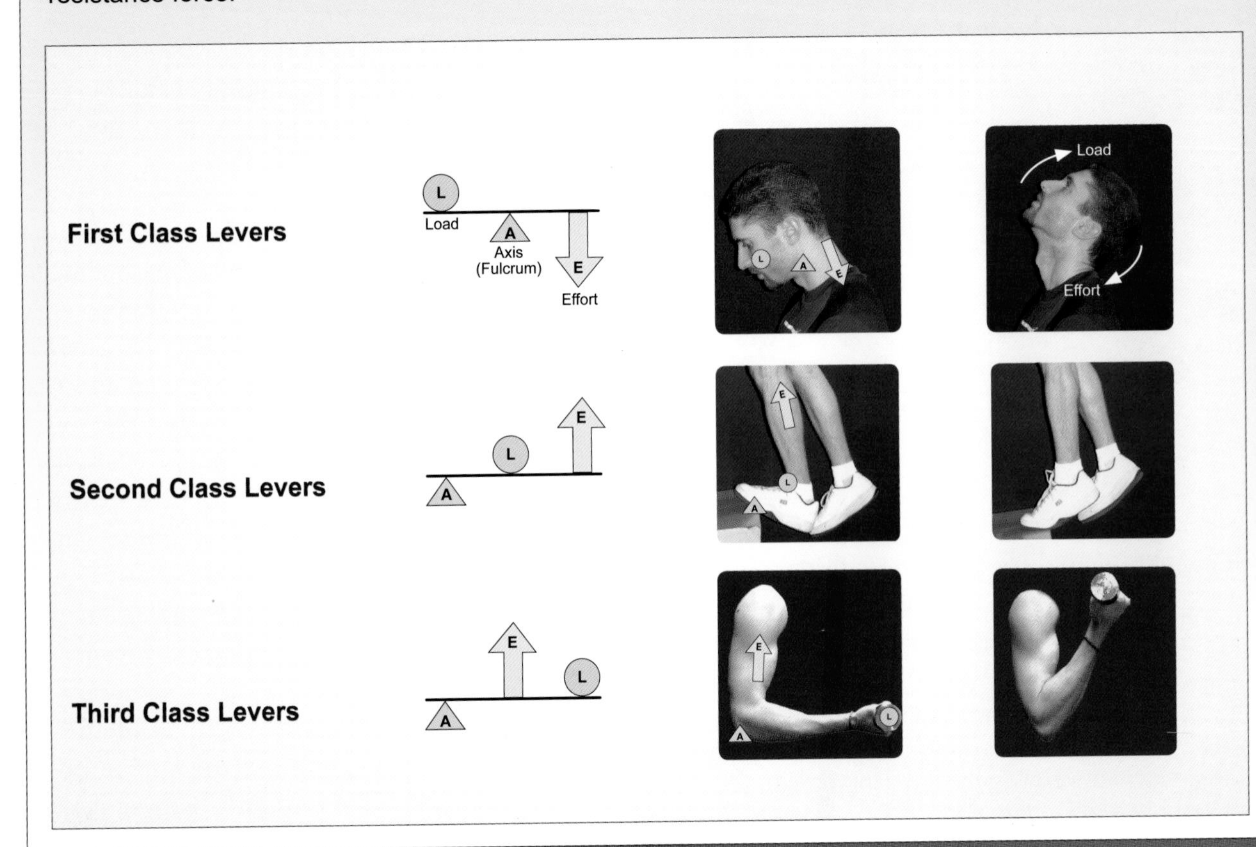

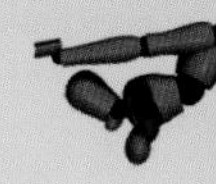

Your Levers at Work

Think of your throwing arm as a lever when you throw a baseball properly. Your elbow becomes a fulcrum, multiplying the speed of your slowly contracting triceps muscle and the forearm muscles. As you throw:

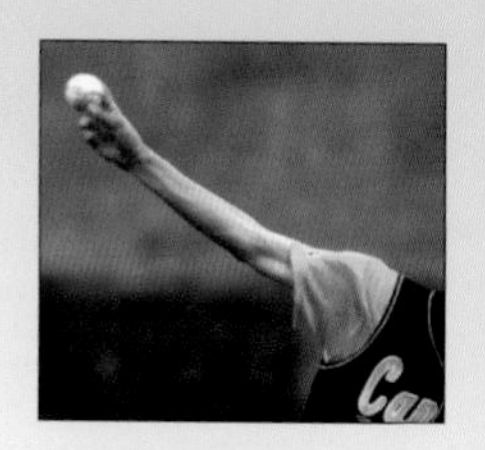

- Bend wrist and fingers (flexors)
- Straighten elbow (triceps)
- Straighten wrist and fingers (extensors)
- Bend elbow (biceps)

To add power to your throw, change the center of gravity during the windup. Shifting your weight to your back leg lowers your center of gravity. As you go through the movement of the pitch, the center of gravity shifts forward and up as your weight is shifted from the back leg to the front leg. A higher pitcher's mound – it is raised by 10 inches – further adds to the ball's speed through the force of gravity.

Forces Represented by Vectors

In biomechanics, physical variables such as time, speed, and force are classified either as scalar quantities or vector quantities. A **scalar quantity** has only magnitude, such as the length of time it takes to run 100 meters or the speed posted on a road sign (e.g., 60 miles per hour). A **vector quantity** has both magnitude and direction. Force is a vector quantity because it has magnitude (large or small) and direction. The force of gravity of an object is always directed down, toward the center of the earth.

Vector quantities are represented by arrows called **vectors**. The end with the straight-line segment is called the tail of the vector, while the end with the arrow head is called the head of the vector (Figure 8.8 A). The head of a vector points in the direction of the variable (e.g., force) the vector represents. The length of the vector is proportional to the magnitude of the variable. Vectors can be added together using the head-to-tail method. To add Vector B to Vector A, a vector identical to Vector B (same length and direction) is drawn with its tail beginning at the head of Vector A. The resultant vector, the sum of Vector A and Vector B, is directed from the tail of Vector A to the head of Vector B (Figure 8.8 and Figure 8.9).

When force (F) vectors are indicated on a stick figure, they are drawn pointing in the direction they act upon the body. By convention, gravity and air resistance are drawn acting from the center of mass (Figure 8.9).

Net Force

The sum of all the acting forces is the **net force**. When all acting forces are balanced, or cancel each other out, the net force is zero and the body remains in its original state of motion (Figure 8.9 A). When a net force is present, the body moves in the direction of the net force with an acceleration

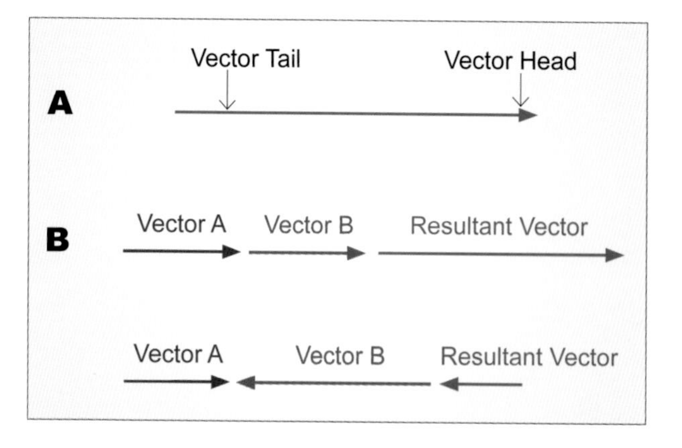

Figure 8.8 Simple vector algebra. **A.** A vector and its components. **B.** A resultant vector is based on vector composition, which is done by adding or subtracting their magnitudes.

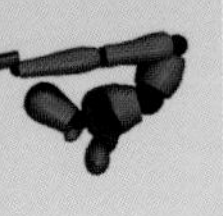

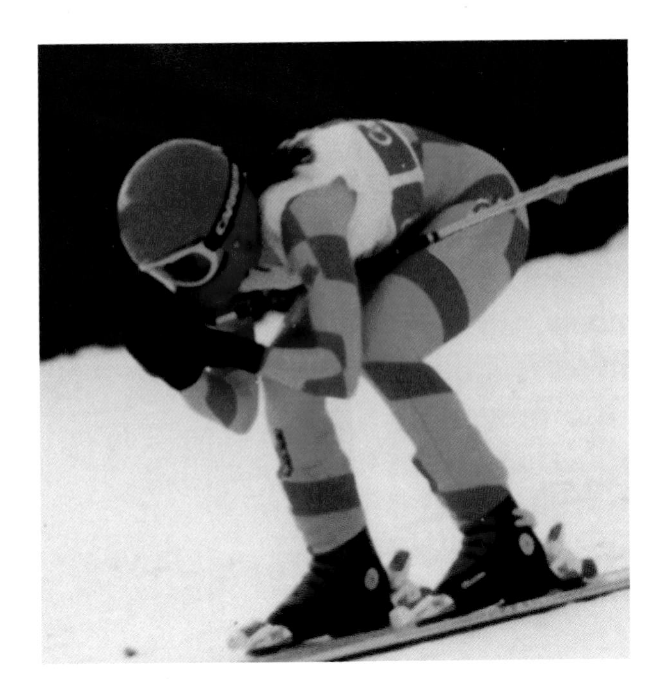

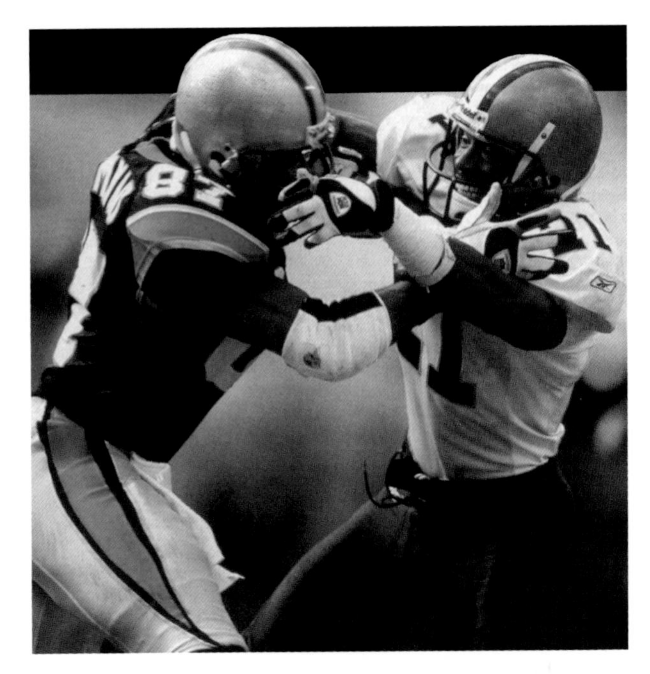

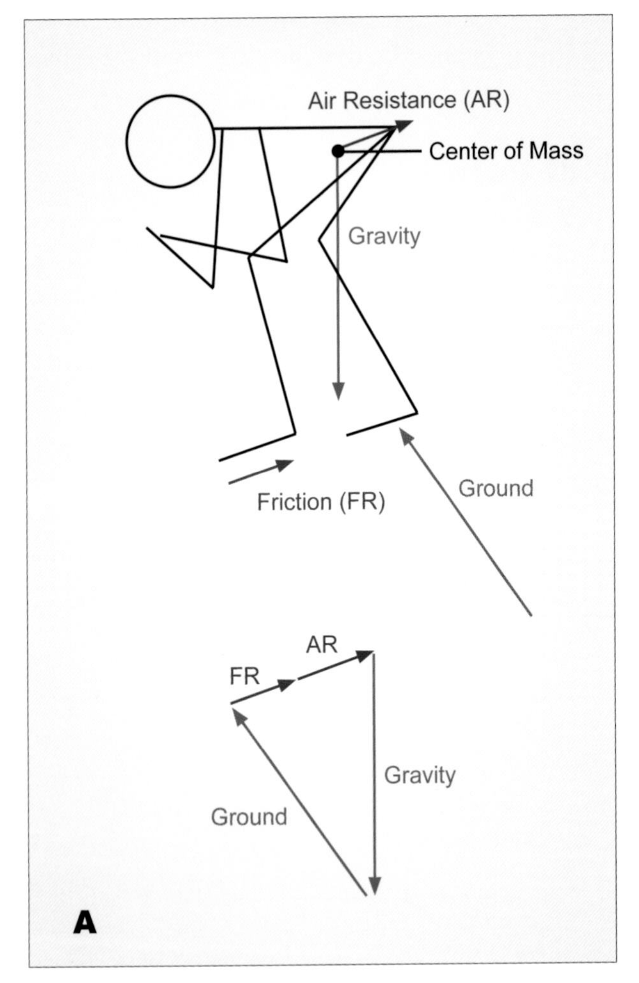

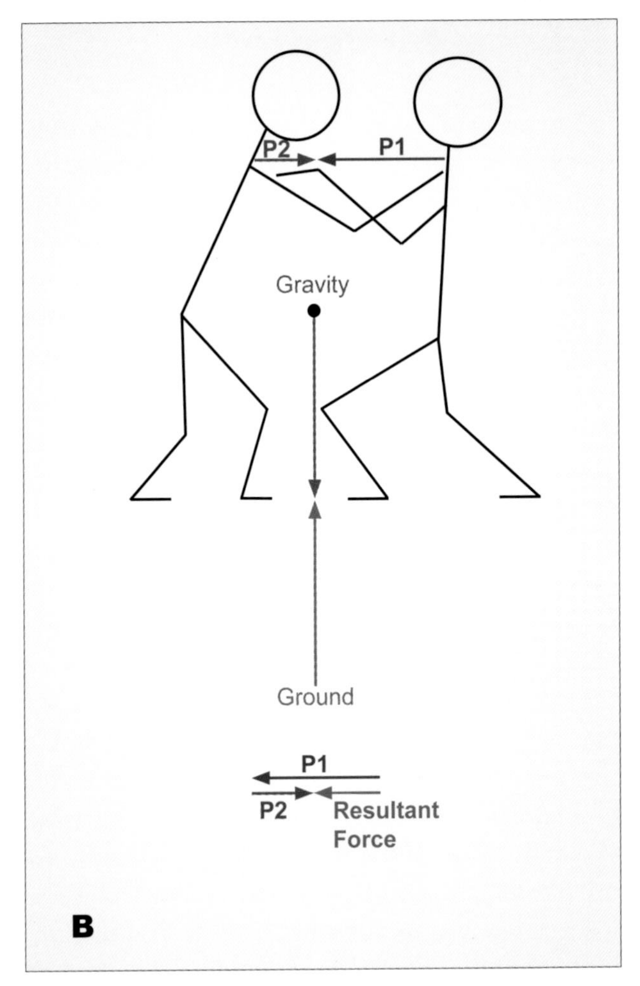

Figure 8.9 Calculating net external force using free body diagrams. **A.** The resultant vector is zero; therefore the skier is not accelerating. **B.** Since Player 1 (P1) is stronger than Player 2 (P2), the resultant vector between the linemen pushing on each other is not zero.

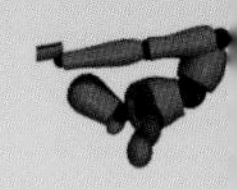

Center of Mass

The point around which the body's mass is equally distributed in all directions is known as **center of mass**, or center of gravity (CG). The CG of a perfectly symmetrical object of homogeneous density is at the exact center of the object. For example, the CG of a bowling ball or golf ball is at its geometric center. If the object is a homogeneous ring (such as a hula hoop), the CG is located in the hollow center of the ring.

Your center of mass is not always found inside the body (as in the case of the skater). In general, it is located about 6 inches (15 cm) above the groin area at approximately 55 percent of standing height in females and 57 percent in males.

The location of CG in the human body is of interest because a body behaves as though all of its mass were concentrated at the CG. Therefore, the force of gravity acting on this point of mass would be the same as the force of gravity acting on the total body. Or when the human body acts as a projectile, as in a long jump, the body's CG follows a parabolic trajectory, regardless of what the various segments of the body do while in the air.

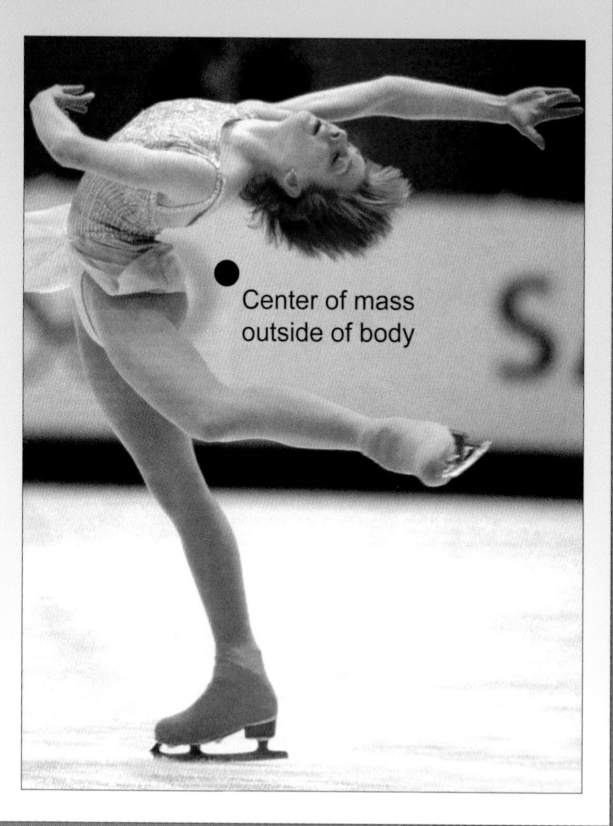

that is proportional to the magnitude of the net force (Figure 8.9 B).

Mass and Inertia Concepts

All objects have matter. The measure of how much matter an object has is its **mass**. Do you know your mass in pounds and kilograms? Where is your center of mass? (For answers, see boxes *Center of Mass* and *Weight Versus Mass*.)

Because objects have mass, they are also reluctant to change whatever they are doing. In other words, they are reluctant to change their state of motion from rest to motion, or to moving faster or slower, or to slowing down to rest. This property of objects is called **inertia**. Compared with a soccer ball, a tennis ball has less mass and therefore less inertia. If both are on the ground and have no motion, which ball would be easier to kick and therefore change its state of motion? If both were traveling at the same velocity, which one would you rather stop (i.e., change its state of motion from moving to rest)?

Rotating objects also have a reluctance to change their state of angular motion: from rest to rotation, or to rotating faster or slower, or to slowing down back to rest. The inertia of rotating objects is measured by their **moment of inertia**, and it depends upon their mass and how their mass is distributed about their axis of rotation. It is more difficult to change the state of rotation of a soccer ball, compared with a tennis ball, because it is more massive and its mass is found farther away from any axis of rotation (i.e., the diameter of the soccer ball is larger). Similarly, layout dives are harder to perform than the same dive in the tuck position because the athlete's body parts are farther away from the rotating axis (which passes through the athlete's center of mass), giving the layout diver a greater moment of inertia (Figure 8.20 A, page 191).

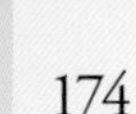

Weight Versus Mass

There is a difference between mass (m) and weight (W). Mass is a measure of inertia, while weight is a measure of the force of gravity (g) acting on the body. Mass is measured in kilograms (kg), while weight is measured in Newtons (N). A person's weight varies directly with the magnitude of the acceleration caused by gravity (9.8 m/s^2). Thus in space where there is no acceleration experienced due to gravity, we weigh 0 N but have the same mass as we do on earth.

To calculate weight, the following formula is used:

$$W = m \times g$$

Gravity

Gravity is the force of attraction between two bodies, the magnitude of which is proportional to their masses and inversely proportional to the square of the distance between them.

For sporting activities (anywhere except outer space), gravity therefore represents a force of attraction between the masses of the athlete and the earth, which varies in magnitude according to the location on the earth. The closer the athlete is to the center of the earth (polar regions, sea level), the greater the force of attraction. The farther the athlete is from the center of the earth (equator, mountains), the less the force of attraction.

At the 1968 Olympic Games, Bob Beamon became the one human on earth who could "fly." In the light air of 7,349-foot-high Mexico City, Beamon jumped longer than any other human in the history of track and field. His 8.9-meter jump was not broken until two decades later.

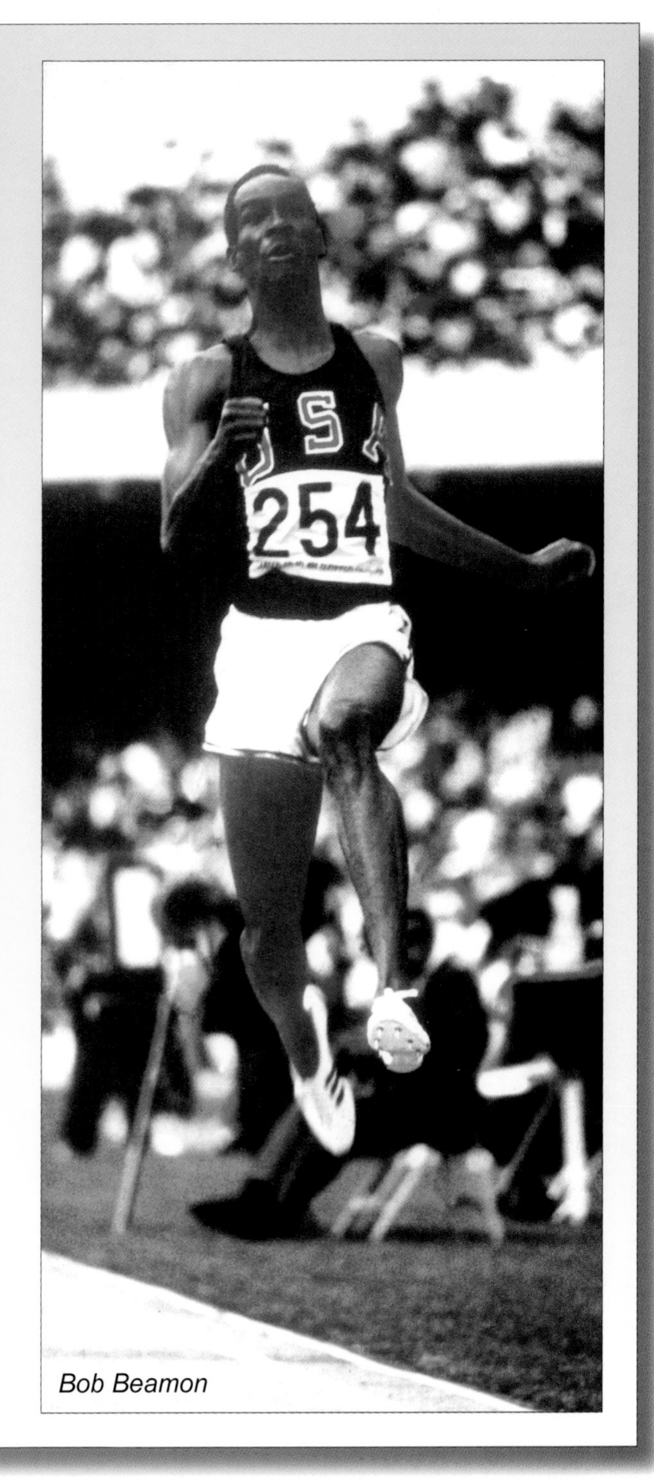

Bob Beamon

Newton's First Law of Motion: Inertia

Newton's first law of motion describes the relationship between inertia and force. It states: objects will not change their state of motion (i.e., they will continue to be at rest, or move with a constant velocity or in uniform circular motion about a fixed axis of rotation) unless acted on by an unbalanced external force (or moment of force). Thus, an object at rest will tend to stay at rest, and an object in motion will tend to stay in motion.

Football linemen, because of their large mass,

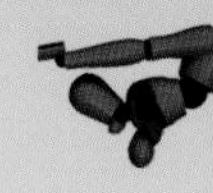

are difficult to move out of the way. A large force is required to change their resting state because of their large inertia. Similarly, once linemen are in motion it is difficult to stop them. Just ask any quarterback! Contrast this with young gymnasts who, because of their small mass (and thus inertia), require smaller amounts of force to manipulate their bodies during spotting.

Force and Acceleration Concepts

If external forces could overcome inertia and change the state of motion of a body, what would the relationship between the amount of force and the resulting change in motion be? Newton's second law of motion describes the relationship underlying this question.

Newton's Second Law of Motion: Acceleration

Newton's second law of motion states that for linear movements, the acceleration (a) a body experiences is directly proportional to the force (F) causing it and takes place in the same direction as the force (F = m x a, where m is the mass of the body) (Figure 8.10). For angular movements, the angular acceleration of a body is directly proportional to the moment of force causing it and takes place in the same direction as the moment of force.

Sprinters must experience a large external unbalanced force acting on their body mass at the start of a race in order to accelerate down the track. Similarly, at the end of the race, sprinters again experience a large unbalanced force but in the opposite direction to decelerate their bodies (m). When body checking, one hockey player applies an external unbalanced force into the opponent, accelerating the opponent into the boards. Divers experience a moment of force on their bodies when making contact with the diving board, thereby increasing the angular acceleration about their axis of rotation (which passes through their center of mass).

The various relationships between force, mass, and acceleration are shown in Figure 8.10.

Impulse, Impact, and Momentum Concepts

Another approach to quantifying the relationship between the external unbalanced forces and the resulting motion is to describe the amount of motion gained or lost by the body. During a race, a sprinter gains motion at the beginning of the race, maintains this motion during the middle portion, and loses this motion after crossing the finish line. While we cannot "see" the accelerations, we can "see" the changes in motion caused by the application of external unbalanced force, thereby indicating the motion gained at the beginning and lost at the end of the race.

The product of a body's mass and its velocity is called **momentum**. Momentum is created by an **impulse**, the application of an internal force over a period of time. Momentum is lost through **impact**, the application of an external force over a period of time.

Impulse and impact are both associated with bodies changing their state of motion (speeding up, slowing down, changing directions) by experiencing large accelerations over relatively short periods (usually less than one second). Consider the changes in speed and direction in the broken-field running of a halfback in football, or a base runner trying to steal second base, or the movements of a dynamic basketball guard. Also consider collisions with other players (football tackles, hockey checks) or with the environment (landings in gymnastics). For most of these activities, the change in momentum is quick, and the time of force application is limited and often cannot be manipulated. Therefore, most changes in momentum in sport really depend upon the magnitude of the net external force acting on the body.

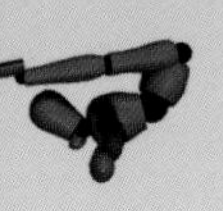

A

The greater the soccer player's force applied to a soccer ball that has the same mass, the greater the ball's acceleration.

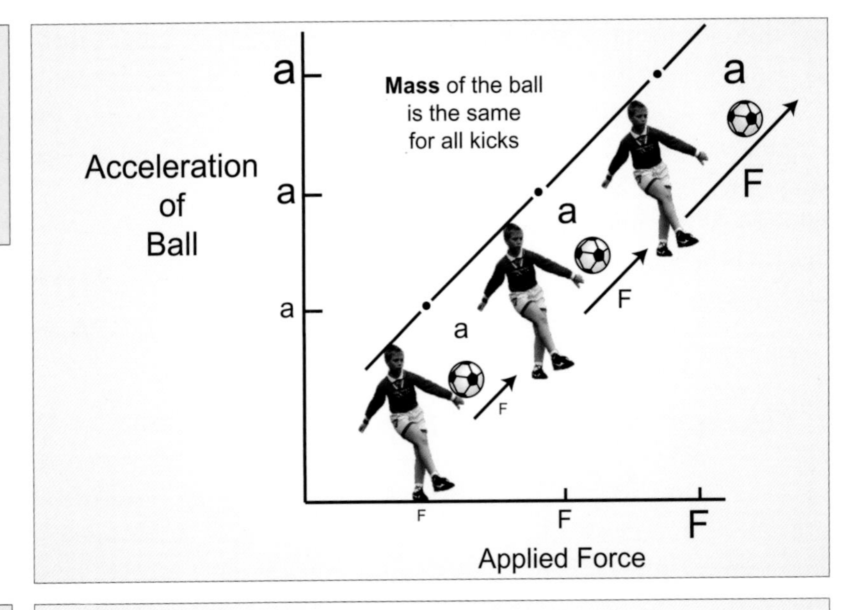

B

As the mass of the soccer ball increases, it experiences less acceleration from a kick that has the same (constant) force.

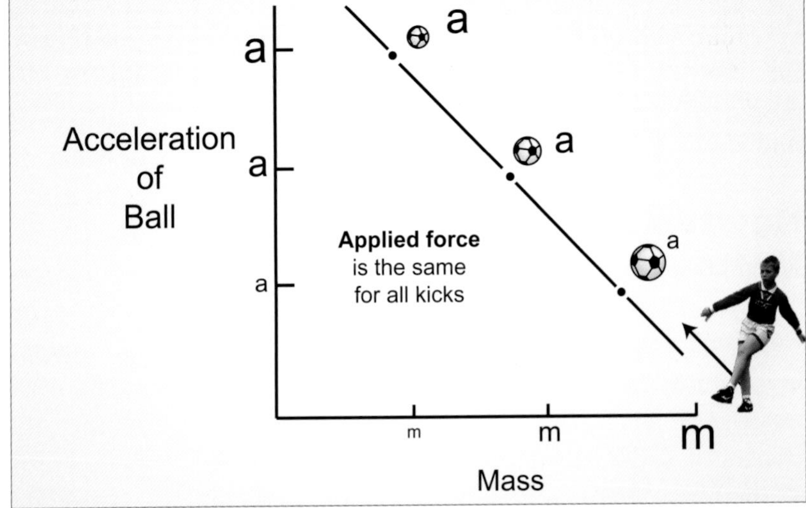

C

As the mass of the soccer ball increases, the soccer player must generate an increased force to kick the ball if it is to assume the same (constant) acceleration.

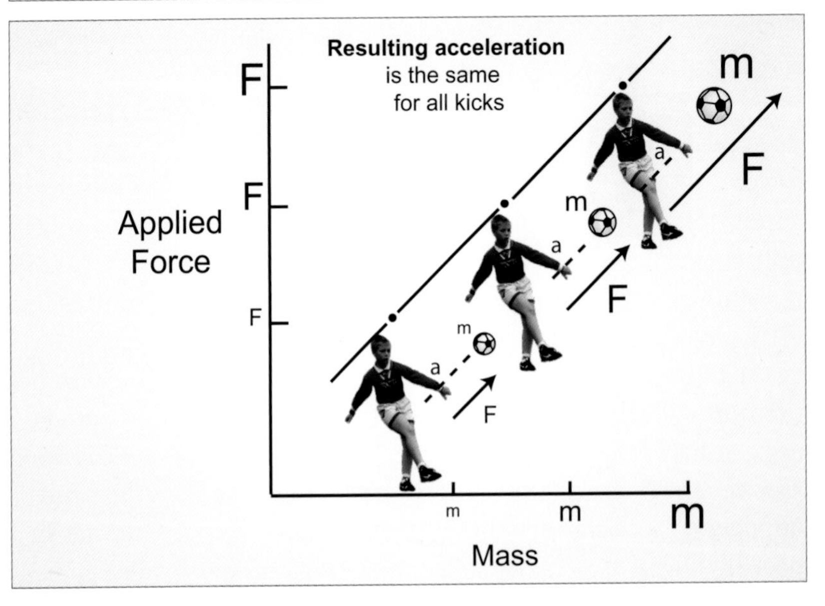

Figure 8.10 Relationships between force, mass, and acceleration.

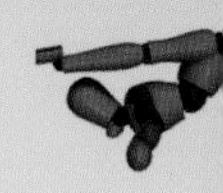

For a sprinter, the time during which each foot is in contact with the ground is limited and decreases with increased running speed. To increase impulse, a sprinter must increase the net external force per step. This implies reducing any retarding forces associated with initial foot contact with the ground and maximizing the propulsive forces during the push-off phase. Many sports skills have similar requirements, including all forms of running, jumping, striking, and throwing skills.

On the other hand, collision or impact skills can sometimes manipulate the time of contact and reduce the magnitude of the external force. In gymnastics landings, athletes can flex the joints of their lower limbs (ankles, knees, hips) to increase the time over which external impact forces from the ground act on their bodies and hence decrease the force. Hockey players can lean into a body check, which increases the time during which they can attempt to resist external checking forces. Similarly, when catching, ball players are able to cradle the ball, thereby increasing the time available to eliminate its momentum and reducing the force exerted by the ball on the athletes' hands. This concept illustrates what is commonly called having "soft hands" in sport.

Action–Reaction Concept

From where do the external forces that affect a sprinter, hockey player, and diver arise? Each of these athletes generates internal muscle forces, the sum of which interacts with their surroundings through some body part (often a foot). At every contact point where the resultant internal force is exerted, an external force from the surroundings is exerted back onto the body simultaneously. These two forces on the two different bodies are equal in magnitude but opposite in direction. This is Newton's third law of motion.

Newton's Third Law of Motion: Reaction

Newton's third law of motion, **action–reaction** principle, states that "every action has an equal and opposite reaction." This law refers to the way in which forces act against each other. The sprinter exerts force onto the blocks, and simultaneously the blocks exert a force back onto the sprinter (Figure 8.11). The force from the blocks is the external force required to accelerate the sprinter. However, the magnitude and direction of this reaction force is completely under the sprinter's control, as it is simply the mirror image of the force resulting from the sum of all the athlete's internal muscle actions.

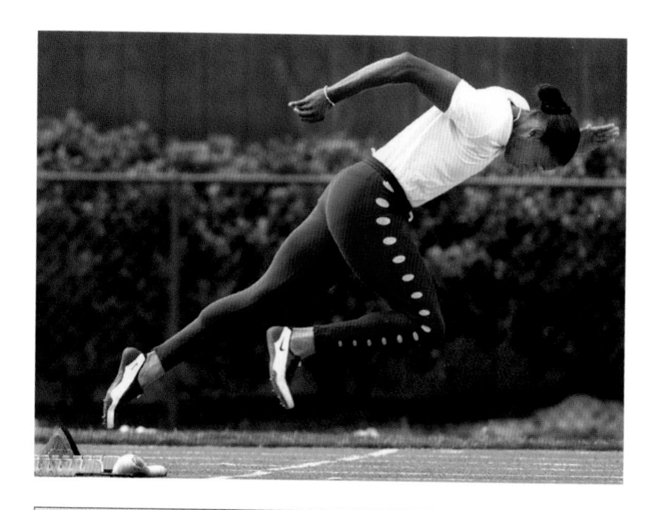

Figure 8.11 The force from the blocks is the external force required to accelerate the sprinter through internal muscle actions.

Newton's action–reaction principle applies to various forms of human movement. Several examples are provided in the box *I Push, You Push: Newton's Third Law of Motion in Action.*

Projectile Motion

Simply stated, any airborne object, including the human body, is a **projectile.** The center of mass of a projectile will follow a **parabolic path** whenever gravity is the only external force acting on the object. Under this condition, the parabolic path followed is determined only as a function of the projectile's takeoff velocity, both magnitude and direction, and acceleration due to gravity (Figure 8.12). If other external forces, such as air resistance,

I Push, You Push: Newton's Third Law of Motion in Action

In walking, an athlete moves the left leg and the right arm forward simultaneously. This results in the hips and shoulders twisting in opposite directions around the body's longitudinal axis. Similarly, a runner twists the upper and lower parts of the body and uses countermovements of the legs and arms. This achieves muscle forces approximately on the same plane when pushing off with either the right or the left leg and prevents twisting of the entire body. At the same time the stride length can be increased by twisting the hips. In cross-country skiing, the forward thrust is achieved through the countermovement of the poles in relation to the leg movements.

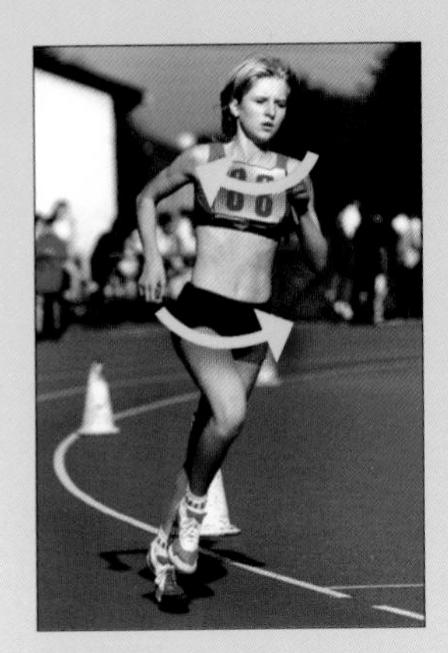

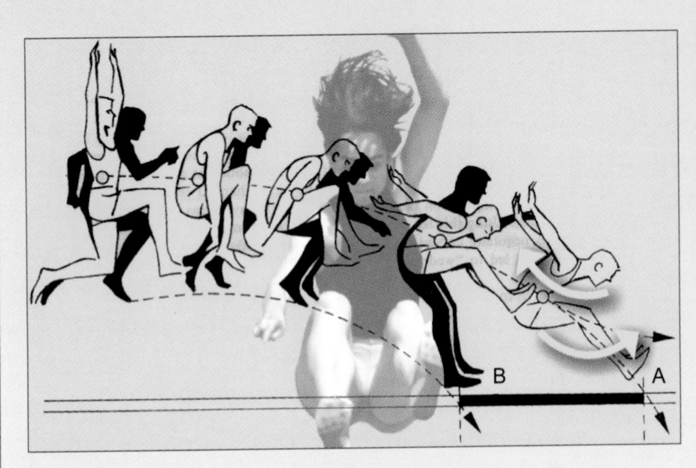

In athletic jumping events it is important to bring the body into a proper landing posture by applying appropriate action and reaction body movements. In the long jump, for instance, the jumper is initially extended. The upper part of the body is then brought forward around the hip joints, causing an action. The principle of reaction causes the lower part of the body to bend forward around the hip joints at the same time in order to achieve the longest possible jump (Athlete A). Poorer results are obtained by the athlete who is less skilled in following this principle (Athlete B).

Effective application of the action–reaction principle is also made in throwing and kicking. In handball, for example, the throwing action is carried out by moving the shoulder forward along with the throwing arm – action. To prevent the whole body from twisting, which is important for good throwing accuracy, the athlete twists the hips forward in the opposite direction – reaction. This also engages the powerful trunk muscles, which significantly increases the power of the throw.

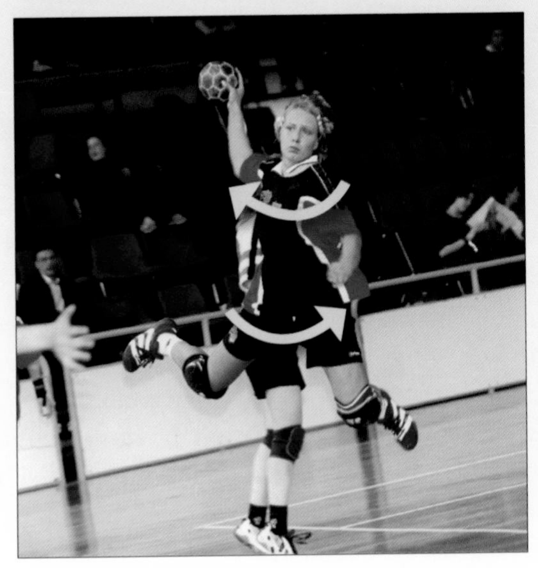

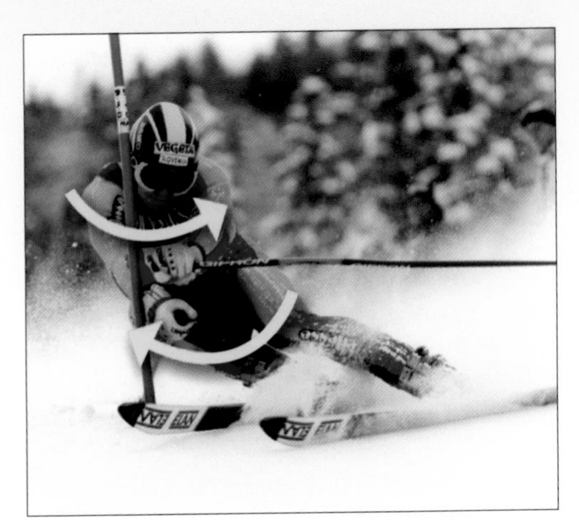

Twisting the upper part of the body in the opposite direction to that of the lower part of the body is the most natural way of negotiating the gates in slalom skiing.

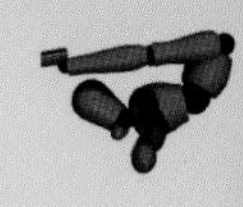

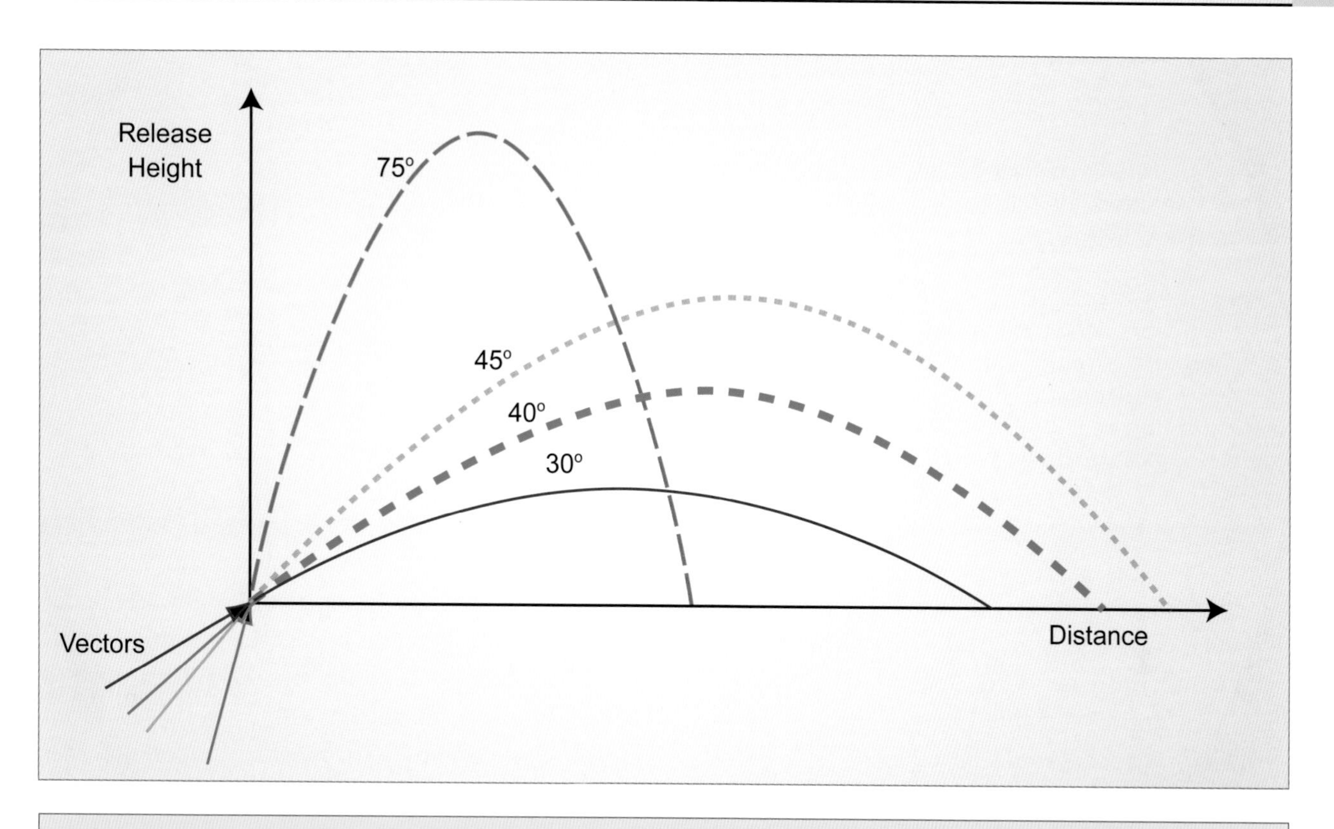

Figure 8.12 Four projection paths at various angles with vectors. A baseball thrown at a 45-degree angle maximizes the landing distance.

act on the object, then the flight path is altered accordingly.

Skills involving some form of projectile have one of three objectives. A high jumper, for example, seeks the maximum vertical distance, or **height**, for the body. A javelin thrower, by contrast, tries to realize a maximum horizontal distance, or **range**. Still others, such as basketball, involve projectiles that seek **accuracy**.

Maximizing Height and Range

Can we determine the conditions under which a projectile will attain a maximum height or range? Using the equations given in the box *Projectile Motion Equations*, we can deduce the following criteria for objects that take off and land at the same height:

1. To maximize the vertical distance (height) a projectile will achieve, one must maximize the takeoff velocity and take off vertically (since the maximum sine value is 1 and occurs at a 90-degree angle). Thus, high jumpers try to jump as vertically as possible, a difficult task given the high approach velocities they attain.
2. To maximize the horizontal distance (range) a projectile will achieve, one must maximize takeoff velocity and take off at an angle of 45 degrees to the horizontal (since the maximum sine value is 1 and occurs at a 90-degree angle, and half of 90 degrees is 45 degrees). Baseball throws from the outfield as well as many throwing events in athletics (javelin, hammer, discus) try to achieve a takeoff angle of 45 degrees (Figure 8.12).

Taking Off and Landing at Different Heights

Most sport activities involve taking off and landing at different heights (basketball jump shots, gymnastics dismounts).

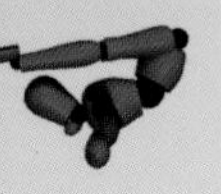

Projectile Motion Equations

For projectiles that take off and land at the same height (or close enough) and for which air resistance can be ignored, the following equations describe the vertical (height) and horizontal (range) distances the projectile will traverse.

For

- v = magnitude of the takeoff velocity
- θ = the takeoff angle with respect to the horizontal
- g = the acceleration due to gravity (a constant) = 9.8 m/s^2

then

Maximum Height $= \dfrac{(v \sin\theta)^2}{2g}$

Maximum Range $= \dfrac{v^2 \sin(2\theta)}{g}$

The range a projectile will travel will increase if the takeoff height is greater than the landing height and decrease if the takeoff height is less than the landing height. Objects that are to be thrown or struck should be released as high off the ground as possible by stretching all possible body parts. If the human body is the projectile, then a higher center of mass can be achieved by elongating the body at takeoff and by raising as many body parts as possible that are not involved in accelerating the body. Golf shots taken from elevated tees travel farther, mainly because the shot is airborne for a longer period of time and can travel farther horizontally. Similarly, the elevated pitcher's mound, through the force of gravity, adds to the speed of the ball.

Air Resistance

Air resistance is another force acting on the projectile. As such, it will change the state of motion of the projectile and its path. The effects of air resistance on objects are discussed in the next section.

Optimizing Range

Of the four factors affecting projectile motion (takeoff velocity, takeoff angle, difference in takeoff and landing heights, and air resistance), which is the most important in maximizing horizontal distance? Each factor does ***not*** work in isolation. Increasing the takeoff height compared with the landing height lowers the optimal takeoff angle of 45 degrees. Skills that take advantage of air resistance in increasing range also have a lower optimal takeoff angle. In most instances, however, increasing the magnitude of the takeoff velocity gains the greatest increase in horizontal distance.

For any projectile activity there are certain constraints, such as an athlete's height and air resistance. Given these constraints, scientists and coaches should be able to predict the optimal takeoff angle for any given magnitude of velocity. As athletes get stronger and improve their technique, these values change.

Fluid Dynamics

All athletic events take place in a fluid environment, whether in water (underwater hockey), in air (cycling, sprinting), or in a combination of both (water polo, swimming). Some activities are largely unaffected (walking, gymnastics, dancing) by the fluid environment in which they occur, while for other activities and objects this environment is very important (running, cycling, skiing, speedskating, surfing, swimming, ping-pong, badminton shuttlecocks, baseballs, softballs, footballs, javelins).

Knowledge of the forces generated by the environment affects our understanding of how these skills are to be performed (i.e., which factors

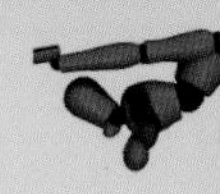

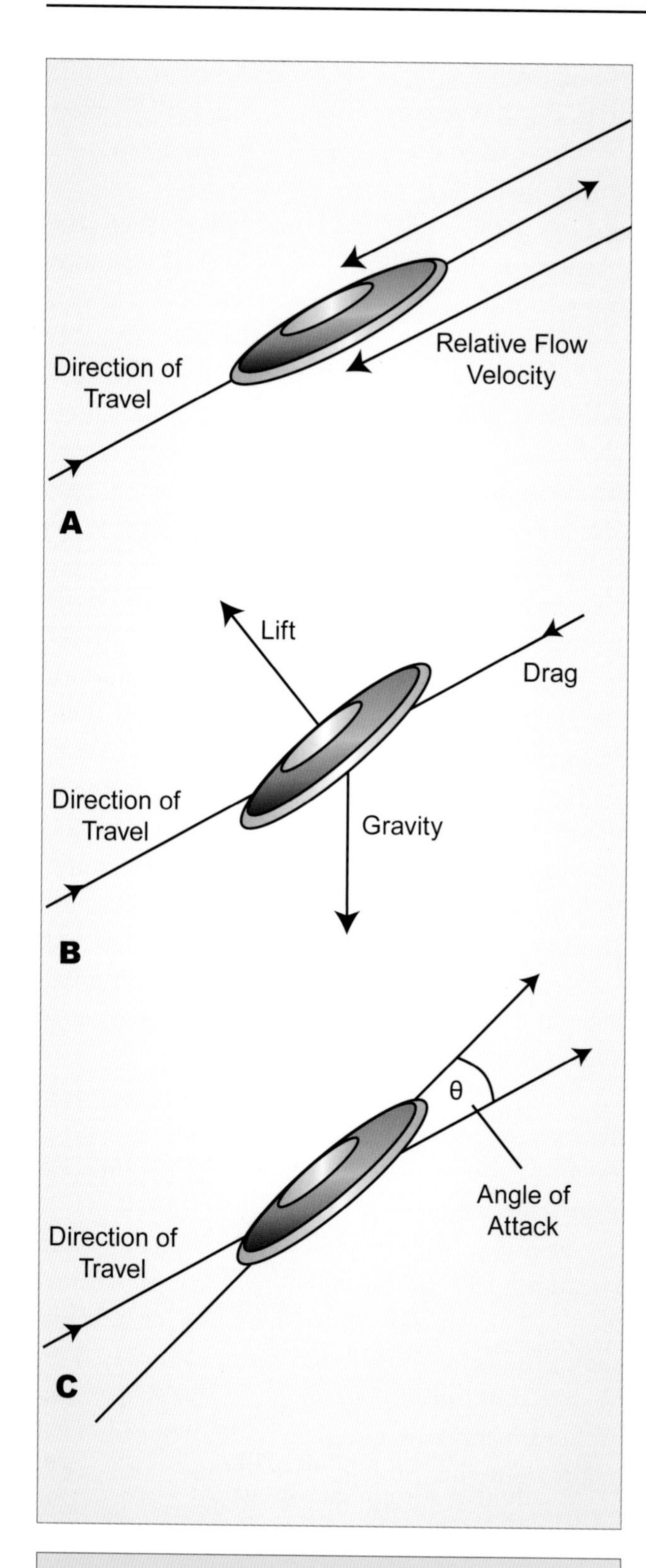

Figure 8.13 Effects of air resistance on a discus. **A.** Discus with direction of travel and relative flow velocity vectors superimposed. **B.** Free body diagram of discus, with lift, drag, and gravity vectors. **C.** Angle of attack (θ, is the angle between the direction of travel and the longitudinal axis of the discus).

affect them; Figures 8.13 and 8.14) and thus how they are taught and learned. For example, why does a cyclist pedal behind another in a race? What is "drafting" to a long-distance runner? Why does a ski racer adopt an egg position but a ski jumper lean toward a prone position in flight? Why do swimmers "spiral" their hands through their underwater stroking? And what makes a curveball curve? These questions are answered in this section.

> **Did You Know the Air Around You Is a Fluid?**
>
> A fluid is a substance that flows – liquid or gas. When you move, you cause the air to flow around you. And, because air resists motion, it slows you down.

Fluid dynamics studies the forces and their effects on human movement through different environments. Fluid forces include **drag force** and **lift force**. Drag and lift forces are perpendicular to each other, produce different effects, are affected by different factors, and have unique applications to various sports movements. All fluid forces depend upon the flow velocity (i.e., the motion of the fluid flowing past an object or the motion of the object through the fluid). Both concepts refer to the same variable, namely, the relative motion between the object and the fluid (Figure 8.13 A). In this section, only fluid forces acting in the air (**aerodynamics**) will be examined. **Hydrodynamics** (fluid forces acting in the water) is beyond the scope of this text.

Fluid Drag Forces: The Dynamics of Air

When cycling, we feel the air against our bodies acting directly opposite to our direction of motion. The faster we cycle, the greater the resistance. Intuitively, we know that if we flex at the hips and waist, presenting less surface area to the air, there is less resistance. The type of fluid force we

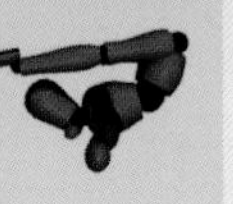

are feeling is called **drag**. Although this force is acting on all surfaces of our bodies and the bicycle, we often simplify its representation by drawing a single vector acting at the center of mass of the system (Figure 8.13 B).

There are two main sources of drag: form and skin friction. **Profile** or **form drag** is caused by the size of the object (or person) and the **air turbulence** produced by its shape as it moves through the air. **Skin-friction drag,** also known as **surface drag**, is caused by the surface roughness of the object (or person) as it moves through the air.

Both skin-friction and profile (form) drag are proportional to the relative flow velocity, cross-sectional area, shape of the object, smoothness of the surface, and density of the liquid.

Skin-friction Drag

The fluid tending to rub (shear) along the surface of the body causes skin-friction drag (i.e., a friction force) parallel and opposite to the flow velocity. The layer of fluid next to the skin sticks to the body; however, the next layer is towed along and therefore slides relative to the innermost layer. The third layer is towed by the second and in turn tows the fourth layer. Eventually, a layer of fluid is reached in which no sliding occurs. The region of relative motion between adjacent layers of fluid is called the **boundary layer.** Two types of flow can occur within the boundary layer: **laminar flow** and **turbulent flow.**

If an object is small, streamlined, smooth, and relatively slow, then laminar flow will occur within the boundary layer. Laminar flow is a smooth, layered flow pattern of a fluid around an object, with no wake or other disturbance. Large bodies with rough textured surfaces will have greater skin-friction drag. Most human activities move too fast to allow laminar flow to occur. Therefore, surface skin drag is not the source of most of the drag encountered in sport activities.

Profile Drag

Profile drag is the main form of drag in skiing, cycling, running, and all projectile events. Profile drag is the resistive drag against the object (Newton's third law of motion). It is characterized by turbulent flow in which the pressure on the leading surface of a body is greater than the pressure on the trailing surface. It is also known as pressure drag or form drag.

The velocity of air flow past the object is too fast for the air to follow the contour of the trailing side of the object, causing a "back flow" to occur at the surface of the object. This causes the boundary layer to separate from the surface contour, resulting in the formation of a large, turbulent low-pressure zone behind the object. This region of low pressure, which is continually formed as the object moves through the fluid, contains eddies that must be pulled along with the object, increasing the amount of work done on the object.

Because drag increases as the square of speed, an object moving 10 times faster will produce 100 times more drag. In high-speed sports (skiing, cycling, bobsledding), where a fraction of a second decides who finishes first, athletes attempt to reduce drag as much as possible by streamlining their bodies to reduce their cross-sectional area (Figure 8.14).

Skiers in their low drag position can increase their velocity by as much as 50 percent – reaching downhill speeds of over 80 miles (130 km) per hour (Figure 8.14 A).

Sledding while supine decreases form drag. The luger's feet cut through the air first, presenting the smallest possible frontal surface area. This allows the air to flow much more smoothly over the body and head. The sleigh is also shaped for minimum form drag and maximum speed. The nylon skintight, rubberized bodysuit along with special "speed boots" decreases lugers' friction drag. The smooth, tightly woven surface of the suit reduces turbulence by allowing air to slide over it much more easily than it would over conventional clothing or even bare skin (Figure 8.14 B).

Bending parallel to the ice, arm(s) behind the back, decreases the form drag of a speedskater. The speedskater's "crouch" minimizes frontal surface

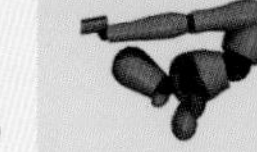

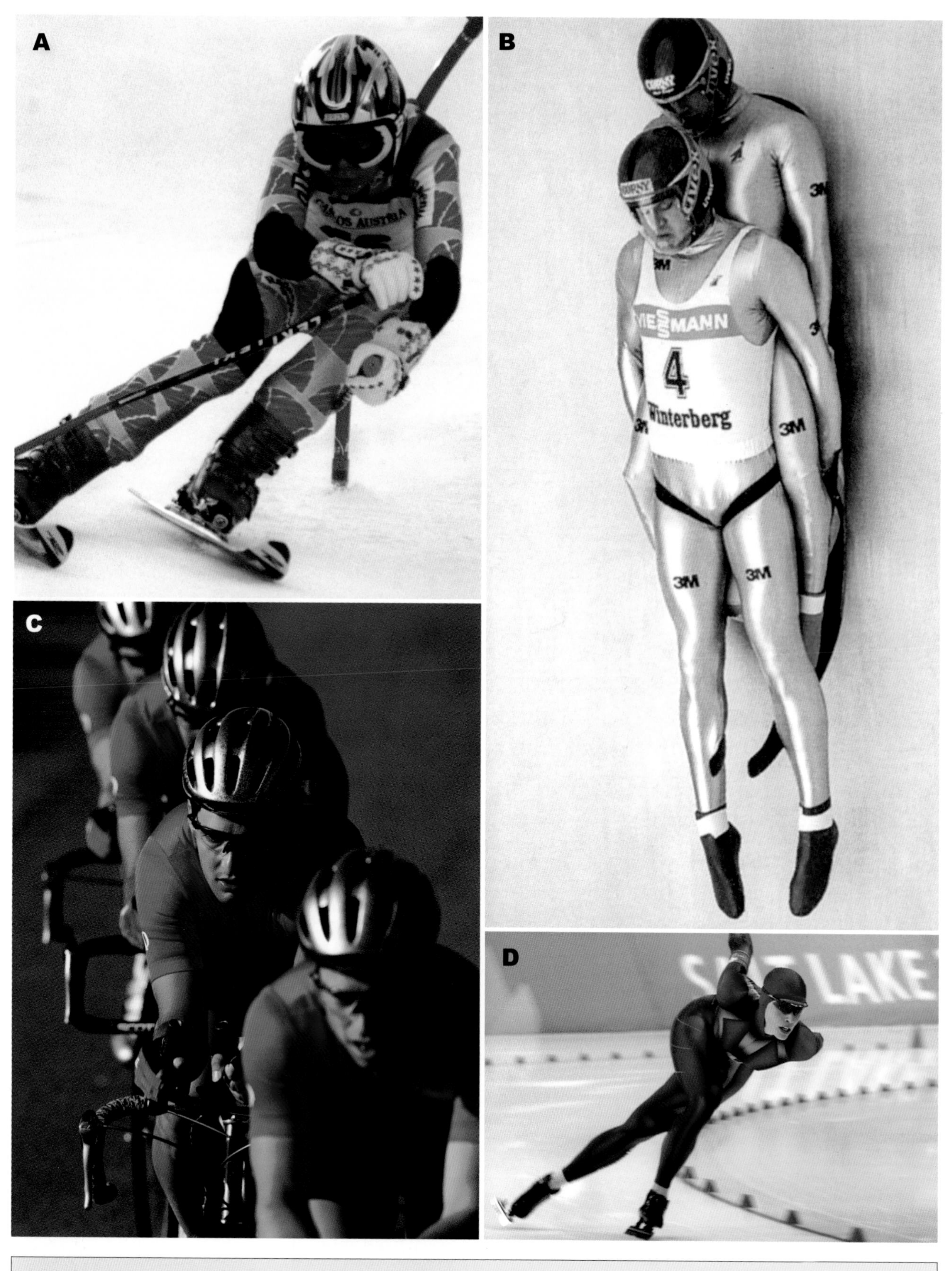

Figure 8.14 Drag forces generated by the environment have an effect on how various skills are performed most effectively.

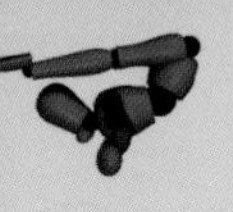

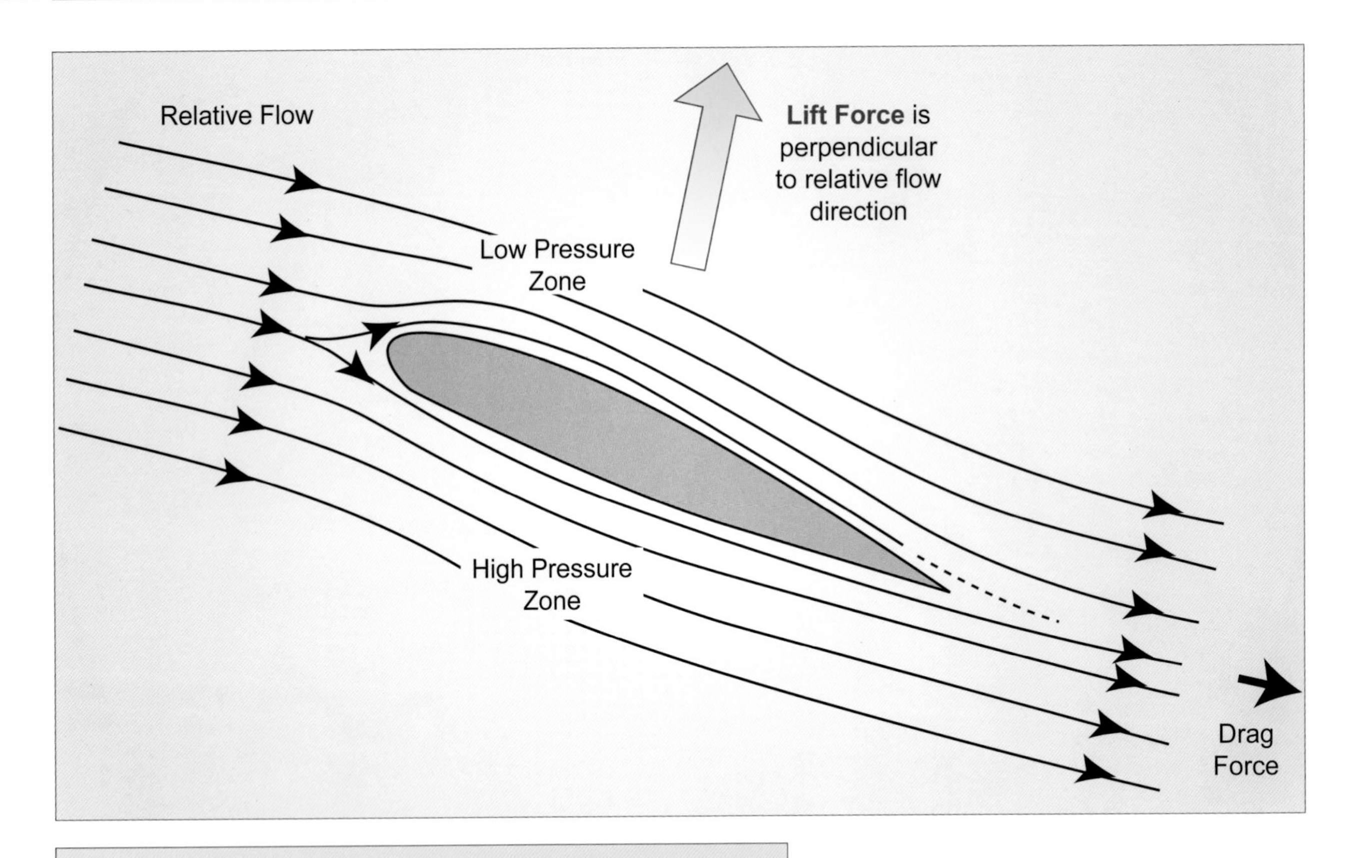

Figure 8.15 Aerodynamic lift force acting on an airfoil (wing).

area, thus significantly reducing wind resistance, and the position of the arms reduces turbulence, letting air flow more smoothly around the body (Figure 8.14 D).

Fluid Lift Forces

Fluid lift forces are always directed perpendicular to the flow velocity (not parallel as with drag forces). These lift forces can be directed (a) upward (discus, javelin, Frisbee, ski jumpers, tennis balls, water skiers), (b) downward (racing cars, sinker ball in baseball, or topspin in tennis), or (c) sideways (curveball in baseball).

How does lift occur? Consider the cross-section of an airfoil (a wing-shaped object) (Figure 8.15). Air flows faster over the upper curved surface than the lower flat surface, such that the difference in velocity across the surfaces results in a pressure difference between the two sides. The pressure difference results in a force directed from the high-pressure side to the low-pressure side. The inverse relationship between flow velocity and pressure is **Bernoulli's principle.** The external force resulting from the pressure difference is perpendicular to flow velocity direction and can thus change the motion of the object (Newton's first and second laws of motion).

Angle of Attack

The tilt of an object relative to the flow velocity is defined as the **angle of attack** (Figure 8.13 C). The angle of attack can mimic the effects of an airfoil by changing the pressure difference across

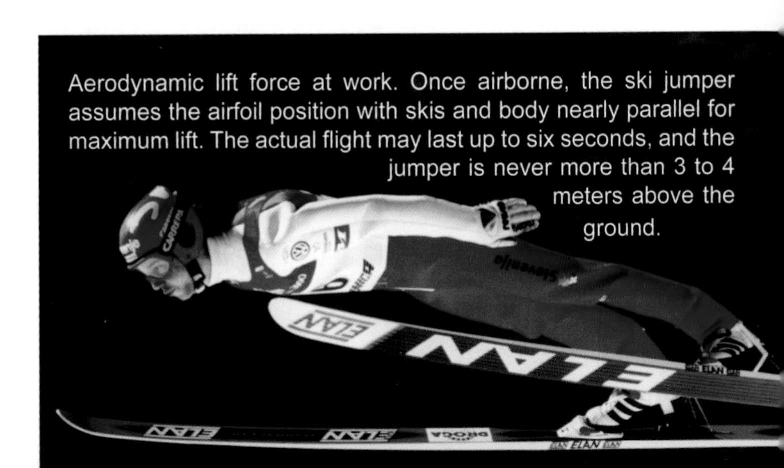

Aerodynamic lift force at work. Once airborne, the ski jumper assumes the airfoil position with skis and body nearly parallel for maximum lift. The actual flight may last up to six seconds, and the jumper is never more than 3 to 4 meters above the ground.

Why a Curveball Curves

The pitcher holds the index and middle fingers close together along the seams of the ball and twists the hand while releasing the ball to give it a very fast spin – approximately 1,800 revolutions per minute. The ball revolves 15 times in the less than 1/2 second it takes to reach the plate.

The ball's 108 stitches pull a thin layer of air with them as they spin. That layer makes the air on the bottom of the ball flow faster than the air at the top of the ball, which produces the curve ball (i.e., Magnus effect at work).

Split finger fastballs, sliders, and screw balls all rely on different kinds of spin – and the Magnus effect – to change direction.

A major league pitcher can make a baseball curve up to approximately 17 inches (43 cm) from its straight path on its way to the plate.

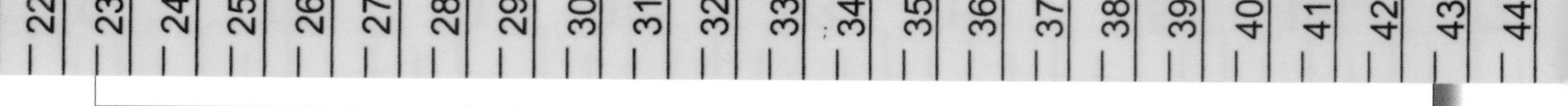

the surfaces of the object. It is a function of the shape of an object and the flow velocity.

The angle of attack may change throughout the flight, which means the amount of lift will change as well. If the angle of attack increases too much, it approaches a critical maximum angle beyond which the lift force suddenly decreases as the drag force becomes dominant. At the critical angle, called the stall angle, the object falls earthward with no further forward motion. Frisbees, discuses, javelins, and airplanes all experience changing angles of attack.

The Magnus Effect

Any spinning projectile generates a lift force. A rotating body carries a layer of fluid with it as it spins. This boundary layer interacts with the fluid through which the body travels, such that if the layer is in the opposite direction to the flow velocity, the air stagnates and there is a zone of increased pressure. If the boundary layer is in the same direction, there is a zone of decreased pressure created. The net difference in the pressure on opposite sides of the body constitutes a force that changes the direction of the body along the pressure gradient.

Take an object that is spinning about an axis not aligned with the flow velocity vector (perpendicular is best), unlike a football in which the spinning axis and flow velocity are coincident. The pressure difference across opposite sides of such an object is such that changes in its flight path can be generated by a type of force known as a **Magnus force**, and the whole mechanism, the **Magnus effect**. The changes in path are always perpendicular to the flow velocity of the projectile.

Topspin restricts the horizontal distance a projectile will travel, with no loss in takeoff velocity. On the other hand, underspin or backspin will increase the horizontal distance, time in the air, or accuracy (golf, tennis, soccer, basketball) for a given takeoff velocity.

For sidespins, a ball will curve toward the spinning side. More curve ("break") is noticed the longer the ball is airborne.

The Magnus effect is seen most readily in tennis, golf, ping-pong, and baseball (see box *Why a Curveball Curves*). In these activities, the projectile is small in size and mass, and it can be given large takeoff velocities and high spin rates,

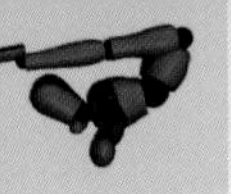

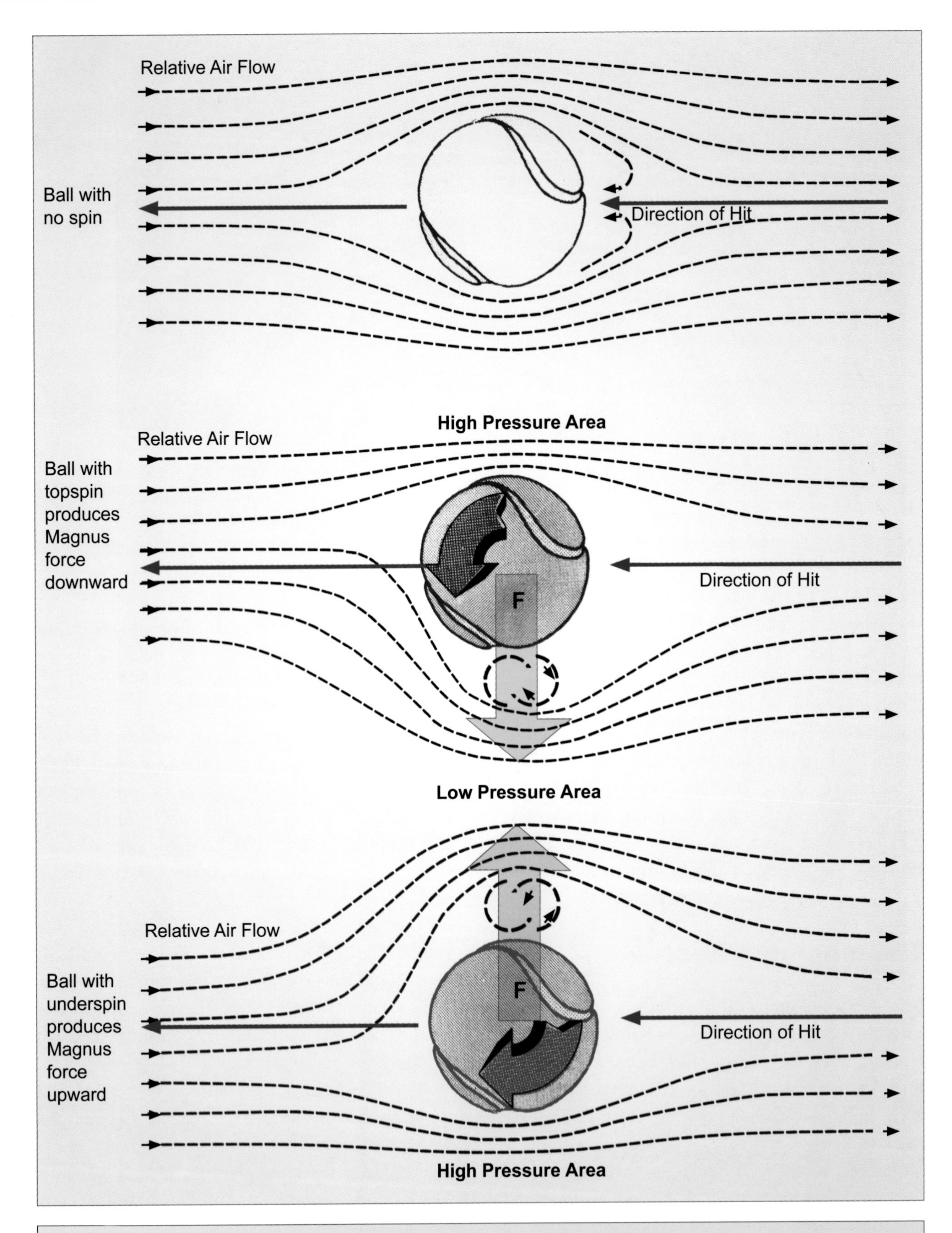

Figure 8.16 The uneven surface of a spinning tennis ball creates a Magnus force (F). The Magnus force is directed from high to low pressure.

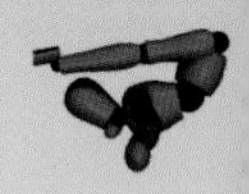

all of which positively influence the Magnus force.

The uneven surface of a tennis ball pulls a thin layer of air along with it when it spins (Figure 8.16). That makes the air on one side of the ball flow faster (and more smoothly) than on the other side – it's like the spinning blades of a fan creating a breeze. The faster flow causes the air pressure on that side of the ball to drop – and the ball drops or curves into the area of lower air pressure.

Body Balance and Stability Control

Balance is a very important factor in athletic performance. In general, it depends upon the location of an athlete's center of mass and how stable that center of mass is. Stick figures are very useful tools in indicating body balance throughout an athletic performance (Figure 8.9, page 172).

Equilibrium

Equilibrium describes the state of a system that is not experiencing any change in its direction or speed. There are two states of equilibrium, static and dynamic. **Static equilibrium** describes the state of a system that is at rest. **Dynamic equilibrium** describes the state of a system that is moving with constant velocity (unchanging speed and direction). In Figure 8.18, the gymnast, lineman, and sprinter are in static equilibrium, while the kayaker, skier, and cyclist may be in dynamic equilibrium as long as their velocity is not changing.

Balance

The process whereby the body's state of equilibrium is controlled for a given purpose is called **balance**. To control the state of equilibrium, we constantly (and often unconsciously) manipulate two factors. The first factor is our *base of support*, which is the area defined by the points of contact between the body and the surface supporting it. The second factor is the location of our *line of gravity*, which is an imaginary vertical line that passes through the center of mass. If the line of gravity passes through some part of the body's base of support, then the body will be balanced (Figure 8.17).

Stability

Stability is a relative term and is a measure of the ease or difficulty with which equilibrium can be disturbed. A net external force is required to overcome the static equilibrium of a sprinter in the starting blocks or the dynamic equilibrium of a running back. A net external moment of force would be required to tip over a gymnast performing a handstand or to overturn a canoe or kayak.

At some critical time within most performances there is a trade-off between **maximizing stability** and **acquiring speed off a mark**. For example, sprinters must be able to move quickly at the start signal (i.e., to go into motion), and therefore it is desirable to be in an unstable equilibrium state. On the other hand, a football lineman or wrestler must be able to resist any external forces and thus strives to be in a state of stable equilibrium.

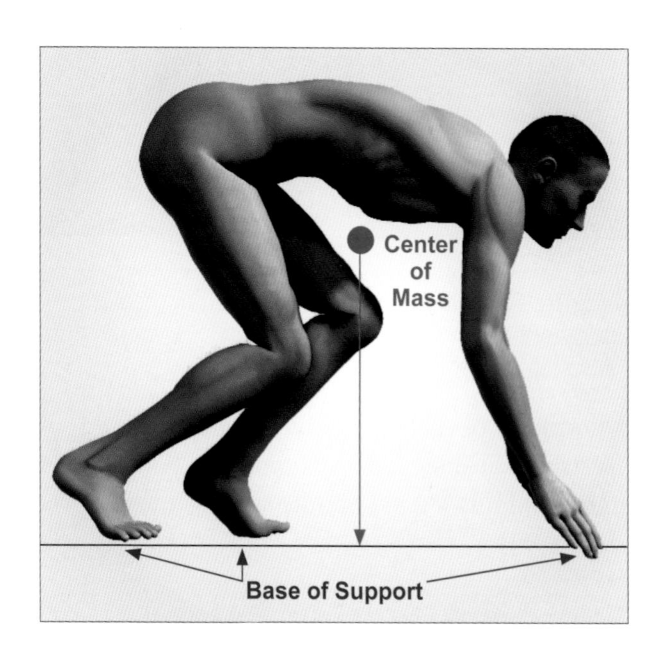

Figure 8.17 Factors affecting balance.

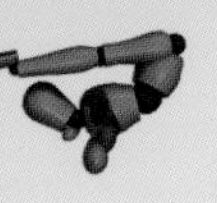

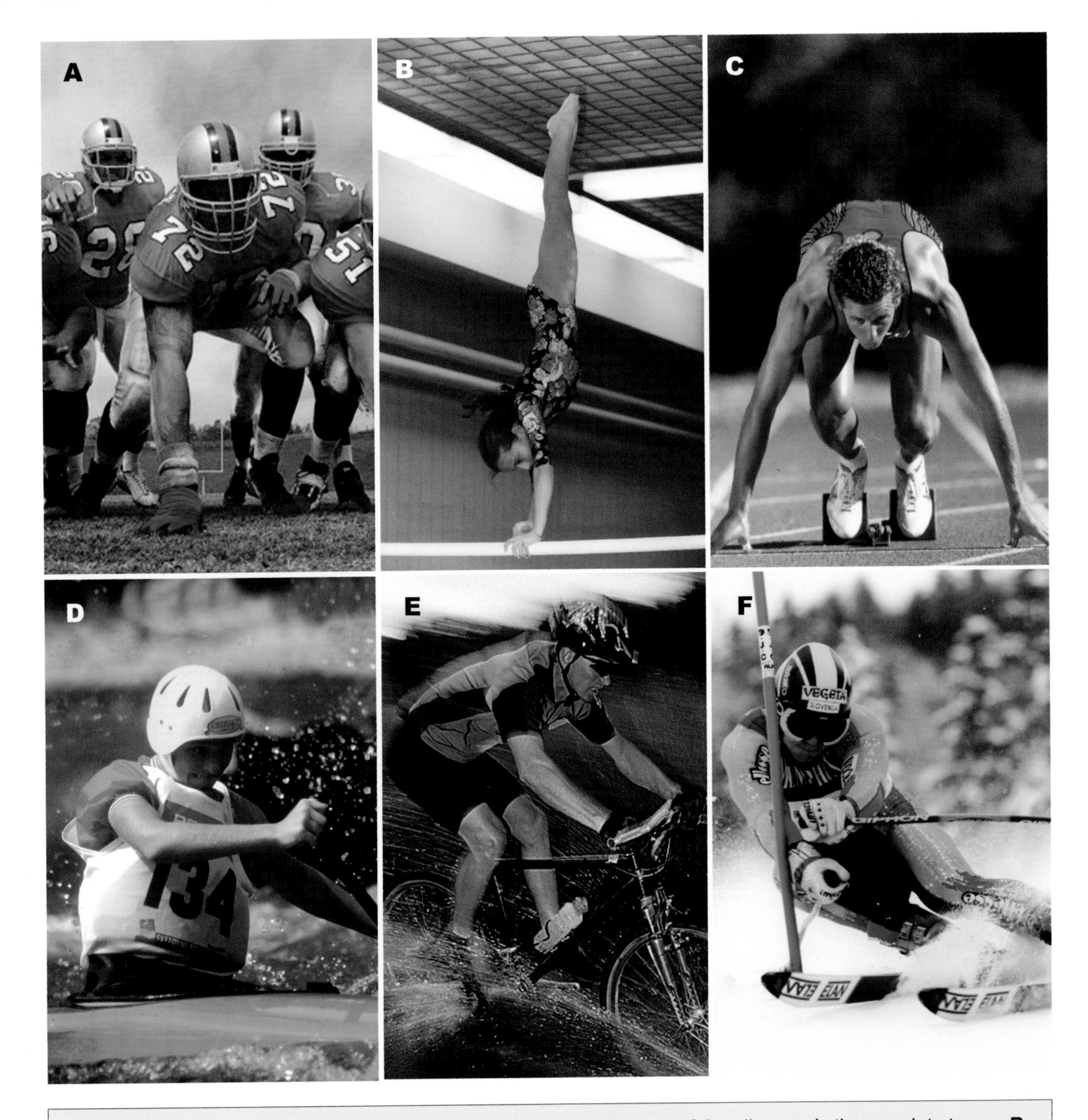

Figure 8.18 Maintaining equilibrium and balance. Static equilibrium of **A.** a lineman's three-point stance; **B.** a gymnastics element; and **C.** a sprint start. Dynamic equilibrium of **D.** a kayaker; **E.** a cyclist; and **F.** a skier.

Knowledge of the ways stability can be altered, or the factors influencing it, is therefore pertinent to understanding a good performance in most sports skills.

Factors Affecting Balance

To *increase* the stability in a static equilibrium an athlete must:

(1) increase the base of support (Figure 8.18 A and B; lineman versus gymnast);

(2) increase the inertia (mass, moment of inertia) of the body – larger forces and moments of force would be required to move the body (Figure 8.18 A and B; lineman versus gymnast);

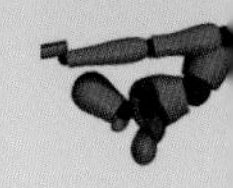

(3) decrease the vertical distance between the center of mass and the base of support (Figure 8.18 B and C; gymnast versus sprinter); and

(4) increase the distance between the point where a vertical line from the center of mass intersects the base of support and the outside edge of the base of support (Figure 8.18 A and C; lineman versus sprinter).

To *increase* stability in dynamic equilibrium an athlete must:

(1) enlarge the body's base of support in the direction of external horizontal forces, which may be given or received (hockey checks);

(2) adopt a starting position in which the center of pressure is close to the edge of the base of support whenever quick acceleration is important (kayaker, cyclist, or skier who wishes to turn quickly);

(3) lean backward but keep normal frictional forces high to prevent slipping when slowing down or reversing directions in running; and

(4) use reflex movements to help regain loss of balance when tripping or falling (windmill action of arms of gymnasts falling off a beam) or to create a new base of support. The athlete can also use the angular momentum created and perform a roll, thereby increasing the time required to exert the necessary force to regain an upright body posture (also temporarily increasing frictional forces between body and ground).

Angular Kinetics

Angular kinetics is concerned with the generation of rotations about an axis of rotation and the control of these rotations. All objects possess inertia and do not wish to start rotating, or if rotating, to change the quantity of rotation they have. However, if an external moment of force is applied to the object, then it will experience an angular acceleration, which results in a new state of motion (Figure 8.6 B, page 168). The greater the applied moment of force (action), the greater the change in the angular acceleration (reaction). This is another example of Newton's third law of motion: for every moment of force applied to one object, an equal moment of force is applied back to the other object at the same time.

The somersault serves as a good example of angular kinetics. It is found extensively in diving, freestyle skiing, and gymnastics. For all these skills, the somersaulting motion is generated while the athlete is on the ground.

Off-center External Forces

Any external force that acts away from the body's center of mass will create a moment of force acting on the total body. This is so because all bodies, when airborne, rotate about an axis passing through their center of mass. Usually the off-center force is a reaction force from the ground or equipment (e.g., diving board), resulting from the internal muscle forces generated by the athlete.

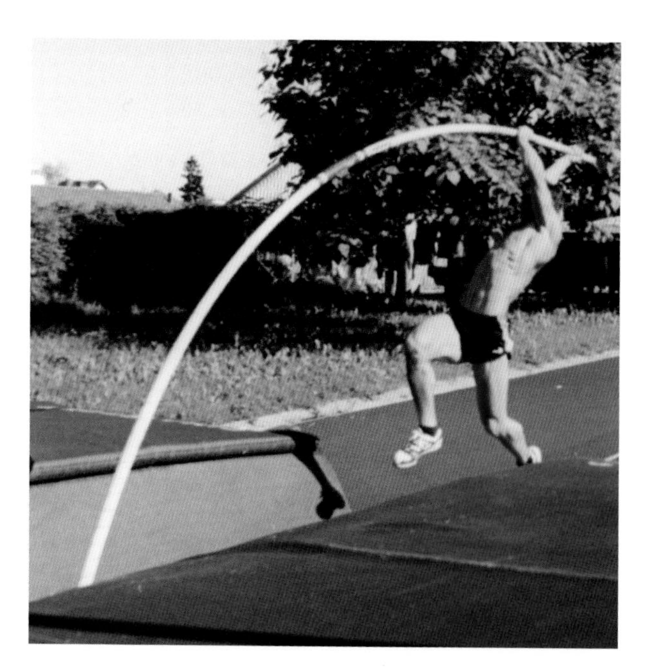

Figure 8.19 A pole-vaulter's movement exhibits rotation about the pivot point created by the planted pole.

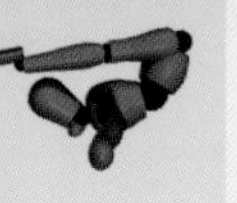

However, if an athlete has forward momentum (e.g., running) and a pivot point is created, then some or all of the linear motion can be transferred into angular motion. Consider a pole-vaulter (Figure 8.19) who, upon planting his or her pole, creates a pivot point and rotates about that point. Similarly, how about the unfortunate runner whose foot gets caught in a hole in the ground and whose body rotates forward about that pivot point?

Conservation of Momentum Within the Body

It is essential for athletes to make good use of the principle of conservation of momentum in turns, twists, and spins occurring in many sports. The mechanical properties of the human body permit great flexibility of its links to change the body form. In many movements, athletes can make skillful use of the fact that they can alter the magnitude of their mass moment of inertia during rotation. This applies to both the control of the rotation and to the successful execution of various complex forms of rotation in general.

Rotations While Airborne

Rotations in many sports are produced while the body is in contact with the ground. The initiated rotations will continue when the body is airborne. In the flight phase when the body can be regarded as a free moving system, angular velocity can be effectively controlled by skillfully changing the body posture and hence the mass moment of inertia. Once the body is airborne, only gravity and air resistance are acting on the body. Gravity acts through the body's center of mass and cannot create a moment of force. Therefore, the amount of angular motion athletes have upon leaving the ground, their angular momentum, cannot be changed once airborne. An athlete's angular momentum is said to be conserved, constant, or uniform while airborne. This phenomenon is referred to as the **conservation of angular momentum.**

However, somersaulting athletes can change their body shape while airborne. Changes in body shape will decrease/increase their moment of inertia about the somersaulting axis, which will change their general resistance to rotating. If the moment of inertia decreases, then an athlete's body will have less reluctance to rotating and will begin to rotate faster (increased angular velocity). If the moment of inertia increases, then the body will have greater reluctance to rotating and will begin to rotate more slowly (decreased angular velocity). New motion is not being created or destroyed, but the speed with which the athlete is rotating changes with changes in the moment of inertia.

For example, in diving, athletes can perform a somersaulting dive in a layout, pike, or tuck position (decreasing moments of inertia about the body's sagittal axis) (Figure 8.20). Given an equal amount of angular momentum upon leaving the diving board, the angular velocity of these dives will be slow in the layout position (Figure 8.20 A), faster in the pike position (Figure 8.20 B), and fastest in the tuck position (Figure 8.20 C).

By changing their body posture during the final stages of the dive, divers have to control their angular velocity in such a manner that when entering the water their bodies have the lowest angular velocity. Only in this way is splashing reduced to a minimum.

The same phenomenon occurs in gymnastics and freestyle skiing. Similarly, in figure skating, athletes can change their moment of inertia about their vertical axis by going into the spin or jump with their arms and free legs as far away as possible from their axis of rotation. The spin or rotation of their jumps is increased by bringing their arms and legs tightly to the body's longitudinal axis of rotation (Figure 8.21).

Coaches have to be aware that rotations are generated and dissipated on the ground only. The illusions of changing rotational speeds are associated with changes in moments of inertia and not the amount of angular motion generated.

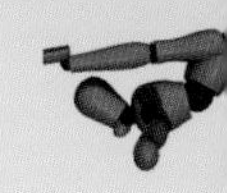

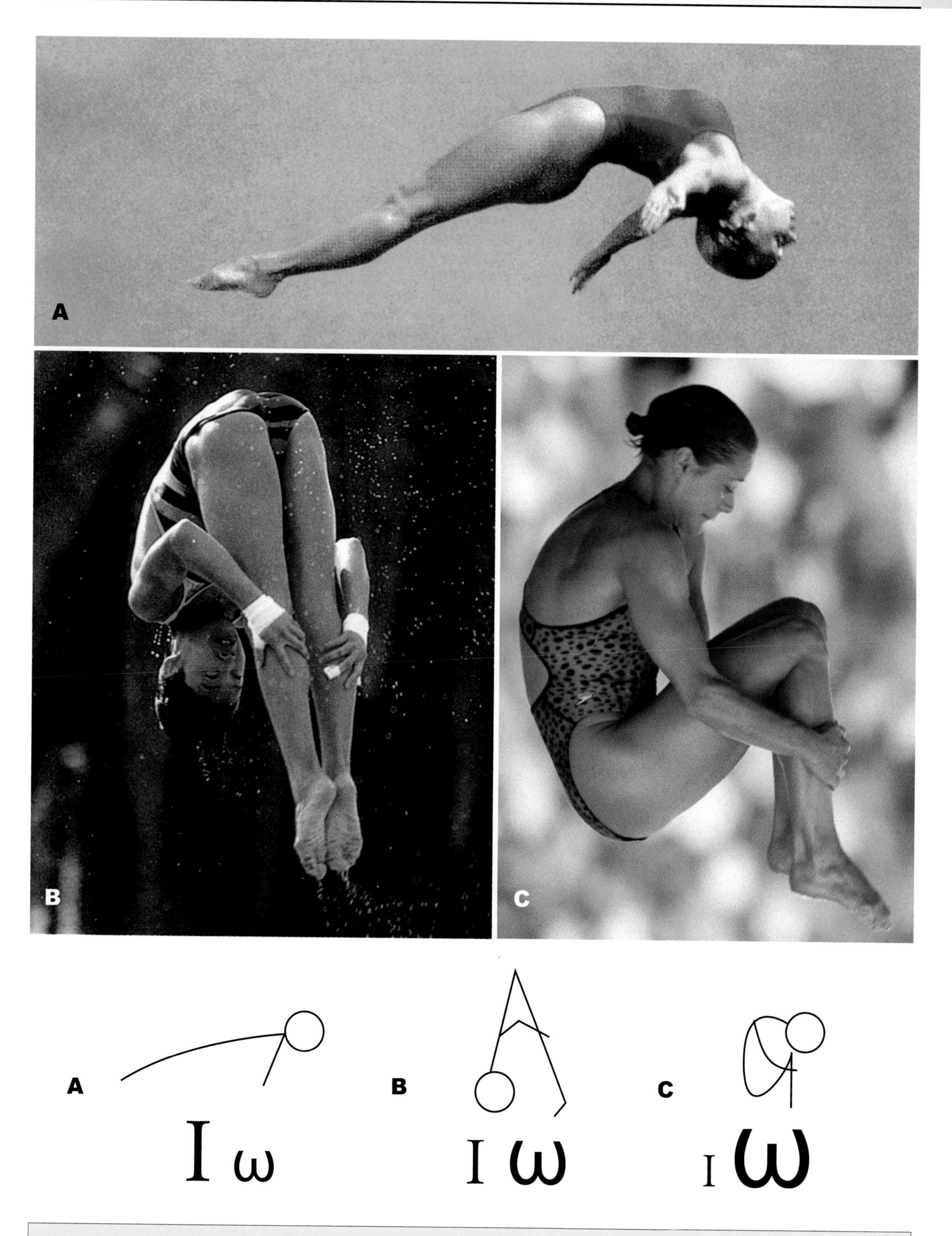

Figure 8.20 The inverse relationship between moment of inertia (I) and angular velocity (ω) for the **A.** layout; **B.** pike; and **C.** tuck position of a somersault in diving.

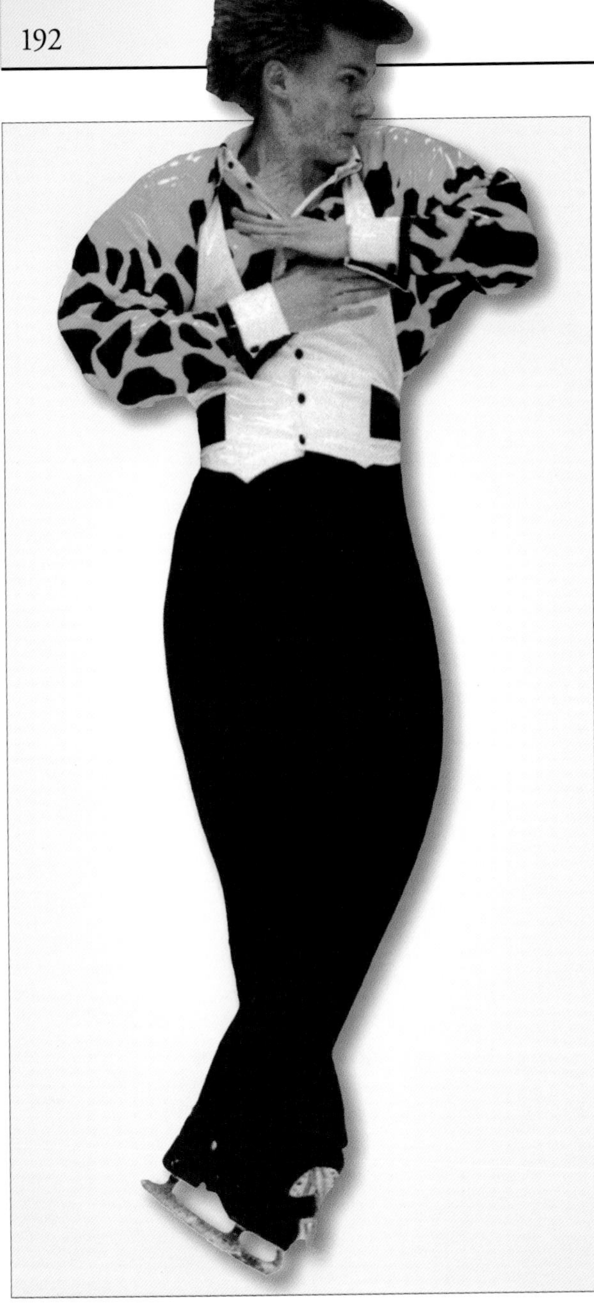

Figure 8.21 Figure skaters bring their arms in tight to the body to maintain high angular velocity during spins and jumps.

Qualitative Analysis of Human Motion

Qualitative analysis is the study of human motion, in the absence of measuring, by observing a movement and applying biomechanical principles in assessing a performance. A qualitative analysis is a subjective and yet systematic evaluation of a movement or skill. It is based on direct visual observation of movement or its video recording. Although movements may be too fast to observe the skill accurately, this technique allows the instructor or coach to discover movement tendencies and to provide the athlete with immediate valuable feedback. This feedback is movement specific and greatly superior to nonspecific jargon-infected feedback such as "don't fall," "rotate more," and "jump higher."

The qualitative approach suggested here is generic. In this approach, the coach is asked to consider the objective of the skill, to analyze the skill biomechanically by identifying phases of the skill and the key criteria and movement patterns, to decide how the observation will be done, and to prepare, in advance, corrections for commonly occurring performance errors (Figure 8.22).

A qualitative analysis is dependent on the constraints or limitations of an event or performer. For example, rules, physical boundaries, equipment requirements, and the environment can all place constraints upon an event. Basketball is played on a specified court, with a ball of specified size, and with an established set of rules. Other constraints arise because of human limitations (such as body build, strength, power, endurance, and flexibility), skill level of the athlete and opponent, and any movement requirements that may precede or follow the skill. However, the generic qualitative analysis is independent of the nature of the skill, whether it is open or closed, discrete or continuous (for more on types of skills see Chapter 11).

Most importantly, however, the qualitative approach to movement analysis is based on instructors' thorough understanding of the movement or skill they are evaluating. This understanding comes from their vast experience with coaching or instructing the activity. Only then will they be able to assess accurately what is wrong or right in the performer's execution of the movement. It takes years of experience to develop a critical eye for correct assessment of techniques and their subtleties.

Qualitative analysis is based on a simple model

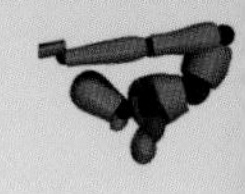

that integrates the four major aspects of quality instruction: preparation, observation, evaluation, and error correction (Figure 8.22).

Skill Objective

An objective can be described for all skills. It may be as simple as throwing an opponent in judo or blocking an oncoming lineman in football. Secondary objectives may also exist, referring to the speed of the movement or the accuracy required. Skills with similar overall objectives will be governed by similar biomechanical principles, which in turn should simplify the analysis process for different skills.

For example, the performance purpose of many skills is to throw, strike, or kick an object for maximum horizontal distance (range). The mechanical purpose of these skills is therefore to release, strike, or impart to the object – at the instant of takeoff – a maximal takeoff velocity at the optimal angle of release (Figure 8.12, page 179). Accomplishing these biomechanical criteria will satisfy the performance objective.

Analyzing a Skill

Divide the Skill into Phases

All skills, whether discrete or continuous, can be

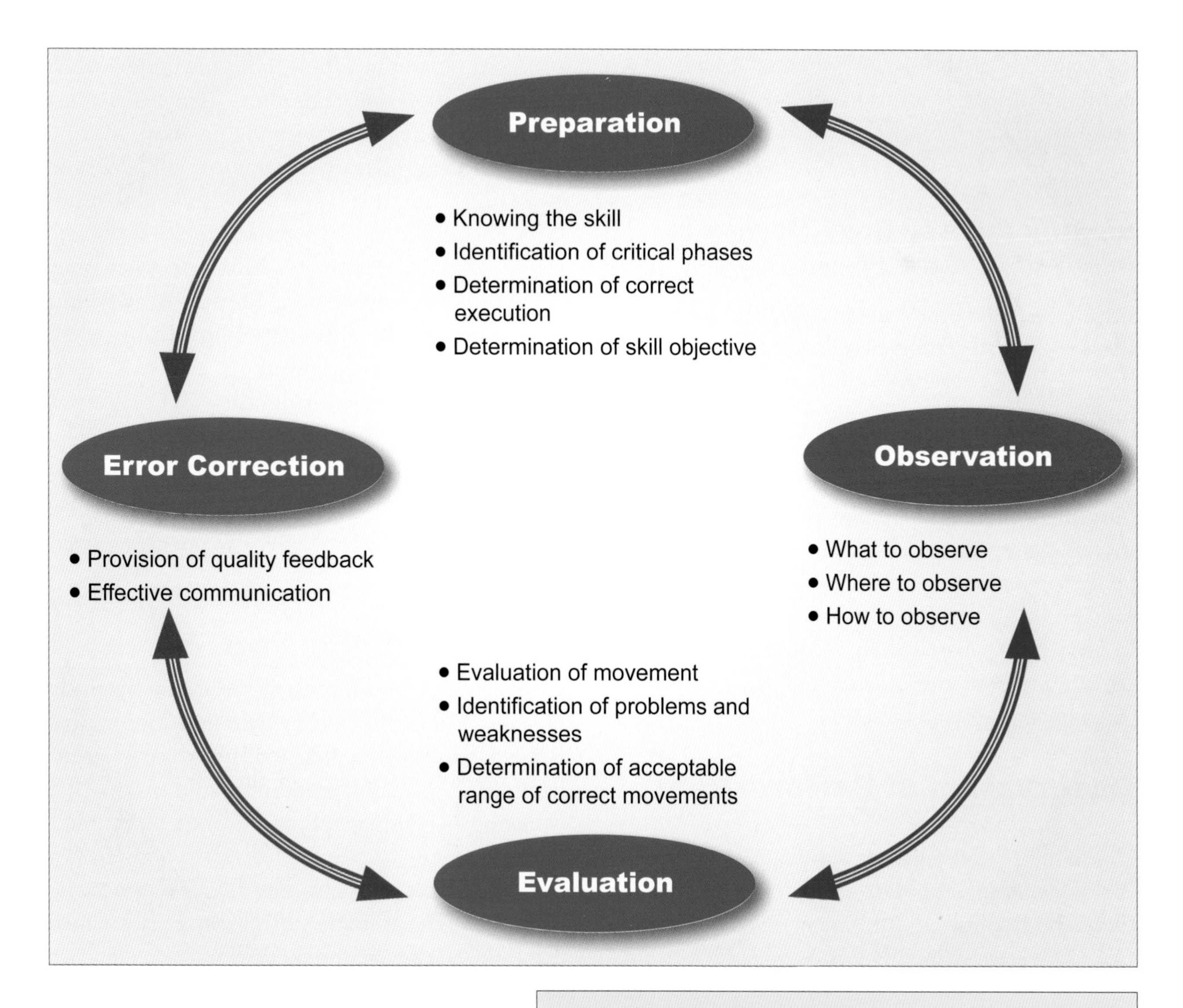

Figure 8.22 The integrated model of qualitative analysis.

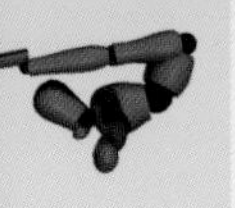

divided into phases or subroutines (for more on subroutines see Chapter 11). These phases should make sense to the coach, as far as how he or she teaches the skill and how the sport defines the skill. One suggestion is that each phase relate to a change in the athlete's state of motion (i.e., any time an acceleration occurs). Common names for phases include preparation, execution, and follow-through, although many skills include takeoff, airborne, and landing phases, or push and pull phases.

Determine the Biomechanical Criteria for Each Phase

For each phase, identify the biomechanical criteria that cause the specific movement patterns associated with the performance of a skill. For example, in the execution phase, shot-putters must maximize the velocity of the shot prior to takeoff.

Identify the Key Body Movements Involved in Each Phase

List the key body movements for each phase (i.e., those segmental actions that should be performed, that can be observed, and that satisfy the biomechanical criteria for that phase). Execution of these movements contributes directly to successfully accomplishing the biomechanical purpose of the discrete phase, and ultimately, the overall performance of the event. For example, in the preparatory phase of the soccer kick, the foot of the stance leg is placed beside the ball. In throwing a baseball in from the outfield, a sequence of body movements from the foot to the throwing arm should be seen.

Observation of Performance

Observing performances is a difficult task. Often, the skills occur too fast to see specific detail. Other body parts or equipment may block the view. There are many distractions on the playing field (weather, other players, time pressures) that may potentially interfere with a coach's ability to observe an athlete's performance. To observe effectively, an observation plan must be prepared before arriving at the playing field. The plan identifies what, why, where, and how observation of the athlete's performance will occur.

What, Why, and Where to Observe

Before going to practice, a coach or instructor must identify the skill, or parts thereof, that he or she wishes to observe, and why. Specific elements of this observation plan include the phase of the skill to be observed, body movements, and related biomechanical criteria. Knowing what and why helps a coach stay organized with respect to observing the skills of all players.

Furthermore, knowledge of what will be observed determines the conditions under which the observation will take place. The coach must decide upon his or her viewing position, making sure that the athlete's body actions will be visible. Sometimes multiple views of the skill from different angles will be required to see all of the movements. For example, while a side view may be optimal for observing a runner, an overhead view might reveal important information when analyzing a discus thrower. In any case, it is important to keep the surroundings as uncluttered as possible and to minimize distractions. The instructor should estimate how many times the skill has to be viewed – enough to obtain an idea of "normal" performance, but not enough to elicit fatigue.

How to Observe

Coaches must use all of their senses to effectively observe a performance. Although our visual sense is dominant, information that is heard (timing of footfalls, breathing rhythms) or felt (spotting in gymnastics) should not be ignored. A thorough instructor will directly observe not only the athlete but also any tracks or traces he or she may have made during the performance (e.g., ski tracks, figure skating traces). Coaches often ask an athlete questions to confirm their observations, and if possible, videotape

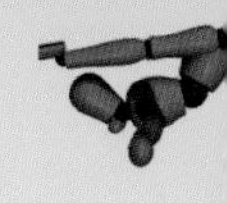

the observation, using slow motion replay to examine fast and/or small movement details that may otherwise be missed.

In general, any observation should begin with an analysis of the whole skill. The coach can then zoom in on the phase and body movements on which he or she really wishes to focus. An athlete must be given an adequate warm-up before demonstrating a particular movement to ensure a *normal* performance. When the athlete is ready, the coach should record his or her observations and/or provide immediate and specific feedback to the performer.

Error Detection and Correction

There are many reasons why athletes make errors. Sometimes the errors are psychological in nature, such as a lapse in concentration or fear of execution, or result from an error in judgment. Other errors occur as a result of lack of strength, power, endurance, or flexibility or because of poor habits. However, errors in technical performance can often be traced to athletes not maximizing or optimizing the biomechanical variables critical to the skill. In this case, coaches must be able to understand the biomechanics of the skill, identify which criteria are not being optimized, and direct their corrections to these biomechanical variables. Performing a biomechanical analysis beforehand will aid every technique used for error detection and correction.

In all cases, the coach must make corrections while keeping the athlete's physical and mental abilities, and the level of competition, in mind.

Error Detection

The most common technique for error detection is visual, by using direct observation, analyzing videos, or observing traces or marks left by the athlete. Visual observation improves with practice. However, performing a biomechanical analysis of the skill beforehand will improve the chances of spotting where the error is occurring, particularly concerning the phases of the skill and body parts used. Other error detection techniques include observing the outcome (placement of a golf shot) or follow-through (end of the tennis stroke), using a chart or checklist, or asking the athletes what they felt about their performance. The first two indicate which biomechanical variable was *not* performed well and therefore suggest a phase or body part(s) on which to focus. The latter two are also useful if a prior biomechanical analysis has been done because they will help athletes and coaches concentrate on critical variables.

One method to avoid is comparison with an ideal form or mental model. While these comparisons may be useful in conceptualizing a skill, everyone has a different body build (skeletal and muscular), which directly affects how he or she will look when performing a skill. By concentrating on the biomechanical variables, athletes will explore with their own bodies how to optimize these criteria. They will be able to concentrate on factors that are under their control and not be drawn into adopting others' idiosyncrasies.

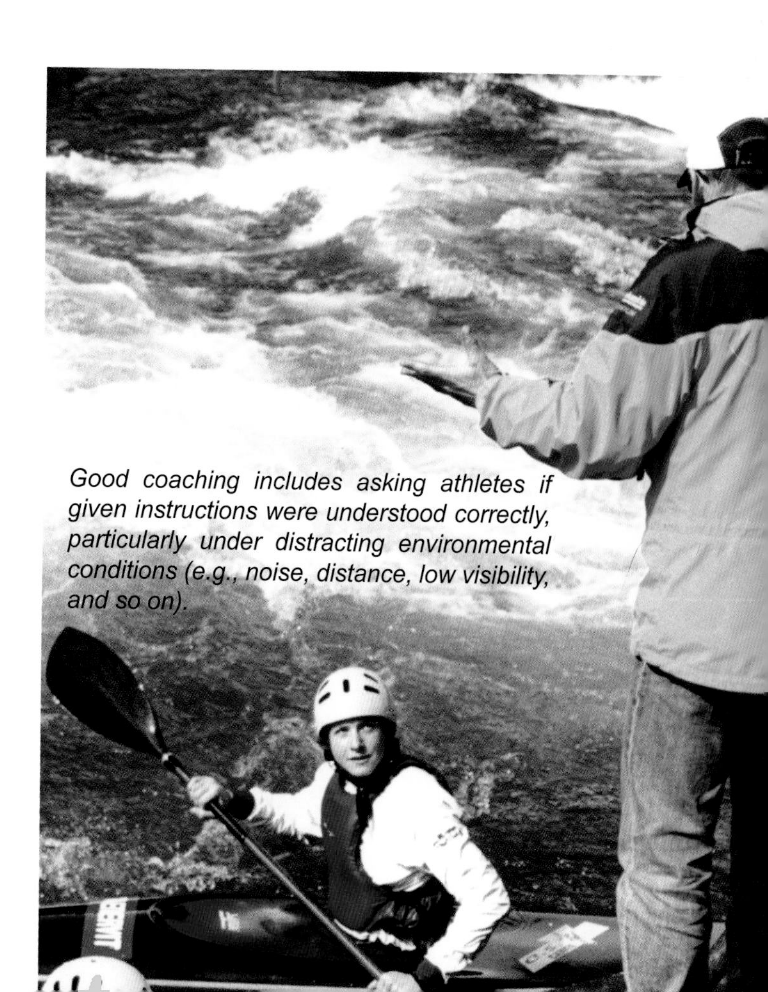

Good coaching includes asking athletes if given instructions were understood correctly, particularly under distracting environmental conditions (e.g., noise, distance, low visibility, and so on).

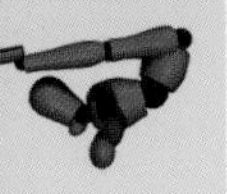

Error Correction

Error correction is usually done verbally, although visual feedback (video, demonstration), repetition (drills), or mental imagery may also be used. In all cases, corrections are being made to body part movements related directly to a biomechanical variable that satisfies the performance objective of the skill. If several errors have occurred, then begin with the earliest error, as this mistake may have introduced other errors in later stages of the skill. Correct only one or two faults before re-observing the skill. Accept that error correction is a multistep ongoing process.

Good error correction is a communication skill as well as a biomechanical skill. When correcting, coaches should use positive and specific language appropriate to the age, developmental level, and competitive level of their athletes. Conscientious instructors ask for feedback to check if the correction instructions were received as intended, and they try to minimize any distractions in the environment before correcting any errors. Good coaches are also familiar with the latest technology and use it in their coaching (Figure 8.23).

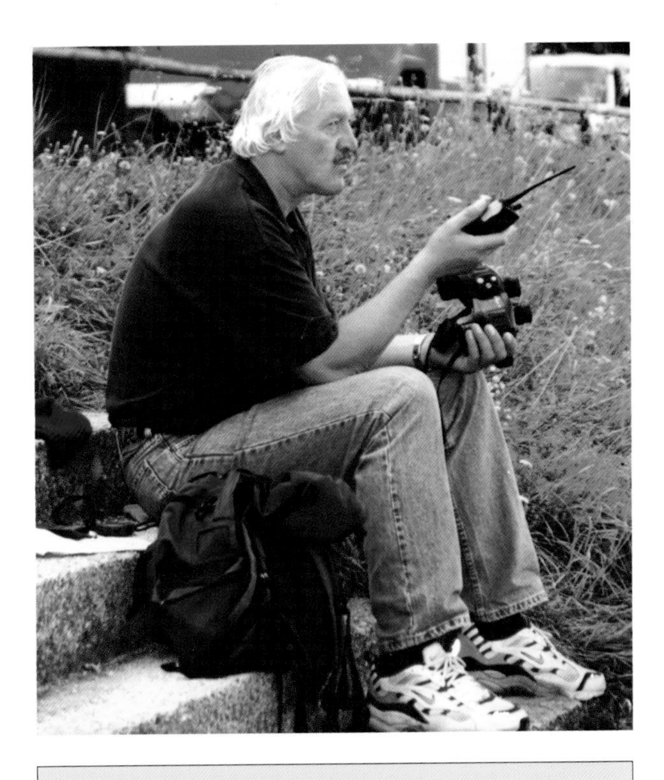

Figure 8.23 In sports where there is a considerable distance between the coach and the athlete, a walkie talkie or other long-range communication device comes in very handy.

Summary

The focus of this chapter was biomechanics, or the *physics* of human movement. The major goal of research in the area of sport biomechanics is to help athletes optimize performance by describing human movement from both a kinematic and dynamic perspective. Biomechanists study movement with the aid of three computer-generated biomechanical models – the particle, stick figure, and rigid segment body models.

Motion in the human body, whether it's linear, angular, or general, is the result of the application of an external force (a push or pull). Newton's three laws of motion describe the relationships between inertia, force, mass, and acceleration. The fluid (i.e., air or water) through which an object or athlete moves generates drag and lift forces. Laws such as Bernoulli's principle and the Magnus effect influence characteristics of projectiles in flight (e.g., the path of a javelin or the spin on a tennis ball). When athletes are in flight, they can control their angular velocity by changing their body positions in the air. An object or athlete not experiencing any change in direction or acceleration is said to be in a state of equilibrium.

Coaches and athletes use qualitative analysis to evaluate skills for the purpose of detecting and correcting errors. A knowledge of biomechanical principles helps a coach determine the source of performance errors and how best to correct them.

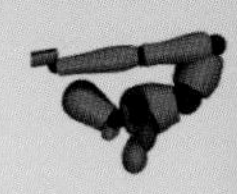

Key Terms

acceleration
action–reaction
aerodynamics
angle of attack
angular acceleration
angular displacement
angular kinetics
angular motion (rotation)
angular velocity
axis of rotation
balance
Bernoulli's principle
biomechanics
boundary layer
center of mass (gravity)
composite diagram
conservation of angular momentum
curvilinear motion
displacement
drag
drag force
dynamic equilibrium
equilibrium
first class lever
fulcrum
general motion
gravity
hydrodynamics
impact
impulse
inertia
kinematics
kinetics
laminar flow
lever
lift force
linear motion
Magnus effect
Magnus force
mass
moment arm
moment of force (torque)
moment of inertia
momentum
net force
Newton's first law
Newton's second law
Newton's third law
parabolic path
particle model
profile (form) drag
projectile
qualitative analysis
quantitative analysis
range
rectilinear motion
rigid body segment model
scalar quantity
second class lever
skin-friction (surface) drag
stability
static equilibrium
stick figure model
third class lever
translation
turbulent flow
vector
vector quantity
velocity

Discussion Questions

1. Define biomechanics. What other disciplines can benefit from studies in biomechanics?
2. Discuss three ways in which biomechanics can be helpful to teachers and coaches.
3. Apply each of Newton's three laws of motion to a skill, or portion thereof, relevant to a sport of your choice. Be specific in identifying forces, masses, accelerations, and so on.
4. Briefly discuss how you would advise an athlete to maximize impulse and minimize the harmful effects of impact in a specific sport.
5. What factors affect the horizontal distance a projectile will travel? Which is most important?
6. Select a sports skill in which a light object is thrown. Discuss the effects air resistance will have on the projectile path of this object.
7. Identify three ways in which athletes decrease drag forces acting against their bodies.
8. Identify two sports skills in which lift forces have a large effect on the resulting motion. Explain this effect.
9. Differentiate between equilibrium, stability, and balance.
10. In a sport of your choosing, identify how an athlete maintains or loses his or her balance during the execution of a skill specific to that sport.
11. Identify the four aspects of qualitative analysis and apply them to a sports skill of interest to you.

In This Chapter:

CHAPTER 9

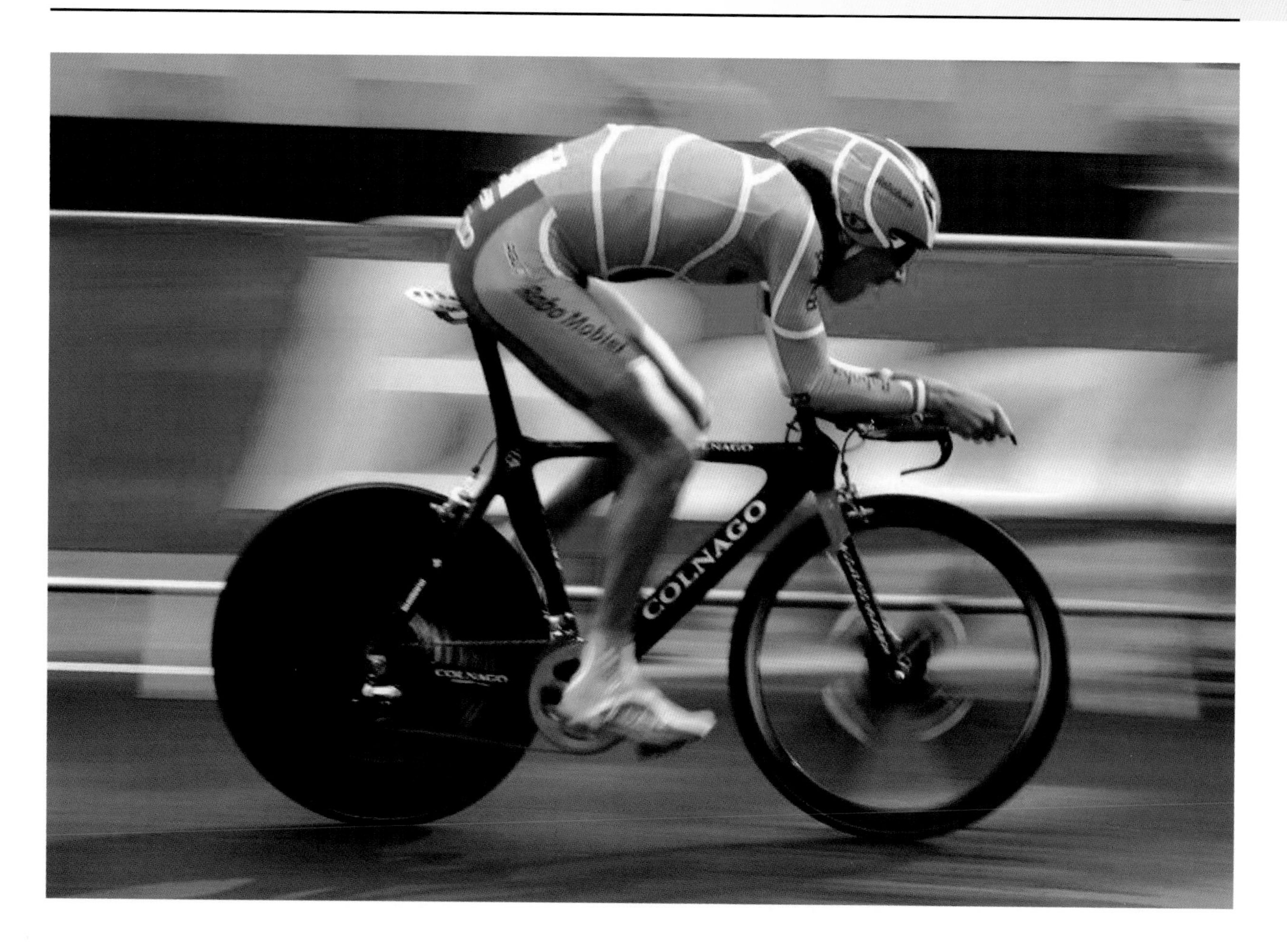

Technology and Sport

After completing this chapter you should be able to:

- describe the role of technology in the refinement of sport;
- explain how technology has led to changes in sports equipment;
- discuss the pros and cons of technological advancements in sport;
- recognize that not all technological advancement is for the better.

In many ways, technology and sport have grown and matured together. Some argue that elite sport mirrors the larger technoculture and the high-tech revolution in all areas of society. Modern sport grew from roots within the industrial revolution. Technology changed methods of production from craft-based systems to an unskilled assembly line. This allowed for more leisure time, which encouraged people to participate in leisure activities, including sport. New sports were invented, such as soccer and football. Inventions like the bicycle were at first considered toys of the rich. But assembly-line production of the new equipment soon made it affordable to a large portion of the population.

Obviously, with new equipment came new opportunities for competition. Bicycle races were held within the first year of its invention. Other innovations such as artificial ice surfaces occurred at the same time, allowing growth of related sports. Artificial ice allowed ice hockey to be played in areas that weren't cold enough to have natural ice.

So, did athletes seek out technology to improve performance? Or did new technologies drive athletes to go swifter, higher, and stronger? This is a tough question. It can be argued that the increased emphasis on performance came *before* the invention and introduction of many sport technologies.

Although the pace of new sports being invented has slowed dramatically, technology has played a huge role in the refinement of existing sports. Advancements in engineering, materials, and manufacturing techniques in other areas have allowed sports equipment to progress to more complex designs, which in turn has allowed better performances in all sports.

Even with all these advancements, it is interesting to recognize the tension that exists between the technological landscapes of North America and the *paradox of performance* in elite sport. The paradox of performance describes the condition where elite athletes are encouraged to improve their performances but are restricted in terms of the means by which they may do so. Race car drivers may be able to go faster by putting different tires on their cars, or by eliminating drag by altering the car body, but the rules restrict such changes. Many professional sports now restrict technologies of all kinds, and sport is one of the only spheres in Western societies where there is an effort to prevent too many technological innovations. It would be difficult to imagine, for instance, desiring a computer that functioned less quickly and efficiently and that required more effort than the current model to complete a given task.

Defining Technology

Technology is very difficult to define, and we often use the word in multiple ways. It is synonymous with science and rational thought, encompassing every little gadget we've ever held in wonder in our hands. It is the collective machinery that powers Western societies and the microchips that power our personal computers. In this chapter, the term *technology* is used to describe any tangible, conceptual, or procedural element of modern sport and exercise science aimed at progress.

Areas of Technological Advancement

Technological advancements have been made in many different areas of sport. These innovations have led to changes in the shape and size of equipment as well as the materials used to make equipment and clothing. Mechanical devices that make athletes faster and more efficient have been invented and refined. Technology has also increased our ability to measure sport performance. And don't forget, you take advantage of technology every time you turn on the television to watch your favorite sport.

Drag and Aerodynamics

Resistance to movement is called **drag** (see Chapter 8 for more on fluid drag forces). As drag increases, more power or energy is required to travel at a given speed. In the case of objects that are thrown, increased drag will result in a decreased flight distance. Since most sports involve traveling through air or water in some way, it is important to reduce drag as much as possible to achieve a peak performance.

What a Drag!

You may remember from Chapter 8 that **profile drag** is the result of the shape of an object. An object's shape can be changed to decrease the amount of profile drag, a process known as **streamlining**.

The other type of drag is **surface drag**, or friction. As an object travels through a fluid, the molecules of the fluid rub and catch on the surface, again increasing drag. Different surface textures result in different amounts of surface drag.

The study of objects moving relative to a fluid, such as air, is called **aerodynamics**. Aerodynamics has played a large role in the development of many sports, including the javelin (see box *Liftoff*). The javelin presents an interesting situation because aerodynamics must be taken into account for three reasons. The first is obviously the minimization of drag to increase the distance of the flight. The second is that javelins need to produce some **lift** to stay aloft longer and therefore increase the distance traveled. Since generating lift causes increases in drag, a balance needs to be found. The third factor is that the rules state the javelin must contact the ground with the tip first.

Shape and Size

Over the years, technology has played a role in refining the shape of many types of sports equipment. Observation of fish and marine mammals showed naval architects the importance of streamlining.

Liftoff

Much research was carried out on the flight of javelins in the 1960s and 1970s, including work done at the U.S. Army Ballistic Research Laboratory. A device was constructed that used compressed air to fire javelins at preset velocities and release angles. In addition, wind-tunnel work and high-speed filming of javelin throws were used to better understand the flight of a javelin and how changes in design could be used to increase the distance of a throw.

Similar work in the former Soviet Bloc states, combined with improved throwing biomechanics and training, culminated in the July 1984 world-record throw by East German Uwe Hohn of 104.80 meters (343.83 feet). This world record prompted the International Amateur Athletic Federation (IAAF) to institute rule changes to cause the javelin to underperform. The primary goal of the rule changes was to move the javelin's center of mass farther away from the center of pressure, causing the tip of the javelin to return to a downward-pointing position more quickly following its release by the thrower. World's best distances immediately fell in 1986 after the introduction of the "new rules" javelin. However, the latest world-record throws (98.48 meters [323.10 feet] for men and 71.70 meters [235.24 feet] for women, as of 2007) are approaching the distances of the old javelins.

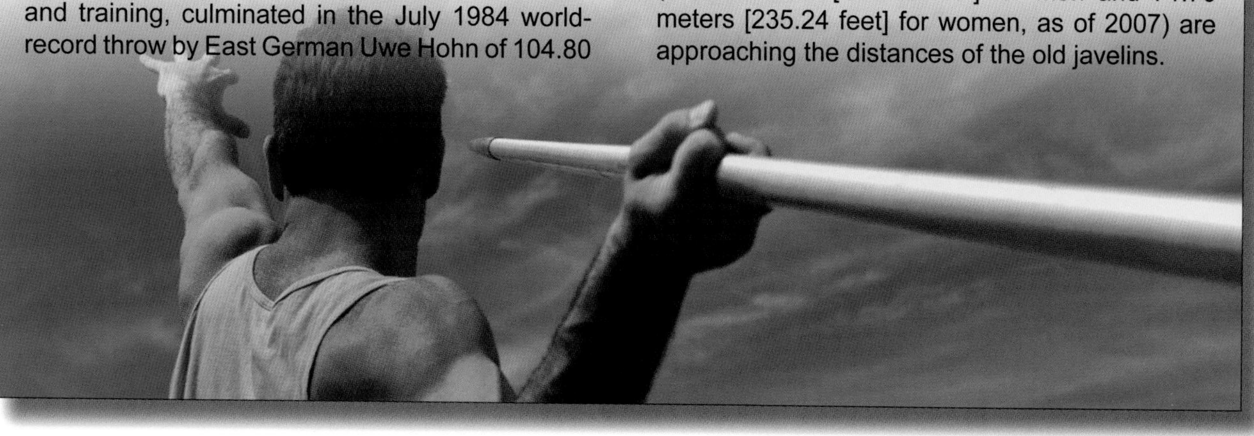

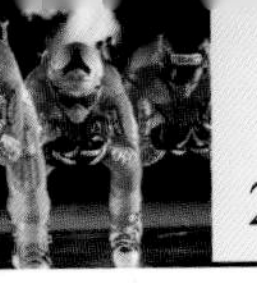

Altering the shape of boats and ships to reduce drag resulted in higher speeds. A good example of this knowledge was the shipbuilding practices of the Vikings. Their warships, known as longboats, were very narrow so they could reach as high a speed as possible, giving the Vikings the element of surprise during raids. They used wider ships to transport cargo.

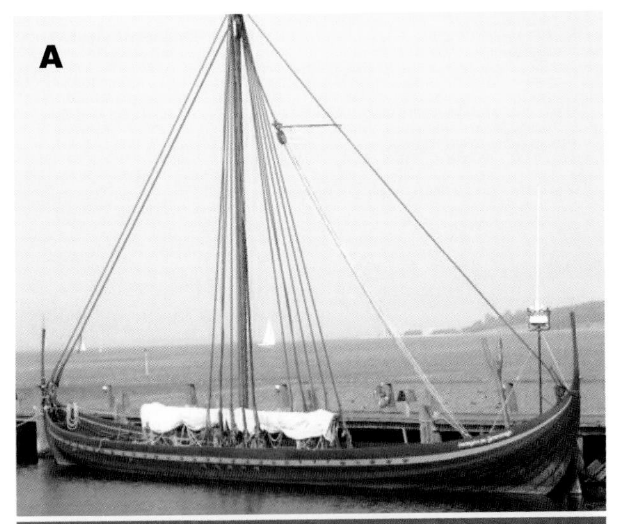

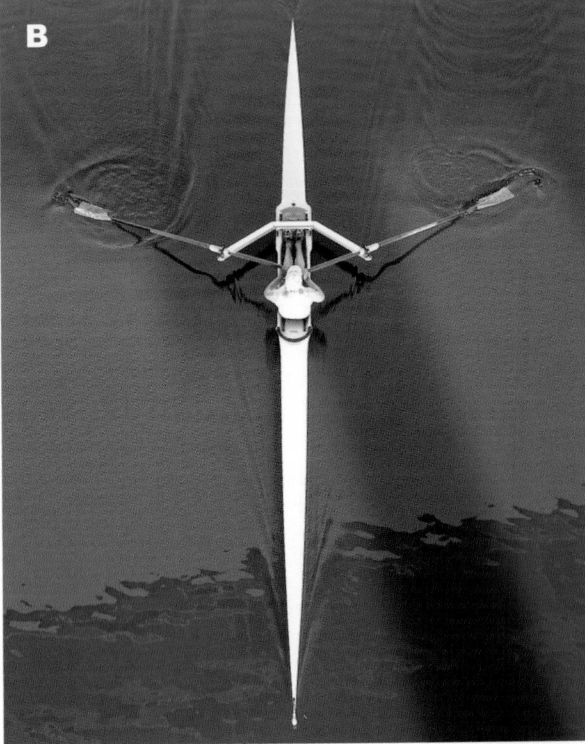

Figure 9.1 Longer and narrower boats reduce water drag and increase potential speed. **A.** Viking longboat. **B.** Single rowing scull.

As the sport of rowing began to grow in the mid-1800s, boat builders used these principles to construct longer and narrower boats (Figure 9.1). The hulls of the boats were made smooth to further decrease the water drag and increase potential speed. Coupled with the development of outriggers that moved the oarlocks farther away from the rower, racing rowing boats (known as shells for their eggshell-like fragility) became quite distinct in appearance. A single scull (one-person boat) was very narrow, with a width of about 1 foot (0.3 meters) and a length of 25 to 28 feet (7.5 to 8.5 meters). Interestingly, since the late 1800s there has been little change in the dimensions and overall appearance of racing shells.

Objects moving through the air are also subject to drag, which reduces the speed at which they can travel. However, unlike boats in water, air drag is not as obvious at low speeds. Early cars and airplanes were completely unstreamlined. It wasn't until many years after the initial development of cars and airplanes that an emphasis was placed on changing their shape to make them travel through the air more easily. For passenger cars, streamlining was not done on a regular basis until the 1980s.

In sports where higher speed of movement occurs, such as cycling (up to 60 mph; 90 km/h; downhill skiing (75 mph; 120 km/h), and speedskating (37 mph; 60 km/h), **air (wind) resistance** plays a large role in success. Air resistance can be reduced in two ways. One is to reduce the profile drag through streamlining; another is to decrease the frontal surface area of the athlete or equipment (Figure 9.2).

In the past 20 years, much time has been spent on decreasing profile drag in bicycles. Both the shape of the bicycle and wheels and the position of the cyclist have been altered to lower air resistance. Using aerodynamic wheels can cut up to one minute from an Olympic-distance 40-km (25-mile) time trial. An aerodynamic frame can cut another one or two minutes from the time. Considering that about two minutes separated 1st from 10th place at the 2004 Olympic time trial, there are significant advantages to using aerodynamic equipment.

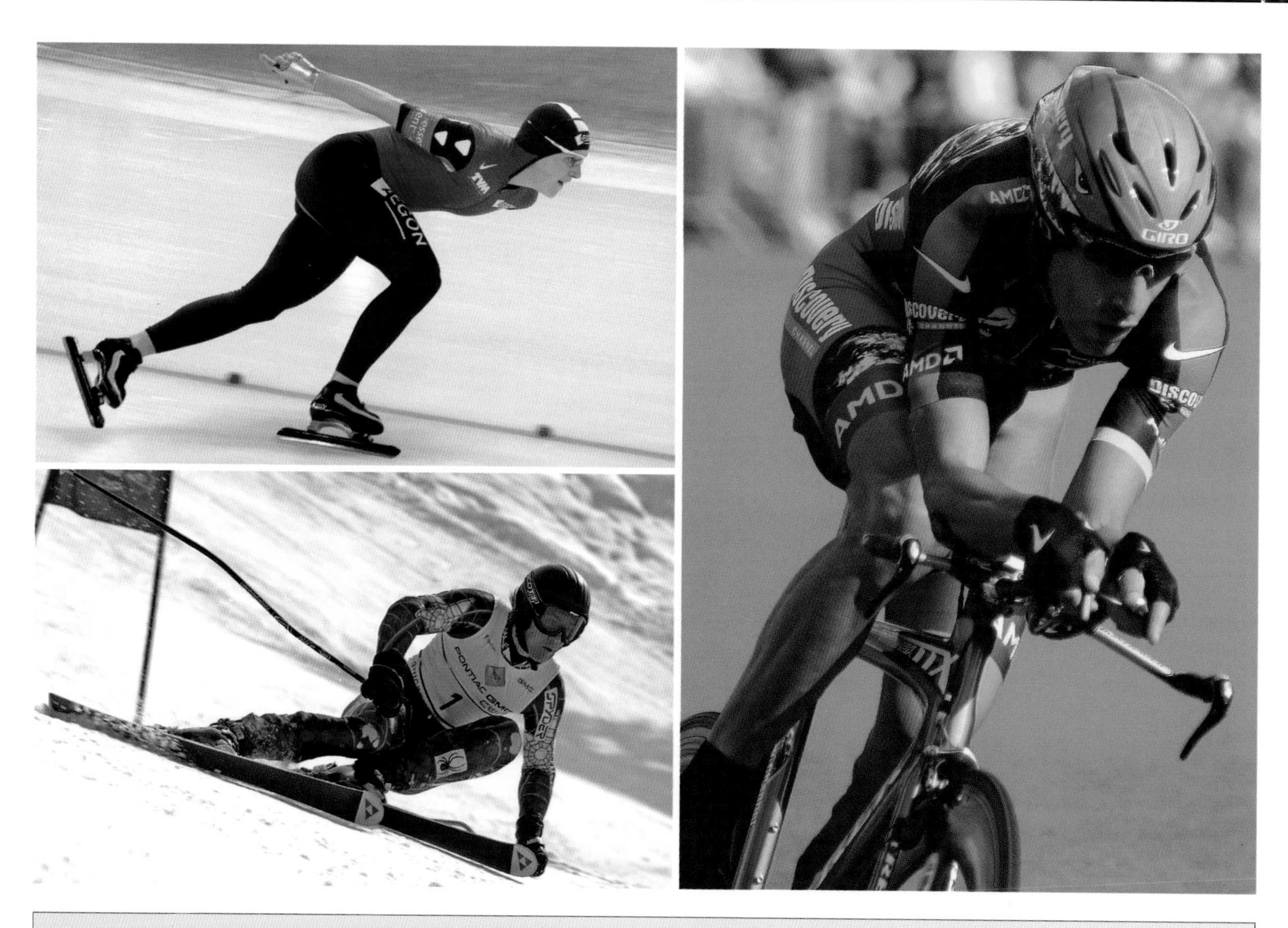

Figure 9.2 In sports where higher speed of movement is critical for success, air resistance can be minimized by reducing profile drag through streamlining or by reducing the frontal surface area of the athlete or equipment. As a result, athletes often adopt a more crouched-over position.

Body Position

In cycling, speedskating, and downhill skiing, it was quickly recognized that standing or sitting upright had detrimental effect. A more crouched-over position was adopted in all three sports. Racing bicycles were designed with dropped handlebars to allow cyclists to bend their bodies into position, which reduced frontal area. In extreme forms, a recumbent (sitting with legs in front) bicycle was found to decrease the frontal area drastically. In the early 1930s, a recumbent bicycle was used to set the "hour record" (farthest distance ridden in one hour); it hasn't been beaten by a conventional bicycle to date. The international cycling governing body did not recognize the record since it wasn't done on a traditional upright bicycle. The current hour record for recumbents is 86.752 km (53.917 miles).

Altering body position has a significant effect since the body produces much of the profile drag. In cycling, moving from an upright position to an aerodynamic one can reduce 40-km (25-mile) time-trial times by up to six minutes. As a result, many of the top cyclists including Lance Armstrong (seven-time winner of the Tour de France) spend time each year in low-speed wind tunnels perfecting their riding positions. However, there is a trade-off. Often a more aerodynamic position (e.g., more bent over) affects the joint angles at the hips, resulting in lower power output from the muscles. In fact, Armstrong had to deal with this problem in 2004, when a consortium of manufacturers spent $250,000 developing a new time-trial bicycle for him. Each change to improve aerodynamic efficiency resulted in decreased sustainable power output. The final result was that Armstrong did not use that bicycle in races but competed with an older one.

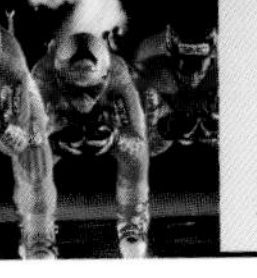

Texture

Surface drag (friction) also contributes to air resistance and water resistance. It may seem counterintuitive, but a slightly rough surface has lower friction drag than a perfectly smooth surface. The dimples on a golf ball are an example. The slightly rough surface traps a single layer of air or water molecules – known as a **boundary layer** – which reduces drag because now the fluid molecules are rubbing against other molecules of the same fluid rather than against different types of molecules. Fluid molecules rubbing against fluid molecules results in much lower friction.

Early attempts at producing racing suits for downhill skiing resulted in suits that were very slippery. In fact, they were considered dangerous because they did not slow a skier after a fall. There was insufficient drag between the suit and the snow to stop the skier from sliding into trees or spectators at high speed. The International Ski Federation banned the suits in the name of safety.

Swimming has benefited in recent years from changes in suit material to reduce surface drag. In conjunction with engineers, Speedo explored the flow of water around the limbs and bodies of swimmers. This research, in addition to observations from nature that sharks and marine mammals have different textured skin in different areas, led Speedo to design new bathing suits. These new bathing suits cover much more of a swimmer's skin and have varied textures (Figure 9.3). In some areas, ridges in the suit run parallel to the water flow. In others, the ridges run perpendicular to the flow so that water attaches to the surface of the suit, reducing surface drag as well as profile drag by decreasing eddies that may form. Manufacturers claim decreases in total drag of about 15 percent.

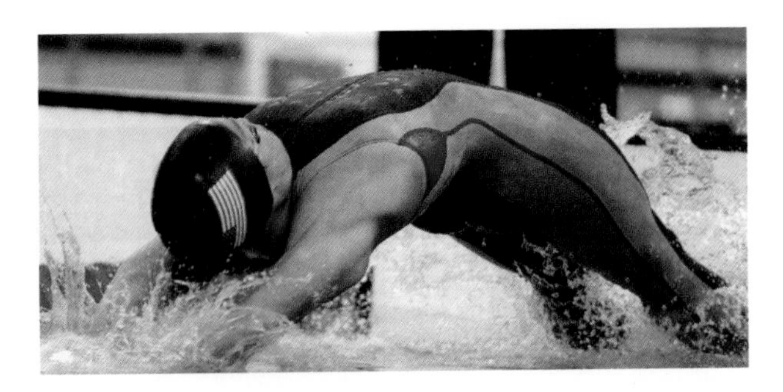

Figure 9.3 As swimmers continue to pursue faster swimming speeds, manufacturers continue to push the envelope with new and improved swimsuit technologies.

Sports Equipment Materials

In about 150 years, sports equipment progressed from wood to iron to steel to aluminum and finally to carbon fiber. This progression resulted from the search for stronger, lighter, and stiffer materials.

Materials in sports equipment can be classified according to strength. However, the term *strength* needs to be used carefully because it can mean many things. There is tensile (or pulling) strength, compressive (or pushing) strength, and shear (or sliding) strength. Different materials possess different maximal resistances to these different domains. If the maximal strength is exceeded, a material may bend or yield to a point where it just breaks.

Most equipment breakages occur because of fatigue, however, not because the maximum strength or stress has been exceeded. Materials can tire. A piece of plastic can be broken if it is bent repeatedly. Each time it is bent it is said to be loaded, or stressed. Note that a **load** doesn't have to cause bending for fatigue to occur. This is particularly true for very stiff materials (e.g., metal titanium) or a composite material (e.g., carbon fiber).

During practice or competition, materials used in the construction of equipment can be repeatedly stressed. Although none of the stresses exceed the materials' maximum strength properties, the sports equipment still fails after accumulation of many loads. As a result, selecting materials for sports equipment is a difficult task, especially considering that lighter materials allow for better performances (consider a lighter tennis racket or hockey stick).

Another factor for a designer to consider is the stiffness of the material. A stiffer material can be considered more efficient for transmitting force

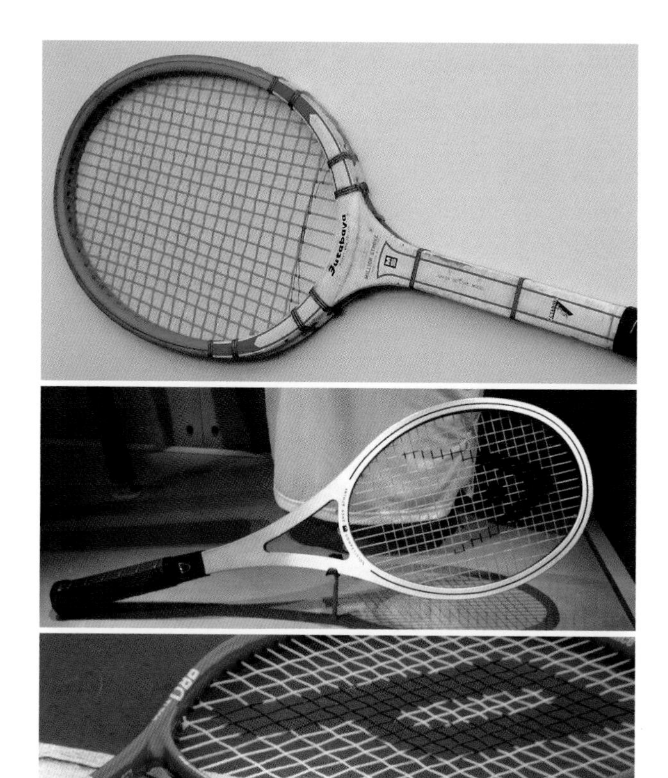

Figure 9.4 Tennis rackets have come a long way from the original wooden designs.

between the athlete and the ground or a ball, since energy is not going into the deformation of the equipment.

These characteristics have led designers and builders from wood to stronger and stiffer materials. The result is that current sports equipment is not only lighter but also much more efficient (Figure 9.4).

From Wood to Aluminum

Wood was the most common material for most sports equipment up until relatively recently. Tennis rackets, hockey sticks, boats, and even bicycles were made of wood for the simple reason that it was readily available and easy to work with. Skilled craftsmen were able to shape different varieties of wood – each with its own characteristics in terms of strength, weight, and stiffness – into many distinct pieces of equipment. The quest for lighter and stronger bicycles was one of the first forces pushing manufacturers into steel. Another benefit of steel is its resistance to environmental effects. Wooden tennis rackets and oars needed elaborate presses to keep them in shape. Steel or aluminum rackets do not need those devices and therefore require less maintenance and attention.

More recently, the changes in materials used in sports equipment have occurred very rapidly. The reasons for these rapid changes are complex but, in general, have occurred very soon after the introduction of newer materials and innovations in the engineering world. Going from steel to aluminum, for example, requires different welding techniques. In addition, the aluminum has to be readily available at a reasonable cost.

Carbon Fiber

The introduction of **carbon fiber** has completely revolutionized equipment manufacturing. It is important to note that it is a composite of two different materials. Carbon fiber is a cloth-like material that is made of strands of carbon. It is held together by a resin, which gives it some of its properties. The composite has strength only in certain directions, depending on the direction that the strands of carbon fiber run through the resin. Building up layers of carbon fiber running in different directions improves overall strength.

Carbon fiber is now used in everything from race cars and bicycles to skates and running shoes. Its primary advantages are twofold: It is light and very stiff. The major downside, other than being difficult to work with, is that it is prone to what is known as **catastrophic failure**. When wood or most metals get close to failure or breakage, they first start to bend. This bending gives warning that the material is about to fail. Carbon fiber composite does not bend prior to breaking. It keeps its properties until it actually breaks.

The best example of catastrophic failure is seen in ice hockey, where carbon fiber sticks

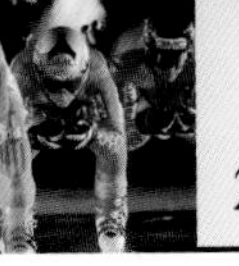

have been breaking with apparently high frequency. Players don't have warning that the sticks are about to break, as with aluminum or wooden sticks. However, the advantages of the lighter and stiffer carbon fiber sticks seem to outweigh the drawbacks for most hockey players (see box *End of an Era*). Catastrophic failure is a major concern in some pieces of equipment such as bicycles. In certain instances, catastrophic failure could result in serious injury or even death. As a result, bicycles tend to be overbuilt, meaning that extra material is used in the frame or wheels in case of high loads.

One benefit that has accompanied this progression in materials is that sports equipment has become cheaper. This allows better access to higher quality equipment, which means more people can participate in sports comfortably and affordably.

Mechanical Devices

Changes in mechanical technology are driven by the need to improve human performance in sport and other physical activities. Humans are relatively constrained in their ability to produce force or speed of movement. We are not as strong as an elephant or as fast as a cheetah. However, through the uses of mechanical devices (tools), we are able to multiply our force- or speed-generating capabilities. A second important factor is the ability of mechanical devices to make our movements more efficient. That is, less energy is required to generate the same force or amount of movement.

In this section, three specific examples of mechanical devices used in sport are described, including a review of their effect on sport performance.

Speedskating: The Clap Skate

Speedskating blades have been fixed in design since the late 1800s. Norwegian skating legend Axel Paulsen developed the first "long blade," which has been in continuous use for more than 120 years.

End of an Era

It was only a matter of time before wooden hockey stick manufacturers felt the effects of the growing popularity of composite sticks. After almost 60 years, hockey equipment icon Sher-Wood will no longer make wooden sticks at its Quebec factory. The company has decided to outsource its production of wooden sticks so it can focus on its composite models.

Composite sticks made from carbon fiber, graphite, Kevlar, and other synthetics are lighter and more flexible. They're also more expensive, costing as much as $300 each for top-of-the-line models. However, players at all levels from peewee to pro are switching to composites. Markets for wooden hockey sticks are falling, and profits are tumbling as a result. Although wooden sticks still make up the bulk of Sher-Wood's sales, it is simply no longer profitable to mass produce the product in Quebec.

Not everyone is convinced that composites are better, though. Although they produce harder shots, composite sticks are inferior to wooden sticks when it comes to shot accuracy and stickhandling. In fact, many proponents of the traditional wooden stick, including some former NHL players, would like to see composite sticks banned. Most current pros, however, appear to disagree. An estimated 95 percent of NHL players are now using composites.

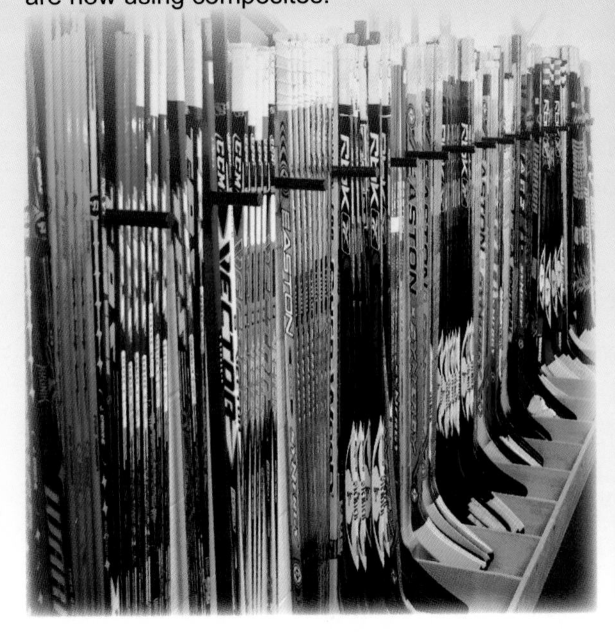

Speedskaters use unrockered skates (i.e., the blade is straight, with no curve at the tip), unlike the skates worn by hockey players and figure skaters. Although unrockered blades glide better because they do not dig as deeply into the ice, they have a distinct disadvantage. When pushing off, if there is any kind of plantar flexion in the ankle joint, the tip of the blade will dig into the ice, greatly increasing the friction and, therefore, making the skater lose speed. Speedskaters have learned to limit plantar flexion by adopting a position in which they sit back on their skates and push off with their heels. These two points must be constantly reinforced in practice or else skaters will plantar flex, slowing the glide of the blades. This corrective technique not only is unnatural for humans when compared with walking, running, or jumping – where we plantar flex strongly before takeoff – it also leads to a loss of power.

It wasn't until the mid-1980s that the problem of limited plantar flexion was examined and a solution proposed. Researchers in the Netherlands were working in two separate areas: speedskating biomechanics and jumping biomechanics. Observations from both groups indicated that speedskaters could generate additional power if they used the powerful plantar flexors in the calves the same way as in running or jumping. The question was how. The Dutch researchers proposed a skate blade that was hinged under the toe. That way the heel could lift up without the tail of the blade leaving the ice and the tip digging in (Figure 9.5).

Even after the theoretical basis was shown, the clap skate was not quickly adopted by elite skaters. It wasn't until a group of top-level skaters began using the blades and showed greater improvements in speed (6.2 percent in one year using the clap skate compared with 2.5 percent using conventional skates) that senior international skaters began to notice. They were concerned that the International Skating Union (ISU) would eventually ban the skates and that they would lose their practiced ability not to plantar flex. Finally, in the winter of 1996-1997, three women on the Dutch national team took the risk. One of the women won the European Championship. This was enough, along with ISU approval, to cause a switchover to the clap skate. By the 1998 Winter Olympics in Nagano, Japan, all the Olympic skaters used clap skates – and all the world records were shattered.

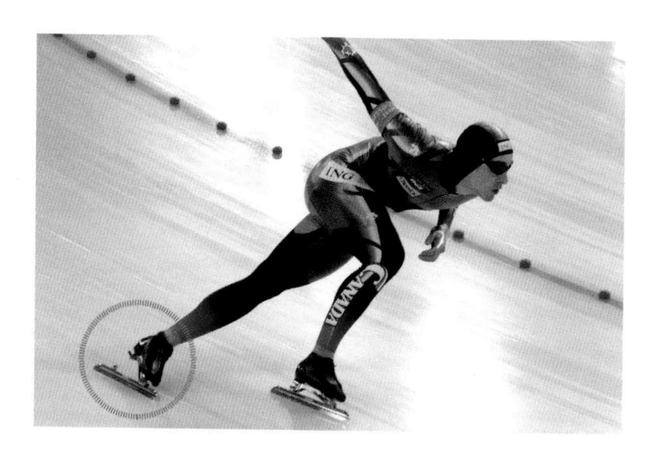

Figure 9.5 The clap skate was eventually adopted by all the top skaters in the world, and world records have been falling ever since.

This is one of the few examples in sport where a theoretical proposal from researchers has led to a technological revolution.

Rowing: Sliding Rigger

Racing shells are fitted with sliding seats. This allows rowers to use their legs as part of the stroke. The legs push the upper body backwards. This backwards movement is transferred through the arms to the oars, which then move the boat. The side effect of this motion is that the body's center of mass moves back and forth in relation to the boat. Since the boat weighs very little compared with the rower, this movement causes the boat speed to vary substantially in the course of a single stroke (think of Newton's third law of motion). One of the technological innovations to overcome this problem was the sliding rigger (the metal support for the oars) (Figure 9.6). In this case, the body stays stationary and the rigger moves. The motion becomes much like a leg press in the weight room. The advantage of little or no movement of the center of mass reduces the variation in boat speed, resulting in higher speeds.

The idea of the sliding rigger was first patented in 1884 by an English engineer. However, it wasn't

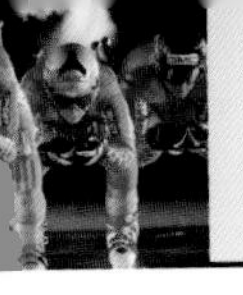

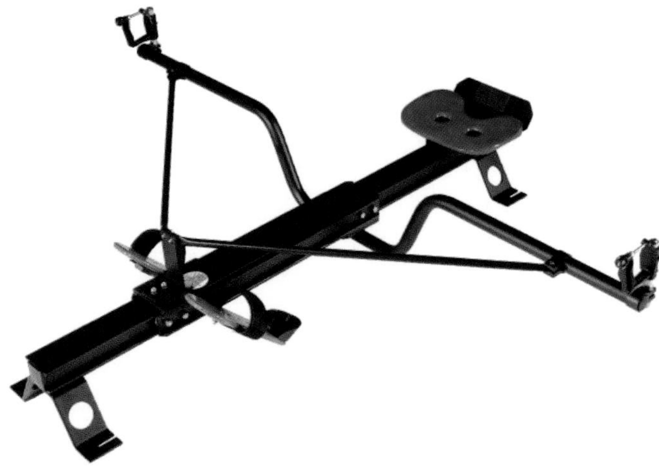

Figure 9.6 Boats outfitted with a sliding rigger are generally faster than conventional sliding seat boats.

until the 1950s that a workable example was built. The boat was found to be faster than conventional sliding seat boats, but the mechanism jammed often and the entire boat was much heavier.

With the advent of lighter construction materials in the 1970s (aluminum and carbon fiber), a raceable lightweight shell was built. Again, it proved faster than all conventional boats. Some comparative tests indicated that rowers using the sliding rigger could significantly increase boat speeds.

The sliding rigger boats were banned by FISA, the international rowing federation. The prevailing feeling was that the new technology would greatly increase the cost of boats, putting poorer rowing countries at a disadvantage.

Athletics: Running Shoes

Much research was conducted in the 1970s and 1980s on running shoes and their ability to prevent overuse injuries such as shin splints. For the most part, the stresses caused by running in terms of foot pronation and high forces on contact were actually made worse by many running shoes. Ground reaction forces, which measure the "shock" of foot contact with the ground, were higher when subjects wore soft running shoes. In fact, some studies indicated it was better to run barefoot on grass or a rubber track.

Consumers, however, were difficult to convince. Most running shoe buyers who intended to run in the shoes felt and continue to feel that soft shoes are better. Manufacturers, of course, kept the consumers happy by making shoes that have air pockets, lower density foam, and other features to soften the contact between the foot and the ground (see box *Smart Footwear*). In addition, devices to limit or prevent pronation were placed in the wrong areas and did nothing to alleviate overuse injuries.

More recently, biomechanists who work in the areas of running have become increasingly convinced that shoes should only serve to protect the feet from sharp rocks and other potential hazards that may cause injury. As well, devices to limit pronation and control the movement of the foot should be eliminated because they often do not work as intended. The biomechanists believe that the foot has evolved well for walking and running.

Smart Footwear

Athletic footwear design has undergone numerous changes over the years in the pursuit of improved performance, from biomechanical shock absorbers and springs to sophisticated "pump" systems. Electronic enhancements can now be added to the list.

The Adidas 1 running shoe is equipped with a battery-powered microprocessor nested in the arch that is capable of making five million calculations per second to adjust cushioning levels automatically during a run. A magnetic sensor in the heel transmits data to the microprocessor to adjust the heel characteristics – firmer for running off-road and softer when running on paved surfaces. This sleek and lightweight shoe comes with a hefty price tag, however, retailing at around $250.

Shoe manufacturers are starting to produce running shoes that reflect this view. However, driven by misinformed consumers, the demand has been limited in the past and will probably not be very high in the near future.

Measurement and Observation

Computers have become part of every aspect of life, including sport. Interestingly, outside of motor sports and sailing, computers remain largely relegated to measurement and observation. Measurement devices such as stopwatches, speedometers, and heart rate monitors are used more for timekeeping and activity analysis than for improving performance. However, speedometers, heart rate monitors, and power-output measurement devices have made training more focused and have allowed athletes to better pace themselves during races.

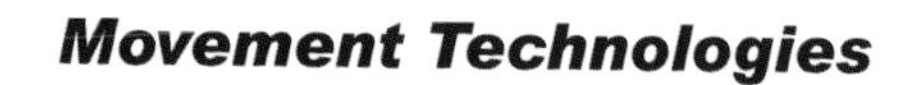

Movement Technologies

Devices and procedures that are designed to assess the form and efficiency of an athlete's body are referred to as **movement technologies**. The most common of such technologies is videotape analysis, although there are much more sophisticated instruments that provide detailed computerized information on an athlete's biomechanics. At the Olympic Training Center in Colorado, for example, swimmers' strokes are evaluated as they swim in an enclosed tank in an effort to identify points in the movement where excess drag is produced.

In general, then, unlike other types of technology, movement technologies are often not visible within the competitive arenas. They are housed in scientific laboratories or present only in practice situations (Figure 9.7).

Finally, besides helping to improve an athlete's existing technique, the data yielded by movement technologies may also facilitate conceptual or stylistic shifts that allow the athlete to compete in a mechanically, aesthetically, and kinesthetically novel manner.

Timing Devices

Timing pieces help define sports. Pre-industrial sports such as tennis, golf, cricket, and baseball do not use any means of timing. However, industrial sports had to be completed in a set amount of time since workers had only limited time available for activity outside of work. In addition, athletes now wanted to know how fast they were running, so stopwatches were used to time events. Until the appearance of computerized electronic stopwatches in the 1950s and 1960s, times for events were gener-

Figure 9.7 In sports where mere tenths of a second can separate victory from defeat, gaining even the slightest advantage during training can determine an athlete's success during competition. Skeleton racers often use wind tunnels to experiment with multiple combinations of shoes, helmets, and technique for optimal aerodynamics.

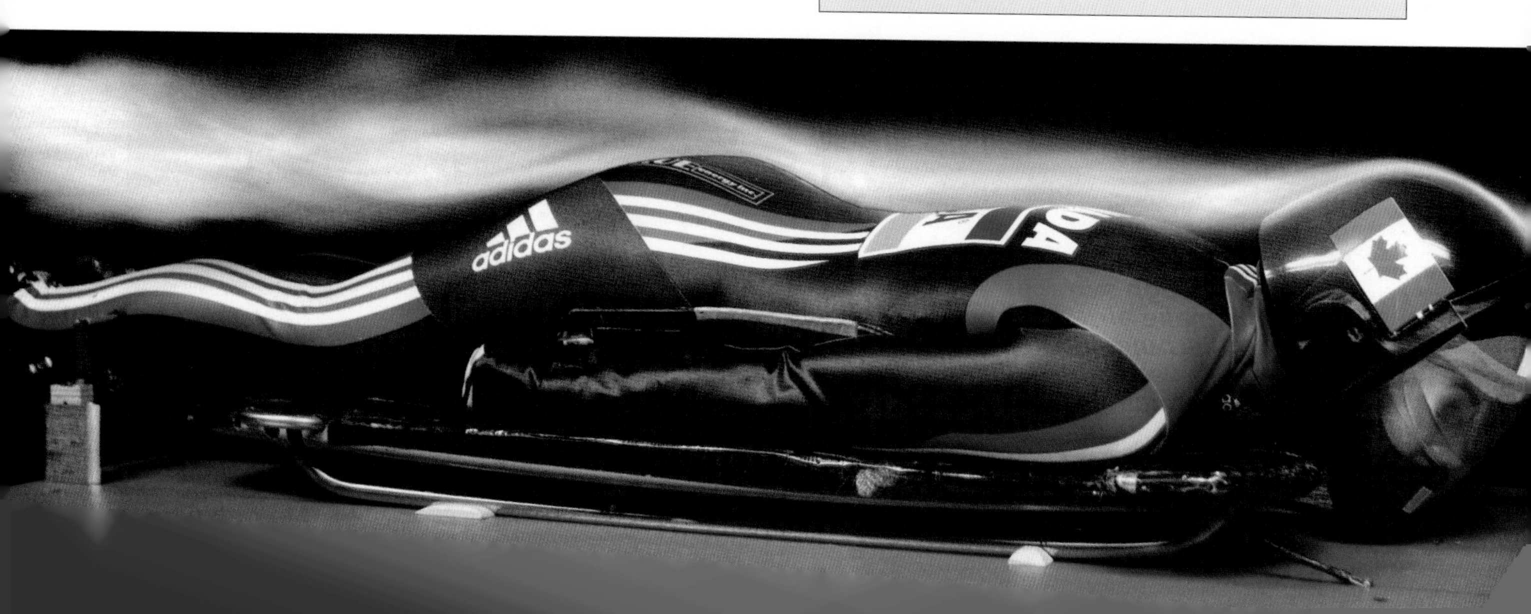

ally measured to the nearest 1/10 of a second. In the first Olympic swimming races that used electronic timing, the equipment was quickly put to the test when a race appeared to be tied at 1/100 of a second. Judges were able to declare a winner by checking the times at a level of 1/1,000 of a second.

Database Technologies

Computers have also made the work of sport scientists much easier and more effective. Researchers are able to collect more data, much more easily than in the past (see box *The Numbers Game*). The data can be quickly analyzed as opposed to the tedious weeks and even months of calculations that had to be done previously. Now athletes working with sport scientists can receive instant feedback on how they are performing and how movements or efforts need to change to improve.

The Numbers Game

What do the Dallas Cowboys do on third downs? How does the quarterback of the New England Patriots react on third-down blitzes? **Database technologies** involve computer innovations that allow athletes and coaches to know everything they need to know about their opponents and themselves.

Database programs have greatly affected the way that many college and most professional coaches and players do their jobs. In the National Football League, for instance, many teams have two or three employees whose job it is to enter the plays that all their opponents run in any given situation; this information is then transformed into a user-friendly database that the coach can use to scout the opponents' tendencies and patterns. Is this taking the human element out of sport? Or is it simply taking advantage of the latest technology to gain an advantage over the opposition?

Electronics

Electronics have changed sport in other ways. Television has become an important part of sport.

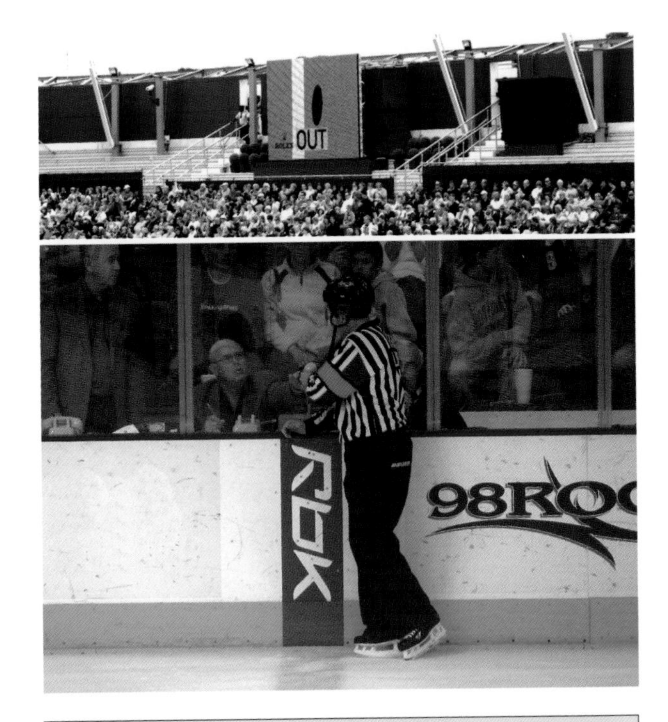

Figure 9.8 The introduction of video recording and instant replay has changed the way sports are officiated. Athletes and fans can now double-check controversial decisions by game officials.

The National Football League (NFL) was one of the first to realize how to utilize the new technology to grow spectator support and financial resources. Numerous rule changes were put into effect to make the game more television-viewer friendly. This has led to a huge growth in viewership for the NFL, which is also very lucrative for broadcasters. Other sports have not adapted as well to television and have suffered as a result.

One unforeseen consequence of television has been the instant replay. The introduction of video recording coupled with the numerous television camera angles used by broadcasters allowed viewers at home to see whether on-field officials made the appropriate calls. This forced many sports to adopt a replay policy that could be used to double-check controversial decisions by game officials (Figure 9.8). For the most part, it has been welcomed by athletes and fans, but it has also made games longer.

It is possible that computers may play a larger role in the future. For example, bicycle manufacturers are working on computers that decide what gear a cyclist should be in, much like an automatic transmission in an automobile. It remains to be seen if these types of technology will be allowed by sports governing bodies, since they diminish the role of the athlete.

The Downside of Technology

Technology in sport does come with certain risks. Changes in technology can make a sport lose its defining attributes, which may or may not be welcomed by the participants or spectators.

Since we will probably never go back to the days of all-natural grass in American football, or cease the use of clipless pedals and two-way radios in the Tour de France, what forms of technology should be allowed and which restricted? Also, who gets to decide how much technology is *too* much? Several arguments against the overuse of sport technologies have been made. Each of these arguments has been used, and will continue to be used, to support restricting various forms of technology in sports.

Access

One problem with allowing any and all sport technologies is that not everyone has access to the latest advancements. A technological "arms race" may drive up costs in the short term very quickly, limiting participation rates in that sport. If success in a sport is determined by what kind of bicycle you can afford, or what kind of bobsled your country can afford, then are high-level competitions really fair?

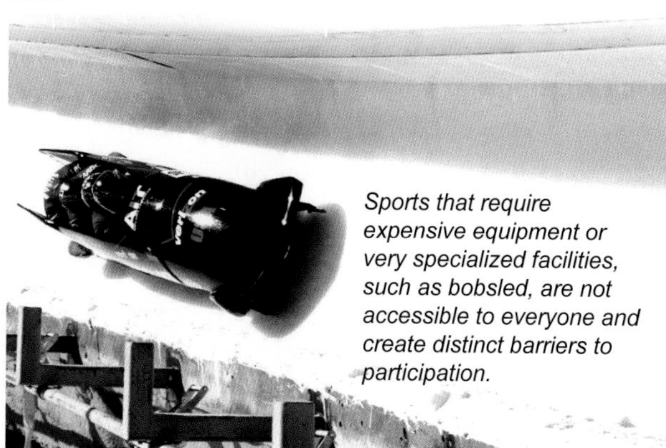

Sports that require expensive equipment or very specialized facilities, such as bobsled, are not accessible to everyone and create distinct barriers to participation.

High-technology training centers can quickly regionalize a sport to the city or town where the training facilities exist. Sports such as ski jumping, bobsled, and luge require very specialized facilities. If extremely high-tech runs and jumps are built, money to build facilities in other parts of the country may not be available. Participation then becomes limited to those from a particular region, and the potential number of new athletes entering the sport is limited.

The Olympics and other international competitions could become contests between the global technological haves and have-nots. Of course, some might argue there is little absolute fairness in sport regardless of technology, and there have always been individual talent differences and differences in access to modern training facilities.

Unintended Risks

Along with issues of access, another major dilemma faced by those involved in sport is how to reconcile the potential benefits of technology with the risks. Technology gives athletes many advantages, and it raises performance levels. However, there are also unintended consequences of sport technologies. For instance, while equipment advancements have decreased the probability of catastrophic injuries, there has been an increase in chronic health problems. So, professional football players may be able to play harder, run faster, and hit harder today, but the effects of hundreds of high-speed collisions over 5 or 10 years may be debilitating. Also, although contemporary football helmets and padding provide far better protection than equipment of previous years, the rehabilitative technologies now available allow athletes to return to competition at the cost of extended bouts of pain and repeated surgeries later on.

Dehumanizing Effects

One of the biggest dilemmas faced by those concerned with the influx of sport technologies is determining which technologies should be allowed in contests and which run counter to

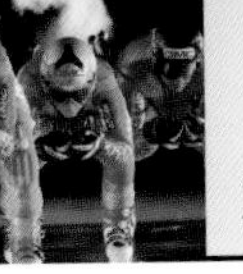

what has often been termed the "human" element of sporting contests (see box *Where Do We Draw the Line?*). If human competitors are fully replaced by competitions between scientists, where the athletes are really just subjects in performance-enhancing experiments, then the results would be troubling. It is doubtful that many people would even watch sporting events where athletes have been thoroughly dehumanized.

De-skilling

The introduction of some technological innovations has resulted in the "de-skilling" of the very activities they were meant to improve. Athletes are often too quick to adopt new technology in the hopes that it will improve performance. Many athletes spend large amounts of money on equipment that may be marginally lighter or stiffer. At the same time, they can be extremely reluctant to work harder or try a new training method. Athletes must be aware that although technology is important, especially at the highest levels, the real deciding factor in winning and losing is going to be the athletes themselves.

The amount of skill required to break world records in many events has been affected as well. For example, the enhanced design of speed skates led to rapidly improved times, and even factors such as Mondo track surfaces can account for valuable seconds each lap compared with older surfaces. The Professional Golfers' Association (PGA) and its players have taken the offensive against the use of new equipment that could compromise constituent parts of the game. The most advanced titanium balls, for example, have been unanimously banned because their extended distance would make many courses obsolete. In fact, the PGA has established an absolute limit of slightly under 300 yards (300 meters) as the maximum flight distance of a ball when struck by a mechanized driving machine. Can you imagine if Tiger Woods were able to use any club and ball he wanted? It could turn moderately long courses into miniature golf!

Where Do We Draw the Line?

Of the countless forms of technology found in sport today, **self-technologies** are perhaps the most obvious. But since they have the potential to fundamentally and often permanently alter an athlete's physical or psychological makeup, many people would argue that self-technologies also represent the most disturbing trend in the technologization of sport.

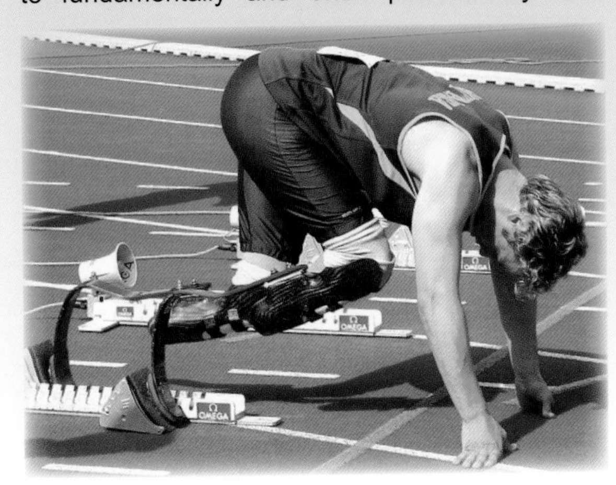

While banned performance-enhancing drugs are the most notorious of these technologies, self-technologies encompass other kinds of athletic innovations, some of which are also controversial. For example, surgical procedures, prosthetic/bionic limbs, sport psychological interventions, and genetic engineering would all be classified as self-technologies. While the presence of certain self-technologies in sport may seem too futuristic (e.g., bionic prostheses, genetic engineering), scientists working on a muscle-building vaccine derived from engineered genes have already recognized the implications of their work for sport.

Summary

The use of modern technology in sport clearly improves performance. Efforts to reduce profile drag and surface drag in sports such as cycling, swimming, and speedskating have resulted in countless world records and personal bests. Many types of sports equipment are now stronger and lighter thanks to advancements in the materials used to make them. And changes in mechanical technology are making the Olympic motto of swifter, higher, stronger a reality for many athletes.

In general, newer technologies raise the cost of sports equipment and facilities, but the costs come down over time as the innovations become more common. The result is that the newer technologies become accessible to a wider variety of athletes. In addition, a newer technology often makes participating in a sport easier for individuals who may not have as much strength or who may have disabilities. Lighter, stronger equipment opens doors for more people to participate in sport.

Not all technological advancements are well received, however. The governing bodies of some sports have intervened and banned certain new technologies. Care must be taken to keep sport "real." There is a fine line between genuine athletic achievement and artificially enhanced performance.

Key Terms

aerodynamics
air (wind) resistance
boundary layer
carbon fiber
catastrophic failure
database technologies
drag
lift
load
movement technologies
profile drag
self-technologies
streamlining
surface drag
technology

Discussion Questions

1. Define the term *drag*, and describe two different types.
2. Explain how technology has changed the javelin and how these changes have affected the sport.
3. How can air (wind) resistance be reduced in sports such as cycling and downhill skiing?
4. What is a boundary layer? Why does it reduce friction?
5. Describe how technology has changed sports equipment manufacturing.
6. What are some of the advantages of technological advancements in sports equipment? Are there any disadvantages?
7. How can mechanical technology improve sport performance? Provide an example.
8. Describe four ways in which computers have changed sport.
9. Explain the downside of technology.
10. Do you think there should be a limit placed on technological advancements in sport? Why or why not?

In This Chapter:

CHAPTER 10

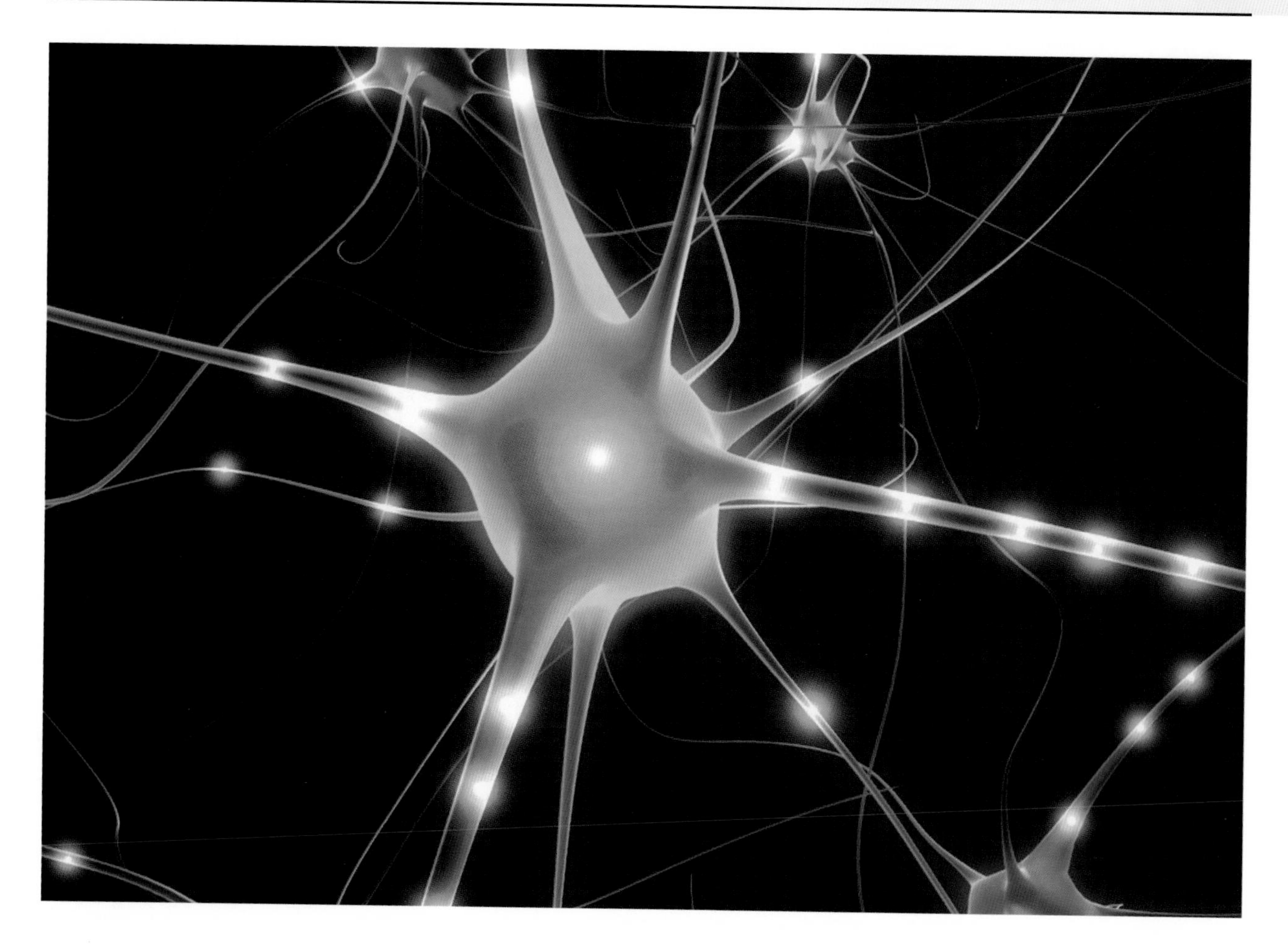

Information Processing in Human Movement

After completing this chapter you should be able to:

- describe the structure and function of the human nervous system as it relates to information processing;
- explain the ways humans perceive and process information;
- demonstrate an understanding of the role of feedback in motor control;
- explain the advantages and disadvantages of closed- and open-loop control systems in motor control.

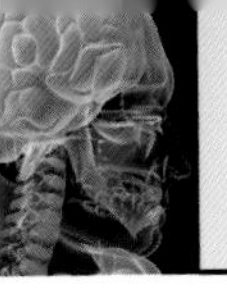

When we view the ease with which people move and execute most skills, it is difficult to appreciate the true complexities of human movement. At a glance, human actions appear simple and perhaps even trivial, but the intricate network and processes underlying motor skills are nothing short of extraordinary. The brain and spinal cord, comprising the **central nervous system (CNS)**, are accepted as the control center for our powerful and far-reaching abilities, whereas the nerve cells and fibers that lie outside the CNS, the **peripheral nervous system (PNS)**, connect the CNS with the rest of the body. The organization and vast capacity of the two systems are often oversimplified to the point that we rarely question how we are able to accomplish a range of movements with the precision we do. We are able to perform not only relatively simple skills such as walking and jumping without much thought but also more complex skills such as those involved in gymnastics and advanced dance steps. Whatever the activity, the colossal network of neurons sending messages to one another from one part of the body to another is responsible in no small part for our ability to sense, respond, and react to the world around us (Figure 10.1).

In today's world of advanced technology, many people marvel at the considerable capabilities of the modern-day computers. Indeed, they are improving so quickly that they often become obsolete within years or even months of their creation. The human brain has often been compared to a computer, with its immense capacity, striking speed, and pinpoint precision. Yet, many consider the computer to be superior in many respects to the human nervous system.

It's a Draw!

Computers have demonstrated extraordinary success in playing chess. In fact, by the early 1990s only the world chess champion and a few others were able to beat the top computer programs like Deep Thought that were able to examine up to 450,000 positions a second. Going one step further in 1996 to showcase the computer's incredible abilities, a match was set up between Garry Kasparov (the world chess champion) and Deep Blue, an IBM supercomputer that took a five-person team six years to build – for the sole purpose of challenging Kasparov to a few games of chess. Deep Blue was able to consider an unbelievable 200 million moves in one second, more than any of its predecessors. The processing speed and efficiency of such supercomputers is mind-boggling, but who eventually came out victorious you might ask? Garry Kasparov, four games to two. Not bad for a *half-witted* human being, wouldn't you say?

In the rematch held a year later (1997) the computer was victorious, whereas in February, 2003, the match ended in a draw. Kasparov finally admitted that computers, indeed, are starting to show some "signs of intelligence."

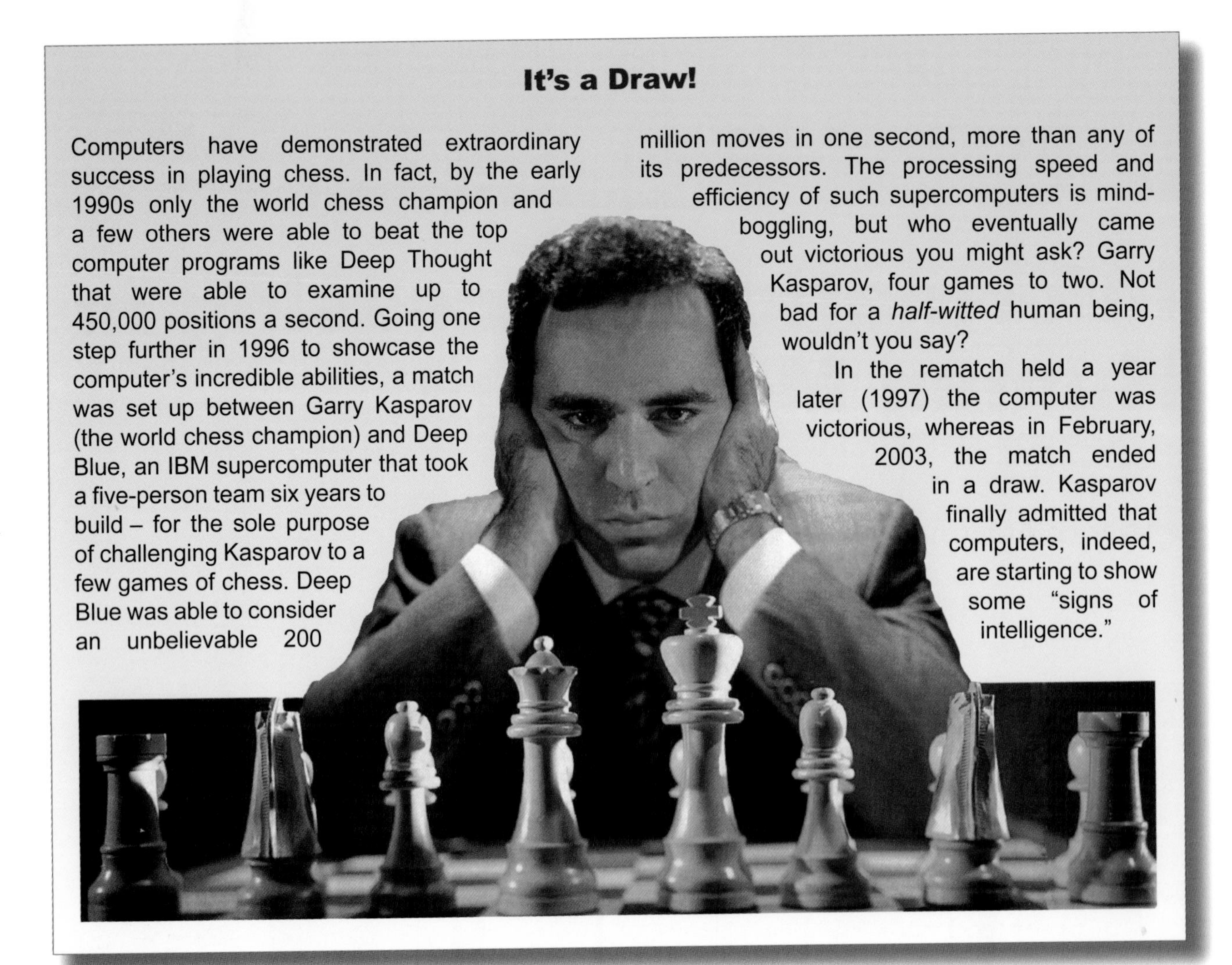

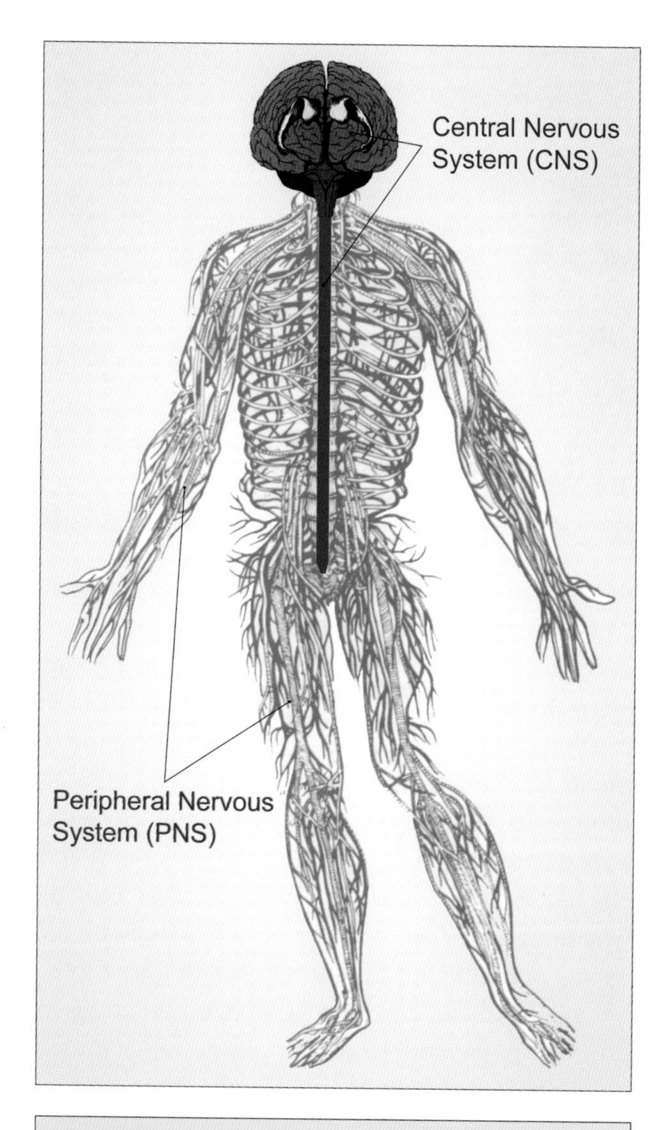

Figure 10.1 The central and peripheral nervous systems.

While it is true that modern computers are capable of carrying out logical tasks (such as solving equations in higher mathematics) in a fraction of the time it would take most individuals to do so, we must not forget that it was the brilliance of the human mind that allowed for the creation of this splendid technology. The fact that any individual is able to claim victory against a machine with such speed and capacity only solidifies the astonishing competency of the human brain itself (see box *It's a Draw!*). So the next time you find yourself driving along the information superhighway, remind yourself how it came to be.

The human body and its nervous system have many parts that cohesively work together to maintain control by sending messages to one another. What are the mechanisms that keep these messages flowing? How do humans process information? What effects do attention and memory have on human processing and performance? The answers to these and other questions to follow should shed light on the marvel of the human body, its capabilities, and its numerous abilities to perform an almost limitless number of motor skills.

Introduction to the Structure and Function of the Nervous System

How is it that a champion chess master is able to plan several moves ahead, or that a tennis player can plan many shots in advance during a point? What processes underlie an individual's ability to perceive, respond to, and execute certain movements and actions? The answer lies in the human brain. But nervous activity is not solely achieved by the brain; rather, in conjunction with the spinal cord and nerves, a complex system is set up whereby vast interconnecting pathways integrate and control the actions of the entire body from head to toe. How the nervous system accomplishes such a remarkable feat is the subject of the brief overview that follows.

The Neuron and Its Function

Types of Neurons

Neurons (nerve cells) are the fundamental functional and structural units of the nervous system that allow information to travel throughout the body to various destinations. There are three general categories of neurons that carry neural information between the brain, spinal cord, and muscles. **Afferent neurons** carry signals *to* the brain or spinal cord and are also referred to as **sensory neurons. Efferent neurons**, or **motor neurons**, carry signals *from* the brain or spinal

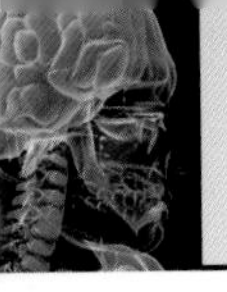

A Giant on Maximum and Minimum Scales

The external appearance of the human brain conceals its true complexity. Approximately 15 billion neurons are concentrated within the 85 cubic inches of the brain, the largest number located in the cortex numbering 10 billion (a value over two and a half times the number of inhabitants on the globe).

At only 1/8 of an inch thick, the cortex may seem insignificant in size, but if all of its numerous folds and clefts were spread out, it would approximate the dimensions of a newspaper page bustling with neurons. Another staggering fact is that all the nerve fibers link to form a network four times greater than the distance between the earth and the moon. Now that's maximum use of space!

cord (Figure 10.2). A third category of neurons, the **interneurons**, originate or terminate in the brain or spinal cord.

Every neuron is composed of many parts, each of which serves a particular purpose. The **dendrites** extend from the **cell body** (which houses the cell nucleus) as branch-like fibers and serve as the centers for stimuli by receiving messages. The **axon** exists as a single extension from the cell body and functions to transmit and carry messages to its **terminal endings**, numbering in the thousands, along to the dendrites of other neurons (Figure 10.3).

Some axons also have a fatty covering that wraps around the axon, called a **myelin sheath**, that is separated by gaps called **nodes of Ranvier**. This specialized structure of some neurons, such as the motor neurons that innervate muscle fibers, offers an advantage because neural messages travel much faster as the impulse skips from one node to the next (Figure 10.3). Myelin acts as an insulator, similar to the rubber that surrounds electrical wire to prevent leakage of current. This rapid and efficient system allows the body to react quickly whenever and wherever required. Whether you are trying to avoid a hit in football, reacting to a spike in volleyball, or contemplating your next move during a basketball game, the central mechanisms involving neurons are essentially the same.

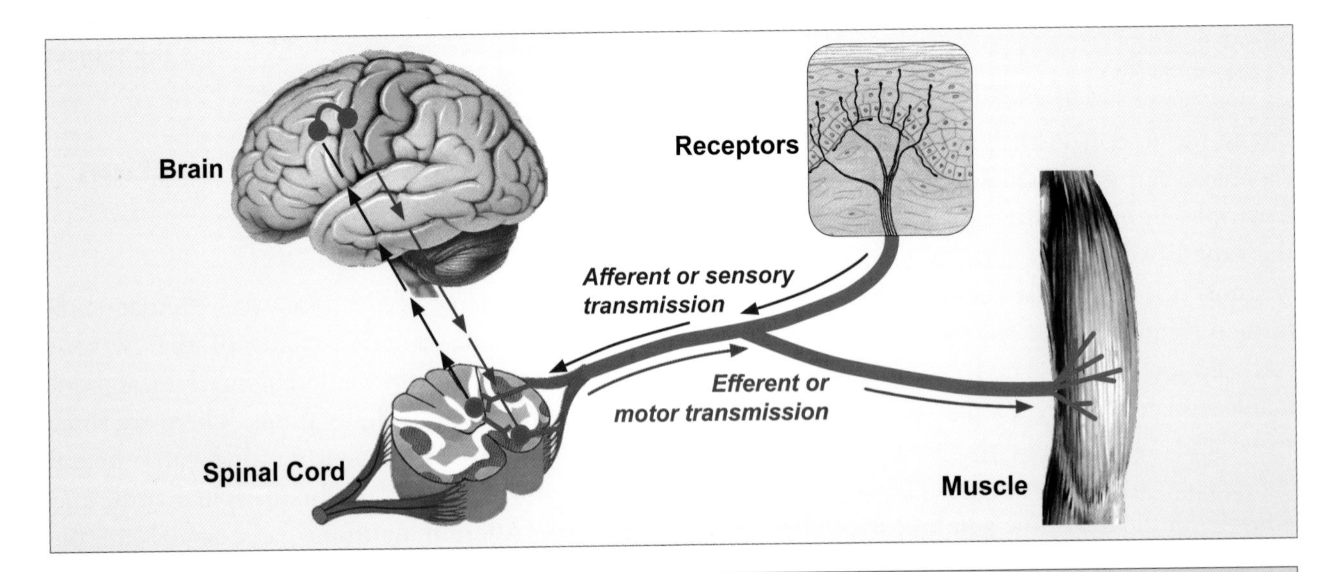

Figure 10.2 The receptors guide the stimulus across a sensory pathway (afferent) network to a specific sensory region of the cortex. Decisions are sent via a motor pathway (efferent) network to muscles and joints for execution.

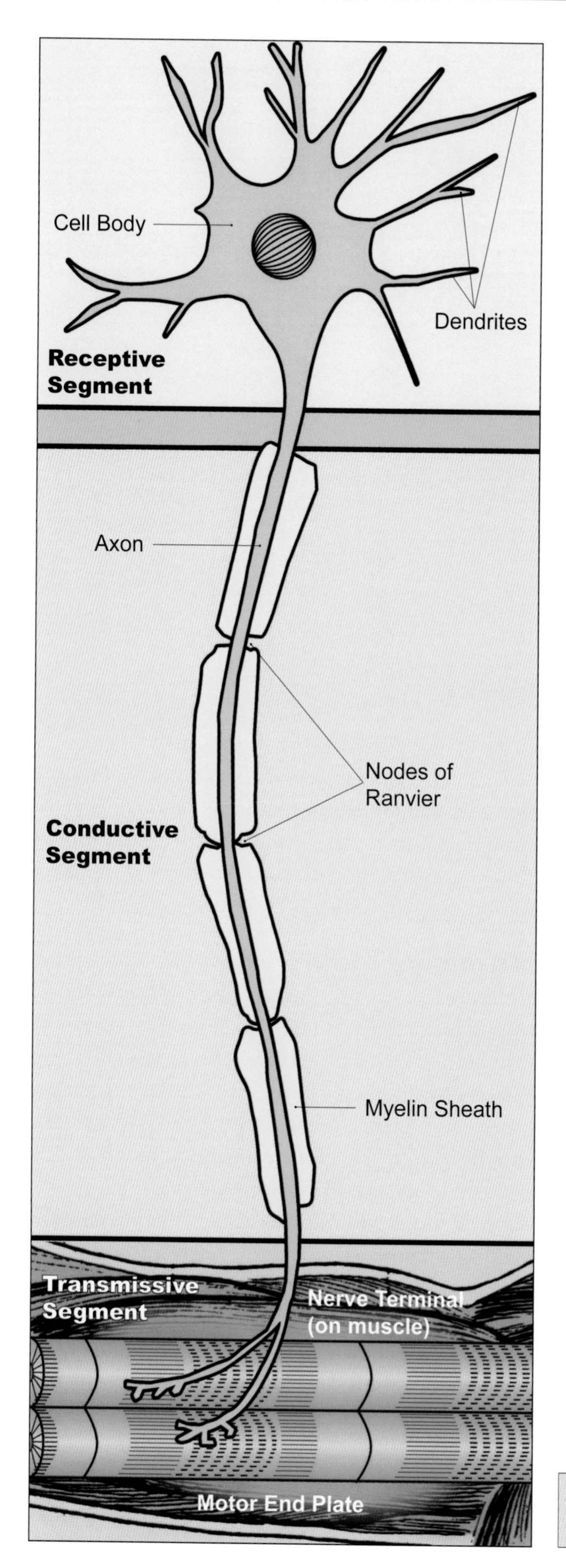

The Neuron's Function

Most neurons contain three functional regions (i.e., **receptive**, **conductive**, and **transmissive segments**), each responsible for a very specific information processing task (Figure 10.3).

Receptive Segment This segment receives a continuous bombardment of synaptic input from numerous other neurons on the receptor site. These inputs are processed and sent further to the conductive region of the neuron, the axon.

Conductive Segment The axon serves as the conductive segment of the neuron. It is specialized for the conduction of neural information in the form of nerve impulses.

Transmissive Segment The axon terminals convert the stimulation of the nerve impulse to release chemical neurotransmitters at its synapses. These chemicals give rise to effective reception of information by another neuron or muscle cell.

Neural Impulses

Our nervous systems can be likened to a railway complex and our brains to a signal tower, although along our sensory pathways, traffic is the law. Neural impulses may be thought of as trains that transport the information necessary for all the activities and actions we carry out, including reading the words in this sentence. They are the language of the nervous system, continually relaying information to the appropriate sensory cells and musculature. But how do these messages find their way along the axons, one neuron to another, without being derailed?

The secret lies with the distribution of ions (charged particles, e.g., sodium and potassium) that are located on both sides of each neuron's cell membrane. The inside of the neuron tends to be negative relative to the outside, while the outside tends to be positive relative to the inside – this

Figure 10.3 Functional organization of a typical neuron.

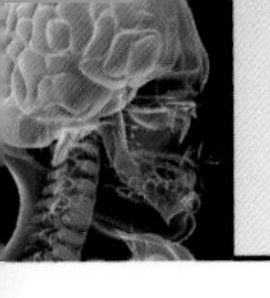

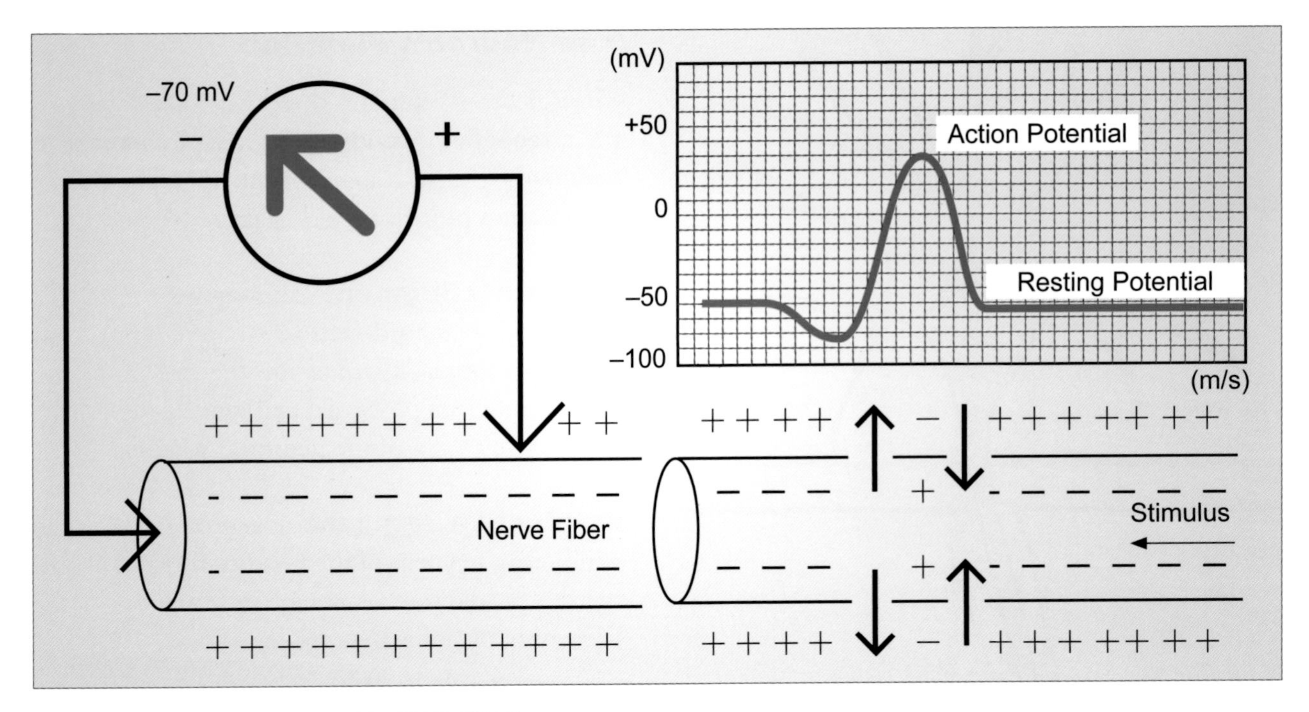

Figure 10.4 Action potential of a neuron.

creates an imbalance of charges, or an electrical potential difference across the cell membrane called a **membrane potential**. This idea may be compared to a battery that has a positive terminal (outside cell) and negative terminal (inside cell).

The situation just described reflects the neuron's resting potential, or state of **polarization** at approximately –70 millivolts (mV). When a stimulus reaches the nerve fiber, positive ions rush into a particular region of the membrane and are then quickly pumped back out to return the neuron to its resting state. This is called an **action potential**, or state of **depolarization**, which reaches its peak at about 40 mV. In a domino effect, the same process is repeated in adjacent areas of the neural membrane until the action potential reaches the end of the cell membrane (Figure 10.4).

The Synapse and Synaptic Transmission

Each axon branches into terminals and at its end forms a junction with another neuron called a **synapse**. Synapses are small – a few billion could fit into a thimble – but their small size says nothing about the very important role they play. Movement of a neural impulse across this junction is called **synaptic transmission**. Although several steps in synaptic transmission have been identified, much about the precise mechanics behind it remains shrouded in mystery.

"All-or-none" Law A synaptic transmission will cause an action potential in the postsynaptic cell as long as its strength is above a minimum threshold level. This characteristic is called the **"all-or-none" law**, and the intensity of the action potential remains constant along the nerve fiber's length. It follows that a stronger stimulus will not give rise to a stronger action potential.

It is useful to explain this phenomenon by making a comparison to the firing of a gun. In order for the gun to be fired successfully, there is a minimum degree to which the trigger must be pulled. Further, when the trigger is pulled past that critical point and the gun fires, it will fire at full force regardless of the force applied to the trigger.

In similar fashion, a neuron will either fire an action potential at full force or it will not fire at all. But while a stronger stimulus will not elicit a stronger action potential, it will cause it to fire at a faster rate. Thus, the rate at which neurons fire provides an indication of the strength of a stimulus.

For example, intense stimuli, those that might result from rapid, powerful movements in the muscles (e.g., golf swing, soccer ball kick, or football throw) or deep bending and stretching in the joints, trigger numerous simultaneous impulses; weaker stimuli, such as those during slow stretching movements, trigger fewer.

The firing rate of action potentials has a limit, just as a gun cannot be fired a second time until the first shot is complete. In other words, an **absolute refractory period** exists (about a millisecond) – a period in which a second action potential is not possible. After this period, neurons enter what is called a **relative refractory period** of several milliseconds, during which a neuron can be fired only by a very strong synaptic transmission (i.e., an elevated threshold level). Although this slight limit exists, rates remain amazingly fast, allowing a batter, for example, to swing at a pitch that seemed to be going outside but instead curved back over the plate.

All synaptic transmissions are not of the same strength, nor do they exert the same effects. In fact, they differ in terms of the chemical transmitter located at the synapse as well as the general function they serve at that synapse. Some transmitters, such as **acetylcholine (Ach)**, have a strong excitatory effect (usually to muscles) and result in a fast response. Others, however, respond more slowly, while still others exert an inhibitory effect. Depending on the particular location and intended function, a variety of transmitters exist, serving to keep the system under precise control.

The preceding discussion has only touched the surface of the complex network that forms the nervous system. If anything, this brief overview was intended to open your eyes to the involved processes that control our every move and guide our perceptions. Without them, you would not be able to turn the pages in this book or even read the words before you.

Information Processing and Decision Making

The goalie starts out of his net, preparing for the oncoming breakaway. As the player draws nearer, the goalie slowly backs in toward the net, following his adversary's every move. The goalie knows that the charging player likes to go to his backhand shot, so he prepares to react to such a move. Indeed, the offensive forward begins the motions of a backhand, but stops halfway, pulls the puck back, and rifles a wrist shot that finds the corner of the net. What was going through the goalie's mind? How did he process the information used to make the decision to move the way he did? Similarly, how does the batter contend with pitches of varying speeds and spins? And what goes through the mind of the tennis player awaiting a powerful serve by her opponent? The ability to sense and respond quickly and with accuracy to such dynamic information in the environment is a crucial component of successful performances.

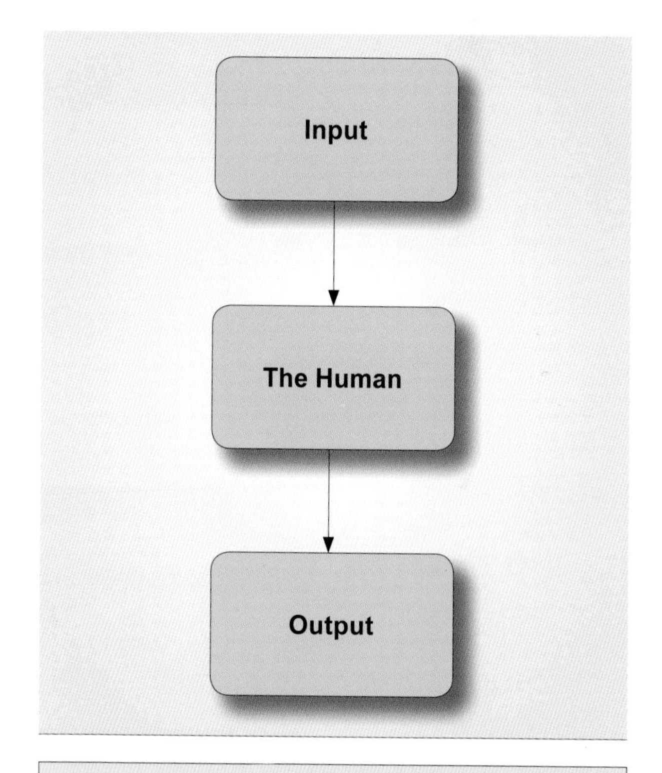

Figure 10.5 The simplest information processing model.

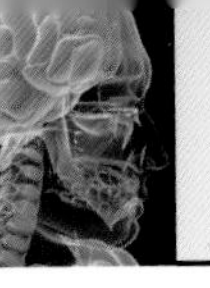

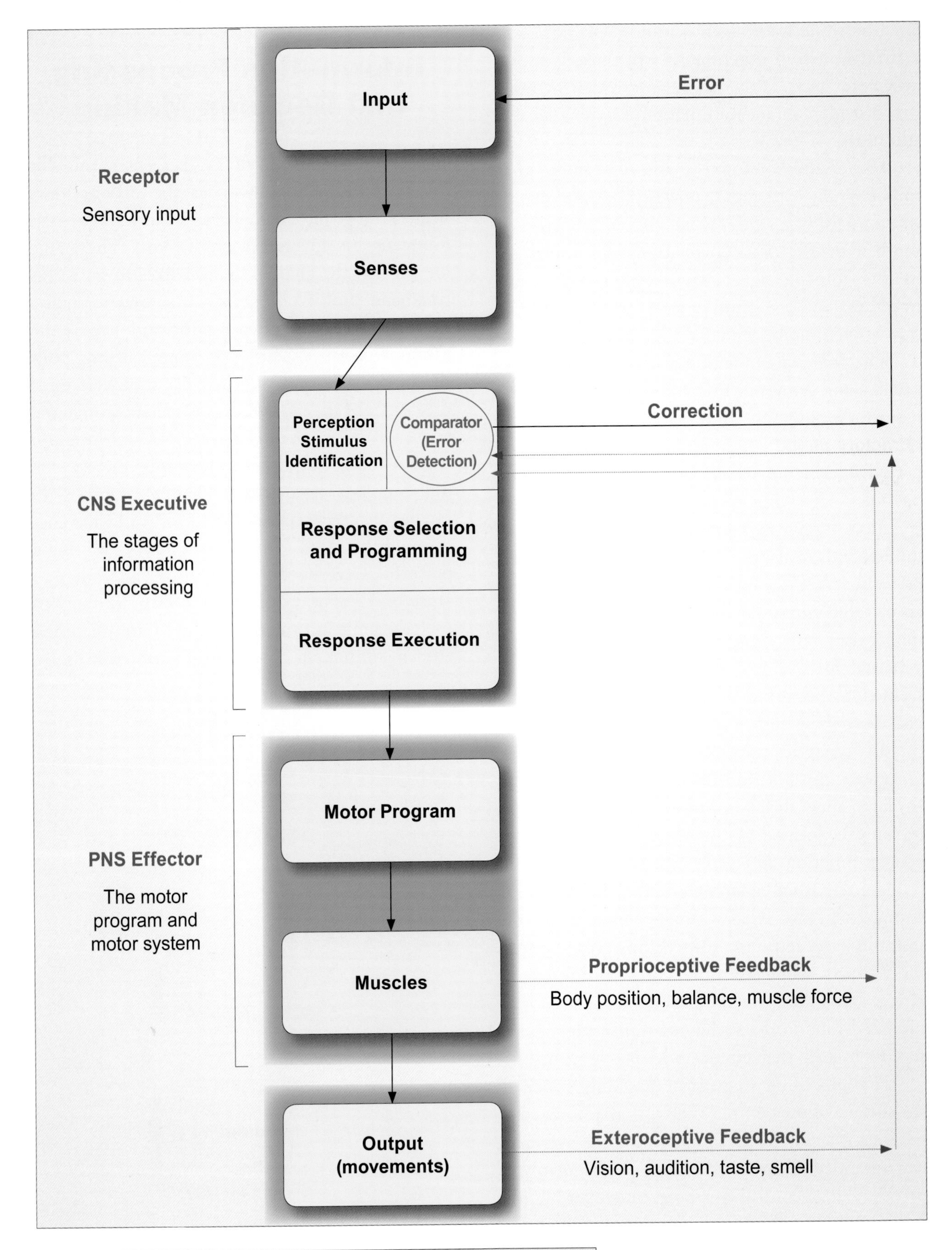

Figure 10.6 A conceptual closed-loop information processing model.

Human beings are often thought to process information in ways similar to a computer. Hence the label **information processing**. Information that is available in the environment provides the input that, after going through several stages of processing, leads to an output of some desired action or movement (Figures 10.5 and 10.6). But what happens at each stage? And what are the processes that allow players to react effectively in a situation that requires a swift decision and a rapid reaction? We will focus on three stages that underlie the processes by which players are able to respond effectively to the demands of their environment.

Information Processing Stages

Stimulus Identification Stage

Whether you are a goalie facing a breakaway or a batter awaiting a pitch, before any real decision can be made, a stimulus must be detected that warrants analysis. Therefore, this first stage is focused on sensing environmental information and determining what it is. Is the pitch a fastball? A curveball? These sensations come from diverse sources including the five classic senses (known as **exteroceptors**) of vision, audition, smell, touch, and taste, as well as a few others such as **proprioception** (the sense of joint movement, muscle tension, orientation, touch, and balance).

This stage is important for providing information about the nature of the environmental stimuli, including patterns of movement, direction, and speed of movement. For example, in order to catch a football successfully, you would need to identify the projection of the ball as well as its direction of motion and relative speed. With this information secured, you have a representation of the stimulus, and the information is prepared so that it can be passed on to the next stage for further processing.

Response Selection Stage

Whereas the first stage deals with the nature of a stimulus and its recognition, this stage is required to generate a response to one's perception of the stimulus, which in turn serves as a stimulus to effector function (which calls upon specific muscles). In other words, there is a translation from perception to a movement or response in the form of a motor program (see discussion on motor programs in Chapter 11), based on the demands of the environment or the intentions of the performer.

An action (i.e., motor program) is selected from among several convenient options. Thus a basketball player may try to decide whether to make a no-look pass to a teammate on a fast break or take off from the free-throw line for a slam dunk. For this reason, the response selection stage can be described as a translation mechanism between what is sensed and what movement is desired.

Response Programming and Execution Stage

This brings us to the final stage of processing, which organizes the selected movement from the prior stage. Of course, before a movement can be executed, many things must first occur: the system must prepare mechanisms in the brainstem and spinal cord, retrieve a motor program that will direct the action, and command the correct muscles to contract in the proper sequence, with the appropriate force, and with suitable timing. For example, it is not enough to simply decide to swing at a pitch; a batter must consider how fast the swing should be, the force that should be applied, and the most appropriate sequence to follow, depending on the pitch and the circumstances of the game.

Feedback in Motor Control

The efficiency of motor control by the human information processing system is based to a large extent on receiving various types of **feedback**. As

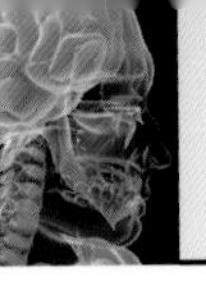

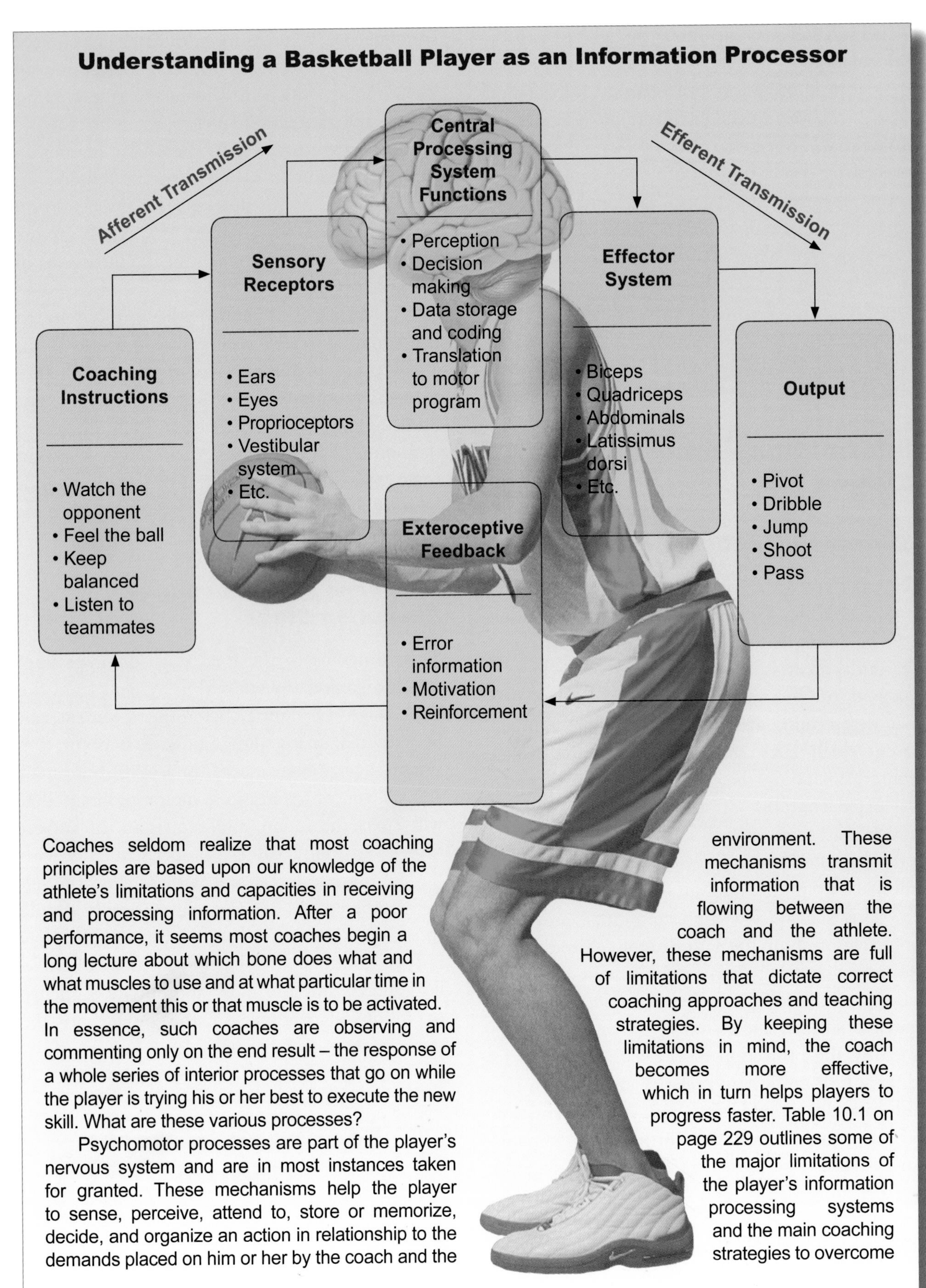

Coaches seldom realize that most coaching principles are based upon our knowledge of the athlete's limitations and capacities in receiving and processing information. After a poor performance, it seems most coaches begin a long lecture about which bone does what and what muscles to use and at what particular time in the movement this or that muscle is to be activated. In essence, such coaches are observing and commenting only on the end result – the response of a whole series of interior processes that go on while the player is trying his or her best to execute the new skill. What are these various processes?

Psychomotor processes are part of the player's nervous system and are in most instances taken for granted. These mechanisms help the player to sense, perceive, attend to, store or memorize, decide, and organize an action in relationship to the demands placed on him or her by the coach and the environment. These mechanisms transmit information that is flowing between the coach and the athlete. However, these mechanisms are full of limitations that dictate correct coaching approaches and teaching strategies. By keeping these limitations in mind, the coach becomes more effective, which in turn helps players to progress faster. Table 10.1 on page 229 outlines some of the major limitations of the player's information processing systems and the main coaching strategies to overcome these limitations.

It is difficult to separate a player's sensory capacities and perceptual processes. What input the athlete actually processes is highly dependent upon the quality of both sensory and perceptual mechanisms.

In practice an athlete is constantly bombarded with stimuli coming in through various senses. These stimuli are provided externally by the coach and internally by proprioceptors (receptors in the muscles, tendons, ligaments, and vestibular apparatus). However, a player's selective attention serves to filter out most of the available information presented. A coach who wants the player to perceive (i.e., hear or see) the right things would have to select and present instructions carefully so that they have a chance of getting through for interpretation and recognition.

Selective attention and short-term memory are limitations of a player's perceptual mechanism that every coach must consider for optimal learning results in practice.

we execute movements, the numerous receptors located throughout our bodies are continually updating the central nervous system about the nature of our actions. When figure skaters take off in attempting a triple axel, how does the feedback received from their senses affect the rest of the jump? Are they able to adjust their body position in the air in order to complete the rotations, or is the jump so routine that it is run off automatically? That is the question we will now consider.

Closed-loop Control System

The human senses perceive stimuli as images from the outside world and sensations from the body's internal environment. These stimuli are the first links in a long cause-and-effect chain of activities in the central nervous system and other interconnected mechanisms. Each sensory cell receives or is sensitive to a specific form of impinging stimuli or energy. The receptors then guide the stimuli across a sensory pathway network to a specific sensory region of the cortex for evaluation.

A process in which a specific reading is continuously compared with a standard value is referred to as a **closed-loop control** system. The system is based on the idea that movements may be planned and adjusted by feedback even during the movement. Therefore, the gymnast who senses a slight loss of balance on the balance beam can make an adjustment that will bring her body back to its desired state to salvage the performance (see box *Closed-loop Control System in Action*).

Several key elements form the basis for closed-loop control: error detection, error correction, and feedback. There is also a **reference of correctness** that specifies the desired value for the system. The resulting movement (output) is fed back and compared to the reference by a **comparator** for error detection and, if necessary, corrected.

A Thermostat Operates Like a Closed-loop Control System

This principle of a closed-loop control system, in which bits of information travel around a circuit from entry to exit, enabling the control reading to be approximated to its standard value, even has applications in technology. The automatic home furnace that has a thermostat set at the desired temperature may serve as an example. The current temperature is continually fed back to this reference, and any difference between the current and desired temperature leads to the furnace turning on or shutting off in order to maintain the desired temperature.

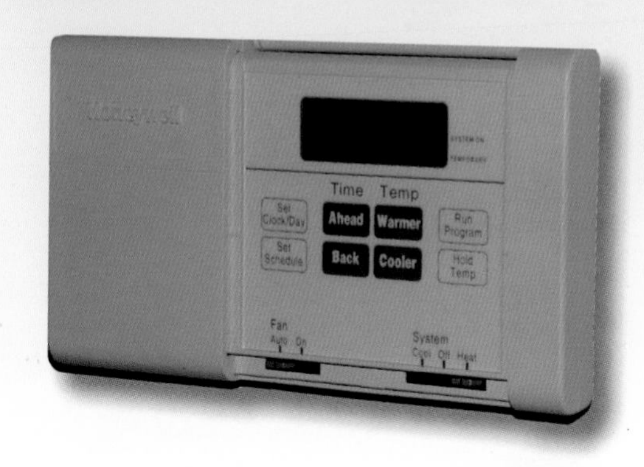

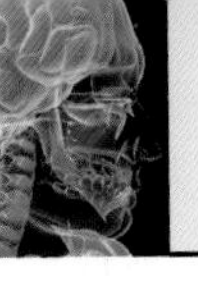

This general process is self-regulating and will continue to maintain the desired movement of the performer.

Advantages of the Closed-loop Control System

Clearly, closed-loop processes offer distinct advantages. Whenever we attempt new skills, we cannot be expected to master them immediately. But the closed-loop control system allows us to perform unpracticed actions, provided that we understand the difference between what we are doing and what is essentially desired (see comparator in Figure 10.6).

Also, the closed-loop control system offers flexibility and adaptability to movement, especially important in tracking skills. Just imagine the limitations to a soccer goalie if all of his or her actions had to be preplanned in advance – reacting to shots and fakes would turn out to be a nightmare. By having the ability to execute a planned movement that may be adjusted according to the situation, we have a great deal more versatility in our movements.

Finally, closed-loop control systems come in really handy in activities requiring precision and accuracy. This may be clearly seen in the shooter who has a strict target to aim at, requiring that movements be continually adjusted and adapted to suit the goal.

Disadvantages of the Closed-loop Control System

However, certain drawbacks do exist with closed-loop control systems. It is generally agreed that such systems do not effectively explain the control of rapid, discrete actions. Because the stages of information processing are an integral component

Closed-loop Control System in Action

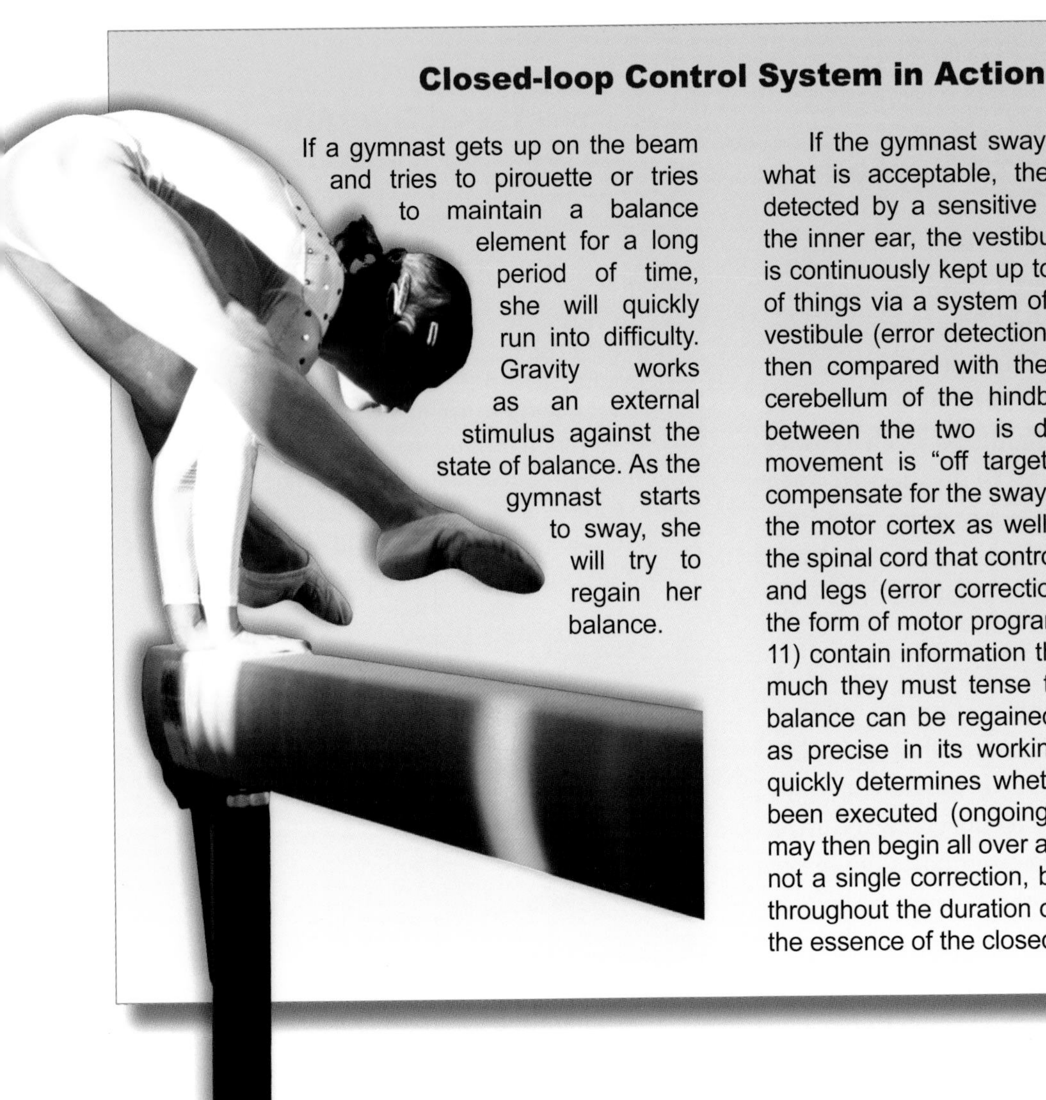

If a gymnast gets up on the beam and tries to pirouette or tries to maintain a balance element for a long period of time, she will quickly run into difficulty. Gravity works as an external stimulus against the state of balance. As the gymnast starts to sway, she will try to regain her balance.

If the gymnast sways significantly more than what is acceptable, the deviation difference is detected by a sensitive measuring instrument in the inner ear, the vestibular apparatus. The brain is continuously kept up to date on the actual state of things via a system of nerves leading from the vestibule (error detection). The incoming data are then compared with the standard values in the cerebellum of the hindbrain, and the difference between the two is determined. If the body movement is "off target," corrective orders that compensate for the swaying movement are sent to the motor cortex as well as to the motor units in the spinal cord that control the muscles in the arms and legs (error correction). These commands in the form of motor programs (discussed in Chapter 11) contain information that tells the muscles how much they must tense to reach the level where balance can be regained. In turn, the vestibule – as precise in its workings as a seismograph – quickly determines whether or not the order has been executed (ongoing feedback). The process may then begin all over again. Thus, the process is not a single correction, but a continuous updating throughout the duration of the movement, which is the essence of the closed-loop control system.

Intrinsic–Extrinsic Feedback Interaction

Luge riders who think they can negotiate the labyrinth of turns by relying solely on their eyes will find themselves at the bottom of the leader board. If they rely on external stimuli (especially visual stimuli) to guide their movements, the extrinsic (outer) regulatory circuit takes over. On the other hand, if luge riders are guided by the intrinsic or inner regulatory circuit, ideally when riding flat on their sleds, we say that their intrinsic (inner) regulatory circuit is at work. Both are important, however, and both play a role in the regulation of their movement down the track.

The intrinsic circuit has an advantage: movements and their corrections can be executed quicker and with more precision (inner or red circuit in Figure 10.6). The muscle feeling, or kinesthetic sense, takes precedence, then, over the eyes (outer or blue circuit in Figure 10.6), and this is often the acknowledged goal in many sporting activities.

of the closed-loop control system, they demand attention as well as time. In fact, each time a correction is deemed necessary, feedback must pass through several processing stages as shown in Figure 10.6. This presents a big limitation. Therefore, although closed-loop control systems may accurately describe relatively slow movements, faster discrete movements (e.g., golf swing, batting in baseball, a quad in skating) once initiated may not properly fall under such control.

Open-loop Control System

Have you ever wondered how figure skaters, gymnasts, and dancers are able to perform routines that run minutes in length without skipping a beat? How is a figure skater able to complete the four rotations required to execute the quad in competition (Figure 10.7 B, page 230)? How is it possible to complete certain skills automatically, without thinking about execution? **Open-loop control** attempts to provide answers to such questions.

The whole concept of the open-loop control system is based on the **motor program** concept, discussed in chapter 11. A motor program is a centrally located structure that defines the essential details of skilled action, before a movement begins, and without the influence of peripheral feedback. This means that certain movements may be structured in advance, enabling automatic execution when initiated.

Whereas a typical closed-loop control system involves feedback and an associated comparator, an open-loop control system is made up of only two main parts – the *executive* and the *effector*. A stimulus (input) reaches the executive, which puts the system into action by choosing a response in the form of a specific motor program and relaying instructions to the effector (specific muscles). It is the job of the effector to carry out the specified instructions automatically. Unlike closed-loop control, the open-loop system will not respond again until the executive is activated anew.

Advantages of the Open-loop Control System

Upon analyzing the basic features of open-loop control and motor programs, certain advantages immediately stand out. First, many movements that are fast and forceful can be produced

Traffic Lights Operate Like an Open-loop Control System

Traffic signals that follow a defined sequence regardless of the conditions on the road are an example of an open-loop control system. Operations and sequencing are specified in advance, so once a motor program has been initiated, it will follow without modification. For this reason, it appears that open-loop control is particularly important in predictable environments, where changes will not require variations in movements once they have been initiated.

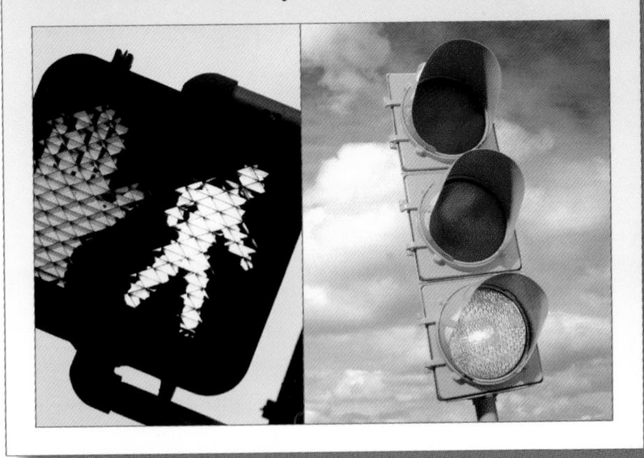

without the need for extensive conscious control. Therefore, we can throw, kick, and swing a golf club as established by a motor program.

Another benefit is the amount of attention that is able to be diverted to other processes. Because feedback does not require processing in the control of movements, a greater amount of attention may be directed to strategy and creativity to enhance performance.

Disadvantages of the Open-loop Control System

Not everything about open-loop control is advantageous, however. As mentioned earlier, open-loop control is not as effective in situations that are unstable and less predictable. In these situations, movements may not be determined effectively in advance, so many movements would suffer without feedback. It follows that the more precise and complex actions would be in need of more extensive well-developed motor programs. Although practice can help develop motor programs so that they do become more elaborate, an open-loop control system is generally more accurate for describing rapid, discrete skills that occur in relatively predictable environments.

Factors Affecting Information Processing

The effectiveness of the learner's information processing depends upon many factors. The most important among them are: (1) the quality of sensory input information reaching the performer's senses; (2) the quality and effectiveness of sensory receptors in relaying information to the CNS; (3) the speed of processing stimulus information, known as reaction time; (4) the ability to anticipate; (5) the capacity to concentrate and attend to stimuli; and (6) the level of arousal and psychological readiness. An overview of characteristics of a learner's information processing mechanisms and appropriate instruction strategies is presented in Table 10.1. A more thorough discussion of these mechanisms is beyond the scope of this textbook.

Summary

It is difficult to appreciate the complexities of human movement, especially when we see the ease with which many actions are performed. The human nervous system, composed of the brain, spinal cord, and nerves, acts as the control center that integrates all of our actions. The numerous parts of the nervous system work together by sending messages to one another with remarkable speed, precision, and capacity, allowing the movements we make to be efficient and accurate. From the dendrites and axons of neurons, to neural impulses that travel a complex route, we are able to sense, react, and respond to stimuli in the world around us – as well as if not better than modern-day computers.

Once information has been sensed by various receptors (exteroceptive or proprioceptive), we must then process this information and decide

Table 10.1 Summary characteristics of a learner's information processing mechanisms and effective instruction strategies.

Mechanism	Limitation	Instruction Strategy
Sensory mechanisms • Exteroceptors • Proprioceptors	• Poor visual skills, such as dynamic visual acuity	• Detect vision problems early
	• Learner does not hear instruction	• Limit the noise in the gym; speak clearly and loudly
	• Learner does not feel the correct position required	• Move the learner's body into the correct position
Perceptual mechanisms	• Limited attention span; can attend to only one major novel point	• Provide only one critical component of a skill at a time
Short-term memory	• Limited capacity	• Provide only limited amount of information; do not overload athlete
	• Significant rate of loss	• Minimize time between demonstration and rehearsal of skill (i.e., practice skill immediately after it has been presented)
	• Subject to easy interference	• Avoid unrelated activities in the gym, such as workers in the background, spectators yelling and commenting, other teams practicing, and so on.
Long-term, or permanent, memory	• Must rehearse/practice to encode and retain information	• Provide continuing rehearsal of skill until it is learned properly
Learner's psychological state	• Arousal and anxiety	• Motivate learner to an optimal arousal level; provide non-threatening learning environment
	• Attention and fatigue	• Avoid practicing new skills when fatigued
	• Boredom	• Introduce new drills to coach same skill

how to respond appropriately. We have a well-developed system that allows us to do this. Information passes through several successive stages of processing (stimulus identification, response selection, and response programming), after which a decision can be made, depending on the information we are given. Reaction time, anticipation, and level of arousal are some of the factors that affect our abilities to respond quickly and accurately to various stimuli.

Our abilities to process information are also dependent on concentration, attention, and memory. Because our attention capacities are limited, we cannot attend to all the stimuli that exist in the environment around us. Therefore, it is important to focus attention on information

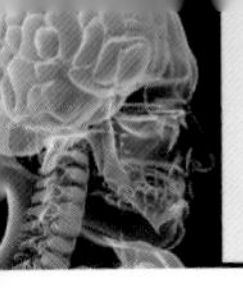

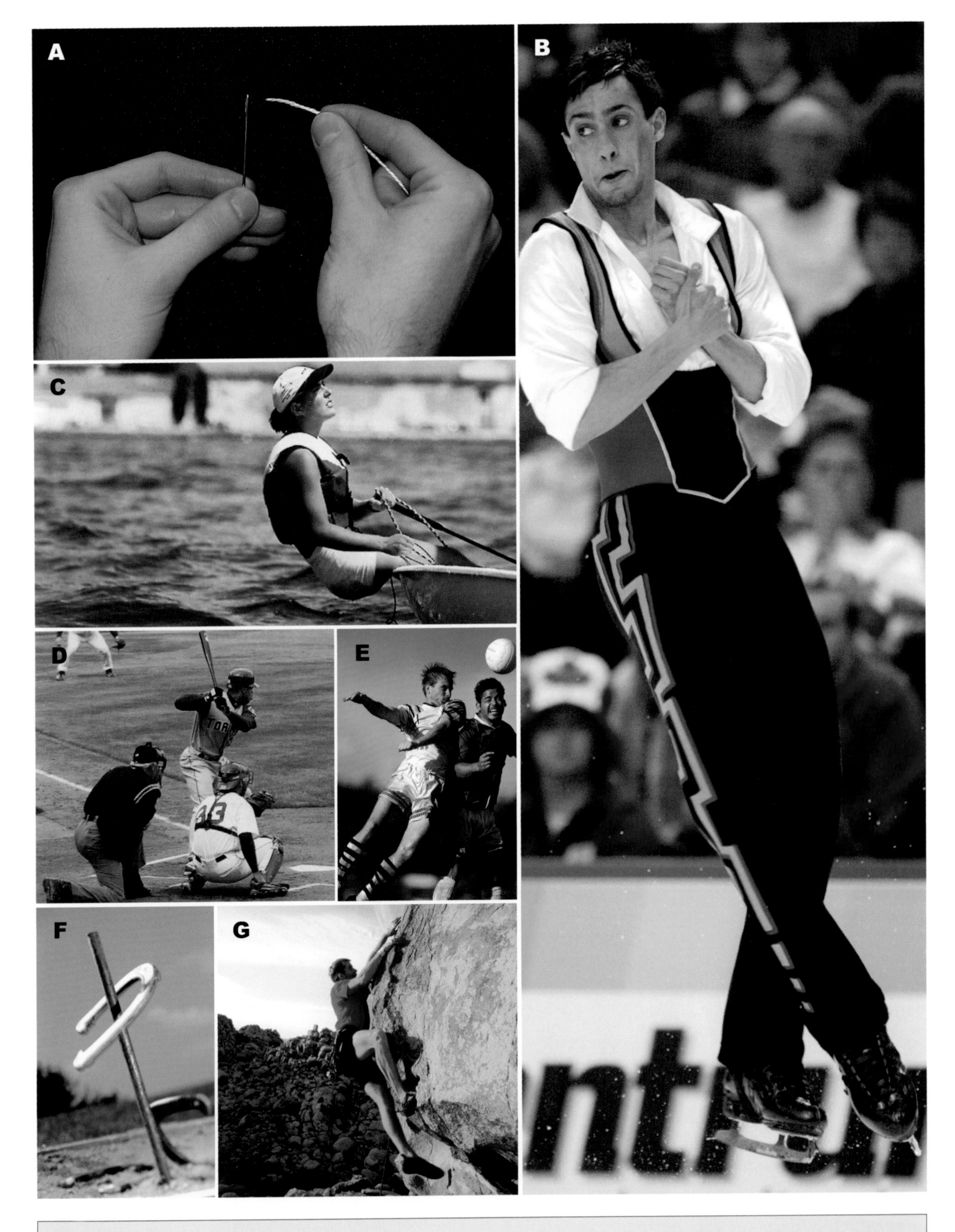

Figure 10.7 What system of motor control is required for: **A.** threading a needle; **B.** figure skating; **C.** sailing; **D.** baseball batting; **E.** soccer; **F.** horseshoe throwing; **G.** rock climbing?

that is most appropriate to the situation, as well as have the ability to shift or broaden this attention as it becomes necessary. In closely contested competitions, concentration can be the defining difference between victory and defeat.

Without memory processes, every movement we attempted would be a new one – we would be forced to relearn numerous skills and movements. Luckily, memory allows us to store, retrieve, and utilize information from past experiences as we need it. Although memory is not always accessed with success, the potential for a limitless amount of information to be stored in long-term memory exists, which acts toward effectively improving future movement performances.

Some of the responses we make in fact result from feedback received through receptors throughout the body that continually update the central nervous system as to how the action is being executed. A closed-loop control system contends that, through feedback mechanisms, responses can be changed and altered even during a movement in order to achieve the desired movement outcome. An open-loop control system is based mainly on motor programs that define movements before they occur and are executed automatically, without feedback. Each theory has its own advantages and disadvantages and is more accurate for describing different types of skills.

Key Terms

absolute refractory period
action potential
afferent neurons
all-or-none law
axon
cell body
central nervous system (CNS)
closed-loop control
conductive segment
cendrites
cepolarization
efferent neurons
feedback
information processing
interneuron
membrane potential
motor neuron
myelin sheath
neuron
nodes of Ranvier
open-loop control
peripheral nervous system (PNS)
polarization
receptive segment
relative refractory period
response programming stage
response selection stage
sensory neuron
stimulus identification stage
synapse
terminal endings
transmissive segment

Discussion Questions

1. What name is given to a nerve cell? What are its major components?

2. Differentiate between afferent and efferent transmission of information.

3. List and briefly describe the three functional regions comprising most nerve cells.

4. Describe the process involved during a change in membrane potential. Why are ions important in the process?

5. Explain the *all-or-none law* as it relates to synaptic transmission.

6. Identify and describe the three information processing stages through which information must pass before a movement is executed.

7. Discuss the major differences between open-loop and closed-loop control. Briefly discuss the advantages of each.

8. For the two information processing mechanisms discussed in this chapter, provide examples of limitations and subsequent instruction strategies to overcome these limitations.

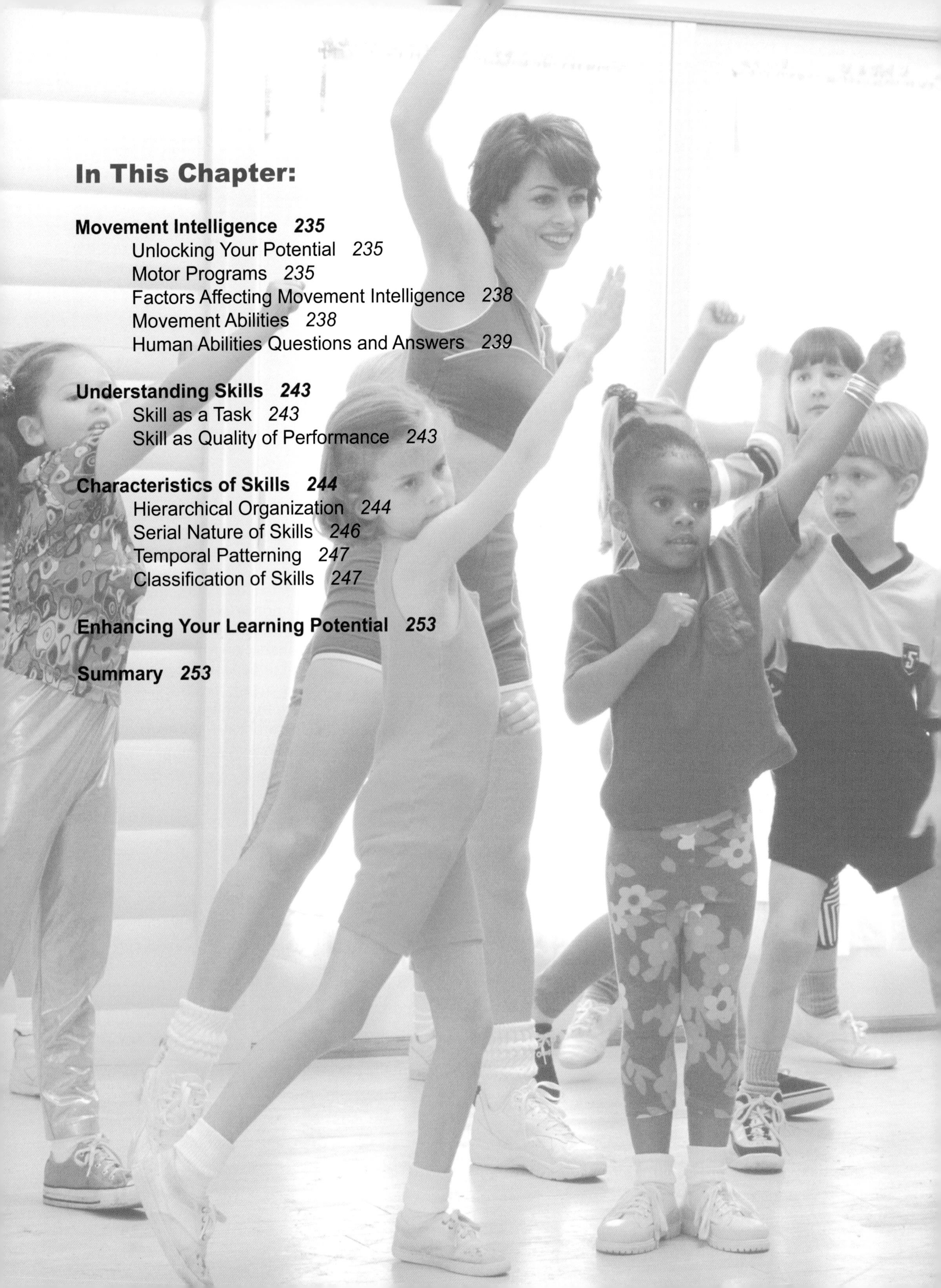

In This Chapter:

CHAPTER 11

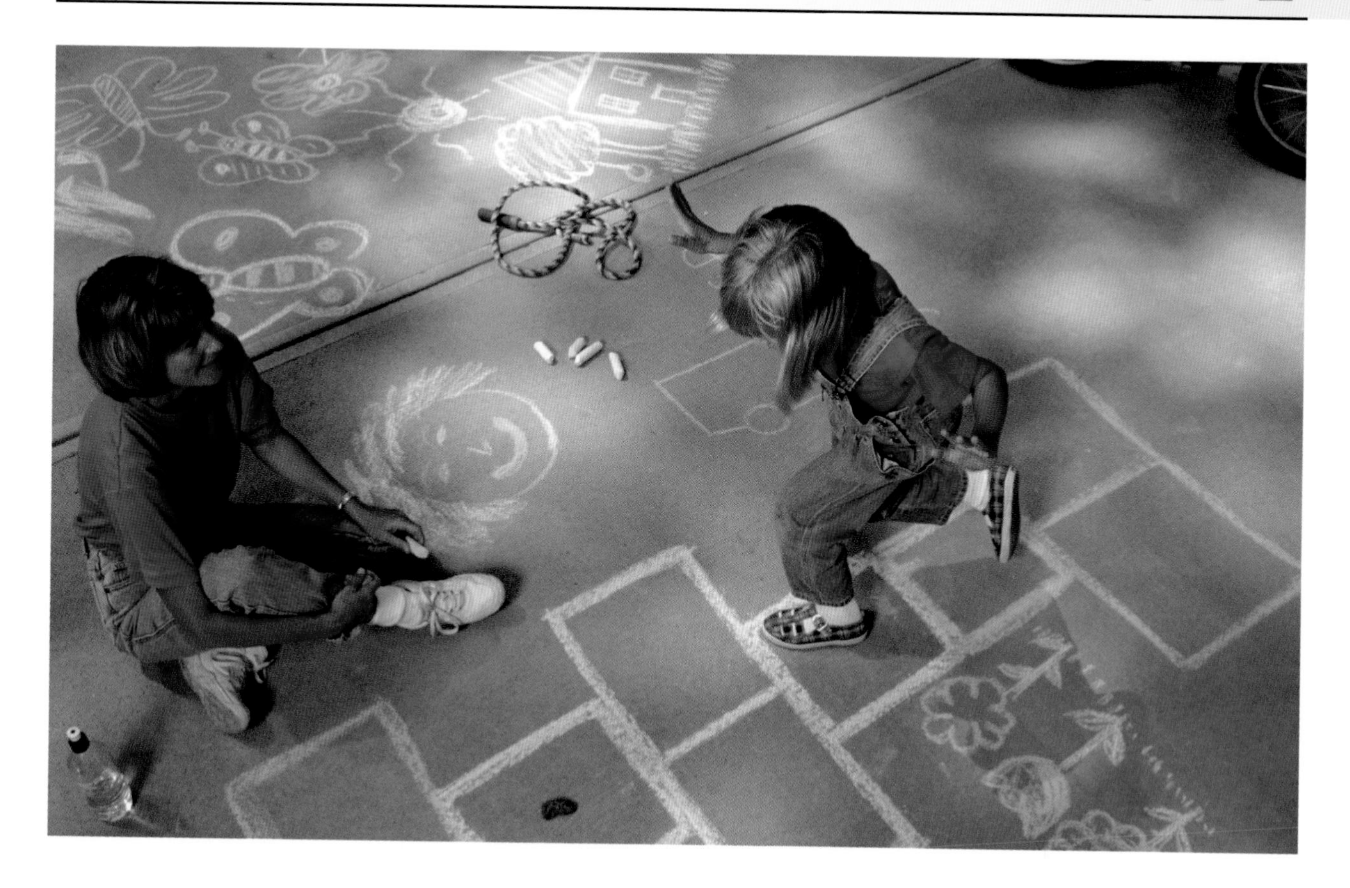

Movement Intelligence: A Vast Store of Motor Programs

After completing this chapter you should be able to:

- explain the concept of movement intelligence in motor skill development;
- describe the rationale for and characteristics of motor programs and movement abilities, and give examples of each;
- discuss the relationship between motor abilities, motor programs, and skills;
- define motor skills and describe their characteristics;
- apply knowledge of the characteristics of a skill to analyze movement;
- explain classification of skills and demonstrate an ability to design learning progression for an open skill.

Whatever activity we may be engaged in, the ability to perform certain skills will always have a bearing on how the activity eventually turns out. Watching others perform skills, and doing so ourselves in various contexts, is a significant part of our lives. During the Winter and Summer Olympic Games and other sporting spectacles, our eyes are glued to the television as we watch, in awe, players and athletes demonstrate an unbelievable level and range of skill. We watch them believing that perhaps we might attain a fraction of their skill, but also so we can share their experiences, if only for a moment.

While Olympic and professional athletes have attained a level of achievement in athletics that most of us will probably never reach, we are all capable of performing the same motor skills they do to one degree or another (Figure 11.1). But many factors will have a significant impact on our ability to execute these skills. All skills share some common characteristics, but they also possess some unique differences that influence learning and performance.

It is no mystery that human skills take many forms. Indeed, the remarkable number of skills we perform is an integral part of not only physical activity and sport but also our daily lives. But the term "skill" is open to several interpretations. We see swimmers execute flip turns at the wall, track athletes clear hurdles with remarkable precision, basketball players shoot jump shots from various positions on the floor, and soccer players head the ball with amazing control. But what are the elements common to these skills? How are skills classified? And what factors affect the learning and execution of these skills? These questions will now be considered in greater detail.

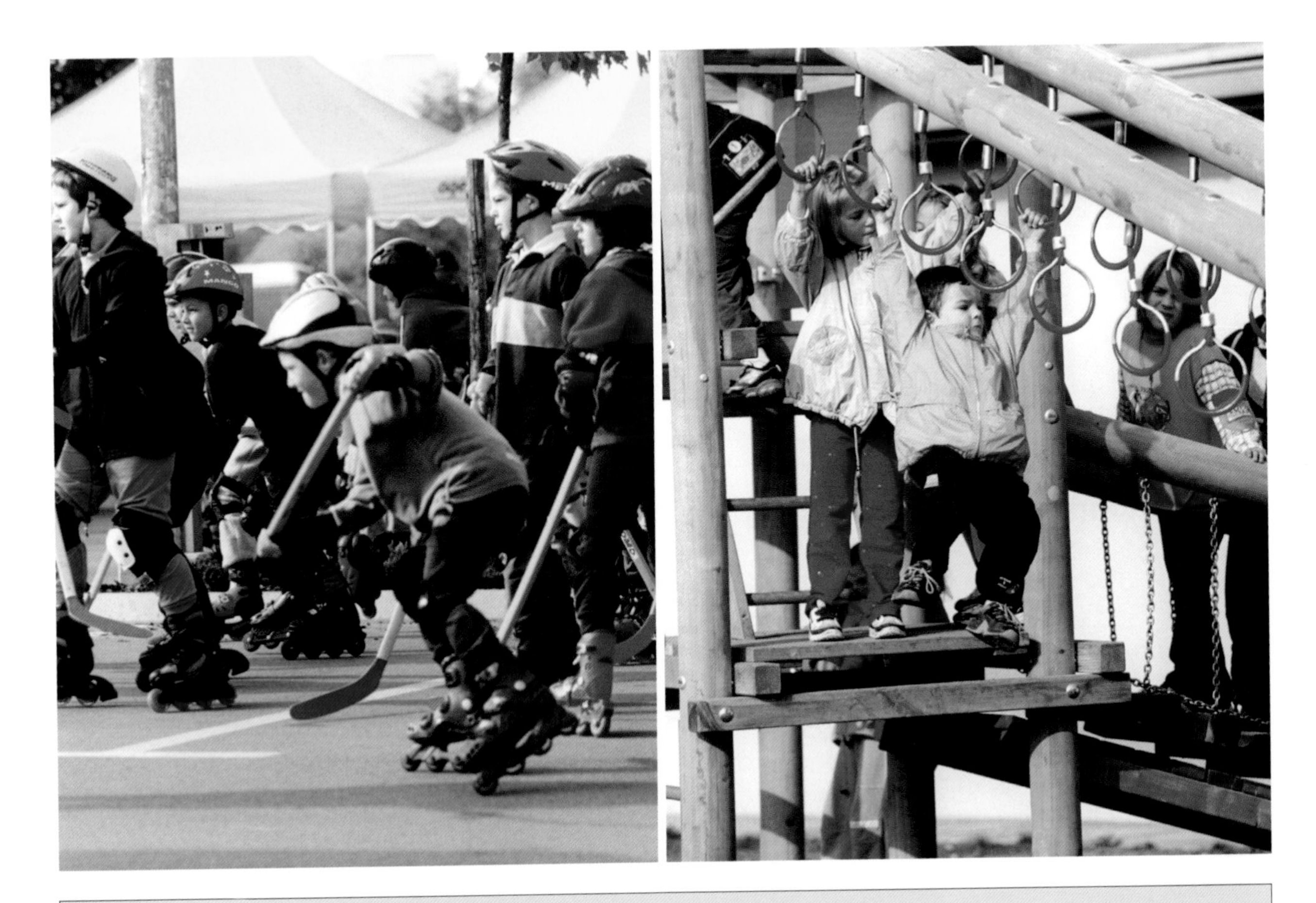

Figure 11.1 In order to attain a high level of achievement in physical activity and sport later in life, it is important to develop a vast repertoire of movement experiences early in life.

Movement Intelligence

Movement intelligence is an aggregate and vast repertoire of movement experiences developed since birth.

We possess the capacity to produce a seemingly endless variety of skills that are inextricably woven into the fabric of our lives. Numerous skills enable us to complete the daily tasks involved with work and school, as well as to participate in many physical activities, all of which offer different and unique challenges. The skills we possess are by no means static elements of our lives; they are continually being enhanced, revised, and adapted through experiences. The ability to learn new skills allows us to improve the way we live in striking ways.

Unlocking Your Potential

Today, we often hear about the many benefits to be had from active living, regular exercise, and a healthy lifestyle. But the advantages of any physical activity depend on some degree of movement intelligence. Participating in activities at an intensity and duration that have a positive impact on our health is greatly enhanced by having a developed skill level. While the advantages offered by physical exercise seem obvious, many individuals may feel uninspired to follow an active lifestyle because they believe their options are limited. Activities such as walking, running, and cycling are undoubtedly effective for improving one's level of fitness, but how attractive are they to the average person? Some might prefer to take part in other nonphysical activities that arouse their interest and that are more fun and enjoyable.

The development of diverse skills can help greatly in this respect. A grasp of the specific skills involved in the activities you would like to pursue will broaden your options, and the possibilities will begin to seem endless. Rather than using the excuse that walking and running are dull and monotonous, you can get out onto the tennis court or take part in a beach volleyball game (or whatever activity you enjoy), displaying your enhanced level of skill with renewed interest and confidence. Being skillful means getting out of physical activity all there is to gain – health, fun, and vitality.

Motor Programs

When learning new skills, we develop movement plans that are eventually stored in memory, known as **motor programs (MPs)**. It is hypothesized that repetitive practice encourages the formation of specialized nerve circuits in the central nervous system that work together when developing a plan for an activity or skill (for more on this topic see Chapter 10). Thus, motor programs emerge as a result of learning.

Motor programs are a set of prestructured muscle commands that, when well developed, allow the performer to carry out the skill automatically. Many skills and movement patterns that must be carried out quickly, almost reflexively, serve as strong evidence for the concept of motor programs. Motor programs also help explain the performances of figure skaters, gymnasts, dancers, and pianists, who must quickly combine together a series of discrete movements into a lengthy program.

Generalized Motor Programs

It is quite possible that developing and storing motor programs for every conceivable movement would place too great a demand on memory. How then do we explain the ability of a performer to meet the ever-changing demands of environmental conditions? In sports, the situations that arise during training and competition and the appropriate actions (motor programs) that must be taken are never exactly the same. In table tennis, for example, every forehand the player hits differs from the one that preceded it. How many motor programs, then, are really needed for the great variety of strokes a table tennis player makes during a rally?

Motor learning scientists have suggested a **generalized** or **dynamic motor program (GMP)**, an alternative to the simple motor program just discussed. The generalized motor program still consists of a stored pattern of movements, but its actual structure is conceived as more abstract. Central to this more general concept is the existence of **parameters**. Some of these parameters are stable and others are more unstable, or changing, depending on the situation in the environment. Parameters specify such things as the order of events or subroutines (see Figures 11.7 and 11.8 for examples of skill hierarchies), the overall duration of the movement, the overall force needed to accomplish the movement, the temporal patterning (explained later in this chapter), and the spatial and temporal order in which the components of the movement are to be executed (explained later in this chapter). An example of a generalized motor program's characteristics and its actions is provided in the box *Table Tennis Forehand in Action.*

When generalized motor programs become well established, they form the basis for automatic and spontaneous movements in sports. They ensure that the athlete's movements, even under different conditions, become supple and adaptable. Well-established generalized motor programs require little or no attention or mental effort, and with experience, their execution becomes fully automatic. A theoretical discussion of this topic is beyond the scope of this textbook.

Movement Intelligence and Motor Programs

Movement intelligence does not refer to any specific ability an individual may inherit. Rather, it is a term that can be used to explain proficiency in performing various skills. Movement intelligence is viewed simply as a vast store or library of motor programs. Like a store or library holding thousands of CDs, each containing numerous tracks, our movement intelligence store is a collection of numerous motor programs, some simple or complex, others fundamental or specialized.

Table Tennis Forehand in Action

The order of events in a table tennis player's forehand serves as an example of a **stable parameter** in the generalized motor program underpinning the stroke. Relative time and relative force to be applied in each stroke are considered stable parameters as well. Both, however, may also have **unstable characteristics** that are easily changed from one stroke to another. These characteristics can be readily adapted to the particular requirements of the rally. To hit one forehand harder than another, the overall force applied must be greater and the overall time taken to carry out the stroke must be faster. Speeding up the sequence of the movements (or subroutines) and increasing the overall force can seemingly be done without altering the stable characteristics of the generalized motor program controlling the player's forehand strokes. The parameters are applied to the generalized motor program in order to specify how a particular forehand is to be expressed.

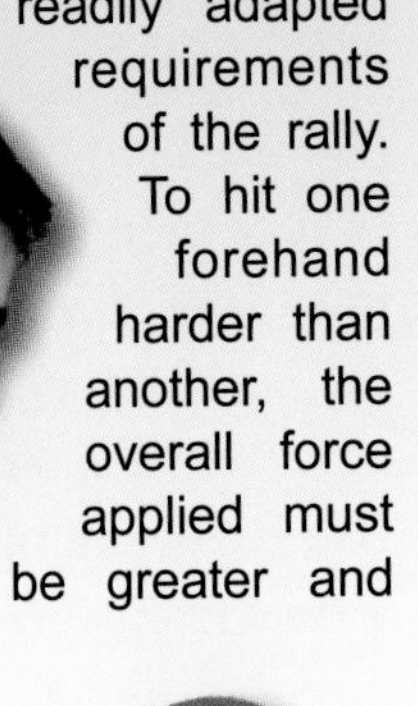

A generalized motor program responsible for the table tennis player's forehand can then be used to perform a large number of similar and yet slightly different forehands by simply adding the appropriate set of movement parameters to the abstract plan of action stored in memory. Armed with a well-developed generalized motor program, the player is ready for the challenges that await him or her during a rally. The execution of forehand strokes becomes fluid and effective under most varied external conditions generated by an opponent.

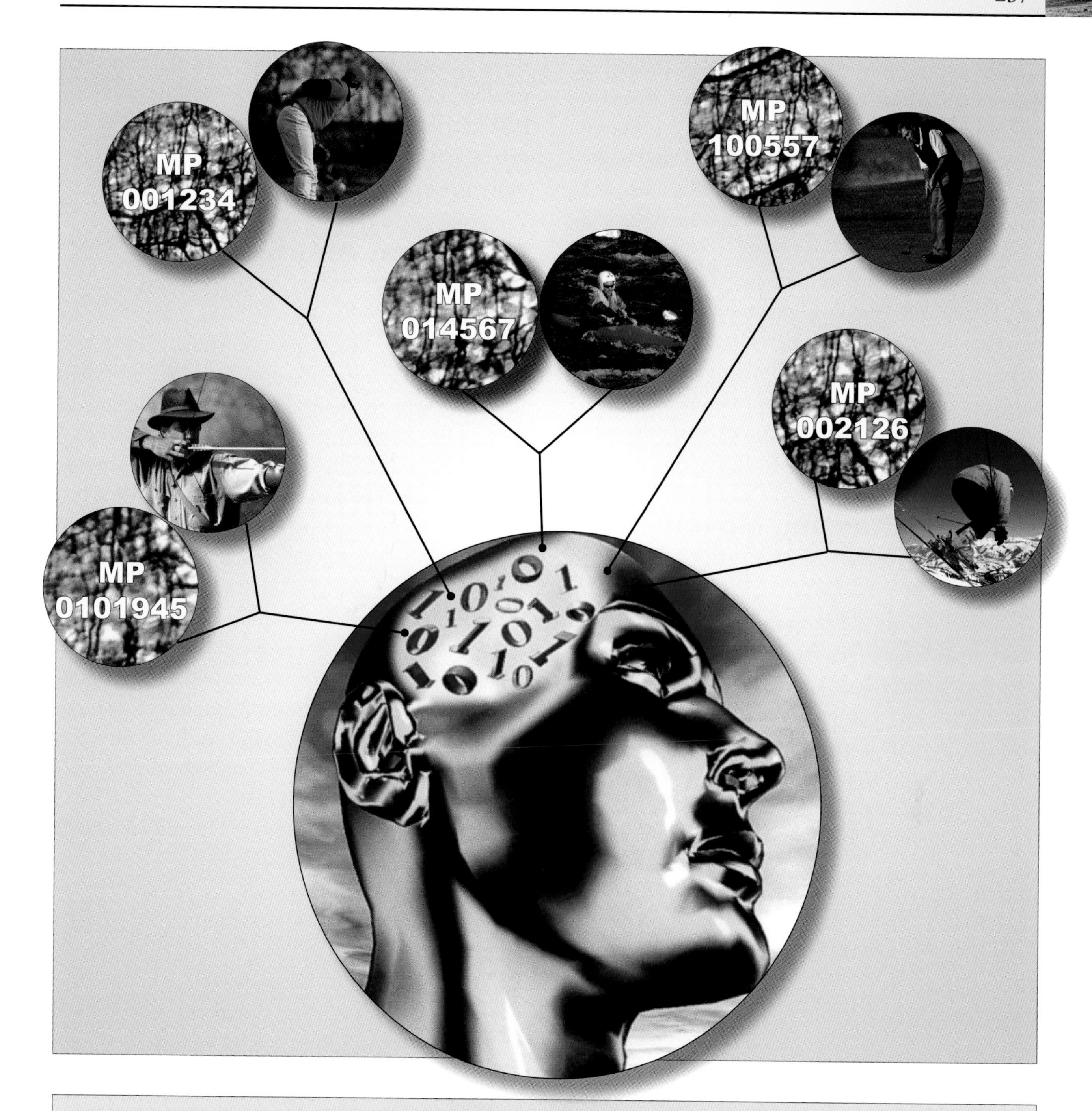

Figure 11.2 Hypothetical example of coded motor programs (MPs) assembled in an individual's motor memory, movement intelligence. Will we ever know how the human brain codes and stores MPs, the blueprints of skills?

Just as you cannot distinguish individual tracks on a CD until it is placed in a CD player, the motor programs stored in our memory through learning cannot be observed directly. But motor programs can be inferred by observing the skills and movement patterns we are capable of performing. In this sense, motor programs can be regarded as the blueprints of the skills we perform. They represent one side of a coin; skills represent the other. Skills are the observable side of the coin; they represent the movements we perform at the swimming pool, on the basketball court, or on the soccer field (Figure 11.2).

Obviously, the number of CDs matters as well.

Greater selection usually makes a larger collection better than a smaller one. Similarly, the degree of motor intelligence you possess has a direct bearing on participation in sports. The larger and more sophisticated your movement intelligence, the more proficient you will be in playing sports at recreational or competitive levels.

It follows that movement intelligence is an active and ongoing process that, through practice, helps individuals develop new specialized movement patterns that will help them adapt to ever more demanding situations in any athletic or recreational environment. Many factors affect the development of movement intelligence.

Factors Affecting Movement Intelligence

The development of movement intelligence depends upon many factors. They include adequate stimulation starting at an early age, opportunities for practice and continuous encouragement, following the right learning progression, expert instruction throughout educational programs, opportunities for practice in community clubs, and the use of quality equipment. However, one factor remains vital for the development of movement intelligence: the inheritance of abilities. In the next section we will look briefly at the question of abilities and their implications for developing movement intelligence.

Movement Abilities

In previous sections we established that motor programs, the blueprints of skills, are active nervous circuits entrenched in the brain and stored in memory. The quality and the effectiveness of these motor programs depend on the presence of underlying motor abilities. In this context **motor or movement abilities** are considered inherited, relatively enduring, and stable traits that serve as the foundation for the development of motor programs. They are the "hardware" that learners bring with them to the learning environment.

For example, balance, speed of reaction, and finger and wrist dexterity are examples of abilities that are important for the development of a variety of motor programs that are outwardly manifested in a badminton smash, a sculling stroke, or a hockey slap shot (Figure 11.3).

A workbench analogy may help in understand-

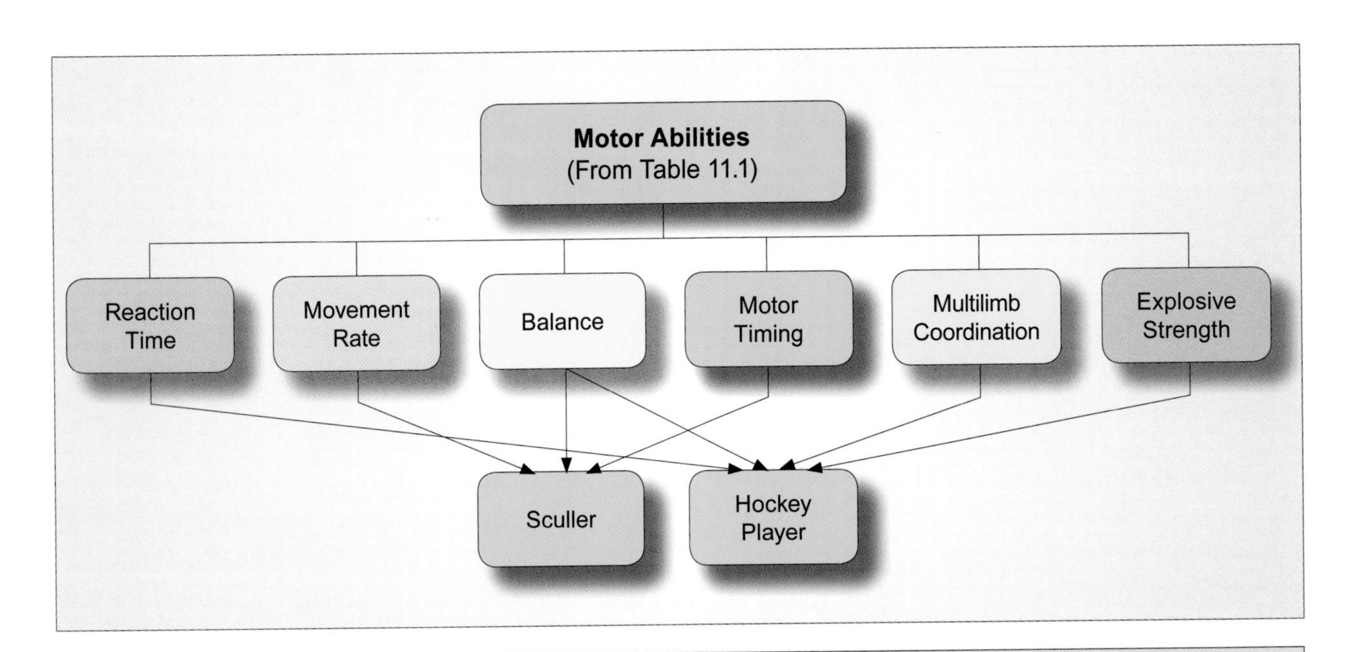

Figure 11.3 Hypothetical model of links indicating abilities underlying performance in two skills, rowing and hockey.

ing the relationship between motor abilities and skills. Motor abilities can be regarded as tools of various kinds used by the carpenter. To build a particular item, such as a table, the carpenter uses several different sets of tools that are highly specialized for cutting, filing, holding in place, drilling, and so on. However, different sets of tools are used for building a shelf. Similarly, the inherited movement abilities are the "tools" used in a variety of combinations to develop and perform skills (Figure 11.3).

Human Abilities Questions and Answers

How many abilities are there?

Relatively limited motor learning research has revealed 26 abilities that have been classified into three major categories as shown in Table 11.1. The first category of abilities deals with perceptual motor abilities, such as reaction time, dexterity, speed of movement, and coordination. The second category of abilities is related to human physical proficiency, such as flexibility, strength, endurance, and balance. The abilities in the third category deal with control of timing, rate of movement, and control of muscle force.

The search for human abilities is far from over. Practice has shown that there may be more abilities than have been identified by laboratory research to date, ranging from visual skills and kinesthetic sensitivity to body configuration. It is expected that future research will identify new abilities that could better explain sport performances of various kinds.

How many abilities do we have?

It is assumed that all individuals possess all of the abilities listed in Table 11.1, albeit to varying degrees. In other words, people differ in the amount or the strength of each ability. For this reason, abilities (or lack thereof) impose limits that influence an individual's potential for success in performing certain skills.

Furthermore, no two individuals have exactly the same pattern of motor abilities. This also explains individual differences in the quality of performance on movement tasks.

Why do people excel at some activities and do poorly in others?

This depends upon the strengths and weaknesses of one's inherited motor abilities (Figure 11.4). A champion sculler, for example, would possess inherited strengths in the particular abilities relevant to sculling (balance, movement rate, motor timing). If the abilities required to play hockey (explosive strength, multilimb coordination) were relatively weak, the same individual would not necessarily excel in hockey and may therefore exhibit less skill as a hockey player (Figure 11.3).

Who are the all-around athletes?

From experience we know there are individuals who perform well in several sports. Because many fundamental abilities are likely common across a variety of sports (balance in Figure 11.3), it is reasonable to assume that **all-around athletes** possess strong abilities that underlie the many sports in which they excel. These athletes differ from the average individuals in the number of abilities in which they are superior. As a result, there are more activities (ball sports, racket sports, contact sports) in which these individuals can achieve success.

Can practice improve motor abilities?

We have stated that human abilities are genetically determined and relatively stable. However, many teachers and coaches believe, based on long-term experience, that intensive ability-specific practice may potentially improve motor abilities. For example, coaches use countless speed drills to enhance the reaction time and agility in players; circus performers practice diligently on various types of swaying equipment to develop better balance; gymnasts improve their dynamic and extent flexibility through range-of-motion-specific practice.

Table 11.1 Human abilities as identified by motor learning research.

A. Perceptual Motor Abilities	**Examples of Skill**
Control Precision: Requires fine, highly controlled muscular adjustments, primarily in situations in which large muscle groups are involved. This ability extends to arm–hand as well as to leg movements.	• Forklift operators who are required to maneuver with careful positioning of the arms and feet.
Multilimb Coordination: The ability to coordinate a number of limb movements simultaneously.	• Batting in baseball, shooting in hockey, or hitting in volleyball.
Response Orientation: Involves quick choices among numerous alternative movements, more-or-less as in choice reaction time.	• Task facing a goalie in soccer, where the type and direction of a shot on goal is uncertain.
Reaction Time: The speed with which a person is able to respond to a stimulus when it appears.	• Starting off the mark quickly in swimming, sprinting, or speedskating.
Speed of Arm Movement: The speed with which a person can make large, discrete arm movements in which accuracy is not the requirement.	• Throwing a shot for maximum distance.
Rate Control: Involves making continuous anticipatory motor adjustments relative to changes in speed and direction of a continuous moving target or object.	• Skiing, snowboarding, or white-water canoeing.
Manual Dexterity: Demonstrated by skillful, well-directed arm–hand movements in manipulating fairly large objects at various speeds.	• Dribbling a basketball or setting in volleyball.
Finger Dexterity: Involves making still-controlled manipulations of small objects involving, primarily, the fingers.	• Threading a needle or assembling parts of a small object.
Arm–Hand Steadiness: The ability to make precise arm–hand positioning movements where strength and speed are minimized.	• Archery and pistol shooting.
Wrist–Finger Speed: Involves the rapid movement of the wrist and fingers, with little or no demand for accuracy.	• Playing the bongo drums and a quick snap of the wrist during a badminton smash.
Aiming: Requires the production of accurate hand movements toward targets at various speeds.	• Throwing a horseshoe or hitting a target with the rapid throw of a dart.

B. Physical Proficiency Abilities	**Examples of Skill**
Explosive Strength: The ability to expend maximum energy in one or a series of explosive acts.	• Performing maximum vertical jumps in volleyball, basketball, or high jump.
Static Strength: The maximum force a person can exert for a brief period.	• Maximum lifts in weightlifting or moving a large object such as a refrigerator.

Continued on next page....

Dynamic Strength: The ability to exert muscular force repeatedly or continuously over time.	• Rock climbing or performing on the still rings in gymnastics.
Trunk Strength: A more dynamic strength factor, specific to the abdominal muscles.	• Performing abdominal curls or crunches, doing leg raises, or holding a position on the parallel bars in gymnastics.
Extent Flexibility: The ability to flex or stretch the trunk and back muscles as far as possible in either a forward, lateral, or backward direction.	• Holding a pose in rhythmic gymnastics or yoga.
Dynamic Flexibility: The ability to make repeated rapid, flexing movements in which the resiliency of the muscles in recovery from stretch or distortion is critical.	• Performing dance or gymnastics routines.
Body Equilibrium: Involves maintaining equilibrium while blindfolded.	• Blindfolded tightrope walking.
Balance with Visual Cues: The ability to maintain total body balance when visual cues are available.	• Performing skills on the balance beam in gymnastics.
Speed of Limb Movement: Underlies tasks in which the arm(s) or leg(s) must be moved quickly, but without a reaction-time stimulus, to minimize movement time.	• Pitching in baseball, shooting in water polo, kicking in soccer, and tap dancing.
Large Body Coordination: The ability to coordinate the simultaneous actions of different parts of the body while making large-body movements.	• Stickhandling in hockey while skating and coordinating the arms and legs while cross-country skiing.
Stamina: The ability to continue maximum effort requiring prolonged exertion over time.	• All endurance events including marathons, cycling, and rowing.

C. General Coordination Abilities	**Examples of Skill**
Movement Rate: Applies more to situations in which a series of movements must be made at a maximum speed.	• Playing the piano, typing, or keyboarding.
Motor Timing: Important for the performance of tasks in which accurately timed movements are essential.	• Most open skill activities, including throwing and receiving a pass in basketball, soccer, or football.
Perceptual Timing: Underlies tasks in which accurate judgments about the course of perceptual events are required.	• Judging the speed and direction of a bounce of the ball in tennis, basketball, or lacrosse.
Force Control: Important for tasks in which force of varying degrees is needed to achieve the desired outcome.	• Playing pool and dancing, figure skating, and gymnastics routines.

Recent research at the University of Toronto has indicated that intensive practice by athletes on the Dynavision board significantly improves a variety of psychomotor abilities at all levels of performance (Figure 11.5).

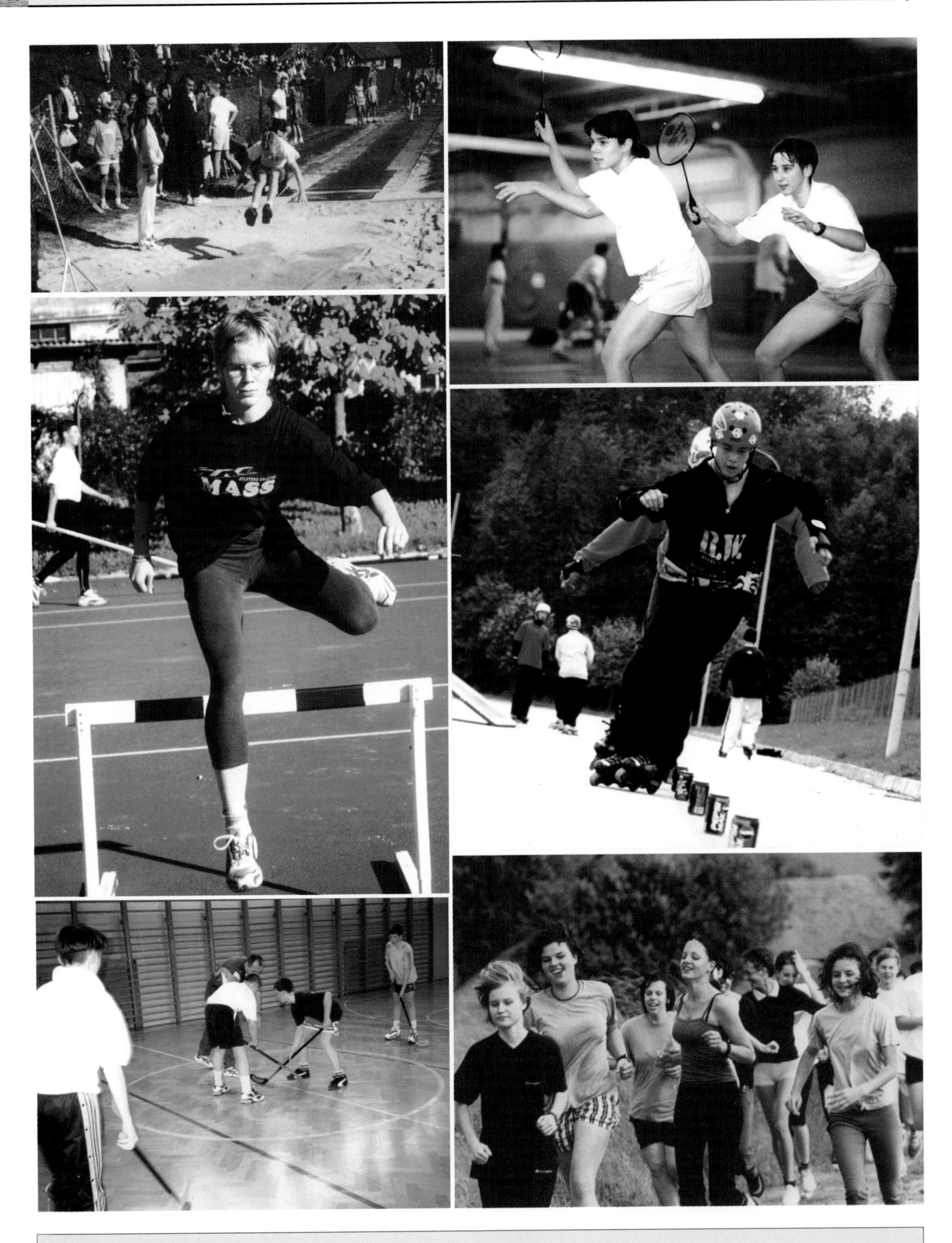

Figure 11.4 A student who has a low skill level in one activity should not be assumed to have a low skill level in another activity: it all depends upon the pattern of inherited abilities.

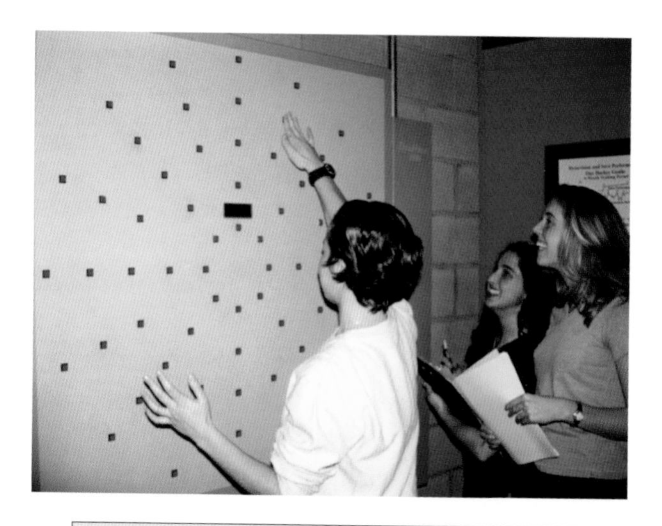

Figure 11.5 Practice on the Dynavision board.

Understanding Skills

Now that we have established the roots of skills, we turn to questions about what skills are, how they may be characterized, and their various types of classification.

The term **skill** can be used in many ways and applied to different scenarios. We will look at skills as tasks and as quality of performance.

Skill as a Task

The use of the term **skill as a task** is quite straightforward and simply denotes "an action or task that requires voluntary body and/or limb movement to achieve a goal." In this context, a skill must be learned, have a purpose, and be performed voluntarily. Serving in table tennis, catching a baseball, jogging, and throwing a Frisbee are all examples of skills defined as tasks.

Skill as Quality of Performance

Skill as quality of performance can be defined as the ability to bring about some end result with maximum certainty and minimum outlay of energy, or of time and energy.

Maximum Certainty

An important feature of this definition is that being skilled involves attaining the performance goal with maximum certainty. Therefore, sinking a long putt in golf on one occasion and missing on all other attempts at the same distance does not constitute a skilled action because the element of luck may have been involved; in other words, making one successful shot does not demonstrate that the shot can be made on other occasions with any certainty.

If your team was down by three points with only three seconds left to play in the game, who would you want to take the final shot of the game – the player who once hit a shot from half court in practice, or the player who hits three-point shots consistently? Obviously, the player who can consistently hit the shot is your pick because he or she has demonstrated the ability to generate the skill reliably over time.

Minimum Energy

The second element in understanding skill as quality of performance is the minimization of energy. If energy is conserved, this allows skilled individuals the opportunity to use their energy at times when it is most needed, or to pace themselves for longer periods of time. Consider the player who expends most of his or her energy early on in the game, only to "run out of gas" in the clutch. Executing skills with minimum energy puts less of a burden on physiological and psychological processes and allows a player to direct more attention to other aspects of the activity, such as creativity and tactical advantages.

Minimum Time

Finally, skilled performers should be able to accomplish their goals in minimum time. Although this may not be true for all activities, some skills are judged almost entirely on the ability to complete a skill in minimum time, such as a 100-meter race, where the person with the fastest time is deemed victorious. Other skills may also be performed successfully if executed rapidly, such as a slap shot in hockey or a punch thrown in boxing; but minimizing time is not the strict goal of all movements. For example, increasing the speed of some skills (e.g., shooting) may lead to less accurate or precise movements. Further, the rapid execution of some movements may affect energy costs by using muscles differently. Therefore, many aspects of skills must be considered when attempting to optimize performance under different conditions.

Characteristics of Skills

Organization and sequence are essential in developing the ability to perform skilled movements. Just try to find an individual who ran before he or she walked, or dunked a basketball before he or she could jump. Obviously some movements precede others, and the specific sequencing of these movements is important to the overall execution of the intended goal.

Hierarchical Organization

A skilled act may be thought of as following a **hierarchical organization pattern**, whereas an unskilled act lacks such organization.

One way to visualize such a hierarchy is by comparison to an organizational chart in which the president is at the top, with lower ranked members located at lower levels. In such an arrangement, the president and the executives direct responsibilities to the lower level members. In a similar way, skills may be characterized by a hierarchy consisting of different levels. The top of a **skill hierarchy** is occupied by the **executive program** (Figure 11.6), the overall purpose of the act, with **subroutines** (components or units of movement) located at lower levels of organization. To put it in simple terms, a skill is directed by an executive program and specific subroutines at various levels of command, which are responsible for carrying out the executive plan.

Executive programs act as a goal, aim, or objective; give direction to skilled acts; order the execution of certain subroutines; and make

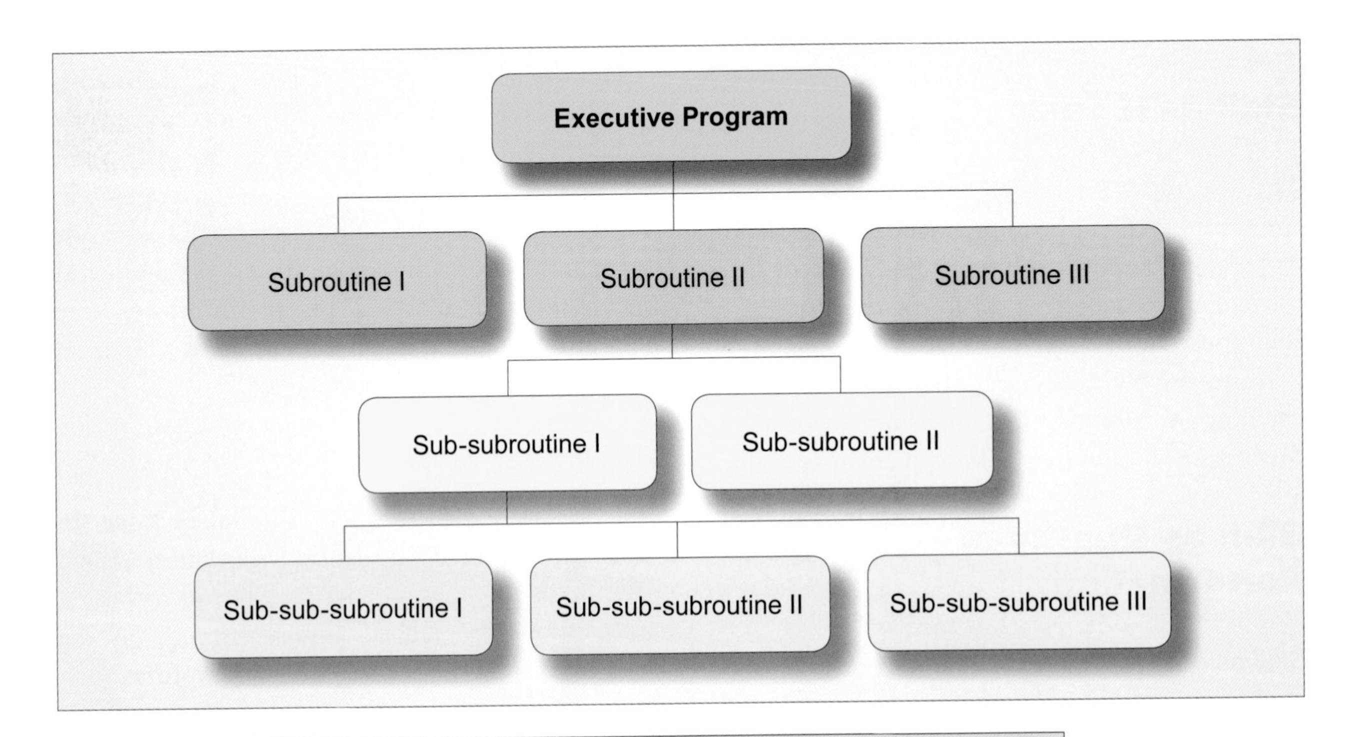

Figure 11.6 A theoretical skill hierarchy showing the executive program and subroutines.

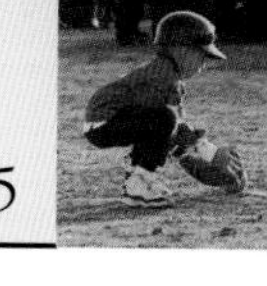

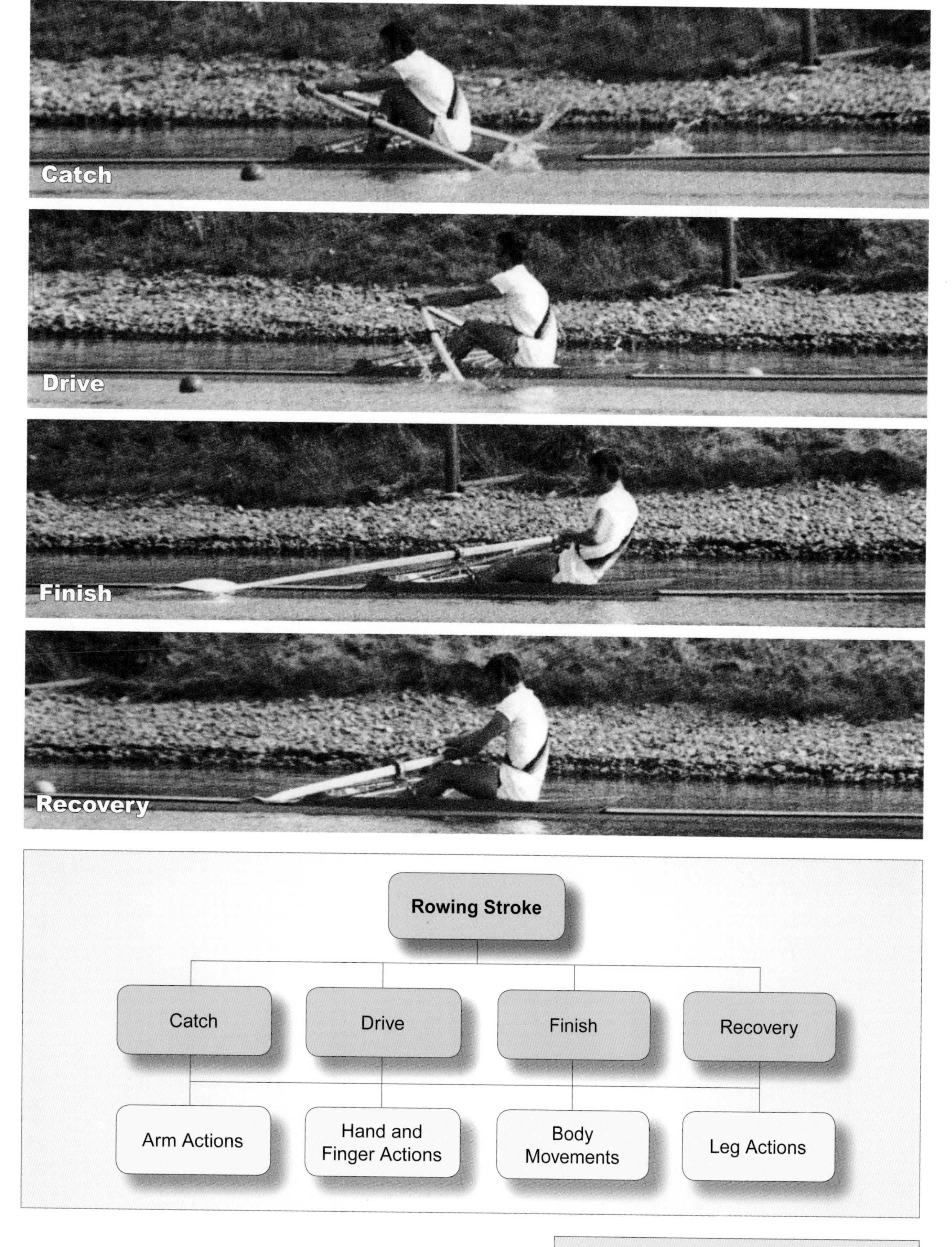

Figure 11.7 A rowing stroke skill hierarchy.

decisions and adaptations that are flexible. However, the executive program, or plan, is dependent upon the sequential execution of subroutines. These subroutines are isolated units of the total executive program, but no less significant. Subroutines on the lowest level of a skill hierarchy are characteristically fixed and will run automatically once the sequence is established. These stereotyped movements are capable of being repeated over and over again unless interrupted or changed by the executive program.

Serial Nature of Skills

Still, a skilled act is serial in nature, meaning the subroutines must follow a particular sequence in order for the executive program to be effectively carried out. A skilled pitcher realizes what sequence produces a good pitch: the motions of the leg kick, hips, shoulders, arms, wrist, and fingers must follow one another during delivery. A coordinated, sequential movement is more productive and often easily distinguished from awkward, uncoordinated movement that is clearly less effective.

A rowing stroke (executive program) consists of four main subroutines – the catch, the pull, the finish, and the recovery – that are further broken down into finer movements of the wrists and fingers, arms, shoulders, torso, and legs (Figure 11.7).

Similarly, most swimming strokes consist of several subroutines such as the kick, arm strokes, and breathing. It is the executive plan that directs the ordering of these units so that the final skilled act may be performed smoothly (Figure 11.8).

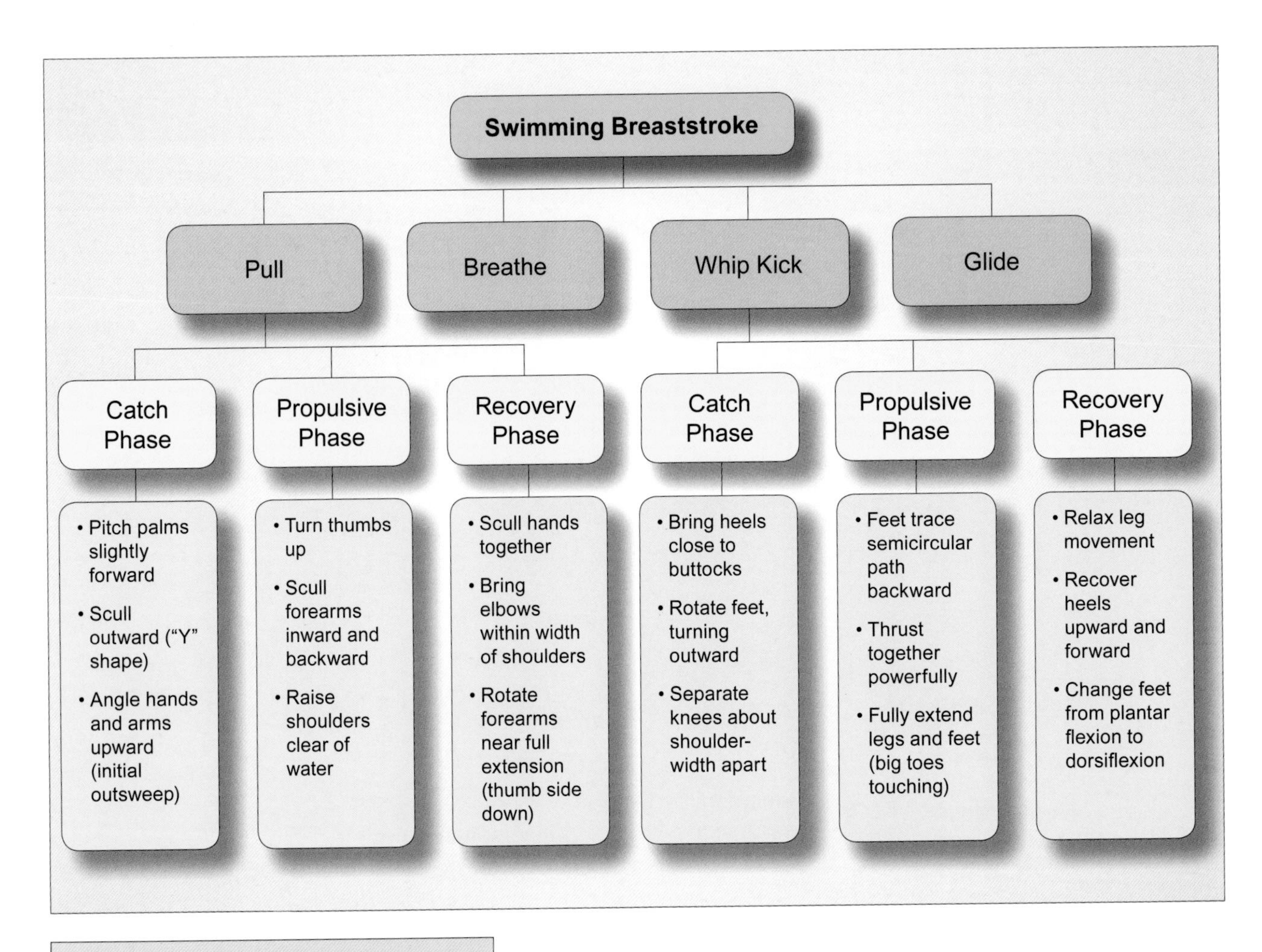

Figure 11.8 Breaststroke skill hierarchy.

Temporal Patterning

The preceding discussion may have painted a simple picture of how skilled acts are executed. In reality, integrating several movement units or components to produce a single movement pattern is more complicated than simply chaining together several separate activities. Anyone who is just learning how to swim can appreciate the difficulty in coordinating all the movements involved with a particular stroke – until the kick, the breathing, and the arm strokes (subroutines) can be well established and correctly organized in the proper coordination pattern, the stroke will not be effective.

The ability to perform a skilled act is closely related to **temporal patterning**, the capacity of the performer to integrate the sequential organization of a movement pattern. This would include the ability to connect successive subroutines smoothly so that a skill may be executed in a flowing, coordinated fashion. A gymnast performing on an apparatus should not string individual exercise components together in an isolated fashion but rather must combine them into a fluid routine or series of elements. A boxer will be more efficient in action when he stops chopping away with straight lefts then rights followed by a left hook. Only when he combines these individual actions together will he be successful.

The inexperienced performer will execute movements in a jerky manner because the timing between related subroutines has not been well established. On the other hand, a skilled individual will most often produce movements in which the transition between each subroutine is shorter as well as smoother, leading to a more successful performance. Once an effective rhythm has been achieved for any movement, the executive program may be carried out with optimal efficiency.

Classification of Skills

Thus far, we have placed skills under one broad heading and discussed them as a single entity. Now, we will consider the various ways that skills may be classified. **Classification systems** allow for a deeper level of understanding of skills, and can directly affect the structuring of the learning environment. Certain training methods and learning strategies may be more appropriate for some skills than others; therefore, methods of instruction can be molded to meet the specific requirements that different activities demand.

Traditional classification systems have focused on classification of activities rather than skills. A common distinction is made between individual, dual, and team sports, but this classification really serves only to provide a description of the number of participants involved. Other classifications of skills include distinctions between summer and winter sports, water and land activities, and contact and noncontact sports. Although such classifications may enable you to differentiate among many activities, a more recent taxonomy provides a more comprehensive and useful way to classify motor skills.

An effective way to classify motor skills is based on the environment in which the skill is to be performed. A skill for which the environment remains stable and predictable is called a *closed skill*. At the opposite end of the continuum are skills for which the environment is variable and unpredictable, called *open skills*. Skills in this case are classified according to the effects of the environment on learning and executing skills and thus include the performer's need to respond to many changes in the environment.

Closed Skills

Closed environments are relatively stable: the surroundings do not change moment to moment. **Closed skills** are correspondingly performed under constant, relatively unchanging conditions, so the movement itself is often the goal of the skill (Figure 11.9). Performers of closed skills will almost certainly benefit from learning to repeat a particular movement pattern with minimal variation involved.

For example, gymnastics routines are performed under controlled conditions and judged by high standards as a result of the

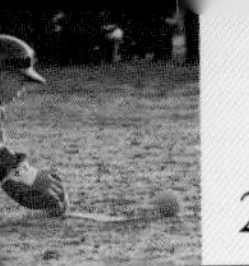

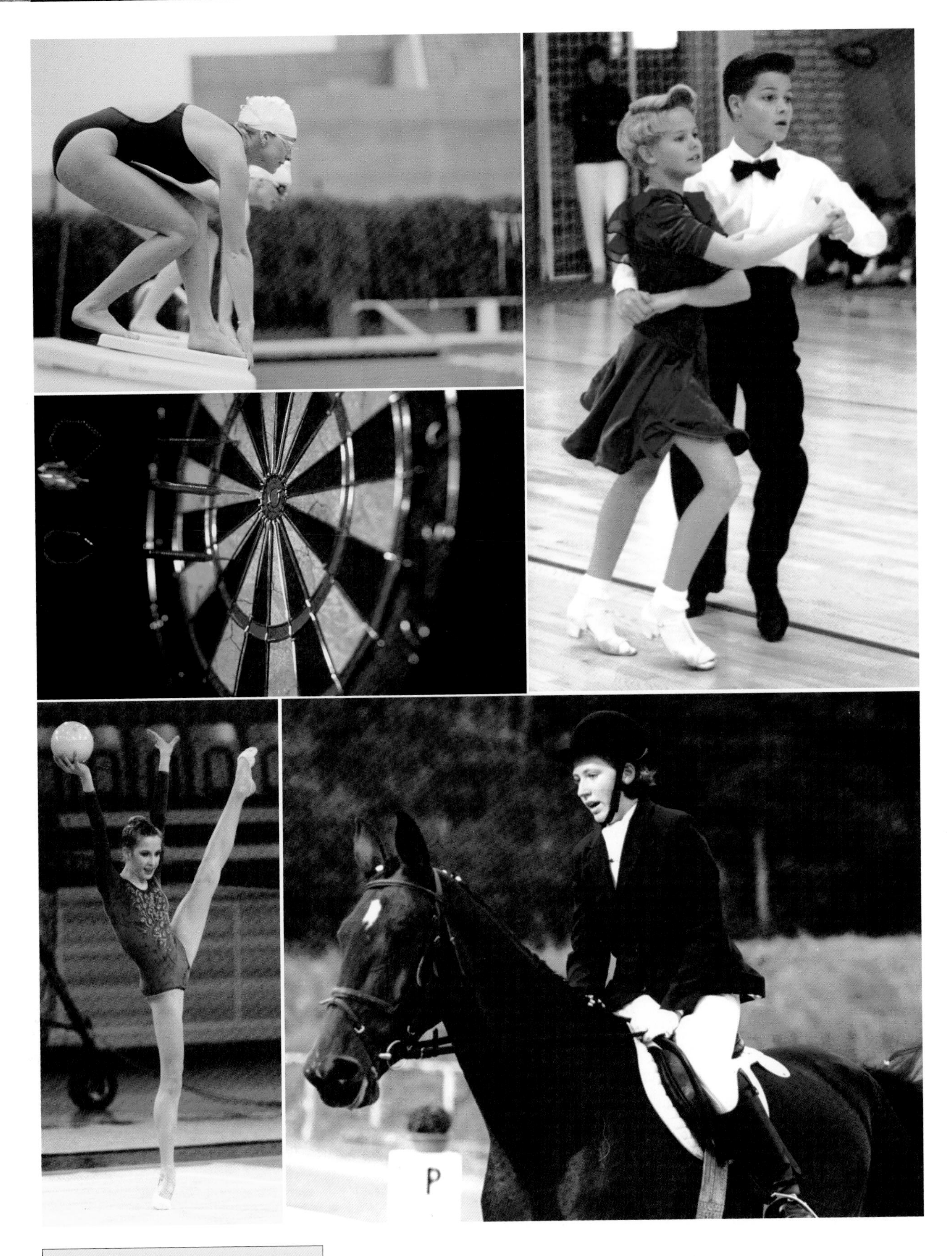

Figure 11.9 Closed motor skills.

predictable environment in which the athletes perform. A similar situation exists in sports such as figure skating, diving, and dance, where precise movements and execution are required for success. Another clear example of a closed skill is bowling. The lanes remain in relatively the same condition from frame to frame, and the pins move only as a result of individual movements in the environment.

Teaching Strategies for Closed Skills In order to develop movements that consistently produce the desired response, it is essential that the learning environment be conducive and that teachers select the proper subroutines. Students should be encouraged to repeat the selected movement pattern consistently without allowing external influences to affect the performance.

Since repetition of specific movement patterns is necessary for success in closed skills, students must learn to block out external distractions. For example, a student must learn to filter out noise when shooting a free throw, or to concentrate on the next shot in bowling regardless of how well a partner is doing.

The learning environment should allow the learner to refine movements more precisely, since the demands on sensation and perception are not as significant to the execution of closed skills. Proprioceptive feedback (also known as muscle sense) can be especially effective for learning closed skills by allowing a student to become more in tune with his or her own body position in space and relative balance. However, this is difficult for the beginner to develop, so the role of a teacher or coach is important in providing early feedback (described in more detail later in the chapter).

Open Skills

Executing **open skills** involves some very different considerations. Open environments are continually changing and require performers to adjust and respond to the environment around them. Because the conditions of the environment tend to be unpredictable from moment to moment, responses cannot be made effectively far in advance (Figure 11.10).

Examples of open motor skills include tennis, basketball, rugby, volleyball, and wrestling, where movements by the performer reflect the changing nature of the environment. Whereas the diver can practice her dives the same way each time, the basketball player is forced to take what is given to him, reacting to the movement of other players and the ball. The ability to anticipate certain events before they actually occur (including scouting reports on players) would certainly make performing open motor skills an easier task. Therefore open skills demand that performers adapt, anticipate, and remain flexible in their responses.

Uncertainties in Open Skills Open skills harbor many uncertainties that make a performer's job very challenging. Team players and those involved in combat sports, for example, may have to deal directly with one or more opponents, their own teammates, and such things as the speed of the ball, the playing surface, and the weather. For the performer, this creates response, spatial, temporal, and tactical uncertainties.

Responding to an opponent's intentions rarely permits the use of the same movement response (or motor program) on two successive attempts. This creates **response uncertainty**. Therefore, it is important that the performer be able to execute many subtle variations of the skill by using a well-developed generalized motor program responsible for the task at hand.

Open skills take place in a temporally and spatially changing environment. In hockey, players must effectively overcome **spatial uncertainty**. To be successful, hockey players must continually move around the ice surface and act in accordance with the puck's spatial location and its speed characteristics, both to a great extent dictated by the opposing team.

In closed environments, skills are mostly self-paced, whereas open skills are externally paced. Again in hockey, players' actions are typically externally paced – they cannot stand in one

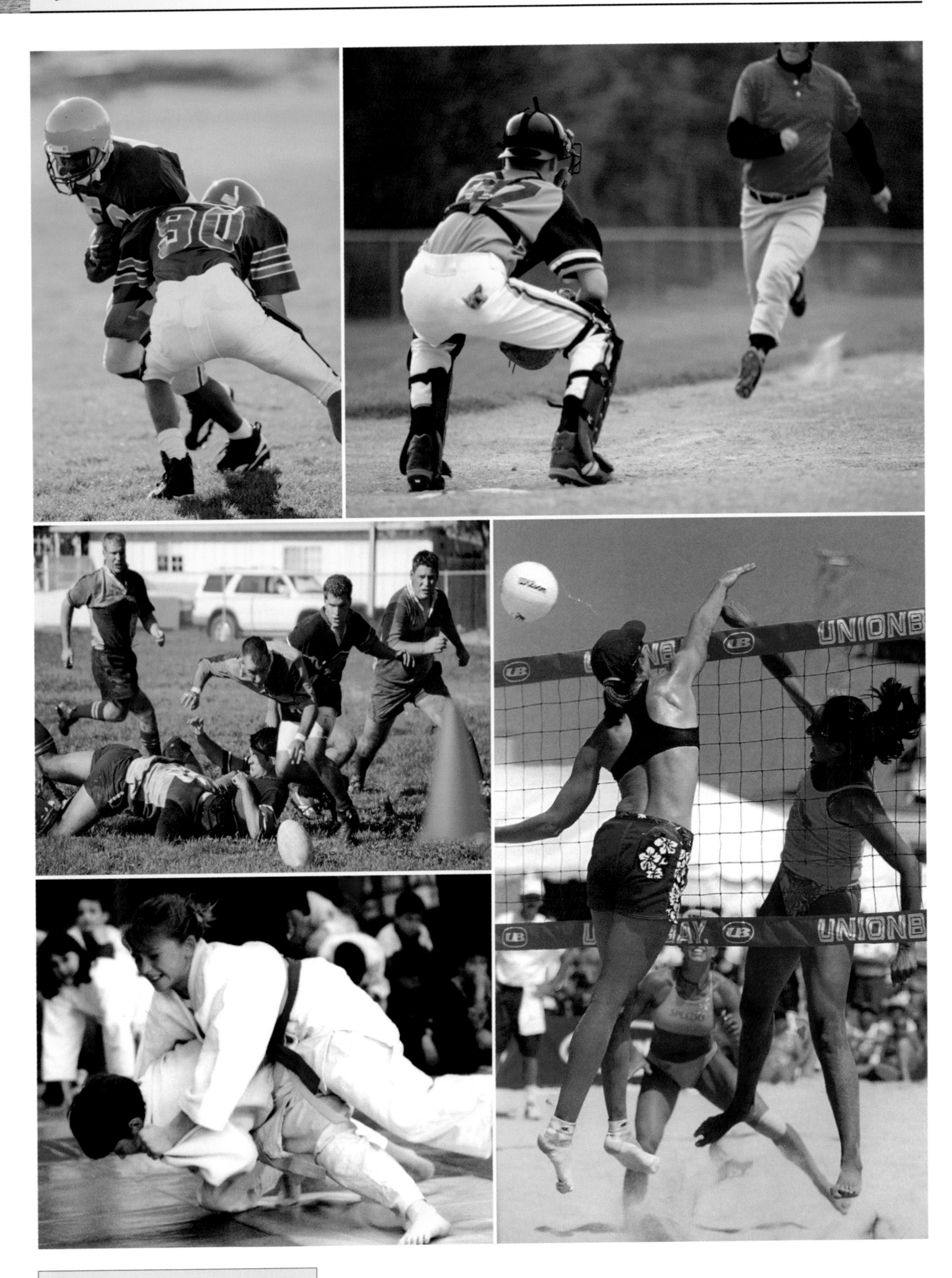

Figure 11.10 Open motor skills.

spot and decide when they will respond to the puck – because they must continuously adjust to the action dictated by the general pace of the game, which is partially influenced by the opposing team's intentions. This creates **temporal uncertainty**.

And finally, all team members must deal with **tactical uncertainty**. For example, a player's actions – losing the puck or unsuccessful coverage of the opponent – might bring about a tactical problem that threatens the interaction between teammates when they are carrying out tactical moves previously rehearsed. Unknown tactical maneuvers by the opponent further increase tactical uncertainties in open skill environments.

Teaching Strategies for Open Skills In order to make the learning of such skills effective, the learning environment should closely approximate the environment in which the skill will take place. In other words, learners should be encouraged to exercise variability and adaptability that more closely approximates the actual environment.

For example, a receiver is not likely to catch the ball in the same area on the football field, just as the quarterback will not throw to the same spot each time. An attempt should be made to incorporate various situations that may arise during the execution of open skills as they unfold. This is not to say that early development of such skills cannot benefit from practicing similar movements over and over again. This may help to establish proper movement patterns early and help to avoid the development of bad habits (which may be difficult to eradicate).

Opponents will often deliberately try to create uncertainty and unpredictability in the environment to gain an advantage. Consider the tennis player who hits a drop shot in the middle of a point, which is returned by the opponent on the other side of the net, but the next shot is a lob that lands just inside the baseline. This makes it more difficult to respond than if the player was able to hit only simple forehands and backhands to an opponent. The player who practices in an environment that provides this kind of uncertainty and variation will benefit from the experience of adjusting to a changing environment. Players should also try to identify patterns in the movement of objects and other players. If you are able to recognize that your opponent's serve (tennis) is slicing out wide or that the rebound (basketball) is coming off the front of the rim, you can better position yourself to return the serve or to get the rebound even though the outcome of the movement may initially be in doubt.

Open–Closed Continuum

While many skills can be placed in one of these two categories, there are certainly others that do not fall specifically under either of them. Some tasks are neither completely open nor closed, so this classification must be considered on a continuum of varying degrees of environmental predictability (Figure 11.11). At first glance, golf might appear to be a clear example of a closed skill – the environment does not change much, and your swing stays fundamentally the same on each type of shot. But what about the effects of the wind or rain on performance? Still other sport tasks may be closed in one situation and open in another. Skiing, for example, may be a closed skill when you are alone on a slope of even grade where your skills may be executed quite routinely. This same task can become an open skill when others arrive on the scene and the slope becomes a little less predictable and has more curves and angles – not to mention changing snow conditions.

Learning Progression Along the Open–Closed Continuum Many sports and activities characteristically change as the context or level of experience changes. What is the advantage of utilizing batting cages and pitching machines for teaching baseball fundamentals in hitting? Obviously, these may help to simplify open skills by performing them initially in a closed environment (e.g., playing tee-ball). Once a certain level of competence has been achieved, the learner may advance to practice with live pitching, and so on, until open skills have been effectively established. Adapting a skill from a closed to an

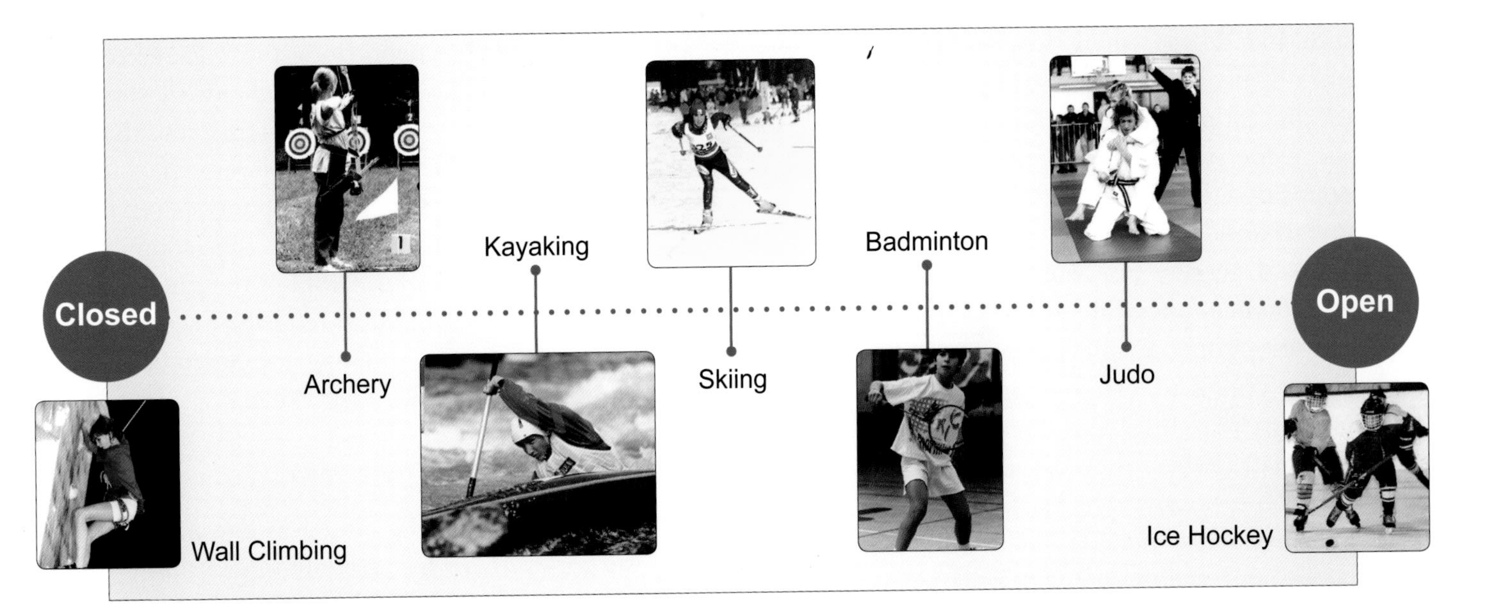

Figure 11.11 Closed and open skills continuum.

open environment provides a good progression for skill development (Figure 11.12).

Reducing the demands of certain task components may serve to reduce the complexity of the skill and various environmental and response uncertainties. Beginning tennis players may utilize ball machines and other devices to practice their ground strokes (see box *Learning Progression in Tennis*); young children may begin their baseball experience by playing tee-ball; and all of us can probably remember the training wheels that accompanied our first bicycles. All these tactics remove a component of uncertainty that serves to simplify a skill until its overall execution becomes more proficient.

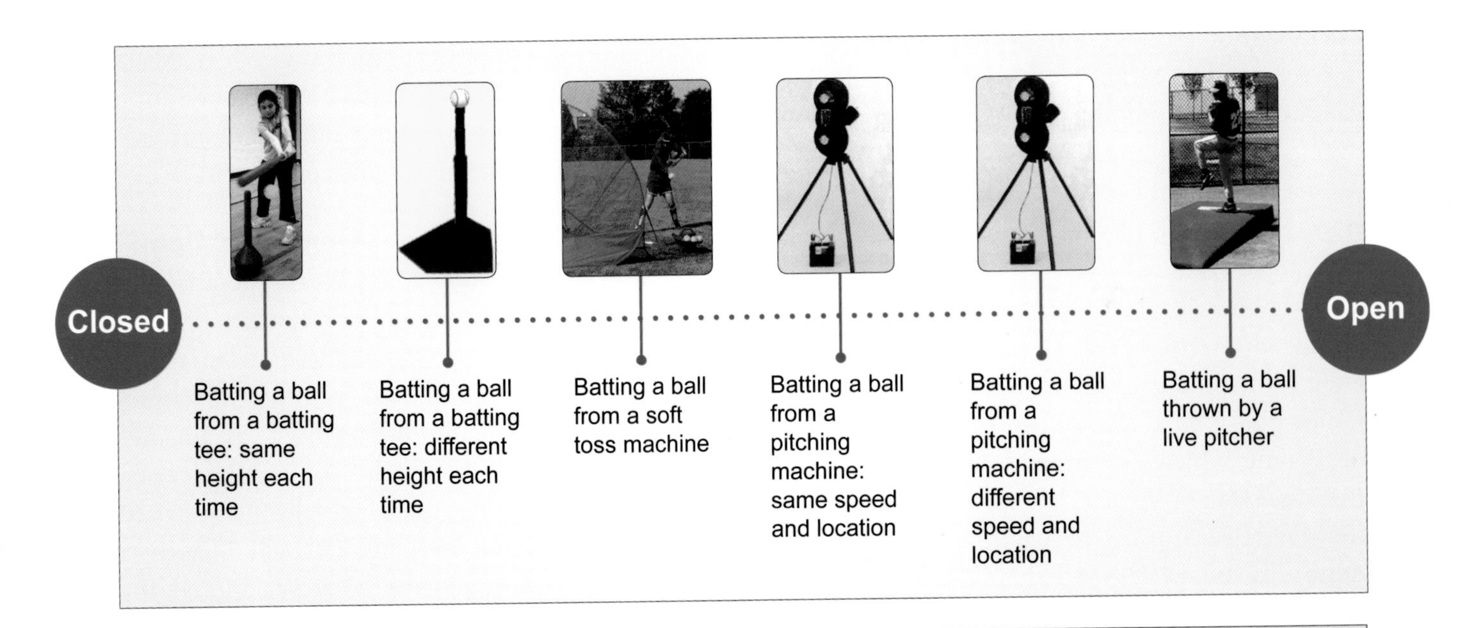

Figure 11.12 Learning progression along the closed and open learning continuum for an open skill: baseball batting.

Learning Progression in Tennis

An effective learning progression for a beginning tennis player may involve several stages:

1. hitting a stationary ball attached to a rubber string or the end of the instructor's stick;
2. hitting balls dropped strategically by a partner or instructor;
3. hitting balls gently thrown by a partner or instructor;
4. playing against a ball-throwing machine: same speed and location each time;
5. playing against a wall;
6. playing against a ball-throwing machine: different speed and location each time;
7. playing with the instructor or partner.

Helping the learner find the correct body or arm position – muscle feeling or kinesthetic sense – is an effective teaching method instructors can use at any stage of a player's development.

Enhancing Your Learning Potential

Many factors affect skill development. Understanding them and their positive and negative effects is essential for optimal achievement and performance.

The structure of our bodies allows us to perform a range of activities and tasks, both simple and complex. The intricate human nervous system and the diverse system of muscles and levers of the human body allow it to perform skills with extreme precision, accuracy, and speed. It is this precise anatomical structure that determines the limits of the human body's vast capabilities. But how the body moves in order to execute skills is another question. A clear understanding of how the body moves most efficiently is a considerable asset when learning and performing skills effectively. Understanding how our bodies grow and develop over time, where our energy comes from, and how the foods we eat affect our health and fitness all positively aid the human body in learning motor skills.

Unfortunately, the human body does not always perform as expected. The occurrence of injuries can greatly affect our ability to execute skills as we would like to, so a healthy body is important to maintaining our level of skill. The ever-increasing occurrence of substance abuse for improving performance in sport is an issue that continually arouses interest and controversy. Is it worth using performance-enhancing drugs to improve one's level of skill? And at what risk? These are examples of some of the issues that negatively affect skill development.

The remainder of the text will attempt to highlight other factors associated with performing skills effectively, including fitness, nutrition, and weight management. These are important factors that make the human body unique and remarkable in its complexity.

Summary

The ability to perform skills affects everything we do. Although some individuals are recognized as being more skilled than others at certain activities, we all have the capacity to perform the same motor skills to varying degrees. Understanding skills and their roots, motor programs, and why they are important to our daily lives is important to getting the most out of life. In order to enjoy the full benefits of active living (including health and enjoyment), a certain level of movement intelligence is necessary. A relatively well-developed movement intelligence allows you to perform a great variety of skills at the intensity and duration that is most beneficial to health and also makes you confident in your physical pursuits.

Skills share common characteristics, but they also have unique differences that influence learning and performance. The skills used in one activity differ from those used in another, just as individuals differ in their capabilities to perform these many skills. But some features remain the same. Skills are organized in a hierarchical pattern that defines the sequential actions that must be followed (subroutines) to execute a performance goal (executive program). This progression of movement units must be integrated to produce a single movement pattern that is smooth, flowing, and coordinated (temporal patterning). All skills may be developed more effectively with an understanding of how they are characterized.

Some skills are performed in open environments that are uncertain and unpredictable. A coach involved with hockey (an open activity) will face different challenges than a gymnastics coach, whose athletes do not face the same degree of variability in a relatively closed environment.

Skills undoubtedly affect most of what we do, and our anatomy, physiology, health, and other behaviors affect our skill development. Gaining an understanding of how our bodies are structured and organized can only enhance our ability to execute skills effectively.

Key Terms

all-around athlete
closed skill
executive program
general coordination abilities
generalized (dynamic) motor program (GMP)
motor program
movement intelligence
open skill
parameter
perceptual motor abilities
physical proficiency abilities
response uncertainty
skill
skill as a task
skill as quality of performance
spatial uncertainty
subroutine
tactical uncertainty
temporal patterning
temporal uncertainty

Discussion Questions

1. Define movement intelligence. How does this concept differ from motor programs and skills?
2. What role do motor abilities play in determining an individual's skill level and performance?
3. Design a four-level skill hierarchy for an activity of your choice.
4. List the three main classifications of human abilities. Then provide three examples of abilities that fall under each category.
5. Using specific examples of abilities, explain what makes someone an all-around athlete.
6. How are skills defined? Identify the main features of this definition.
7. Explain the importance of temporal patterning in performing skills.
8. How have skills traditionally been classified? What taxonomy has been used more recently?
9. Distinguish between closed and open skills. Give examples of each.
10. Why are open and closed skills considered to be a continuum?

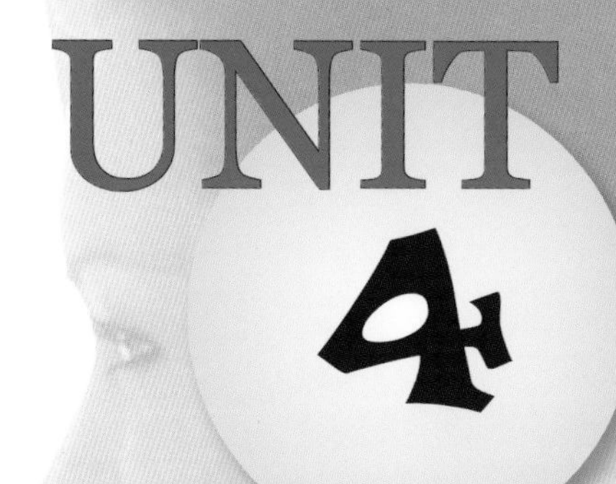

Fitness and Health

- Enhancing Health, Study, Work, and Play Through Physical Fitness
- What's My Score? Evaluation in Kinesiology
- The Nutrition Connection
- Weight Management: Finding a Healthy Balance

In This Chapter:

CHAPTER 12

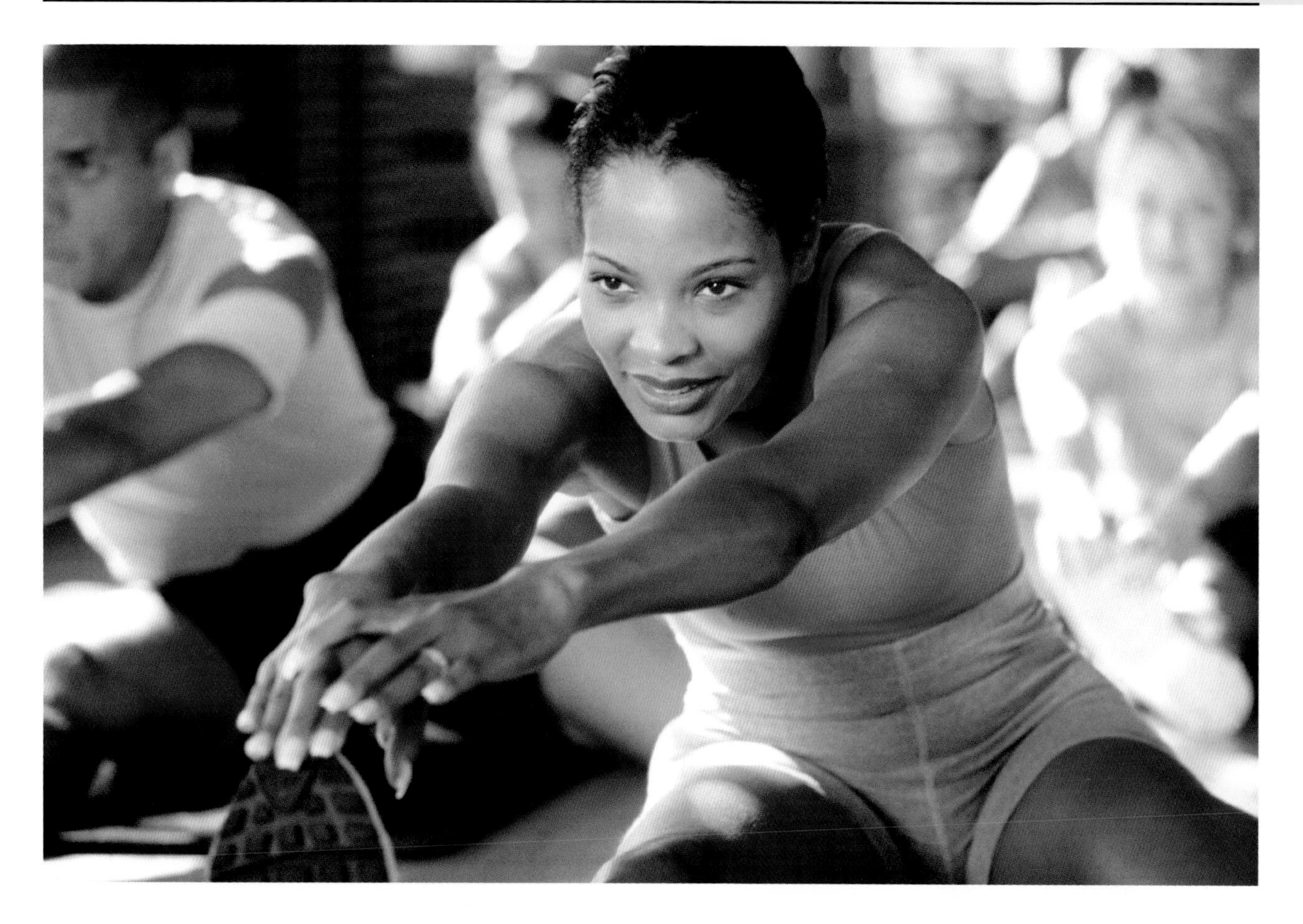

Enhancing Health, Study, Work, and Play Through Physical Fitness

After completing this chapter you should be able to:

- identify and discuss the various components of physical fitness;
- describe the contribution of physical fitness to overall health;
- evaluate the effects of various training methods on performance;
- examine your own physical fitness level and develop an awareness of personal fitness requirements;
- adapt physical fitness and activity programs to address personal needs.

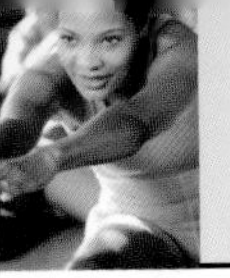

The health, enthusiasm, and creativity of a well-developed personality depend to a great degree upon general fitness levels. Fitness is your functional readiness and level of effectiveness that are required for everything you do. It involves the ability to adapt to the demands and stresses of daily life and is directly related to the amount and intensity of your physical activity. The term fitness is used in many ways and has many dimensions, including physical, emotional, social, and intellectual. The focus of this chapter will be on physical fitness.

Physical fitness is more than just a concept – it is a way of life. It incorporates many components important for health, such as cardiorespiratory endurance; flexibility; muscular strength, power, and endurance; and body composition. Each of these components offers unique benefits and advantages that affect your health in a positive way. Engaging in physical exercise provides numerous benefits that help you control your weight, manage stress, and boost your immune system, as well as protect you against disease. Not only does exercise help you look and feel good, but it allows you to have fun while achieving a state of health and vitality. Fitness need not be boring and monotonous, or restricted to running and cycling; there are many options available, and all you need to do is discover what activities interest you most. Exercise is one of the most important, and indeed, most controllable, factors affecting your general health.

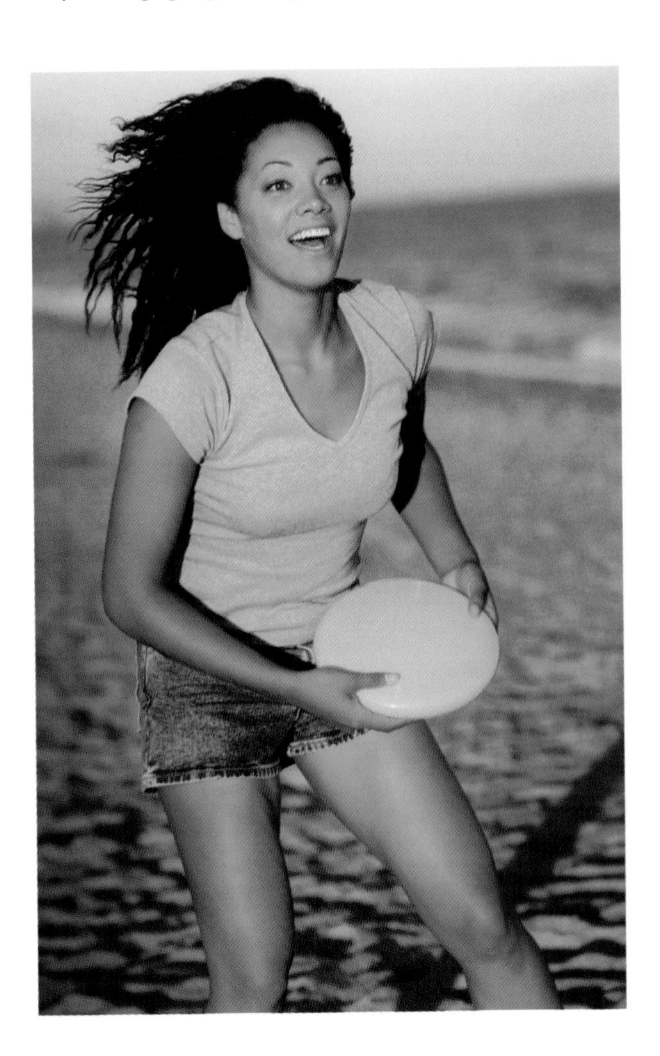

General physical fitness forms the basis for sport-specific fitness and is ultimately related to it. High levels of general fitness are of utmost importance to athletes who strive to achieve high levels of performance. High levels of general fitness constitute important prerequisites for the effective and optimal development of sport-specific fitness. Both develop on the basis of the training principles governing exercise.

In order to get the most out of exercise and physical activity, you need the basic knowledge and an understanding about how to exercise properly and most effectively. This chapter will provide you with concepts related to components of fitness and equip you with basic knowledge governing training principles and their interrelationships.

Definition of Terms

Physical fitness can be defined as the ability of the body to adjust to the demands and stresses of physical effort and is thought to be a measure of one's physical health. In contrast, **physical activity** is defined as "any movement carried out by the skeletal muscles requiring energy." The term **exercise** is considered to be a subset of physical activities that are planned, structured (usually repetitive bodily movements), and designed to improve or maintain physical fitness.

Although physical activity and physical fitness are related measures, physical fitness should be distinguished from physical activity. Physical fitness is an achieved condition that limits the

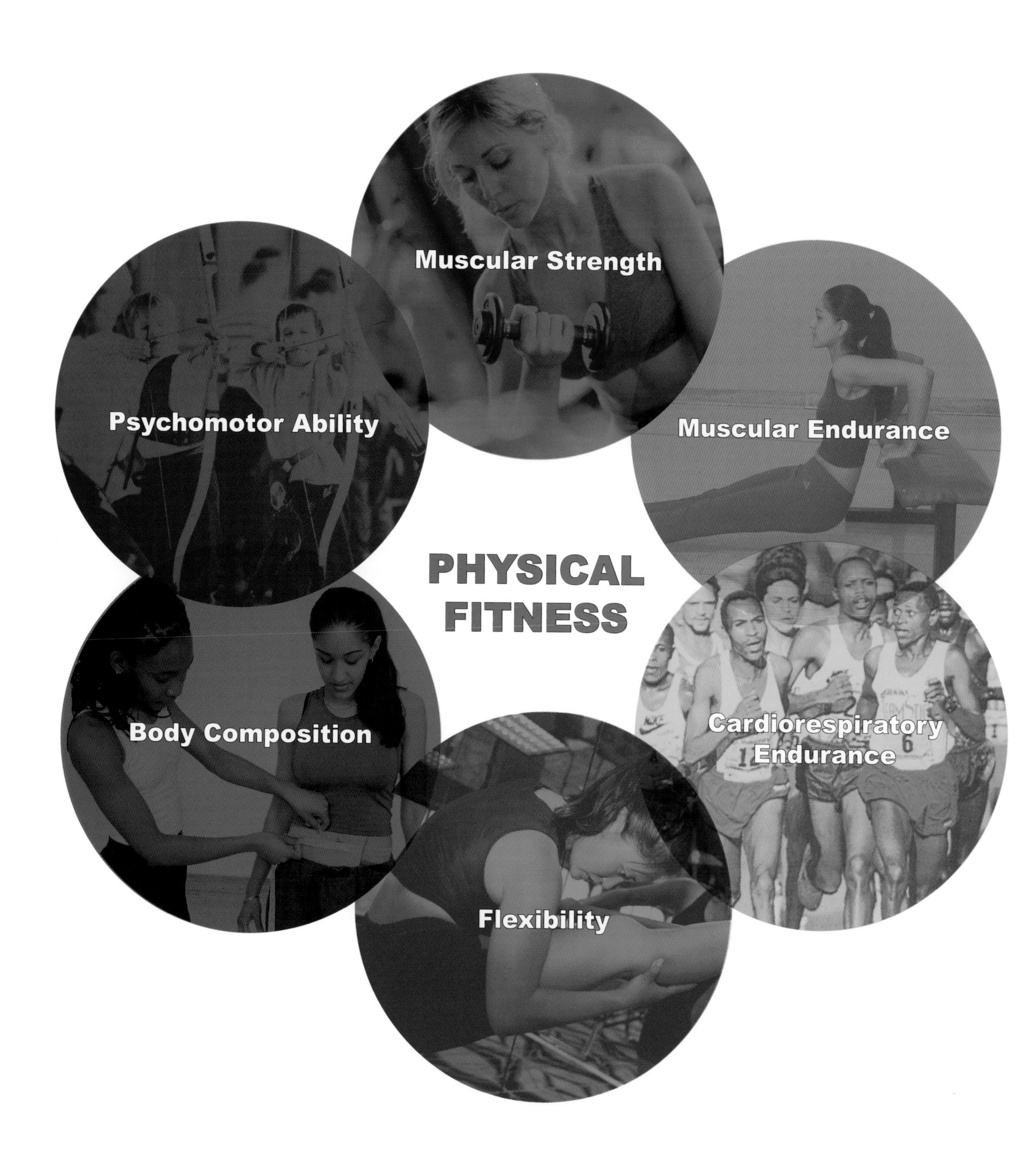

Figure 12.1 The components of physical fitness.

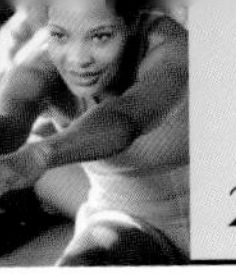

amount of physical activity that can be performed. A physical activity such as walking, cross-country skiing, or swimming might be considered exercise by an unfit person, while considered physical activity by someone who is very fit. The point is that a physical activity–exercise continuum exists. It demonstrates the specific nature of exercise and physical activity. How much activity, what type, how intense, and how often one should exercise are all important questions that should be considered before any exercise program is designed. In what follows, the terms exercise and physical activity are used interchangeably.

Components of Physical Fitness

Physical fitness is achieved when all of the physiological systems of the body are functioning efficiently to meet the physical demands of everyday activities. The components of physical fitness include muscular strength, muscular and cardiorespiratory endurance, flexibility, psychomotor ability, and body composition (Figure 12.1).

Muscular Strength

Muscular strength is commonly measured as a maximal value and can be defined as the ability of a muscle or muscle group to exert force against a resistance. Thus, strength and force are synonymous. The force generated by a muscular contraction may be applied against a movable object, as in weightlifting, or against a fixed object, such as the starting blocks in sprinting. Force is the product of mass times acceleration (F = m·a), and when a force is applied through a distance (D), work (W) is accomplished (W = F·D). It follows that the greater the mass of a muscle, the greater its capability of generating force (see Chapter 5). Think of sports that require great strength. Do the athletes that participate in these sports have large muscles?

Power

As defined in Chapter 5, **power** is the ability to overcome external resistance at a high rate of muscular contraction. It is the force that can be generated at speeds characteristic of the activity to overcome gravity (see discussion on gravity in Chapter 8) and thus accelerate the body or an implement. The ability to exert force is in turn dependent on muscular strength. Thus, power is an important derivative of muscular strength and is decisive in performance in most sports and many recreational activities (Figure 12.2; also see discussion on power in Chapter 5).

Muscular Endurance

Muscular endurance is defined as the ability of

Agonist–Antagonist Training

When planning training, care must be taken to include exercises that stimulate both the agonists (working muscles) and the antagonists (counteracting muscles; see discussion on muscle teamwork in Chapter 4). A program that focuses only on increasing agonist strength tends to shorten the agonist muscles and weaken the antagonist muscles. This results in a change in the proportion of strength between agonists and antagonists, which under normal circumstances is well balanced. This shift in strength equilibrium can result in impaired joint positions and make articular cartilage and muscles (especially the tendons) prone to disease and injury.

Thus, a program that includes exercises to develop the biceps should also include exercises to enhance the triceps; trunk extensor training should be complemented with trunk flexor training. This approach to strength training is referred to as **agonist–antagonist training** (Figure 12.3).

To achieve a balanced development of strength, your strength program must ensure a balance between the training of agonists and antagonists.

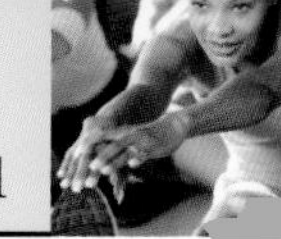

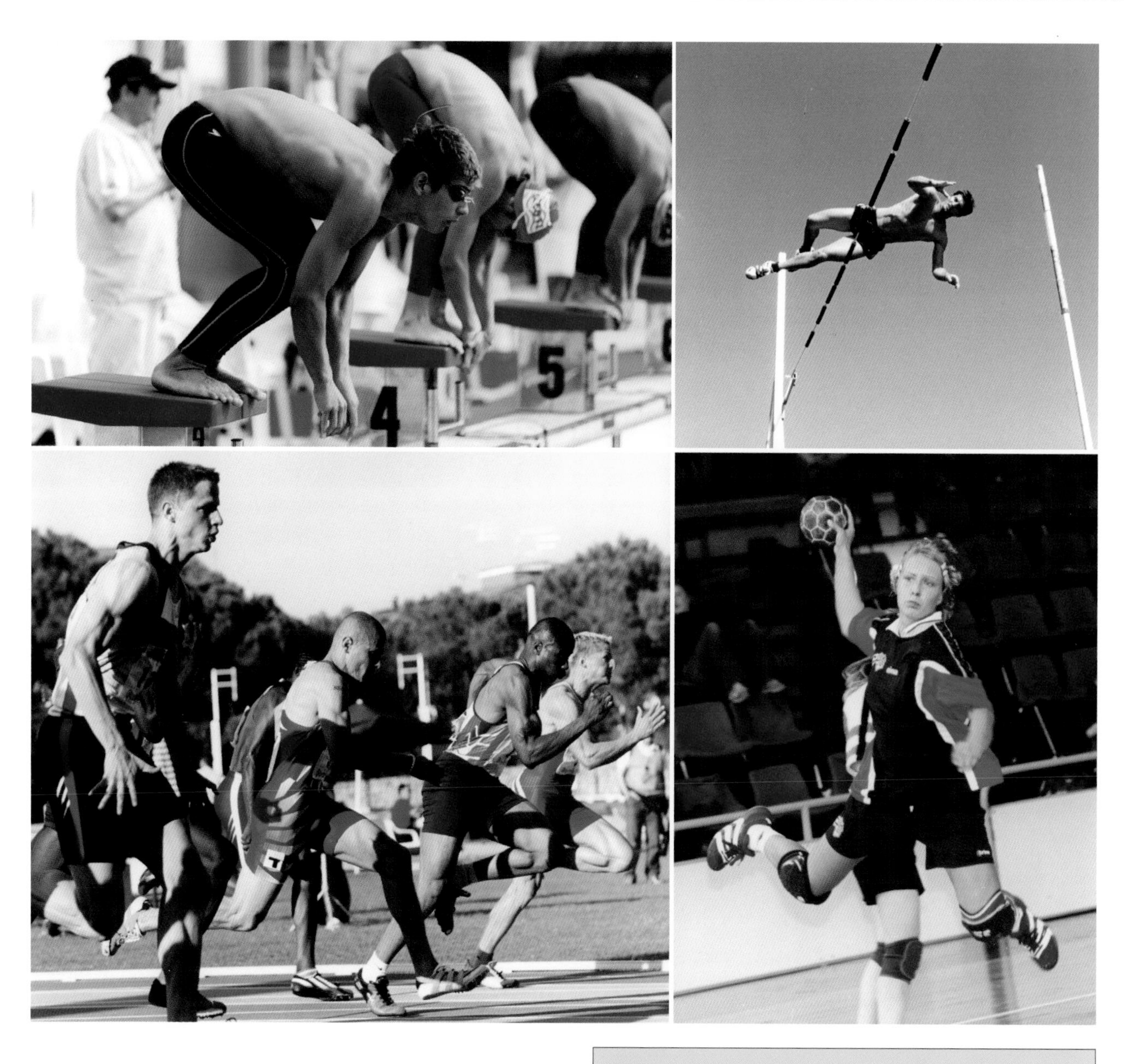

Figure 12.2 Activities requiring explosive power.

a muscle or muscle group to sustain a given level of force (static exercise) or to contract and relax (dynamic exercise) repeatedly at a given resistance. Static exercises involve sustained contractions, which often compromise blood flow. As a result, oxygen is rapidly used up and metabolic by-products accumulate, causing fatigue. Performing a flexed arm hang will provide you with this experience. Your heart and lungs do not have much trouble performing during a flexed arm hang, but your arm muscles (local muscle group) feel a strong burning sensation and fatigue rapidly.

In contrast to static exercises, dynamic exercises involve continuous rhythmical contractions and relaxations that allow for oxygen to be continually delivered to the muscle and metabolic by-products to be removed. Thus, other physiological systems play a greater role, and depending upon intensity, fatigue may take longer to develop. For example, during cycling, in addition to your leg muscles requiring muscular endurance, your cardiorespiratory system is also involved. Exercises that employ large muscle groups for prolonged periods of time such as distance running, cross-country skiing, cycling,

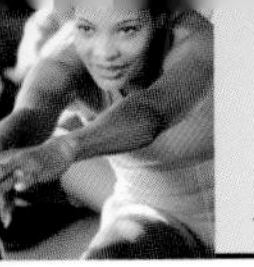

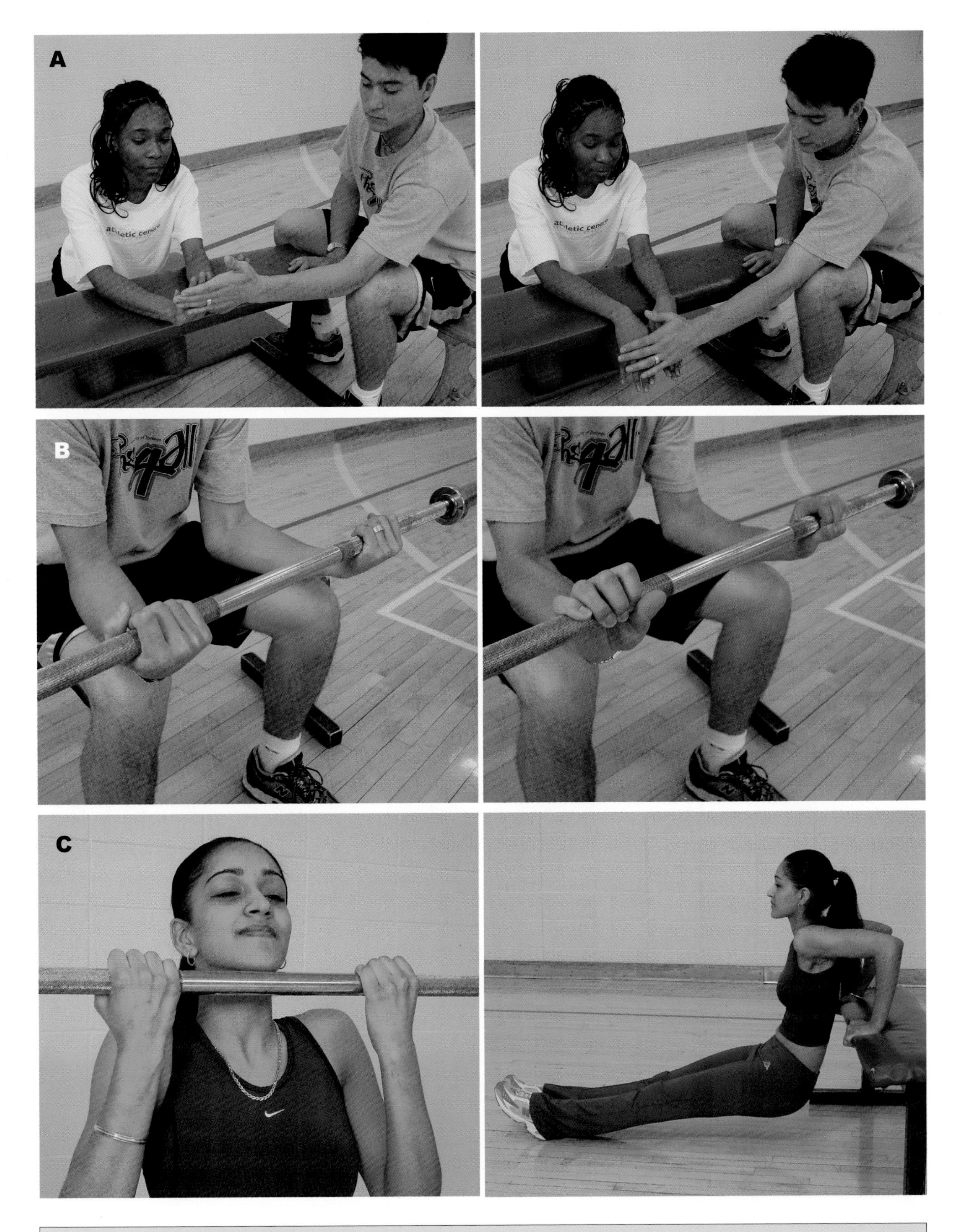

Figure 12.3 Agonist–antagonist training. **A.** Using partner-assisted exercises. **B.** Using free weights. **C.** Using one's own body weight.

or swimming involve cardiorespiratory endurance, another important component of physical fitness (Figure 12.4).

Cardiorespiratory Endurance

As its name implies, **cardiorespiratory** (also called **cardiovascular**) **endurance** or **fitness** involves both the heart (cardio) and the lung (respiratory) systems. A major function of the cardiorespiratory system is to provide oxygen to the tissues. The maximal rate at which the body can take up, transport, and utilize oxygen is known as **aerobic power** or endurance, which is expressed as maximal oxygen uptake, or $\dot{V}O_2max$. $\dot{V}O_2max$ is also the maximal rate of aerobic metabolism and is the single most important criterion of physical fitness (see discussion on aerobic power in Chapter 6).

Cardiorespiratory fitness is the ability to produce energy through an improved delivery of oxygen to the working muscles. It is needed for exertions over relatively longer periods of time, regardless of the activity. It is intimately related to muscular endurance because the working muscles rely on the oxygen supply sent by the pumping heart, delivered via the blood, and used by the muscles. The major improvements or training effects related to cardiorespiratory endurance were discussed in Chapter 6.

Maximal Oxygen Uptake ($\dot{V}O_2max$)

$\dot{V}O_2max$ can be measured, estimated, or predicted in many ways. Measuring the $\dot{V}O_2max$ of a person

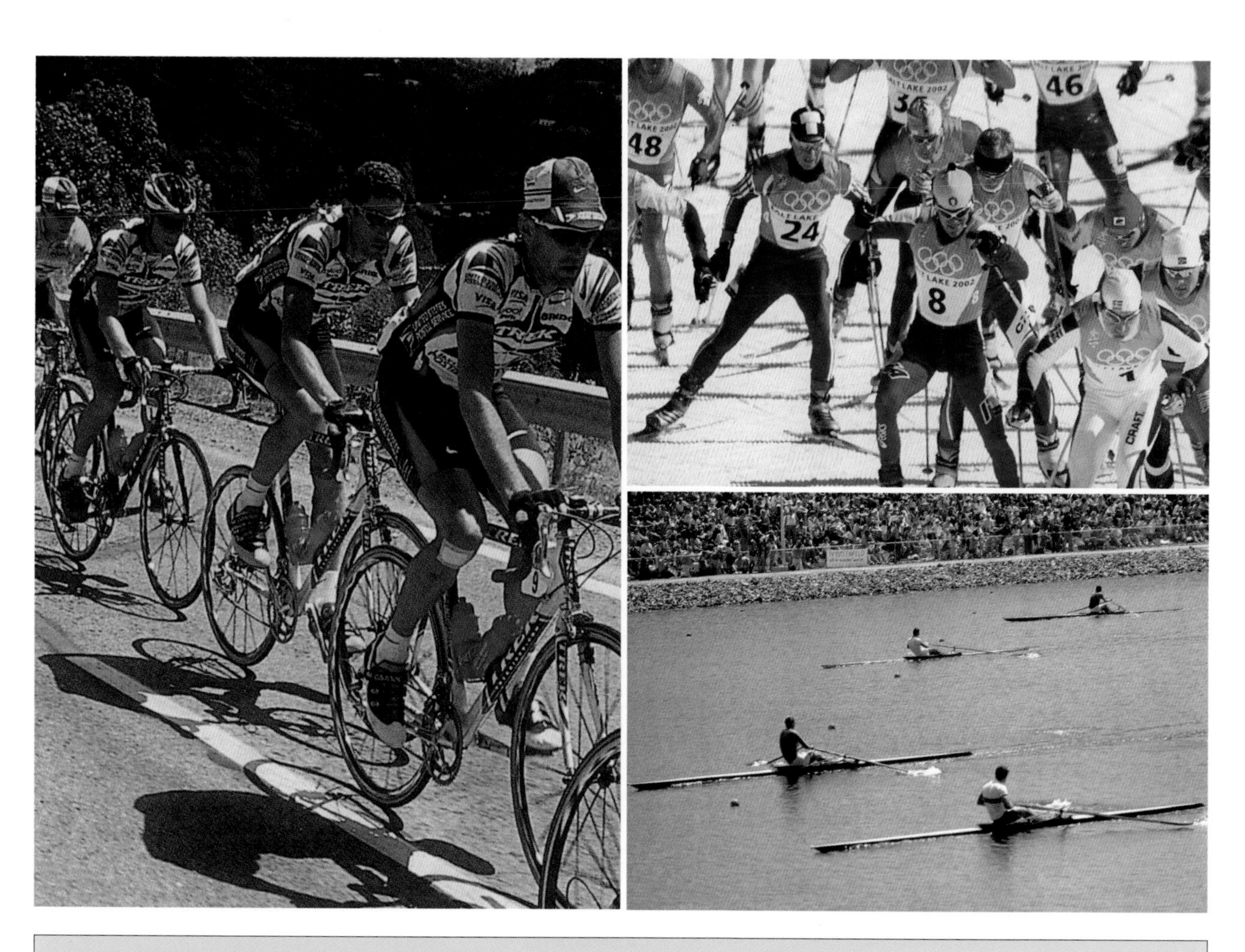

Figure 12.4 Performances in rowing, cycling, and cross-country skiing are based on muscular and cardiovascular endurance.

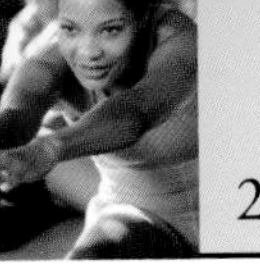

running on a treadmill involves having a person run at a given speed or workload for a few minutes (2 to 3 min) (Figure 12.5) while oxygen uptake, or consumption, is measured over a period of time (2 to 3 min) at each workload. The workload is gradually increased by increasing the speed or the treadmill slope. At each new workload, the individual demand for oxygen increases (i.e., as the workload is increased, more oxygen is taken up by the lungs, delivered by the heart, and utilized by the muscles). However, eventually a point will be reached where the increased workload cannot be supported by an increase in oxygen uptake. Oxygen consumption is said to have reached a plateau, or reached a maximal value. This plateau is known as one's **$\dot{V}O_2$max.**

Prediction of $\dot{V}O_2$max With each new workload, as more oxygen is required, the heart will pump more blood, delivering more oxygen to the exercising muscles. Thus, at each new workload the heart rate will also increase and eventually reach a maximal value. The linear relationship between heart rate and workload that exists over a given workload range is the basis for estimations or predictions of $\dot{V}O_2$max.

Absolute $\dot{V}O_2$max $\dot{V}O_2$ is expressed in an absolute manner as a **volume per unit time**, liters per minute (L/min). In general, an **absolute $\dot{V}O_2$max** measurement is related to mass, especially muscle mass. Larger individuals usually have higher $\dot{V}O_2$max values because of their greater

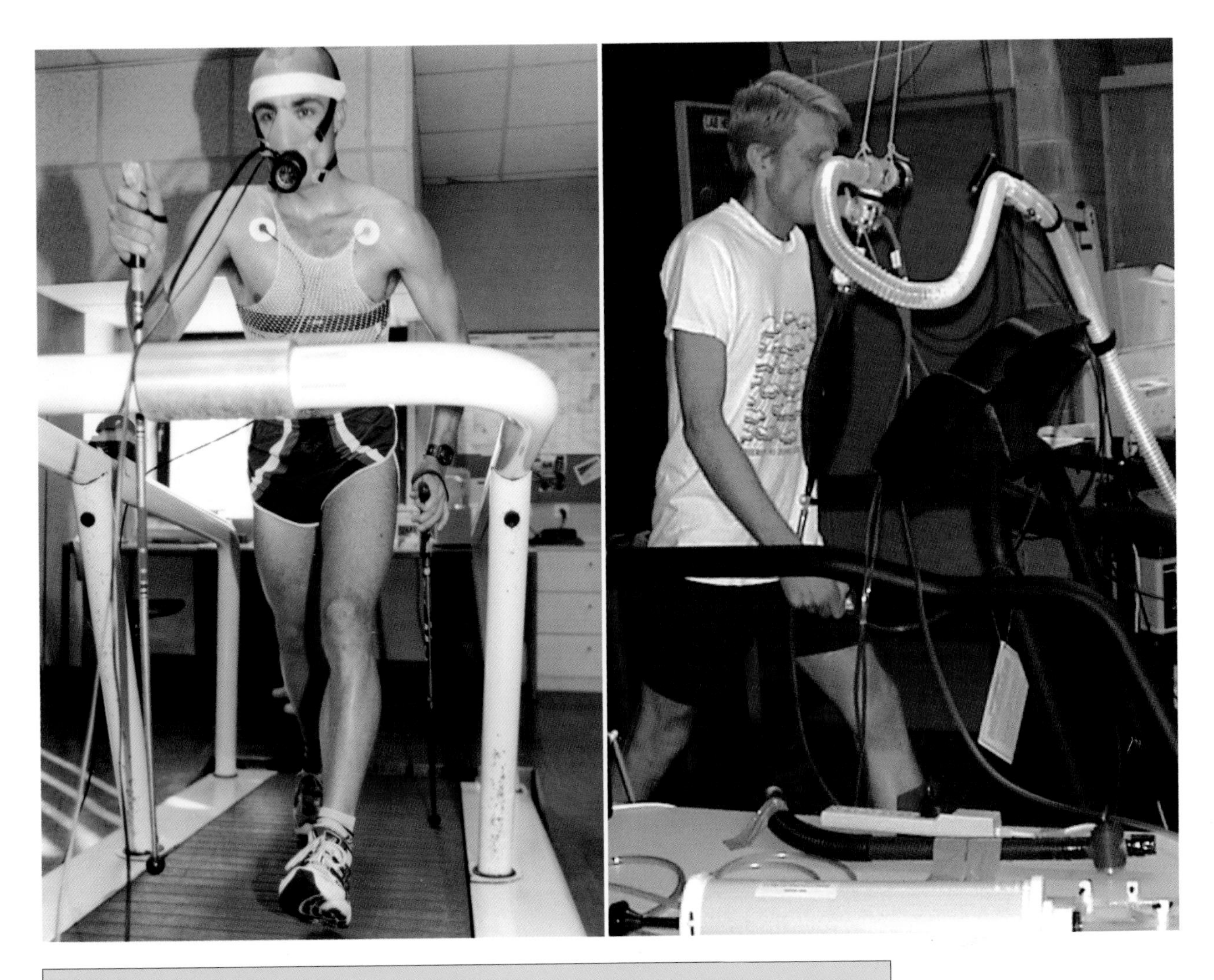

Figure 12.5 Testing for $\dot{V}O_2$max can only be carried out in a laboratory setting.

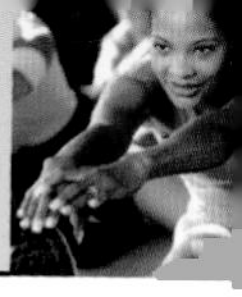

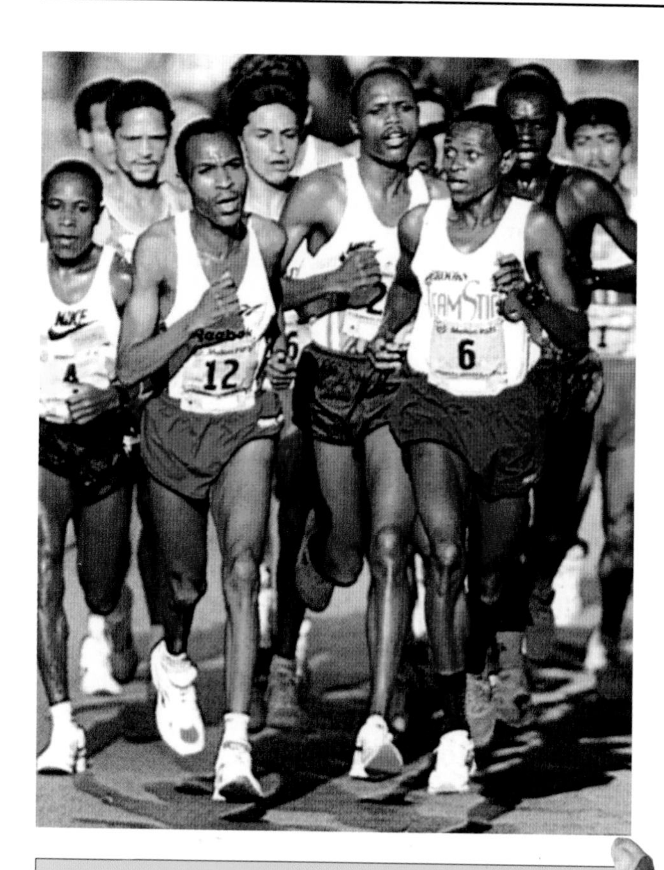

Figure 12.6 Marathon runners are among the best when it comes to relative $\dot{V}O_2max$.

muscle mass. For example, it is not uncommon for elite male rowers, who are generally tall and muscular, to have $\dot{V}O_2max$ values of approximately 6.0 L/min. In contrast, shorter and comparatively slighter runners might have $\dot{V}O_2max$ values of only 4.5 L/min.

Absolute measurements of $\dot{V}O_2max$ are useful for comparison within groups but limited when comparing two groups that differ in mass or body composition.

Relative $\dot{V}O_2max$ To account for differences in mass, $\dot{V}O_2max$ can also be expressed in a relative manner (i.e., in relation to mass expressed in kilograms). Thus, when comparing two athletes playing different sports, it is often useful to divide their absolute $\dot{V}O_2max$ by their mass to obtain **relative $\dot{V}O_2max$** values (Figure 12.6). When $\dot{V}O_2$ is expressed relative to mass, the units used are expressed in **ml/kg/min**, thus indicating the consumed volume of oxygen in milliliters per kilogram of body weight per minute. Using our male rower and runner example, if the rower weighed 90 kg and the runner weighed 68 kg, then both have the same relative $\dot{V}O_2max$, 66 ml/kg/min (this value was obtained by dividing their absolute $\dot{V}O_2max$ by their mass).

Flexibility

Have you ever wondered how gymnasts or ballet dancers perform the splits or arch their spines so far? This type of performance illustrates their ability to perform movements that require a great measure of **flexibility**.

Flexibility is defined as the ability of a joint to move through its full range of motion. Flexibility is determined primarily by joint structure and to a lesser extent by muscle elasticity and length.

Connective tissue is the most important part of muscle in terms of its flexibility. The main structural protein in connective tissues is **collagen**. Collagen fibers provide structure and support to tissues, ligaments, tendons, and joints. Collagen is a **triple helix** that can withstand very high tensile forces. In addition to collagen, another protein known as **elastin** provides an athlete with stretching ability.

A number of factors such as age, sex, and inactivity can affect flexibility. Just compare the level of flexibility of a young and active rhythmic gymnast (Figure 12.7) with that of an elderly person with arthritis. Flexibility promotes good joint health, slows joint deterioration, and generally improves quality of life for most individuals. It may also prevent

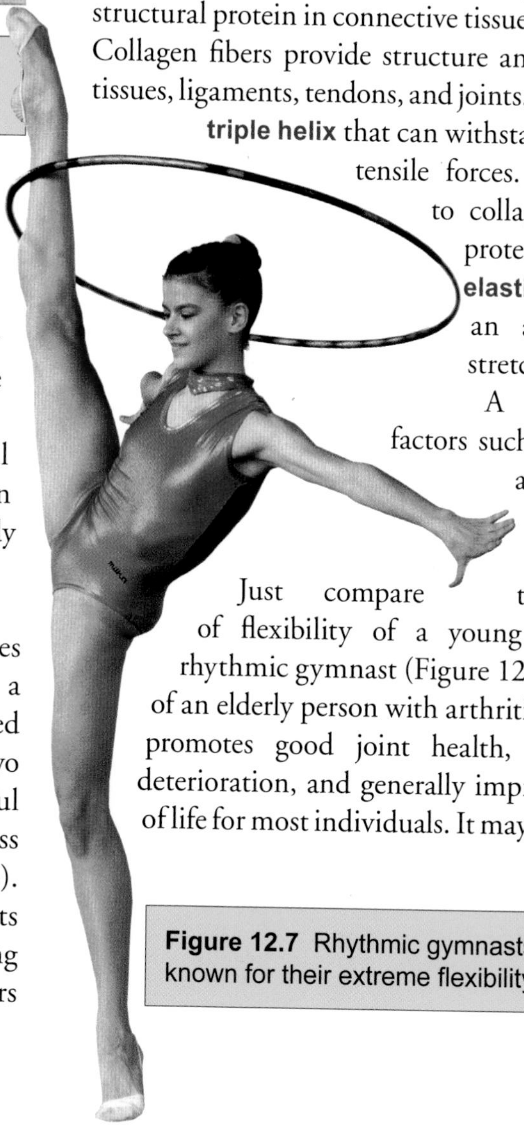

Figure 12.7 Rhythmic gymnasts are known for their extreme flexibility.

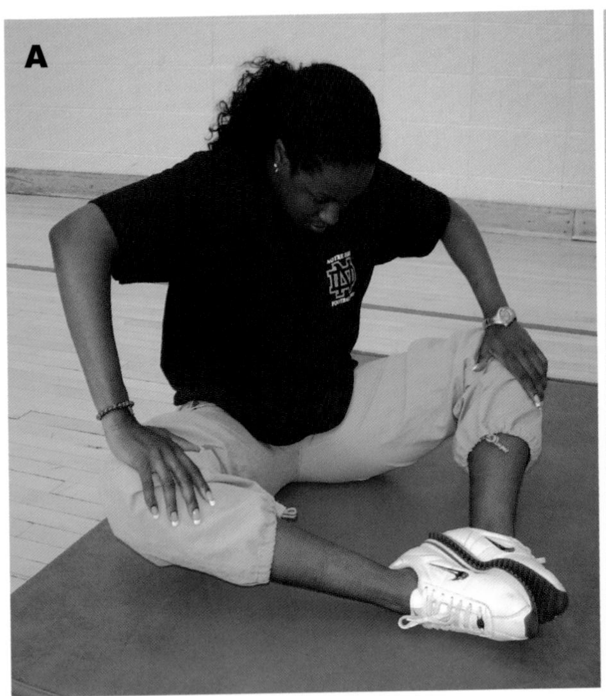

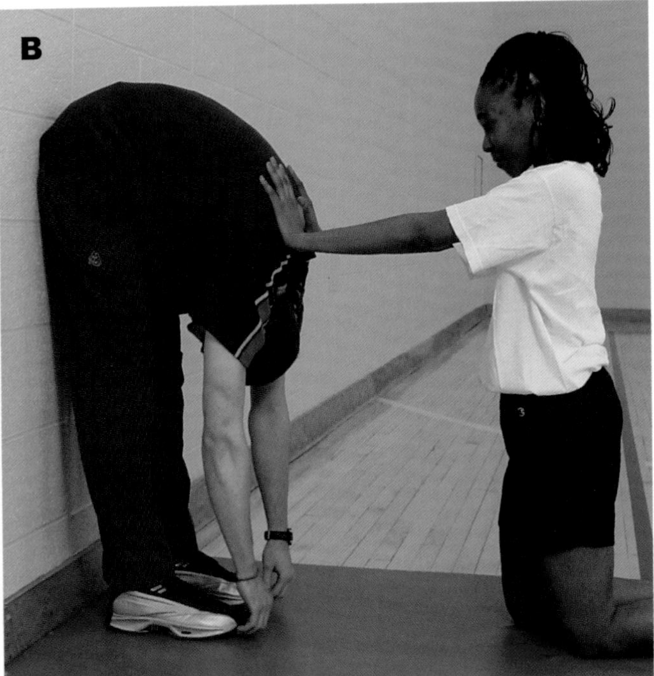

Figure 12.8 A. Active stretching. **B.** Passive stretching.

lower back pain and injuries as well as reduce the frequency and severity of injuries.

Active and Passive Flexibility

Flexibility can be active or passive. **Active flexibility** is the range of movement generated by individual effort, while **passive flexibility** is the range of movement achieved with the help of external forces (a partner, weight, rubber band, and so on). Passive flexibility exercises help achieve a wider range of movement than do active flexibility exercises (Figure 12.8).

Stretching Methods

There are three stretching methods: the static, dynamic, and proprioceptive neuromuscular facilitation methods.

Static Stretching **Static stretching** refers to holding a fully stretched position, such as the splits. Using this method, an athlete slowly relaxes the muscles to be stretched and holds himself/herself in a stretched position for 10 to 30 seconds. The process may be enhanced by an assisting partner. The process is repeated four to six times for maximal efficiency.

Dynamic Stretching **Dynamic** or **ballistic stretching** refers to rapidly moving a joint through its full range of motion, such as the arm of a baseball pitcher. The method involves stretching with repetitive bouncing movements using small intervals, rather than just one pull. An athlete begins the first repetition over a relatively small range of joint motion, gradually increasing the amplitude range, reaching the maximal range after 10 to 20 movements. The process is then repeated three to five times, using body weight or an assisting partner (Figure 12.9).

Prestretching The **prestretching** or **proprioceptive neuromuscular facilitation (PNF)** method exploits the natural protective reflex of the muscle and its tendon sensors – the muscle spindles and Golgi tendon organs. It is regarded as the most efficient stretching method.

The PNF method is carried out in three phases with a partner.

Strength Training and Flexibility

Some exercises may have a dual training effect by developing both strength and flexibility. Arm raising exercises from the mat, for instance, involve little stretching; when performed from the bench, however, the same exercise allows for a far larger range and thus promotes the stretching of the pectoral muscles in particular. Half-knee bends, if overused, cause the quadriceps to shorten; deep-knee bends help stretch them.

It is for this reason that weightlifters, who must often assume very deep squatting positions to clean or snatch heavy loads, have extremely elastic leg muscles. Similarly, competitive swimmers develop extreme flexibility in their shoulder girdles. Such examples show that, under certain conditions, the same exercises may develop both strength and flexibility. However, the movement range around a joint must always be exploited to its full capacity. If not, muscle stretching will not occur; indeed, the muscle may shorten, and strength training may then lead to impaired flexibility. To achieve optimal flexibility through strength training, you must exploit the full range of joint movement that can be achieved during any given exercise.

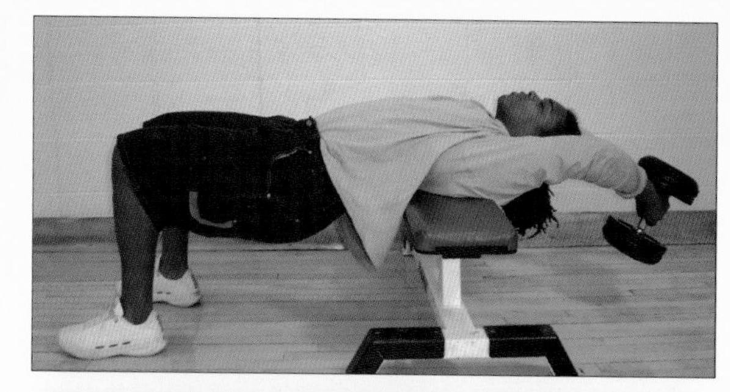

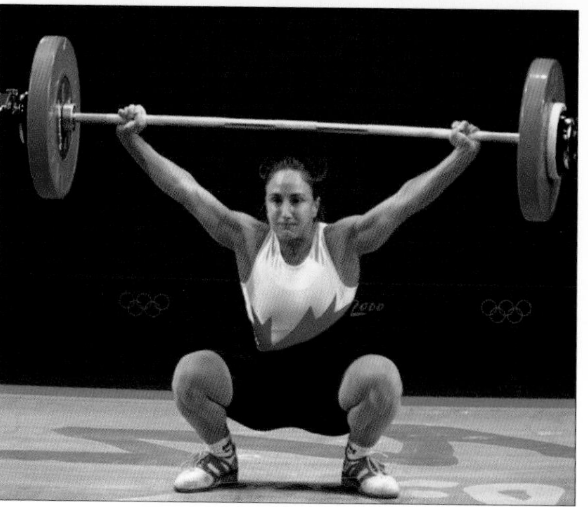

- During the first **active stretching phase**, the muscles to be stretched are actively pulled to the very limit of the movement range. This initial stretching movement should be performed slowly and continuously. This prevents the muscle spindles from initiating the stretching reflex and thus contracting the muscles.

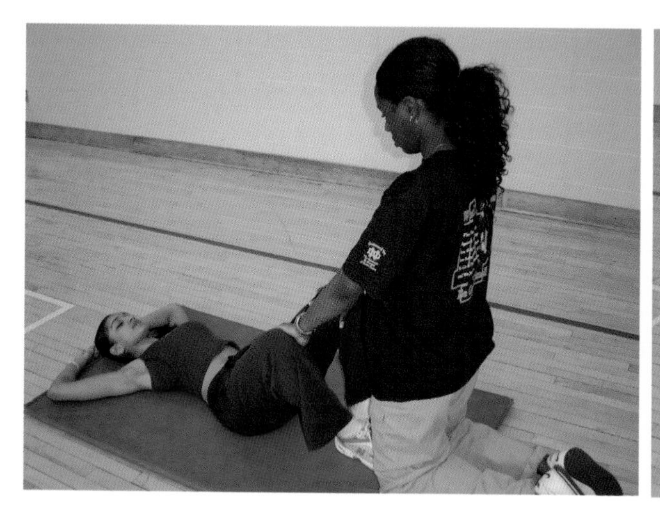

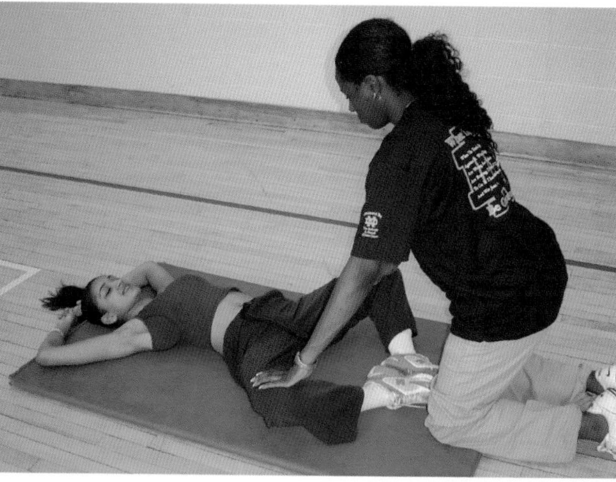

Figure 12.9 Partner-assisted dynamic stretching.

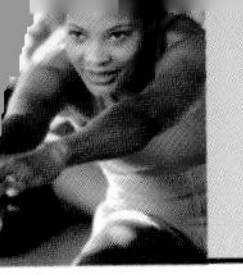

- In the second **pretension phase**, the trainee exerts a full static resistance (a strong isometric contraction) against partner resistance for approximately seven seconds. This causes the Golgi tendon organs to release inhibitory impulses, which in turn cause an involuntary relaxation of the muscles to be stretched.
- In the third **passive stretching phase**, the partner pushes the body further into a stretched position, almost to the point of pain. This final position is then held, with all muscles relaxed, for approximately six seconds. The partner's pressure must be applied slowly and constantly in order to prevent muscle spindles from initiating a reflex contraction, which may cause injury.

Body Composition

Body composition refers to the amounts of body constituents, such as fat, muscle, bone, and other organs, and is regarded as one of the major components of physical fitness. Of particular interest are percentages of lean body mass and fat mass. Typically, an active and physically fit individual has a lower percentage of body fat than an inactive, unfit person. The large number of overweight young people in our society is a cause for concern. Any fitness program, strength or cardiovascular, should be designed with an aim to help reduce body fat. For detailed information about body composition, weight management, and the effects of obesity see Chapter 15.

Psychomotor Ability

Successful athletes appear to move effortlessly. In addition, they can respond easily or readily to changes in their surroundings. To accomplish this, athletes must monitor their environment, collect information, make decisions, and execute their movements. It is their **psychomotor ability** that allows them to complete these tasks quickly and accurately.

A high level of psychomotor ability serves to integrate the workings of the central nervous system with the more physical components of fitness. The body constantly monitors both its internal and external environments, collecting information and making decisions about what is relevant information and what is irrelevant information.

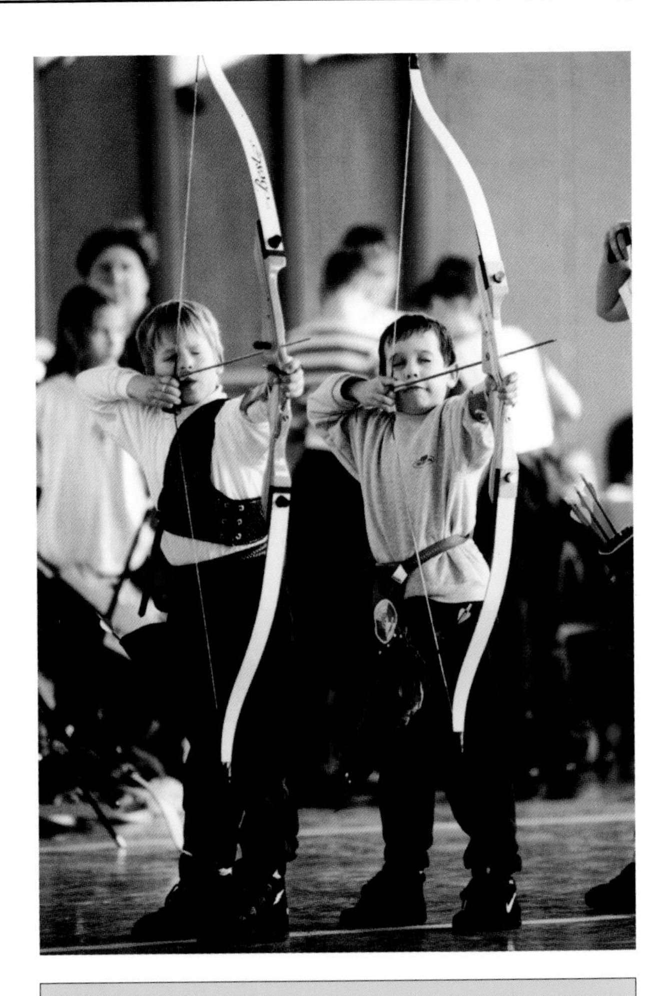

Figure 12.10 Archery requires hand steadiness as well as undivided concentration.

The psychomotor domain may seem an unimportant component of physical fitness; however, it is of utmost importance to effective functioning in all environments.

Psychomotor abilities are many. The most significant ones are reaction time and anticipation, visual skills, hand–eye coordination, perception, attention and concentration, balance, proprioception or muscle feeling, memory processes and recall, and decision making (Figure 12.10). These abilities are presented in more detail in Chapter 11.

Components and Principles of Fitness Programs

Fitness training programs are based on several closely related training components. These components follow well-established training principles that are intended to generate optimal adaptation and performance improvements of trainees. These components and their principles are the subjects of this section of the chapter.

The following interrelated training components should be considered when designing a comprehensive fitness program: training time, frequency of exercise, intensity of exercise, volume of training, work-to-rest ratio, and the type of exercise. Strength training also involves other components vital to effective training: the order of exercises used, number of repetitions per set and number of sets, and the recovery or rest periods between exercises.

Training Components

Training Time

Training time refers to the total time devoted to developing fitness. It is based on duration of each training session and the frequency of training during a week, month, or year.

Training Frequency

Training frequency depends on an individual's goals, abilities, and fitness level. Normally, an athlete undertakes 3 to 10 strength and cardiorespiratory training sessions per week, depending on the needs of his or her particular sports activity.

Depending on the overall goal of fitness training, recreational athletes normally perform 2 to 6 sessions per week. If the goal is to maintain certain levels of fitness, 2 to 3 sessions per week are sufficient; however, if the goal is to reduce weight or to increase strength and/or cardiorespiratory fitness, 4 to 6 sessions are necessary.

Training Volume

Training volume is one of the most important components of training. It refers to the sum total of work performed during a training session or phase of training and is measured in various units depending upon the type of activity. In cyclic movements (walking, running, swimming, and so on), the total distance (e.g., in miles or kilometers) in one workout or several workouts represents the volume of training.

For various strength exercises using body weight, the volume may refer to (a) the number of all repetitions of each exercise (e.g., 20 push-ups) or (b) the sum total of all repetitions during a workout (200 repetitions using 10 different exercises within one circuit training session).

For weightlifting exercises using a barbell, the volume is calculated on the basis of (a) the sum total of all weight lifted per training session (e.g., 4.5 tons using 8 exercises) or (b) the number of repetitions performed with a given load (e.g., 6 x 80 kg, or 3 x 6 x 80 kg).

Training Intensity

Training intensity is probably the most important component of strength training. Generally, it characterizes the degree of stimulation intensity of exercise per unit of time. It is measured in various units depending on the type of activity, as follows:

Distance Covered: meters per second (m/s) and miles or kilometers per hour (mph or km/h) for cyclic activities, such as running, cross-country skiing, and cycling.

Resistance to Be Overcome: pounds (lb) or kilograms (kg) lifted per unit of time (e.g., lb/min; kg/30 min) in weightlifting using barbells, dumbbells, and so on.

Frequency of Movements: rate per unit of time for acyclic activities, such as gymnastics, figure skating, diving, ski jumping, ball games, and so on. (Figure 12.11).

Training intensity is always expressed as a

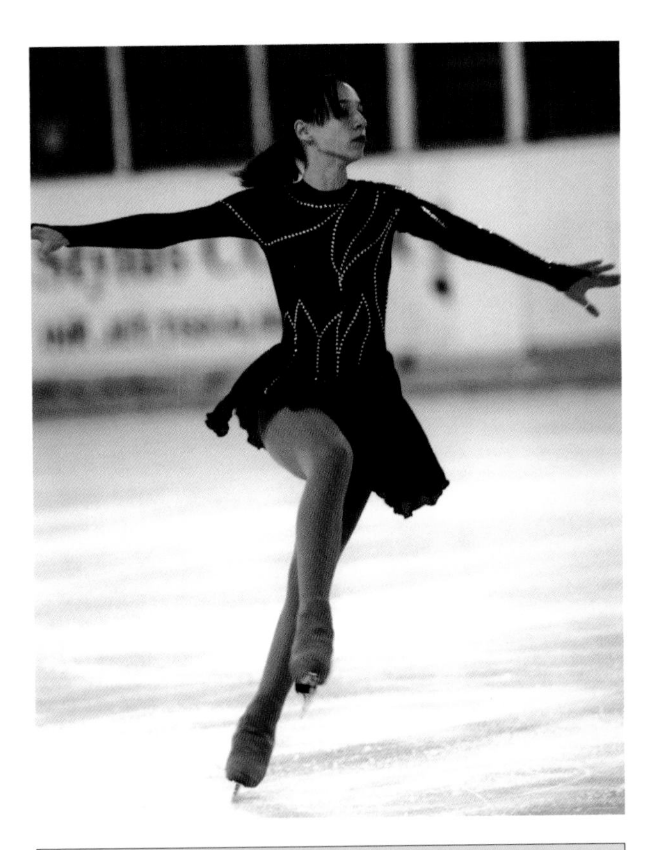

Figure 12.11 In figure skating, the intensity of training is measured by the total number of repetitions of a movement per unit of time (5 min, 10 min, 30 min, and so on).

percentage of a trainee's personal best, or 100 percent performance in the activity, when converted to the units of measurement described previously. This performance becomes the benchmark, the starting point, for defining the various ranges of relative intensities used in planning workouts.

1RM

In strength training, for example, a 100 percent performance expressed in pounds or kilograms is the trainee's maximal performance in one repetition trial (**1RM**) for a specific lift or exercise (for more on 1RM see Chapter 5). The load intensity of strength training expressed as a certain percentage of the 1RM represents an athlete's necessary effort in training. Thus, the 100 percent performance, or 1RM, of the athlete becomes the starting point for defining the various ranges of relative intensities used in the planning of training.

Work-to-Rest Ratio

A **work-to-rest ratio** refers to the relationship between the phases of work and rest during training. It is not possible to work continuously without a break throughout a training session unless the intensity of exercise is relatively low. Generally, the lower the intensity of exercise per unit of time, the shorter the rest periods required by the working trainee. Conversely, the higher the intensity of exercise per unit of time, the longer the rest periods that must be scheduled.

A trainee's heart rate is normally used to determine the length of rest between individual sets and/or series of exercises. Depending upon the fitness level of the trainee, after an incomplete recovery period of about 30 to 180 seconds, the heart rate may drop to about 120 to 140 beats per minute, at which point exercising can resume.

Training intensity must always be considered in connection with the other components of training, such as the volume of exercise and type of exercises used. Some of these relationships are presented in Figure 12.12.

How Much Rest?

In general, training programs (methods) designed to improve endurance require relatively short rests when the intensity of exercise is relatively low. Training programs (methods) designed to improve speed and power require exercising at relatively high intensity levels with extended rest intervals to allow almost complete recovery.

Type of Exercise

The type of physical exercises used in fitness programs is a decisive component for fitness development. Exercises may differ considerably in their spatial and dynamic structure and in their complexity and difficulty. In strength training, for example, multiple possibilities of load selection can be achieved by exercises using an athlete's own body weight, partner exercises (Figure 12.13), and exercise with weights (i.e., dumbbells, round

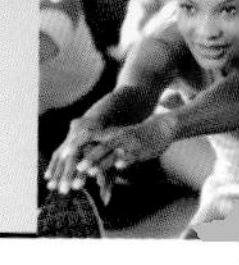

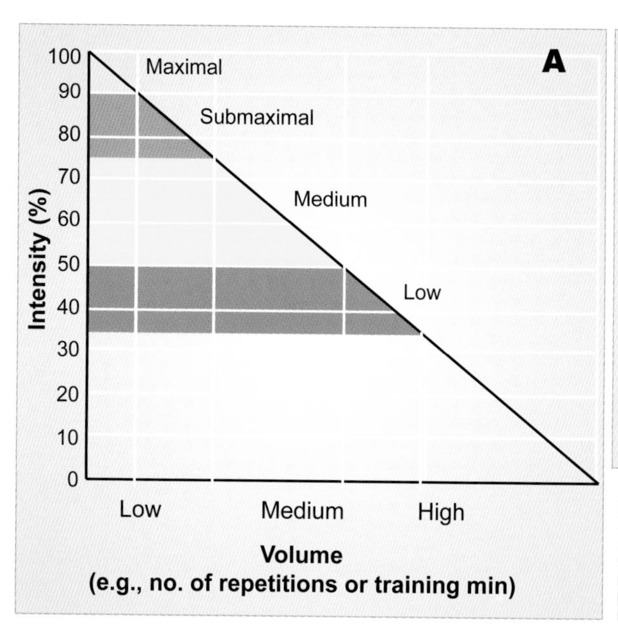

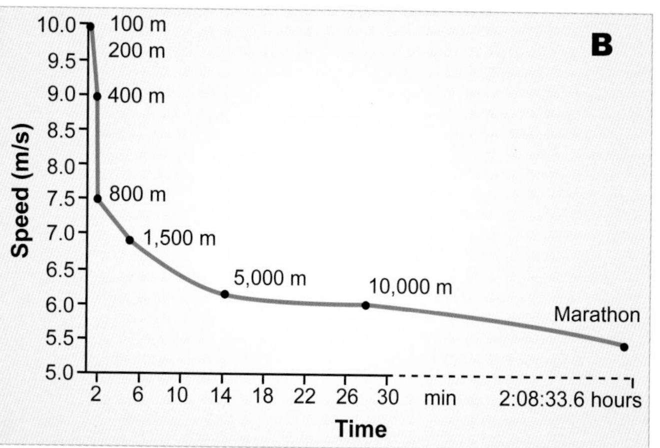

Figure 12.12 Diagrams showing the relationships between **A.** intensity and volume of exercise and **B.** distance/time and speed of running.

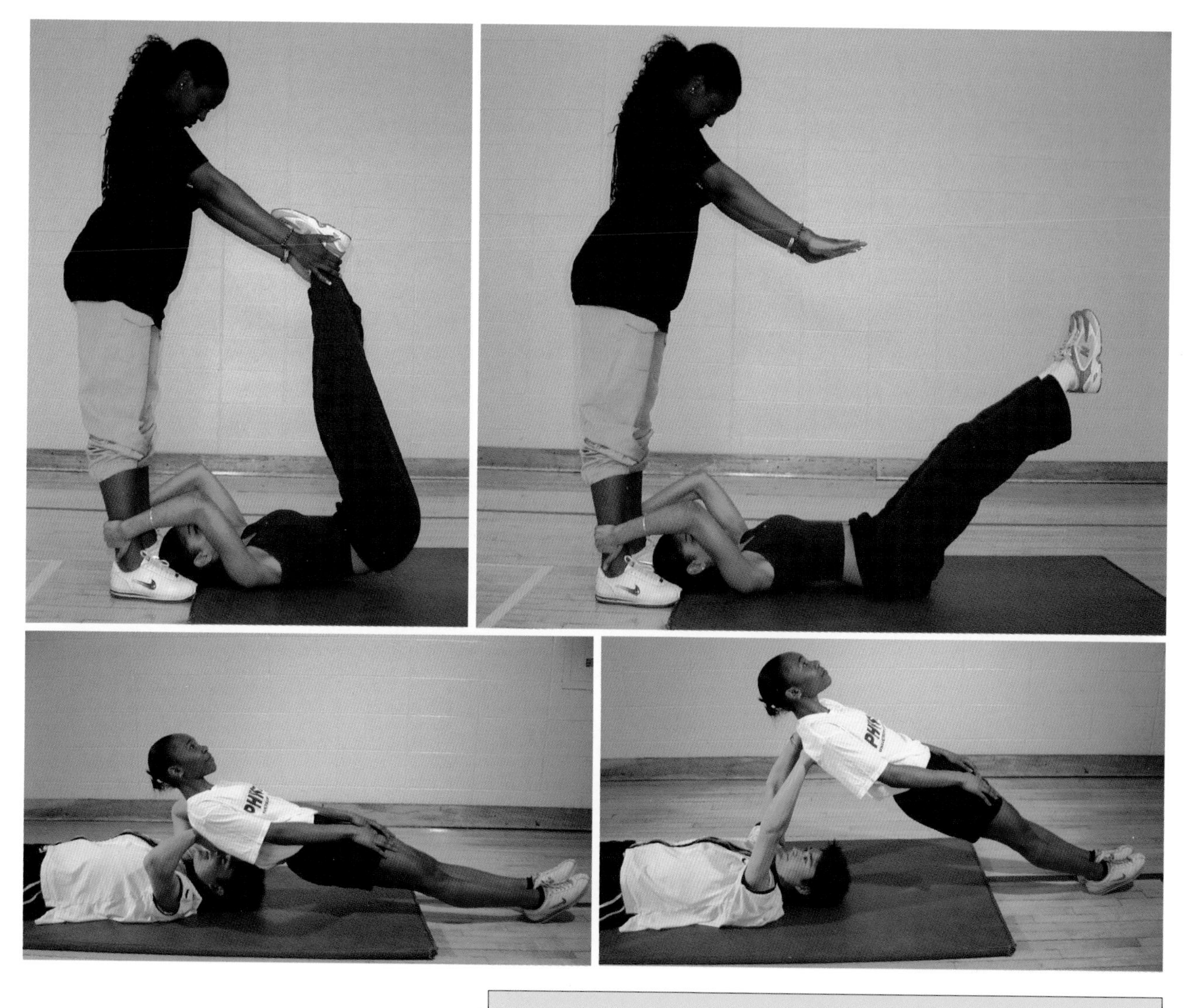

Figure 12.13 Partner exercises are cheap, effective, and fun.

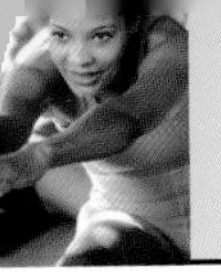

weights, barbells, body weight) and, of course, various strength training machines, such as Nautilus, Universal Gym, and Hercules.

In cardiorespiratory fitness training, one can choose from running on the track, running in parks and on beaches (sand), running the bleachers, hill running, and so on. Each running environment provides different intensity stimuli that can be effectively explored and incorporated in one's fitness program.

Warm-up and Cool-down

Loosening-up and relaxation exercises before training and after training facilitate physical and mental relaxation and also reduce and sometimes eliminate the potentially harmful effects of training (Figure 12.14). The warm-up procedure prepares the body and mind for the exercise activity by:

(1) raising the body temperature, increasing respiration and heart rate, and increasing blood flow, metabolic rate, and oxygen exchange;

(2) increasing range of movement, thus decreasing muscle tension and guarding against muscle, tendon, and ligament strains; and

(3) increasing central nervous system activity, which coordinates the trainee's movements, reduces the time of motor reaction, and improves coordination.

The cool-down procedure is particularly important after vigorous exercising. A proper cool-down helps a trainee recover more quickly by helping physiological systems return to their normal levels faster.

Other Components of Training

Other components of training that must also be considered include exercise speed, number of repetitions and sets, order of exercising, and number of exercises used.

Exercise Speed Exercise speed is particularly important. Lower exercise speeds promote an increase in the muscle diameter (for more on

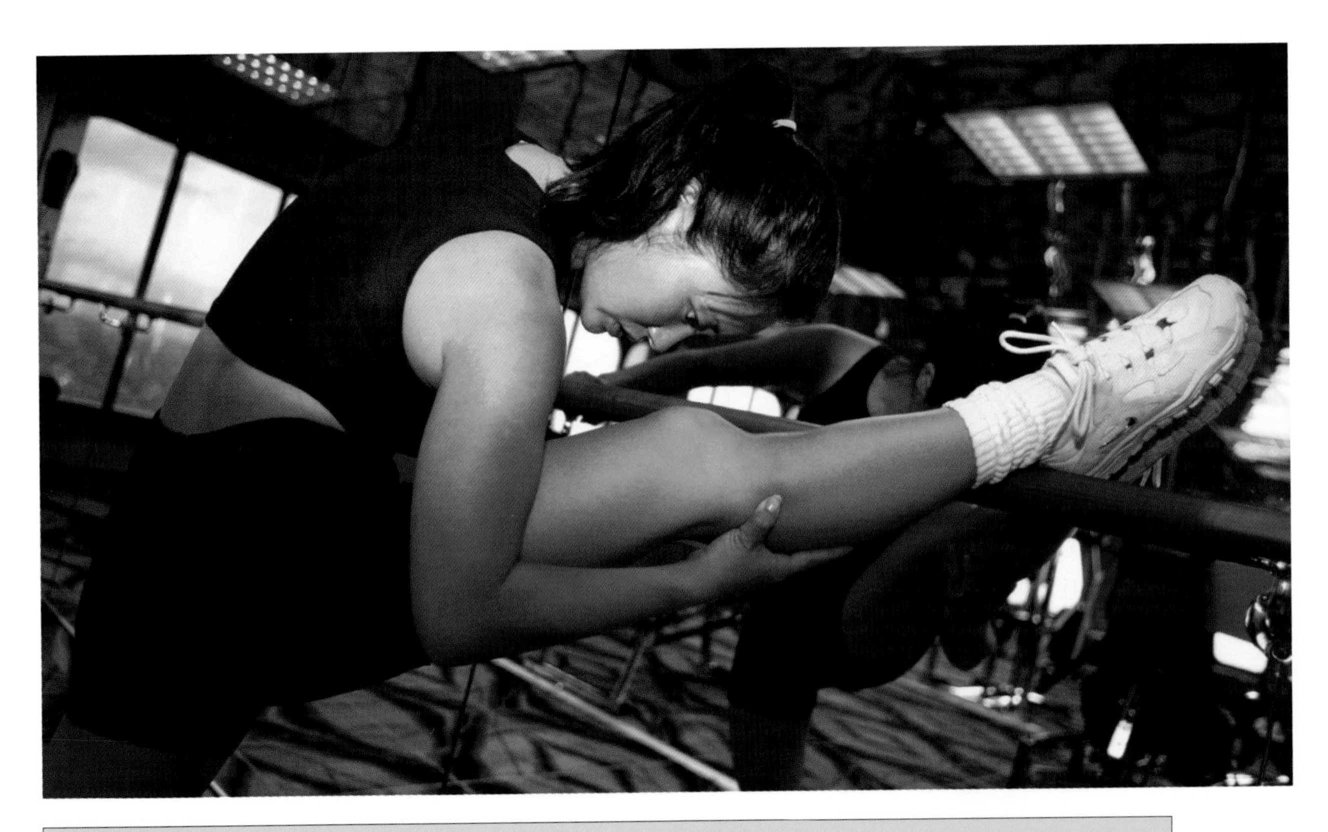

Figure 12.14 Loosening-up exercises are most beneficial after an exhausting exercise session.

muscle hypertrophy see Figure 5.9 in Chapter 5), whereas brisk exercise speeds develop power, or muscular explosiveness.

Number of Repetitions The number of repetitions and sets used is dependent upon the training method chosen and a trainee's performance level and goals. Generally, a lower number of repetitions per set promotes development of maximal strength and power (i.e., 5 to 12 repetitions are recommended for the increase of muscle diameter; 1 to 3 repetitions are sufficient to improve intramuscle coordination). A greater number of repetitions causes fatigue and is suitable for muscle endurance-type training.

Variety of Exercise The variety of exercise and the respective order of exercises within a training session must also be considered. The variety of exercises depends on the overall goal. Recreational athletes seeking to develop all-round strength of as many muscle groups as possible may train with over 40 different strength exercises.

Competitive athletes striving to develop strength capacities that are sport- or event-specific may find 3 to 5 exercises adequate. Weightlifters customarily include 8 to 12 different exercises in their regular training program. In comparison, bodybuilders use the greatest number of exercises by far in their training regimen, as they target almost all muscles of the body.

Principles of Fitness Training

Strength training is a fairly complicated process involving various pedagogical, biological, and psychological principles at many levels. Put into practice, these principles underlie a systematic approach to training and provide the necessary methodological guidelines. They should never be considered in isolation, but must be mastered and applied as a whole. They determine training in all its aspects: content, means, method, and organization. Training principles are not immutable laws, but in as much as they reflect general experience and successful practice, they embody values important to the coaches and athletes alike. Four of the more important training principles are presented in this section.

From Greek Mythology

In his youth, Milon of Croton (disciple of Pythagoras, scholar, and multiple Olympic wrestling champion in ancient Greece) decided to become the strongest man on earth. To achieve this he lifted and carried a calf every day. As the calf grew and became heavier, Milon's body adapted to the growing weight of the animal and became increasingly stronger. When the calf had grown into a bull and Milon a man, he had become the strongest man of his time.

Progressive Resistance or Overload Principle

The **overload principle** is based on a simple observation: new and progressively higher training demands enable athletes to adapt their physical and mental functions to increase performance capacity. After a period of time, an overloaded muscle will increase its strength and at some point the level of stress that was previously considered stressful or an overload will no longer provide an adequate overload stimulus. Thus, what was once an overload has now become a "normal load." To ensure the muscles/systems are being adequately overloaded, resistance should be periodically increased. Hence the principle of **progressive resistance**.

There are various ways of increasing load, depending on one's fitness level and the particular method of training used. For example, training volumes that may be maximal for a beginner may not be sufficient for an advanced athlete even to

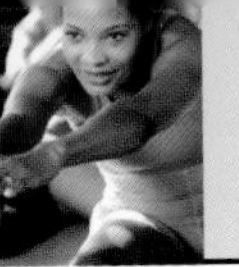

How to Overload

One way to determine whether to increase the load is by judging the number of times a given weight can be lifted before causing fatigue. For example, if one starts lifting 55 pounds (25 kg) 10 times, and after training for a length of time (two to five sessions), one can lift the same weight 15 times, then to increase muscle strength, the load should be increased to what can be lifted maximally (until exhaustion) 10 times. This new weight will most likely be 65 pounds (30 kg). This ensures that the muscles are working in the overload zone and the "signals" that stimulate adaptation are being sent to the muscles.

maintain his or her current performance level or capacity.

Generally speaking, an increase in training load affects all training components. However, training volume and training intensity are of special importance. Training load can be increased gradually or abruptly.

Gradual Load Increase Increasing training load gradually in small steps is recommended for beginners and recreational trainees. The training load is increased from one training cycle to another in small steps. An example is shown in the box *How to Overload.* In general, all training and individual exercises should be performed to the point of fatigue. **Gradual training load increase** also depends on training frequency, volume, and intensity, in that order.

Explosive Load Increase Abrupt or **explosive increase in training load** is especially effective in more serious training for competition. For training athletes, this method provides an important complement to gradual load increase. It requires a substantial increase in volume or intensity of training (or both) from one training cycle to another. Coaching experience has shown that much higher training load demands make explosive load increase highly effective.

Reversibility Principle

This principle implies the avoidance of long interruptions in the training process. Interruptions in training have a negative effect and result in stagnation or even decline of performance (**reversibility**). With a loss of training time, cardiorespiratory and muscular endurance performance decline faster than maximal strength or power performance.

The loss in performance due to training interruption applies to coordination and technical and tactical skills and abilities, as well as to the overall standard of performance, because all these factors are interrelated.

An athlete's training experience also has a bearing on the stagnation process caused by interruption in training. Athletes who have trained over many years are more resistant to performance loss than beginners. Highly trained athletes also tend to make up for loss in performance relatively quickly.

Specificity of Exercise Principle

Coaches often state "you play the way you practice" or "practice does not make perfect, it makes permanent." These statements are true and illustrate the principle of specificity. This principle states that the response(s) to exercise is specific to the nature or type of exercise performed. What this means is that if we wish to increase a particular fitness parameter, we must train that parameter in as specific a manner as possible. The principle of **specificity** applies to the specificity of strength, muscular and cardiorespiratory endurance, coordination, speed of movement, and motor patterns. Specificity should also take into account joint angles, neuromuscular components, and the speed of muscle contraction as well as the type of contraction. The point of this principle is that specific exercises cause specific physiological responses. Several examples of specificity are presented in the box on the following page.

Periodization of Training Principle

Periodization is a systematic division of the training year into periods that allow a coach to

When You Exercise for Performance, Be Specific!

- If you work out by pushing against immovable walls (static contractions), you will get strong at pushing walls but not at lifting weights, which requires dynamic contractions.
- It makes little sense for basketball players to practice shooting at an 8-foot basket if they have to shoot at a 10-foot one in a game.
- Running at 75 percent speed during training may help one learn what to do, but it provides little help when your opponent forces you to run at full speed.
- If one has to lift and/or move a 200-pound (90-kg) opponent, as in rugby, wrestling, or football, it makes little sense to work with a 155-pound (70-kg) dummy during training. Likewise, bench pressing 165 pounds (75 kg) will not be suitable in terms of specific strength demand and will provide little help during a game/event situation.
- Sprinters will do themselves little good if they train by running long distances.
- Sprinters are very good at running sprints or short distances. However, they are generally not very good at playing wide receiver in football because of the specificity of coordination (skill of catching the ball at full speed). In addition, running sprinters are also not very good at swimming sprints. Why? Specificity!

prepare players to perform at their optimum during competition (Table 12.1). There are three major periods in the training year: preparatory (PP), competition (CP), and transition periods (TP).

The individual periods are further subdivided into macrocycles (two to six weeks), microcycles (seven days), daily cycles (one to two training sessions), and training sessions (one to two hours).

The **periodization of training principle** can be applied to longer or shorter training cycles that are typical for high school and university sports schedules. Table 12.2 gives examples of possible periodization variations of different duration. Notice the changing relationships between preparatory and competition phases as the training cycles become shorter.

Preparation Period The prime objective of this period is the development of a high level of fitness on which the trainee can build in future periods. This stage is characterized by a gradual and progressive increase of volume of exercise (overload principle) at medium intensity levels.

Competitive Period One goal in the competitive period (league games, playoffs) is to maintain the level of fitness achieved in the preparation period. Both volume and intensity of fitness work are reduced because the main emphasis of this period is on sport-specific skill and tactics training.

Transition Period The transition period is relatively short, about two to four weeks, and is designed to offer the athlete a necessary break from

Table 12.1 Division of the training season into periods and subperiods.

	Training Period						
Periodization	Transition	Preparation		Competition			
	Transition	General Preparation	Specific Preparation	Pre-competition	Competition	Taper	Playoff

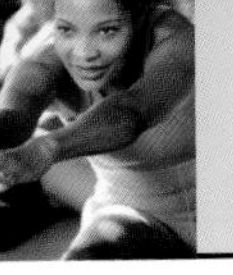

Table 12.2 Periodization of training.

Training Cycle	Training Period			
	Transition (wk)	Preparation (wk)	Competition (wk)	
			1st stage	2nd stage
12 months (52 weeks)	5	32	9	6
8 months (35 weeks)	4	20	5	6
6 months (26 weeks)	3	13	5	5
4 months (18 weeks)	2	8	3	5

Ratio between preparation and competition periods:
12 months approx. 70% : 30%
8 months approx. 65% : 35%
6 months approx. 55% : 45%
4 months approx. 50% : 50%

competition and intensive training. However, it is recommended that this time be used for recreation and circuit training activities to ensure that strength and muscular and cardiorespiratory endurance do not drop significantly.

Designing Fitness Training Programs

The major fitness training methods are presented in Table 12.3. These methods are designed to develop various forms of specific and general fitness. Strength and muscular endurance are developed by strength training methods, whereas aerobic and anaerobic capacity or fitness are developed by cardiovascular training methods. If combined, the two methods can improve overall fitness.

Resistance Training

Station Training

Station or dynamic resistance training promotes the development of strength by using free weights (popular with serious athletes) and strength training exercise machines with constant or variable resistance (popular with recreational athletes). **Station training** refers to the completion of all the sets of one exercise before moving to the next exercise. When performing a series of sets within a station, the same muscle groups are stressed over and over again. The optimal training stimulus for strength development is moderate to high intensity, 60 to 100 percent of 1RM. Therefore, this type of training requires relatively longer breaks between sets. And finally, it is important that any station training program be based on the agonist–antagonist training principle discussed at the beginning of the chapter.

The use of heavy free weights requires excellent lifting techniques, expert spotting, and well-maintained equipment. Since all of these requirements are rarely met in school programs, no further discussion on the method is provided here.

Circuit Training

Circuit training is an exercise program that allows an individual to combine specific exercises to achieve specific fitness goals. It embraces a number of carefully selected exercises designed to work all major muscle groups – legs, abdominals, arms, shoulders, back, and trunk – in one session. This aspect of circuit training is illustrated by the circuit training layout in Figure 12.15.

Table 12.3 An overview of fitness training methods and their effects.

Training Method	Training Effect
Resistance Training	
• Station training	• Strength fitness
• Circuit training	• Strength and muscular endurance fitness
Cardiorespiratory Training	
• Endurance training	• Aerobic fitness
• Fartlek training	• Aerobic fitness
• Interval training	
- extensive interval	• Aerobic* and anaerobic fitness
- intensive interval	• Aerobic and anaerobic* fitness
• Tempo or repetition training	• Activity-specific aerobic and anaerobic fitness
Combination Training	
• Combo circuit training	• Strength* and aerobic fitness
• Cross training	• Cardiorespiratory fitness

* *emphasized fitness development*

A circuit training program is a valuable and effective method of exercising used in many sports. By manipulating training components presented in previous sections, you can improve strength, muscular endurance, and cardiovascular endurance to varying degrees. With creativity and originality, a circuit exercise program can be designed that is difficult enough to challenge athletes at various levels. It can also be easily and very effectively incorporated into school physical education and athletic programs, as well as provide a valuable approach to fitness development for anyone whose objectives are to improve general fitness or lose weight.

Circuit Training Variables The major variables of circuit training programs include the number of exercises, sequence of exercises, number

Guidelines for Designing an Exercise Program

- Set ambitious but realistic goals for each training session; every effort should be made to fulfill them.
- Schedule training sessions, and record the performance achieved.
- Take note of the relationship between load, fatigue, and recovery during the planning and performance stages of training.
- Increase the training load according to training load principles.
- To avoid injury, warm up before training and cool down after exercise.
- Increase the training load properly, bearing in mind the relationship between the various training components. Concentrate on the essentials.
- Train over the whole year for several years. Avoid discontinuation of training, which may lead to stagnation and loss of performance.
- Monitor the quality of performance in each training session.
- Participate regularly in competitive contests. Compare the results achieved with the goals set.

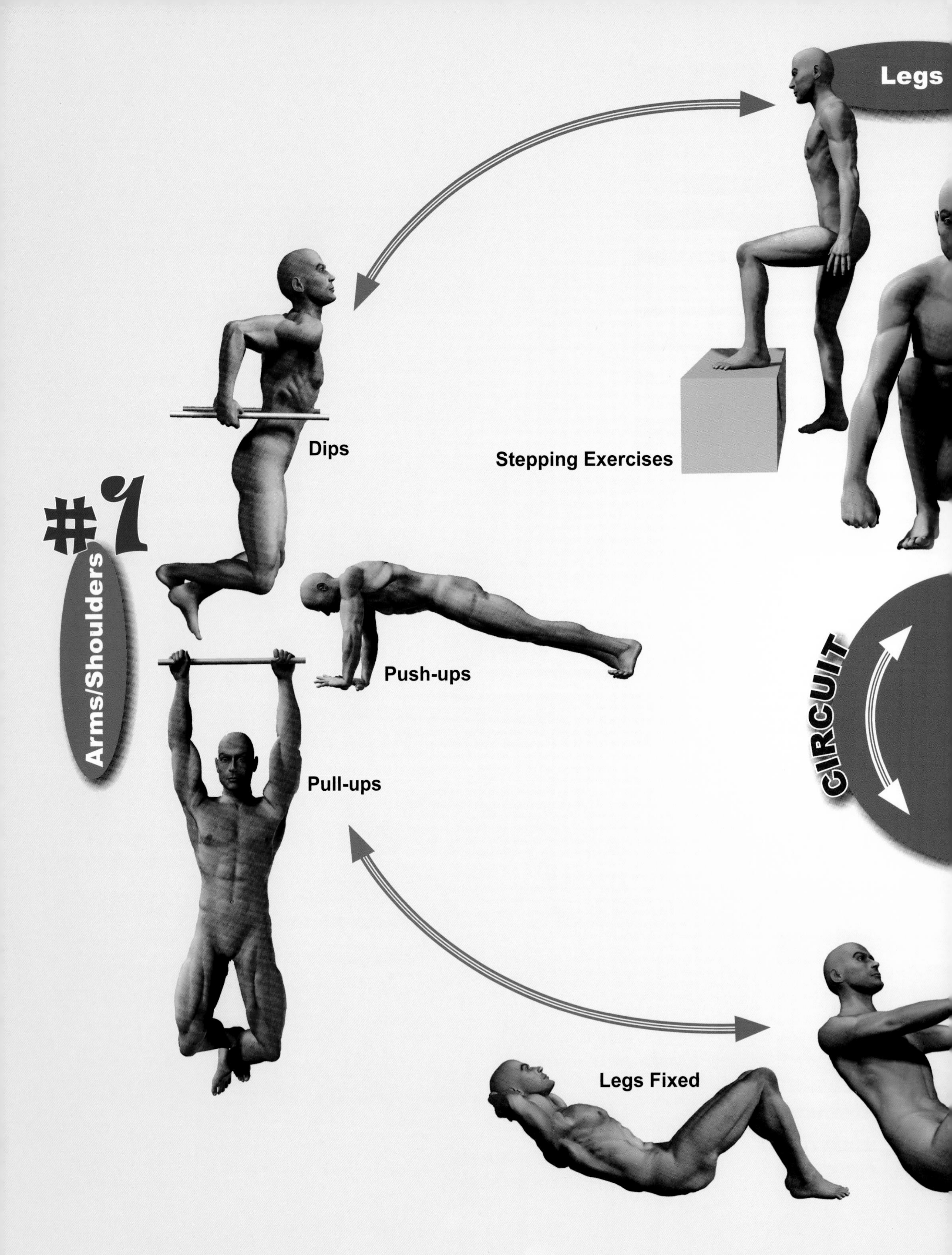
Legs
Dips
Stepping Exercises
#1
Arms/Shoulders
Push-ups
CIRCUIT
Pull-ups
Legs Fixed

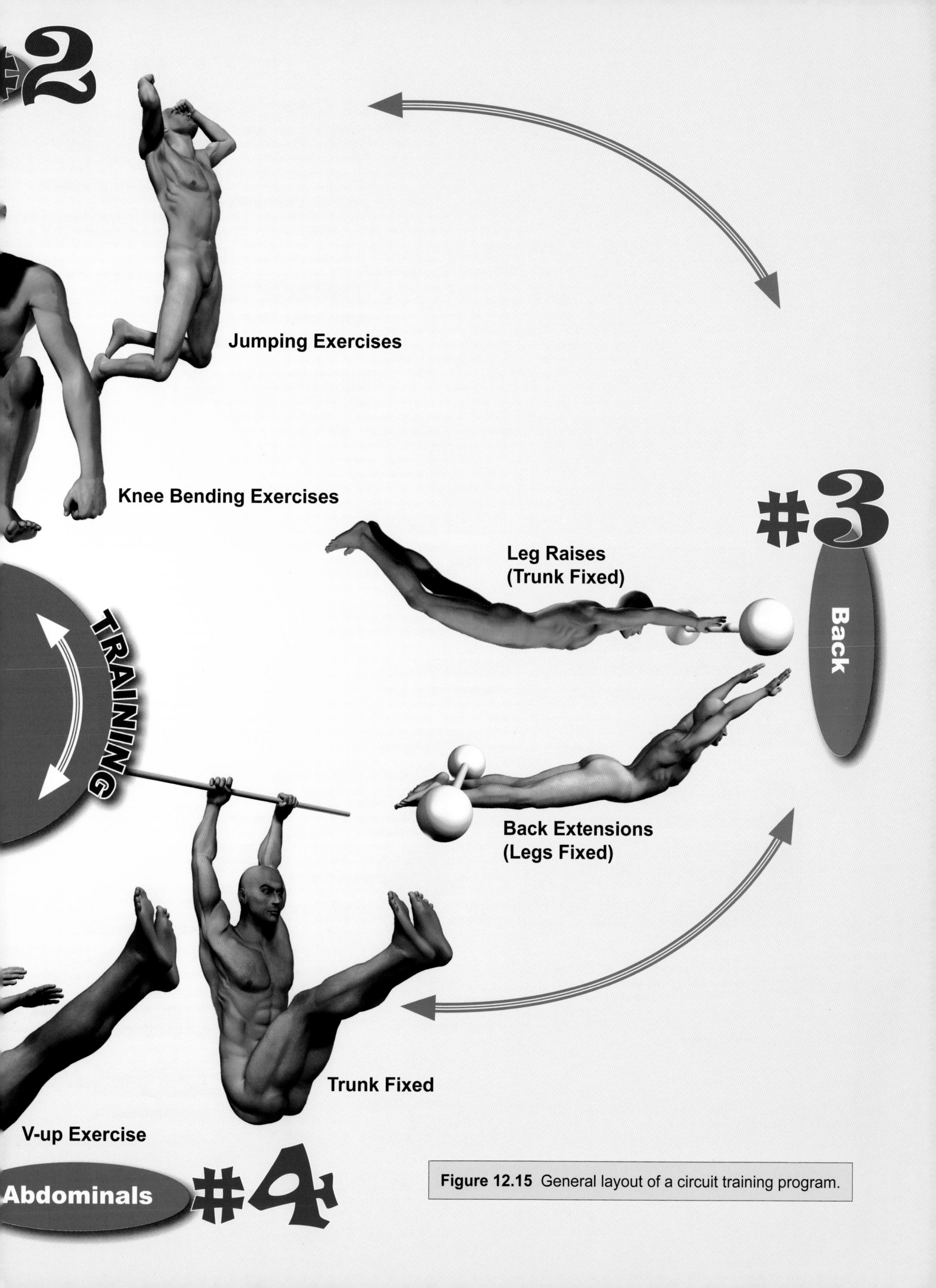

Figure 12.15 General layout of a circuit training program.

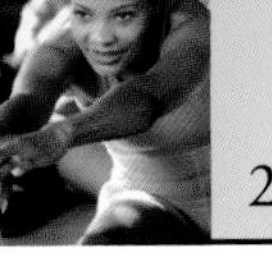

of trips around the circuit, number of repetitions, resistance levels, rest period between sets and circuits, and types of exercises.

- **Number of Stations** The circuit may consist of 6 to 18 stations of different exercises. Circuits with 8 to 12 stations are most popular. In a typical circuit exercise program, each muscle group may be successfully exercised by several different exercises. The number of exercises per muscle group depends on the trainee's needs and the training effect to be achieved.
- **Exercise Sequence** The loading of the main muscle groups changes as the trainee moves from one station to another. The sequence of exercises is arranged so that no two consecutive exercises involve the same muscle group. Thus, a set to develop the arm extensor muscles could be followed by a set to exercise the leg extensors. This, in turn, can be followed by exercises to develop the abdominals, and so on.
- **Number of Laps** A circuit is normally repeated one to three times. Competitive athletes may perform up to six laps during the preparation period.
- **Number of Repetitions and Level of Resistance** The number of repetitions per exercise depends on the objective of training: muscular endurance development requires 8 to 15 repetitions per exercise using 30 to 60 percent resistance; strength development requires 2 to 4 repetitions per exercise at 80 to 90 percent resistance.
- **Recovery Between Exercises** The recovery between exercises and laps depends on the training objectives: for muscular endurance development, relatively short or no recovery is planned (the trainee moves from one exercise station to another with no interruption in exercising); for strength development the rest intervals are longer, allowing good recovery between exercise sets and circuit laps.
- **Types of Exercises** Circuit training can be carried out by using a great variety of means: own body weight, partner-assisted exercises, medicine balls, dumbbells, barbells, and exercise machines.

Popular Circuits The structure of three popular circuit training programs is shown in Table 12.4.

Table 12.4 General structure of three popular circuits designed for general or specific fitness development for school or club programs.

Variation 1
- 10-12 exercise stations
- 30 s on, 30-60 s off (perform as many repetitions as possible in 30 s; followed by 30 s recovery)
- instructor uses whistle to indicate start and end of exercising; commands can be prerecorded
- trainee records number of repetitions achieved/station (example: 15/7)

Variation 2
- 10-12 exercise stations
- 10-15 repetitions at each station
- set exercise time to 10 minutes
- no recovery between stations
- trainee records number of laps and number of exercises achieved in the last lap (example: 2/7)

Variation 3
- 10-12 exercise stations
- 10-15 repetitions at each station
- no recovery between stations
- trainee records total time achieved per circuit (example: 8:27 min)

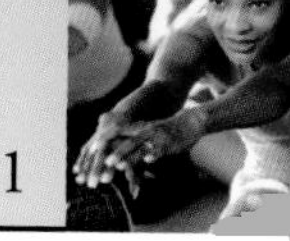

Cardiorespiratory Training

The interaction among the components of training, notably training volume and training intensity, is reflected in the various training methods, which characteristically use different ranges of relative intensity. The transition between these ranges of intensity is fluid and is reflected in the four basic training methods: endurance, Fartlek, interval, and repetition (Figure 12.16).

Endurance Training

Endurance training, also known as **continuous training** or **slow long distance (SLD) training**, involves training at approximately 40 to 60 percent of maximal performance ability over a long distance. Typically, SLD training is carried out without a break (Figure 12.17 A). The intensity and duration of exercise are typically "conversational," whereby the trainees are able to talk without undue respiratory distress.

The physiological benefits derived from SLD training primarily include enhanced aerobic capacity and development of staying power. Psychological benefits include increased determination and self-confidence and the ability to resist fatigue and mobilize oneself for hard sustained work.

The major objective of SLD training is to develop a solid fitness base during the preparatory season. Many athletes use it in the transitory season as well. The SLD training method combined with Fartlek training (Table 12.5), discussed in the next section, forms the bulk of fitness training of many competitive and recreational athletes.

Fartlek Training

Fartlek is an endurance training method used by runners mainly during the preparatory season. It is designed to develop basic endurance using an extremely flexible training program that can be done just about anywhere, any time, and all year.

Table 12.5 Sample training week for a serious high school cross-country program during the preparatory phase of training.

Sunday	Monday	Tuesday	Wednesday	Thursday	Friday	Saturday
Rest	40-60 min SLD	40-50 min Fartlek training	40 min SLD	20-25 min extensive interval	40-50 min SLD	40-50 min Fartlek training

Table 12.6 Sample Fartlek training session for a high school cross-country program.

Preparation Phase	Main Body Phase	Conclusion Phase
• Stretch • 10-min easy run	• 100 m at race pace • 2 min easy • 250 m at fast pace • 3 min easy • 400 m at fast pace • 3 min easy • 50 m at all-out pace • 4 min easy • 300 m at race pace • 3 min easy • 600 m at fast pace	• 10-min easy run • Stretch

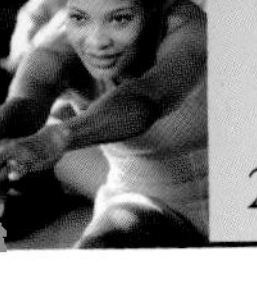

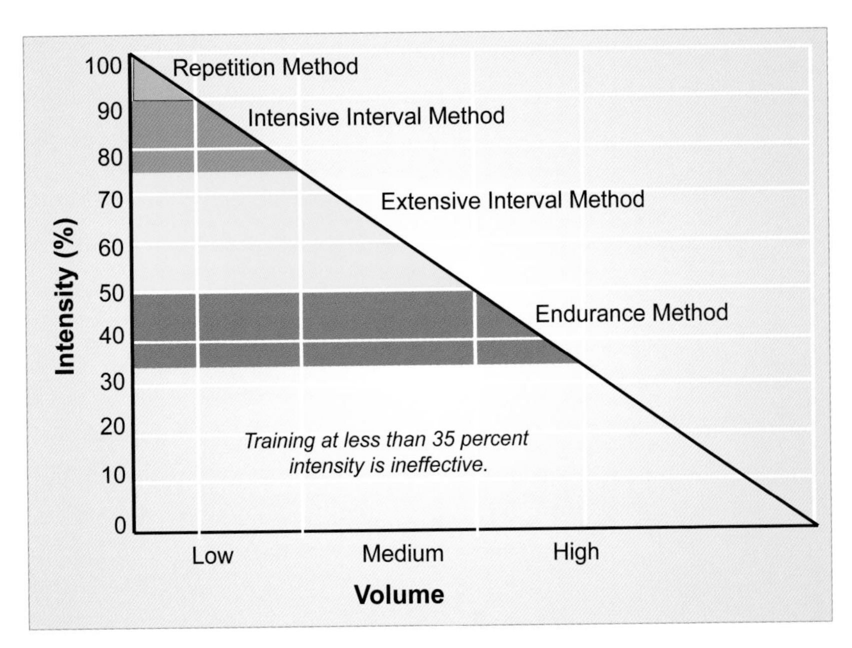

Figure 12.16 Cardiorespiratory training methods as a function of intensity and volume of exercise.

Fartlek combines slow long distance training, pace/tempo training, and interval training. It involves easy running, fast bursts of running of varying lengths, hill running, and running on the beach, in parks, on streets, and so on (Table 12.6). This basic format can also be applied to cycling, swimming, cross-country skiing, and skating. Because it is such a diverse workout, you can create a Fartlek training program for yourself or challenge an exercise partner to come up with a new workout every other week.

Commonly Asked Questions About Fartlek

- ***What's in the name?*** Fartlek is a Swedish word meaning "speed play" or "playing with speed."
- ***How often?*** Once a week almost all year round; more often (two or three times per week) during the preparatory season.
- ***What intensity and how far or how long?*** Depending on your feeling at the time, you can go as fast or as slow for as short or as long as you wish.
- ***What rest?*** For beginners, run slowly until you're breathing comfortably (conversational pace) before starting the next speed surge.
- ***Where?*** Fartlek can be done anywhere and in a variety of different ways.

Interval Training

Aerobic and anaerobic capacity or fitness (discussed in Chapters 6 and 7) are most effectively developed by interval training, which involves the systematic alternation of exertion and recovery. The constant repetition of physical stress causes continuous breakdown of high-energy substances in the working muscles and at the same time generates an ongoing increase in the buildup of fatigue.

We distinguish between extensive and intensive interval training methods.

Extensive Interval This method requires the trainee to carry out a great number of repetitions of selected distance in one session (Figure 12.17 B) with a recovery period equal to the work interval, thereby keeping the work-to-rest ratio (W:R) at 1:1-2 between intervals and 1:2-4 between sets. Each exercise (running, cycling, swimming, or cross-country skiing) is repeated 20 to 30 times. The repetitions are divided into several sets (Figure 12.17 B). The training intensity in the extensive interval method is higher than in the previous two (SLD and Fartlek training). It is between 60 to

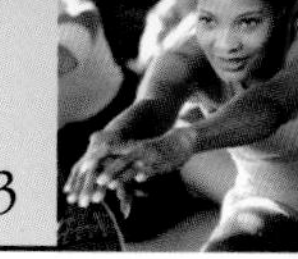

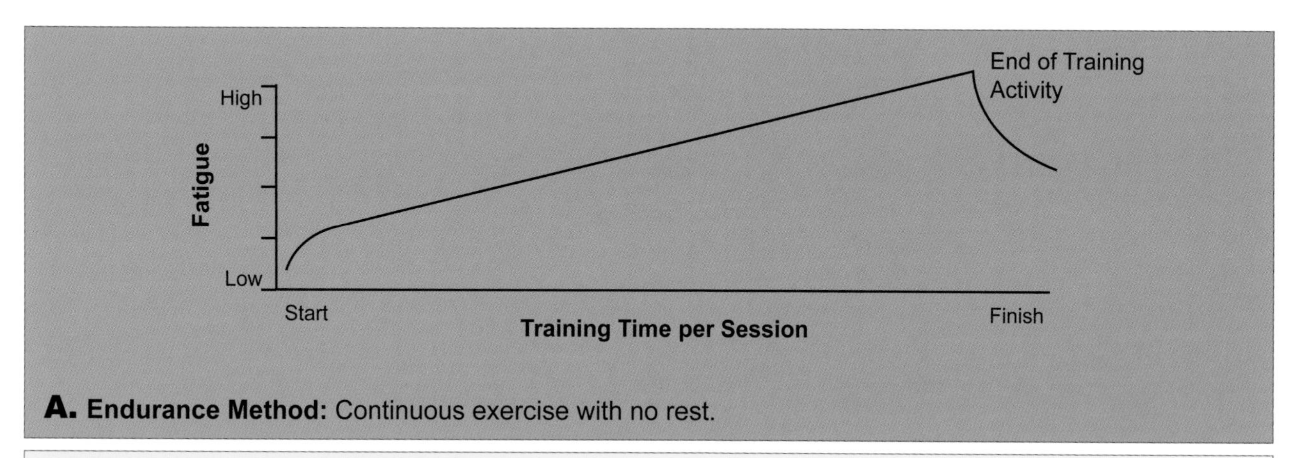

A. Endurance Method: Continuous exercise with no rest.

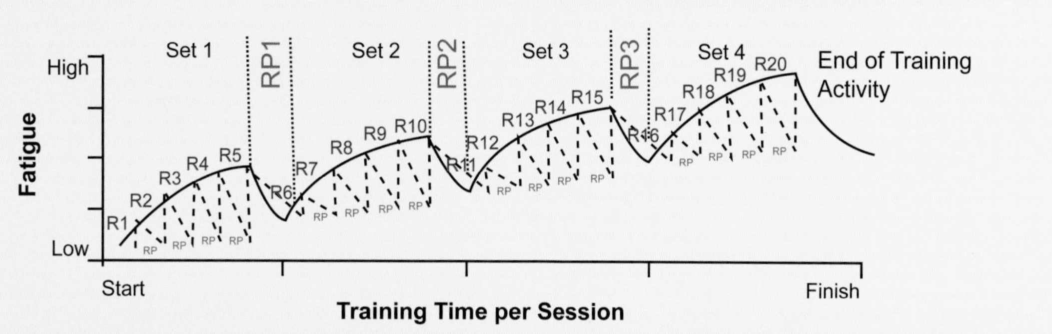

B. Extensive Interval Method: 4 sets of 5 repetitions of exercise; recovery between repetitions and sets.

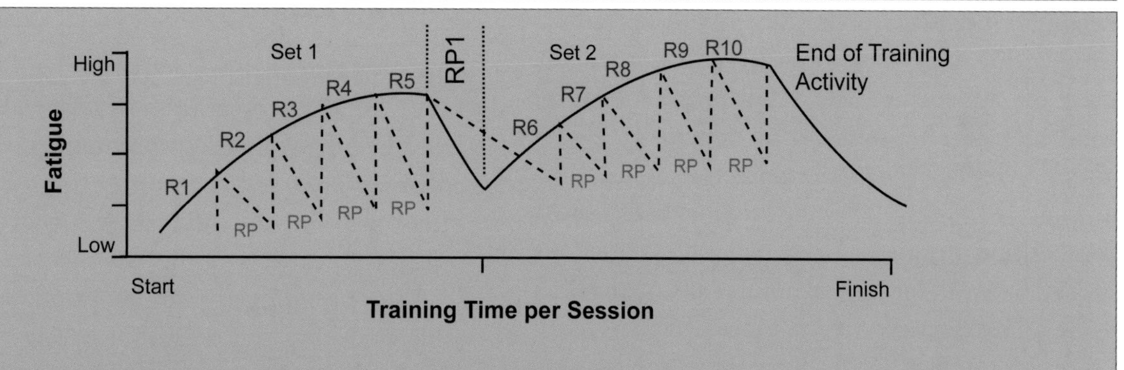

C. Intensive Interval Method: 2 sets of 5 repetitions of exercise; recovery between repetitions and sets.

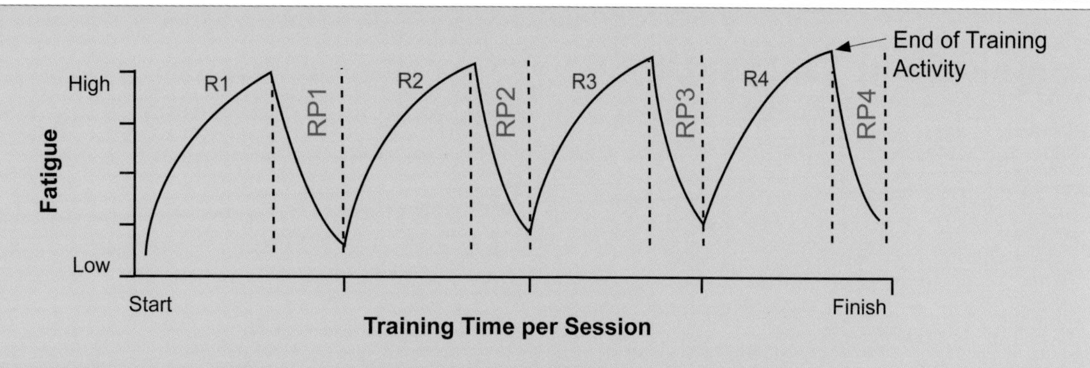

D. Repetition Method: 4 repetitions of exercise with long recovery between each.

Figure 12.17 The number of training intervals (repetitions per set), number of sets, and accumulation of fatigue for the four aerobic/anaerobic fitness training methods (R = repetition; RP = rest period).

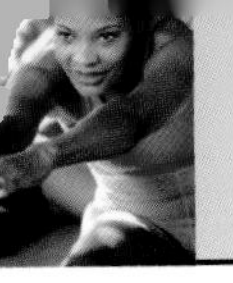

80 percent of the trainee's maximal performance capacity. This method predominately stresses the development of the aerobic energy system.

Intensive Interval This method features an overall lower training volume – each interval is repeated 10 to 20 times – than the extensive interval method, performed at a higher intensity level, 80 to 90 percent of the trainee's maximal performance capacity (Figure 12.17 C). Each interval taxes the individual close to $\dot{V}O_2max$. Therefore it requires longer breaks: W:R is approximately 1:2-3 between intervals and 1:4-6 between sets.

Because intensive interval training is very demanding, it should not be practiced until a solid fitness base of aerobic training has been attained through previously discussed methods.

Repetition Training

Repetition or tempo training is conducted at maximal intensity levels. The method mimics competition pace and intensity and is therefore used by athletes in the final preparations for competition. The duration of exercise at all-out intensity level is normally longer than the ones in interval training. It often extends to the entire competition distance. Long recovery periods are needed between individual bouts, causing the W:R to be approximately 1:5 or longer (Figure 12.17 D). An example of a training week with repetition training is shown in Table 12.7.

Combination Training

Combination training programs offer multiple benefits for the trainee. They simultaneously develop both muscular and cardiorespiratory fitness. These programs are particularly popular with recreational athletes, who use them all year round. Because of their general nature, serious athletes use them only in the transition period.

Combo Circuit Training

In addition to strength exercises, a circuit may include running laps between stations. The distance of the running segment may vary between 50 and 400 meters depending on the available facility and specific needs of the trainee. If, for example, a soccer or football team goes through a circuit program (using partner exercises, Figure 12.18) on the field, each run may involve running once around the track (i.e., 400 meters); in comparison, a basketball team doing the same circuit on a basketball court may run once around the gym, covering only about 80 meters.

Cross Training

Cross training involves activities that offer aerobic fitness benefits similar to those offered by running. In addition, it can also promote total body fitness and may help prevent overuse injuries. Runners often use this method when recovering from injuries.

Cross training is popular among competitive athletes during the transition period. To provide variety and prevent boredom and burnout, recreational athletes use cross training throughout the year.

Aerobic cross training may involve cycling, swimming, cross-country skiing, water running, and skating. **Muscular endurance cross training**

Table 12.7 Sample training week for a serious high school cross-country program during the competition phase of training (one week prior to competition).

Sunday	Monday	Tuesday	Wednesday	Thursday	Friday	Saturday
Rest	40-50 min Fartlek training	40-50 min SLD	40 min extensive interval	20-25 min intensive interval	40-50 min SLD	20-30 min repetition

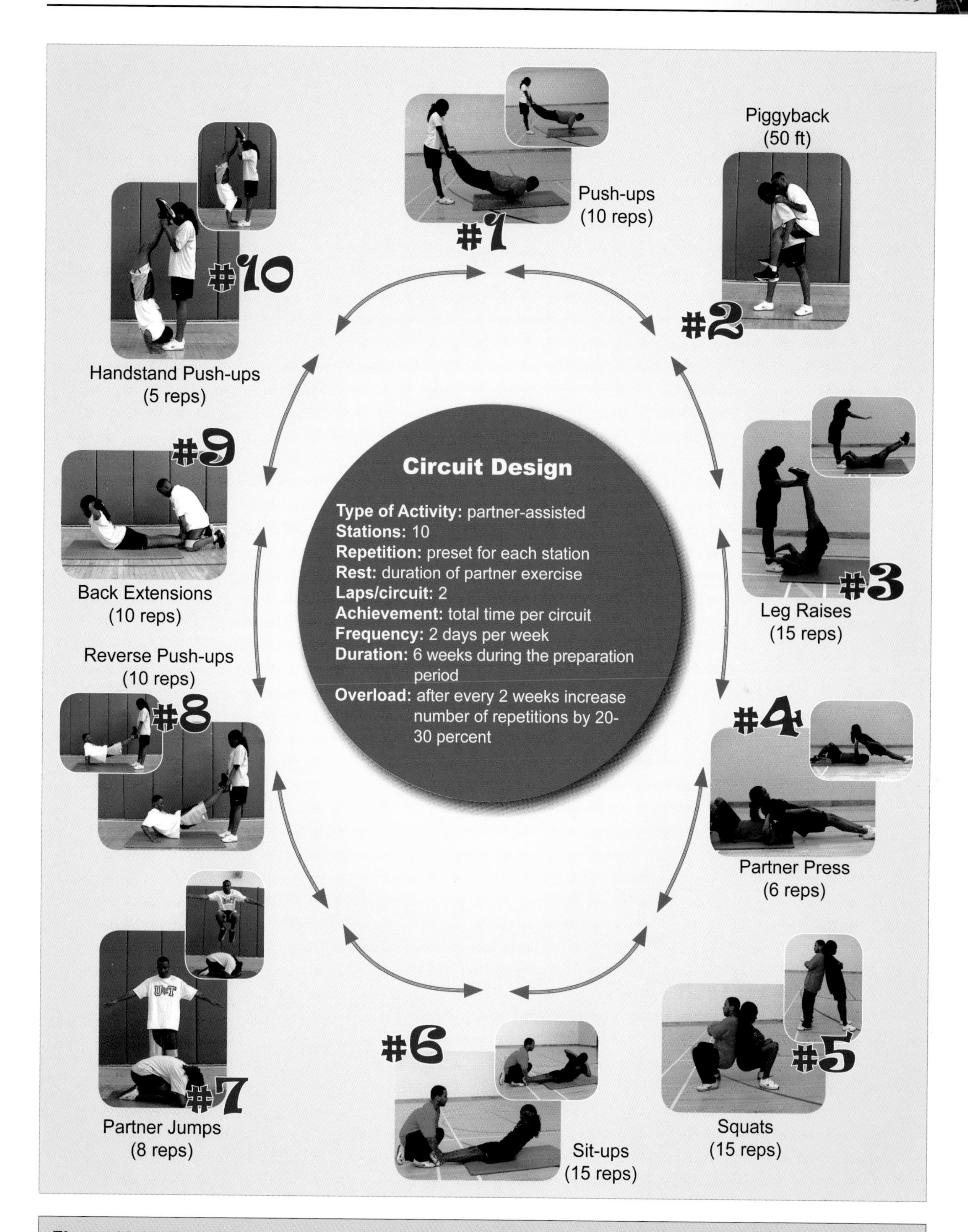

Figure 12.18 Sample circuit with partner-assisted exercises, for high school varsity teams' general fitness development. For partner-assisted exercises, it is important that team members form partner pairs of similar size.

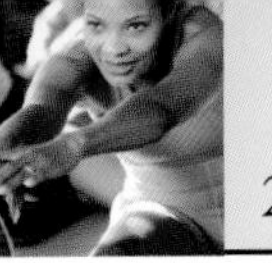

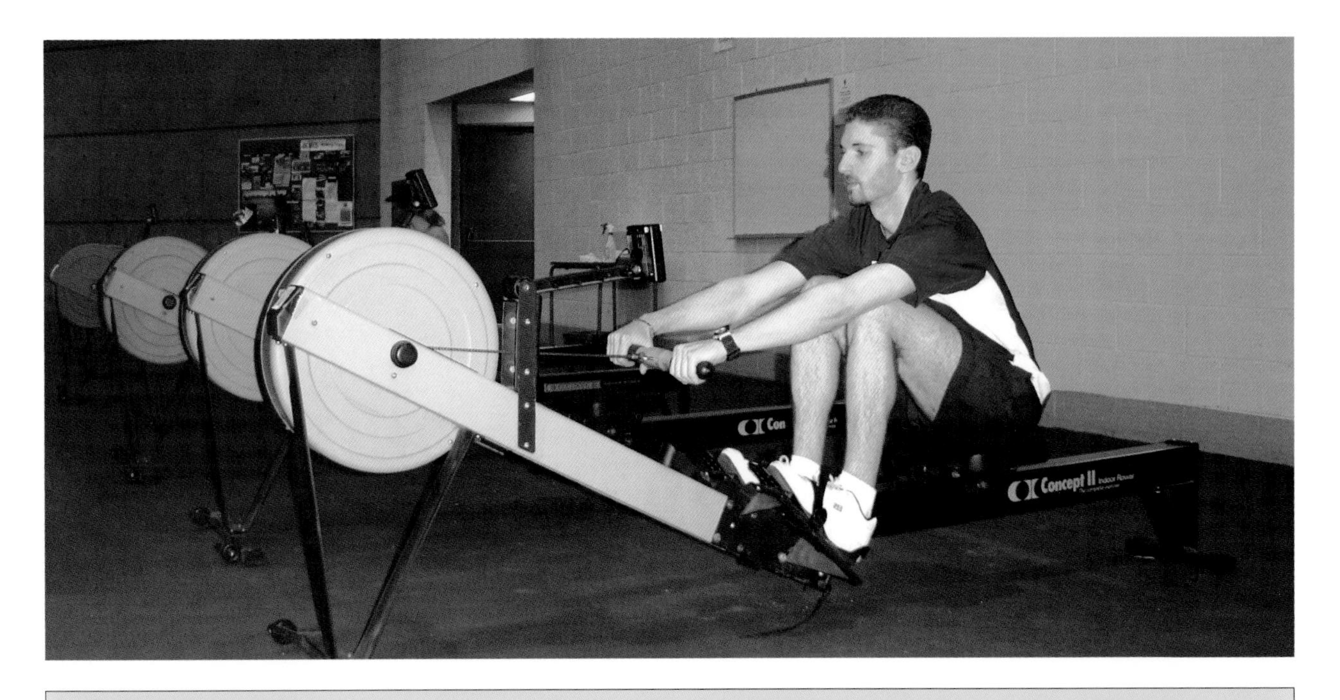

Figure 12.19 Working on a Concept II rowing machine requires little skill but provides great fitness benefits.

may involve working on a rowing machine, StairMaster, cycling ergometer, and NordicTrack (Figure 12.19). **Activity cross training** may involve participating in several different activities (Figure 12.20).

Summary

The concept of physical fitness deals with factors that have a positive impact on your lifestyle, helping to maintain and significantly improve your health through active living. Physical fitness encompasses many components that are important for health, including strength, power, endurance, flexibility, body composition, and psychomotor abilities. Resistance training using free weights, exercise

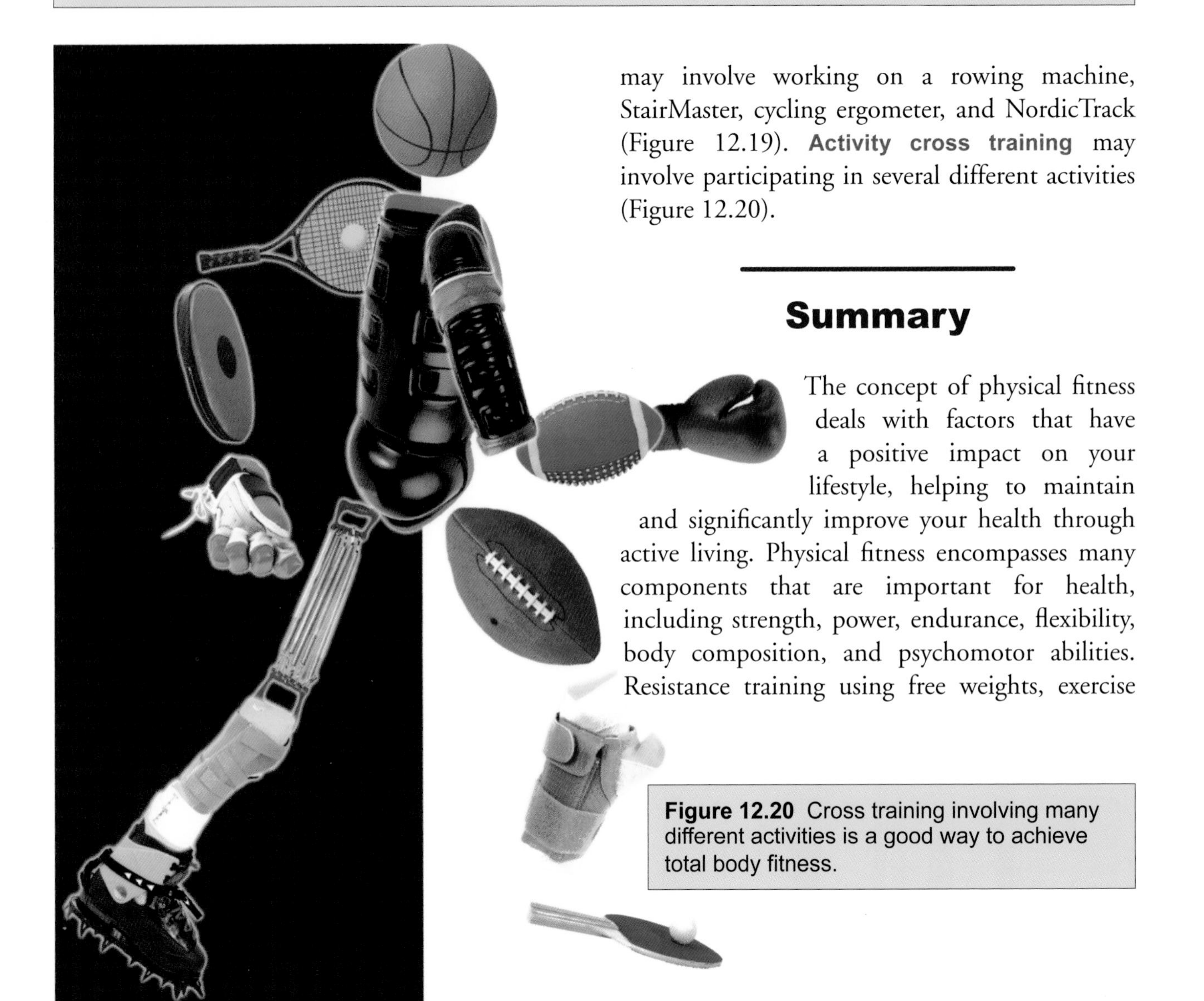

Figure 12.20 Cross training involving many different activities is a good way to achieve total body fitness.

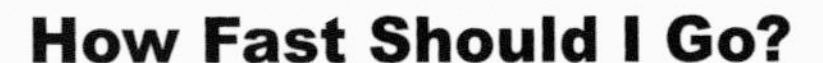

How Fast Should I Go?

How much exercise is enough to maintain or improve health fitness? Two simple measures can be used to answer this question: the breath sound check and the talk test.

If you wish to maintain or improve your general health, moderate-intensity activity is adequate. The **breath sound check** is an easy way to determine when this minimum level of activity has been reached. You want to reach your **ventilatory threshold**, which is the point at which you just start to hear your breathing. In other words, you should be able to hear your breathing when you perform aerobic exercise.

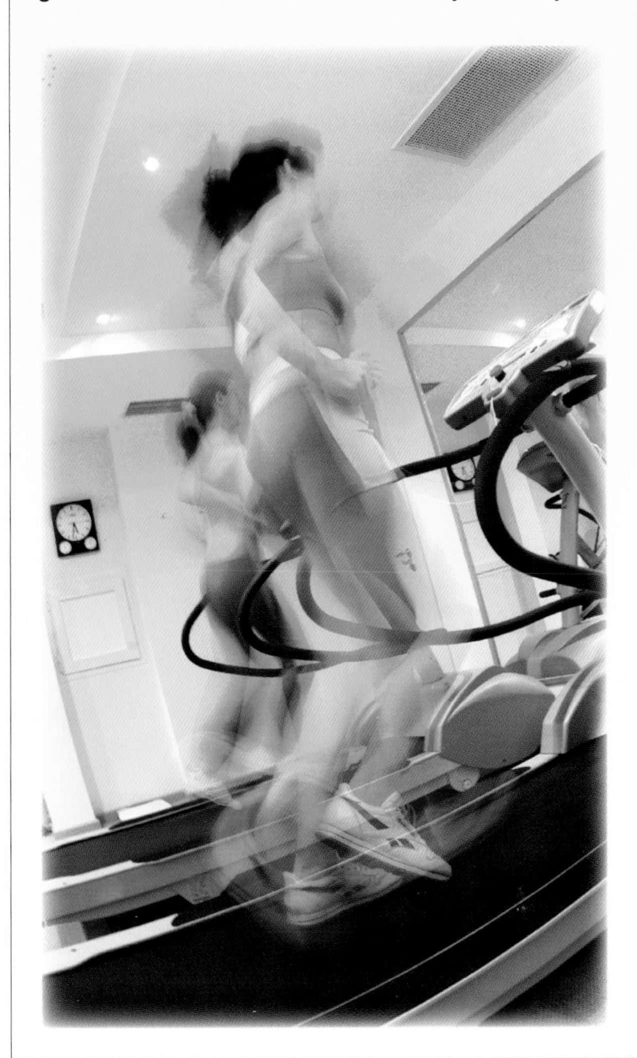

The **talk test** is based on the principle that you should be able to carry on a conversation while exercising. If you find that you have difficulty talking and are out of breath, you are working above the ventilatory threshold and have reached an anaerobic level.

To establish your ventilatory threshold, jog slowly or walk vigorously for one minute. Increase the pace until the sound of your breathing is audible, and maintain the pace that gives you that sound level. If you can hear your breathing and are able to talk, you are at or close to the ventilatory threshold. Individuals who participate regularly in physical activity have higher ventilatory thresholds and are able to do more before breathing sounds become audible, while less active individuals will hear their breathing much sooner.

On the other hand, if you want to participate in more vigorous activities such as hockey, squash, or track and field, you may be interested in rapid gains or larger improvements in your anaerobic threshold. The **anaerobic threshold** is the point at which your body's main source of fuel comes from your short-term energy store, the lactic acid system (see Chapter 6). While working at his level may not improve your health any more than moderate activity, it can improve your performance fitness. Programs designed to improve both health and performance fitness are possible.

machines, your own body weight, or partner-assisted exercises can be used to develop and maintain muscular strength.

One measure of cardiorespiratory endurance is maximal oxygen uptake, or $\dot{V}O_2max$. $\dot{V}O_2max$ represents the maximal volume of oxygen that can be supplied to and consumed by the body and is the most important criterion of physical fitness. Relative $\dot{V}O_2max$ is a useful way of comparing the cardiovascular fitness of athletes across different disciplines. Cardiorespiratory endurance can be enhanced through four different types of training: endurance training, Fartlek, interval training, and repetition or tempo training.

Flexibility, the ability of a joint to move through its full range of motion, can be improved by three methods: static stretching, dynamic stretching, and proprioceptive neuromuscular facilitation

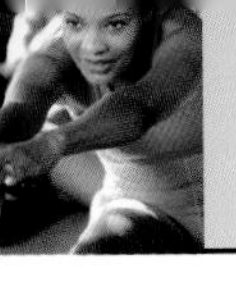

(PNF). PNF is considered the most effective technique. Psychomotor abilities (e.g., reaction time, coordination, concentration, and balance) help an athlete monitor and respond to his or her environment.

When developing a strength or cardiovascular fitness program, several components must be taken into account, such as training time, frequency, volume, and intensity. Work-to-rest ratio depends on the training intensity and describes the amount of rest needed between the phases of a workout. The type of exercise, exercise speed, number of repetitions, and order of performance also must be considered when building an exercise program.

Several important principles offer training guidelines for athletes and coaches. The overload principle specifies that progressive resistance is required to increase performance as a muscle adapts to a given load. On the other hand, if load is decreased or training is interrupted, a loss in fitness gains will result. This outlines the reversibility principle. The principle of specificity requires that exercises be specific to the desired result. For example, a sprinter will not improve performance by running long distance. Finally, the periodization principle allows a coach to divide the training year into three periods (preparation, competition, and transition) and develop training regimens suitable for each stage.

A popular exercise method for both serious and recreational athletes is circuit training. Circuit training combines and manipulates exercises to achieve specific fitness goals. With combination circuit training, gains in strength, muscular endurance, and cardiovascular endurance can be achieved simultaneously.

Knowing how and when to exercise can have a significant impact on how enjoyable and rewarding your experiences are with physical fitness. The secret lies in putting together a fitness plan that is right for you as an individual. By setting realistic goals and following the training principles outlined in this chapter, you are well on your way to a lifetime of rewarding physical activity.

Key Terms

absolute $\dot{V}O_2max$
active flexibility
activity cross training
aerobic cross training
aerobic power ($\dot{V}O_2max$)
agonist–antagonist training
anaerobic threshold
body composition
breath sound check
cardiorespiratory (cardiovascular) endurance
circuit training
collagen
continuous training
dynamic (ballistic) stretching
elastin
endurance training
exercise
explosive training load increase
fartlek
flexibility
gradual load increase
muscular endurance
muscular endurance cross training
muscular strength
passive flexibility
periodization of training principle
physical activity
physical fitness
power
progressive resistance (overload) principle
proprioceptive neuromuscular facilitation (PNF) stretching
psychomotor ability
relative $\dot{V}O_2max$
reversibility principle
slow long distance (SLD) training
specificity of exercise principle
static stretching
station training
talk test
training frequency
training intensity
training time
training volume
ventilatory threshold

Discussion Questions

1. List the components of physical fitness described in this chapter. Explain how each dimension relates to physical fitness.

2. What is antagonist training? Why is it important that antagonist training be incorporated into a strength training schedule?

3. Describe the various methods used to promote muscular strength, muscular endurance, and cardiorespiratory endurance.

4. Distinguish between $\dot{V}O_2max$, absolute $\dot{V}O_2max$, and relative $\dot{V}O_2max$. List the appropriate units of measurement for each.

5. Why is flexibility work important for one's health? What are some of the established flexibility methods? Which of the methods is most effective?

6. Discuss the relevance of psychomotor abilities as a component of fitness.

7. Identify the principles of exercise training and explain how each dimension affects the planning of a fitness program.

8. Identify five components of an effective cardiorespiratory and muscular fitness program. Briefly explain the important characteristics of each component.

9. Describe the elements of a circuit exercise training program. How can you incorporate circuit training into your overall fitness regimen?

10. How can people improve their muscular and cardiorespiratory endurance in one workout?

In This Chapter:

CHAPTER 13

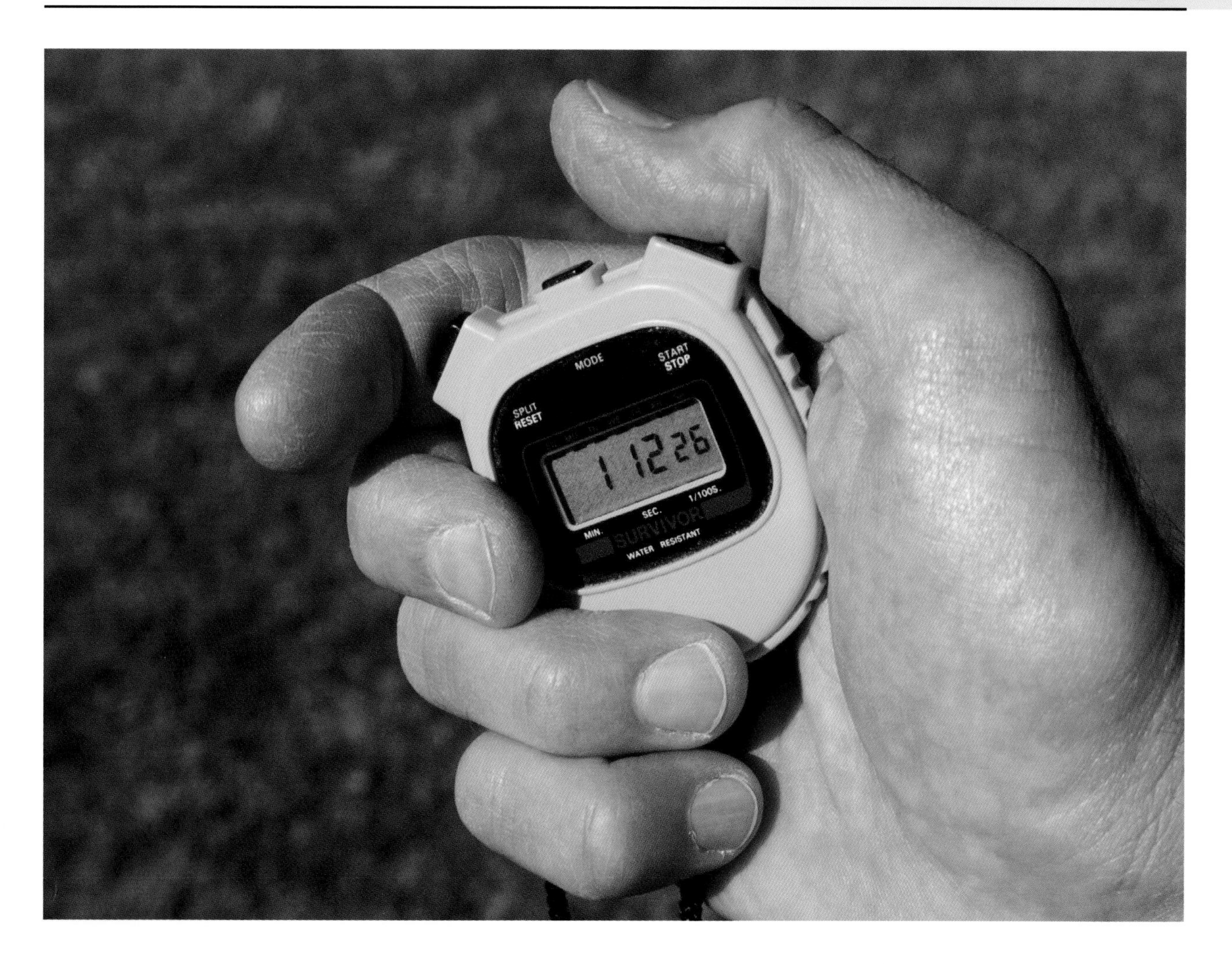

What's My Score? Evaluation in Kinesiology

After completing this chapter you should be able to:

- discuss the usefulness and application of testing, measurement, and evaluation;
- outline the criteria for the evaluation and selection of tests;
- describe a variety of practical and economical tests that are useful to the average physical education teacher and student in various performance areas;
- administer these tests to yourself and others in a reliable and valid manner.

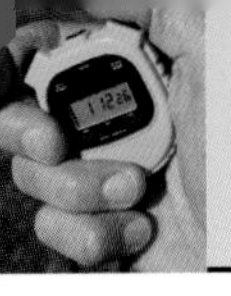

In the field of human performance, testing, measurement, and evaluation serve an important purpose. We all make evaluative decisions on a daily basis, although the soundness of these decisions varies with the information we use to make them. In order to make accurate judgments, we must first accumulate relevant information, organize it, and evaluate this information in order to draw conclusions that support our eventual decisions. During election years, for example, numerous surveys are conducted in order to inform voters about how the candidates are faring in their campaigns. This provides us with relevant information that is applicable to the evaluation and decision process.

What would it be like to go through life without knowing what effect nutrition has on performance, or how smoking affects our health? It seems that virtually everything we do is based on research and testing that has been (or is being) done. Whether we make decisions concerning who we should vote for, what kinds of foods we should eat, what sport to pursue, or how much we should exercise, these decisions are only properly made with the aid of testing, measurement, and evaluation.

In order to effectively gather, sort, analyze, and evaluate relevant information before making a decision, you must determine whether that information is reliable, valid, and objective. Ultimately, the effectiveness of a decision can be traced to the relevance and quality of the information used to make the decision.

Take fitness appraisals as an example. In a society that has become increasingly preoccupied with issues of weight, health, and exercise, obtaining a precise evaluation of your fitness level is becoming correspondingly more important. People want to know how they can improve their health through exercise, which aspects of their fitness should be improved, and where they fit in with the rest of the population. The evaluation you receive from simple field tests (Figure 13.1) or modern laboratories can reveal whether your physical condition is consistent with good health and can help you plan a program that is appropriate for your level of fitness, making exercise more enjoyable and individually rewarding.

Purposes of Testing and Evaluation

Why is it important to have skill and knowledge in performing correct and effective measurement and evaluation? Some of the reasons are illustrated by Kevin's story (see box *Test for Success*). When Kevin decided to use testing to evaluate his performance, this provided him with motivation and the means by which he could easily and objectively monitor his improvement. Using specific tests to monitor your performance can be an ideal way to stay motivated and to work toward continual improvement. However, it is important to remember that the

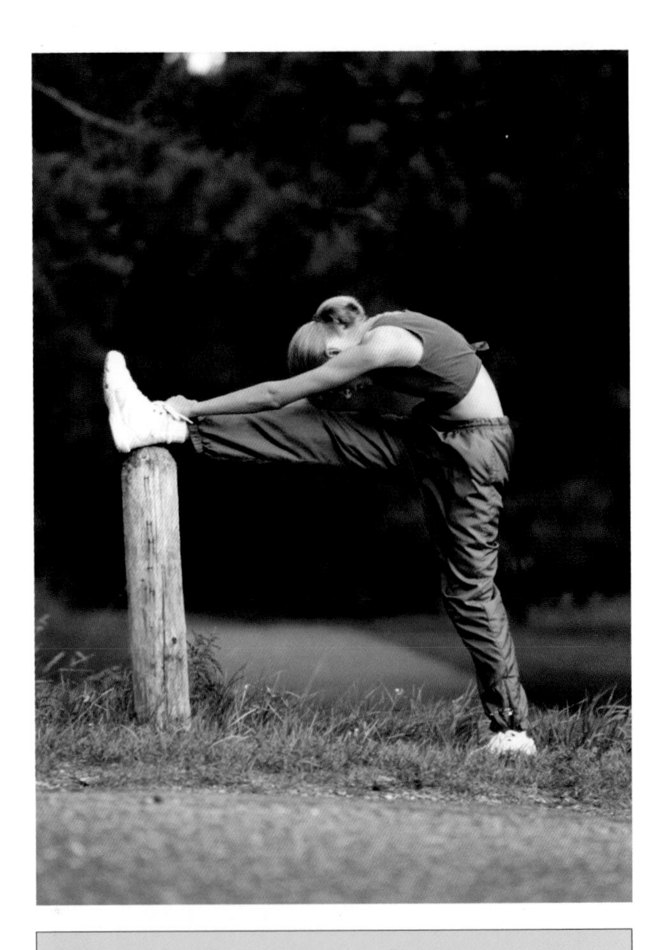

Figure 13.1 Simple tests of flexibility can be good indicators of your general level of fitness.

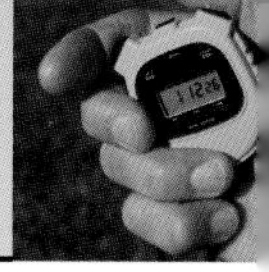

Test for Success

Kevin loved to play basketball. If he wasn't doing homework or watching television, you could be sure he was shooting a few hoops outside in his driveway. But despite his love for the game and his willingness to practice for hours on end, he could not seem to make his high school basketball team. He had tried out for the team the previous two years and was one of the last players to be cut on each occasion. This left Kevin dejected and lacking confidence – he almost considered giving up basketball altogether.

Instead, the season continued and Kevin decided to sit in on a few of the team's practices with the permission of the coach. He watched carefully and made note of some of the tests and drills the team used to evaluate and improve their skills, and he decided that he would use some of them to monitor his own performance during the off-season. When summer came around, Kevin was excited and had renewed interest in pursuing basketball.

Kevin decided to use a free-throw shooting test to begin, since shooting accuracy was one of his primary weaknesses. He simply recorded the number of free-throw shots he could make in 20 attempts. Most players on the team could make at least 14 out of 20 shots, so he set a goal of attaining this base level of achievement. His first day of practice, he only made 11 out of 20 shots. But persistent practice and steady improvement brought with it motivation; after just three and a half weeks, he was consistently making 16 out of 20 free-throw attempts–a higher percentage than many players on the team were shooting. Delighted with his improvement on the free-throw shooting test, he tried out another drill that tested his dribbling ability and ball control. He tested himself with several similar drills in the remaining summer months, until he felt he had improved adequately.

Finally, the basketball season arrived. Kevin was nervous about his chances this year, but the measurement and evaluation process he endured during the summer provided the challenge, stimulation, and confidence he needed to make the team. Kevin tried out for the team and not only made the roster but also cracked the starting lineup just three games into the season. He went on to have a very productive season and became a respected team leader.

most important consideration is the selection of valid tests that are reliable and meet your needs for time and effort.

Although there are many other reasons for testing, we will focus on six general reasons to illustrate its importance to students, teachers, and researchers in the field of physical education and human performance.

Diagnosis

Once a test has been administered, the results may be evaluated to identify deficiencies or weaknesses in the subjects – in other words, to make a **diagnosis.** Whether it be a student, athlete, medical patient, or fitness appraisal subject, one can effectively use testing and measurement to determine areas that need improvement or require special attention.

Placement

One reason for testing and evaluating human performance is for the purpose of **placement.** Initial tests may be used in circumstances where it would be beneficial to group individuals on the basis of their skill level or ability, so that time is spent where it is needed. Grouping individuals together who share a certain characteristic makes the most efficient and effective use of time and energy.

Prediction

Specialized tests have long been used for the **prediction** of future events or results with varying degrees of success. Entrance exams for colleges and universities, personality inventories, and skinfold measurements all propose to predict some aspect of human performance. It is a challenging task to predict future events on the basis of past or present data, but tests and measurements assist us in getting one step closer to doing so accurately.

Motivation

How difficult would it be to get a classroom full of students to hand in assignments if they were not being graded or their marks had no special significance? Very difficult. Most individuals need the proper **motivation** if they are to put forth their full effort, and the measurement and evaluation process provides this challenge and stimulation (Figure 13.2).

Achievement

In order to effectively evaluate an individual's **achievement** level in an instruction or training program, it is necessary to establish a set of objectives that accurately and objectively measure it. In accomplishing this task, you must make use of the measurement and evaluation process, which will indicate how an individual has fared at a particular task.

Program Evaluation

With increasing competition for funds and resources, **program evaluation** is becoming more useful and something of a necessity. Program evaluations allow superiors to determine (according to established standards) whether or not a particular program has successfully achieved its objectives. For example, if you request increased funds for your fitness program, you must first demonstrate that the program is resulting in the improved fitness of your clients.

Norms – Your Reference Perspective

Humans are social beings, so we like to know how we compare to those around us. It sometimes isn't enough to know how we placed – we want to know who finished ahead of and behind us. Standardized tests often provide such information. For example, in order to evaluate your level of explosive power, a vertical jump test is administered. Your results are compared with **norm-referenced standards (norms)** that have been established after numerous previous trials, and you are able to obtain results that reflect your level of achievement relative to a clearly defined subgroup (e.g., people of the same age, sex, or class). In other words, you are able to determine how your performance compares with other males or females of the same age.

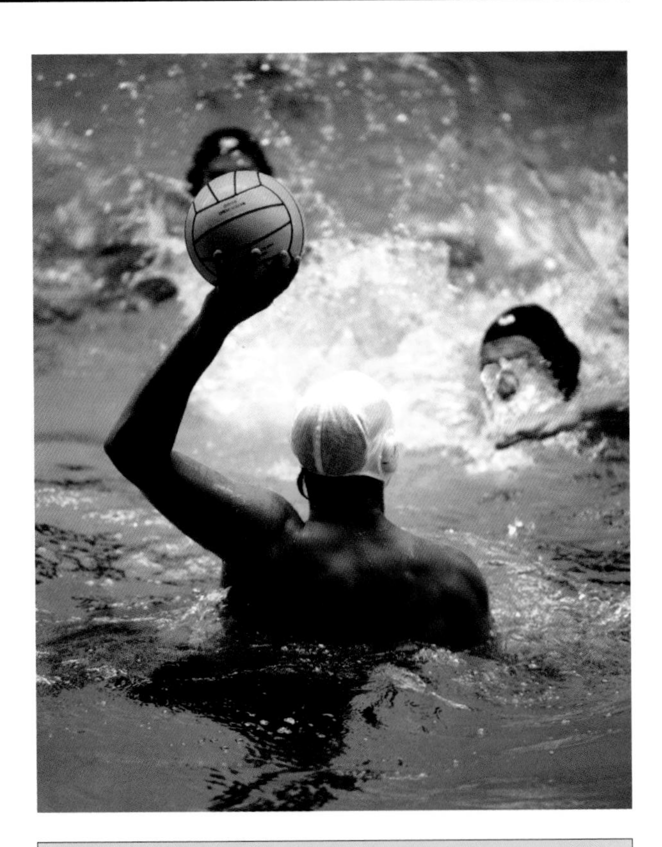

Figure 13.2 When we know our performance is being evaluated, we are motivated to put forth our best effort.

Norms can serve many purposes. A major benefit of using norms is that individuals can be effectively compared on a specific task with others who share important characteristics such as age and sex. For an athlete or coach who is interested in athletic talent identification, norms can provide him or her with an indication of whose performance is above average and who is perhaps

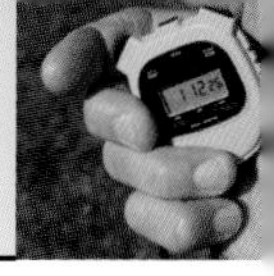

better suited for a different activity. Norms can also provide you with an indication of where improvements need to be made and where most of your efforts should be directed during training. They give you a starting reference point from which your performances can be compared.

Reliability and Validity

Reliability and validity are essential to testing, measurement, and evaluation. Testing involves careful planning in order to obtain results that are consistent and accurate (Figure 13.3). Thus, you must look for accuracy and consistency when making measurements, and the proper choice of instrument is the first major consideration. It is therefore necessary that you understand how to properly use a testing instrument, as well as to have some knowledge about the quality of the measurements it generates. A test or instrument that fails to demonstrate precision and reproducibility runs the risk of yielding faulty results.

Reliability

Reliability refers to the consistency or repeatability of test scores, data, or observations. A test is reliable if measurements are the same (or approximately the same) each time the test is administered to the same individual. This ensures that the test results are dependable and consistent. For example, if you test a student's running speed over a 50-foot (15-meter) distance each hour for four hours, you would expect similar (not exact) results for each trial.

Validity

Whereas reliability refers to the consistency of test scores or data, validity is a characteristic of the instrument or test being used. **Validity** is the degree of truthfulness of a test score, referring to the extent to which a test measures what it proposes to measure. Most people would agree that sit-ups are a valid measure of abdominal muscular endurance. But do sit-ups measure upper body strength? Obviously not. In order to be deemed valid, a test must thus be reliable and relevant and measure what it reports to measure.

Reliability and Validity

Both *reliability* and *validity* must be present if results are to be accurate and meaningful. A test can sometimes be valid in one circumstance but not in another, or reliable but not valid. For example, although total body weight is a reliable measure from day to day, it is not a valid measure of body fatness since the body is composed of tissues other than fat. Thus, it is incorrect to equate total body weight with body fatness. Always consider issues of reliability and validity when conducting tests or interpreting results.

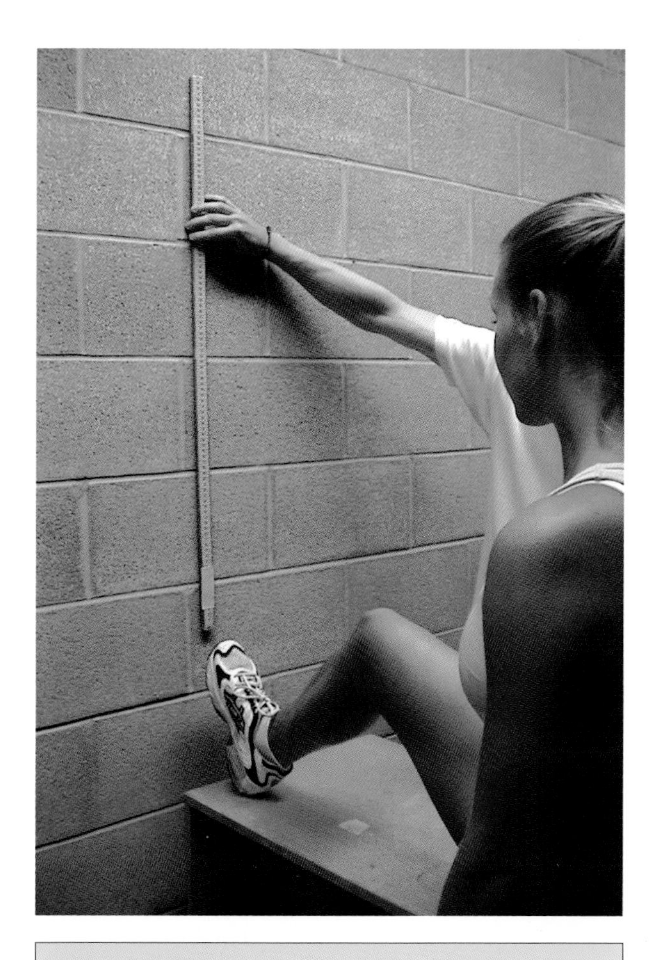

Figure 13.3 When administering any test, accuracy and consistency are required to produce reliable results.

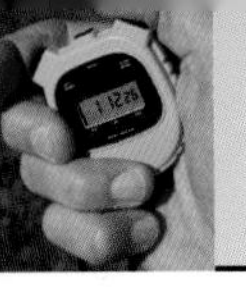

Assessing Physical Fitness

Attaining and maintaining a high level of physical fitness has various documented benefits that support leading an active lifestyle. This has led many people to begin exercise programs directed at improving their strength, endurance, agility, flexibility, body composition, and general quality of life. But how do you accurately determine your level of fitness? You may have seen, or experienced firsthand, fitness appraisals being done at health clubs or universities involving step tests or treadmills for endurance, grip strength tests, and sit-and-reach tests for flexibility, for example. But what do these tests actually measure? Do they provide you with an accurate indication of your actual level of physical fitness? It's important to set goals for yourself that make sense for you – fitness appraisals can be beneficial in this respect. This section will help you become more familiar with the various ways fitness is measured, how you can use the results of these tests to make personal changes in your life, and how you can administer these tests in a reliable and valid manner. Understanding the components of physical fitness (see Chapter 12) and how they can be measured will go a long way in assisting you in your own pursuit of physical fitness and health.

Measuring Aerobic Capacity

Cardiorespiratory endurance is a key component of physical fitness. It is what we are usually referring to when we say that someone is in "good shape" or "physically fit." The concept of cardiorespiratory endurance reflects an individual's aerobic capacity or aerobic power – in other words, the ability to supply oxygen to working muscles during physical exertion (see Chapter 6).

The most accurate and reliable measure of cardiorespiratory function is **maximal oxygen consumption**, or **$\dot{V}O_2$max**, which is a measure of the amount of oxygen consumed per kilogram of body weight per minute of exercise. Measurement of aerobic capacity in the laboratory often involves a maximal exercise test on an ergometer (usually a treadmill or stationary cycle) in which the subject works at progressively increasing loads (intensity) until reaching exhaustion. Other reliable and valid testing protocols have been developed for estimating (predicting) $\dot{V}O_2$max; they are calculated from measurements of maximal or submaximal exercise performance or submaximal heart rate. These **laboratory tests**, however, are rigorous and time consuming, and they often require expensive equipment such as gas analyzers, ergometers, and computerized metabolic systems. This puts lab testing of aerobic power out of reach for most schools.

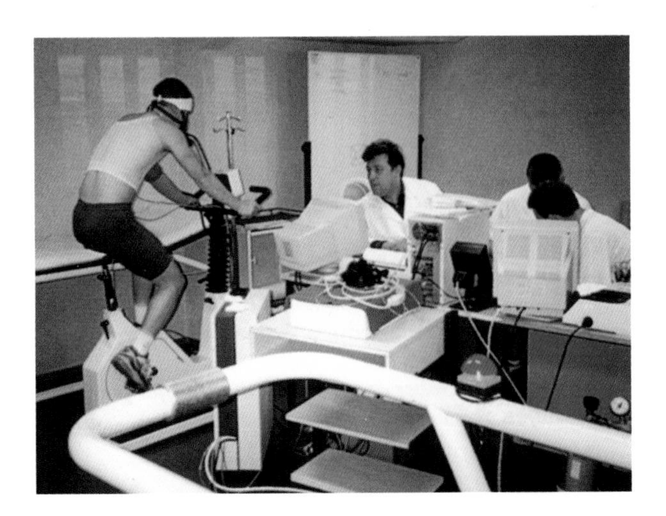

Other simpler and more practical **field tests** have been devised to measure cardiorespiratory function. Popular field tests include running and step tests. **Running tests** require subjects to run a prescribed distance or run for a predetermined length of time; the time required to cover the distance and the distance covered in the allotted time, respectively, are the measurements used to evaluate aerobic capacity. The **step tests** involve stepping up and down steps of a certain height at a particular rate for an established period of time. Aerobic capacity is then estimated from the heart rate response or recovery heart rate following the activity – an individual with high aerobic power will return more quickly to a lower heart rate than a less "fit" individual. Make note of the fact that

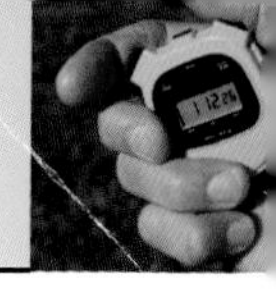

many step tests were devised for use by individuals of college age or above.

It is important when using field tests to employ standard distances, timers, and recording procedures for the most accurate results.

12-Minute Run–Walk Test

This test is satisfactory for both males and females from junior high school to college. Little equipment is required – a stopwatch, whistle, and distance markers are really all you need to complete the test. However, a course of specified distance will make counting the number of laps completed an easier task; the number of laps can then be easily multiplied by the course distance. Distance markers can also be used effectively to divide the course into quarters or eighths so that the tester can quickly and accurately determine the distance covered after 12 minutes have elapsed.

The goal of the test is simply to run or walk (or both) around the course as many times as possible in 12 minutes following the starting signal from behind a designated starting line. A spotter assigned to each runner should maintain an accurate count of each lap completed by the subject until the stop signal is given after 12 minutes. The runner should keep track of laps as well. The distance covered is calculated by multiplying the number of laps completed by the distance of each lap (including the incomplete lap). Spotter and subject can then reverse roles to complete the testing. If 12 minutes seems too long for a particular age level, 9-minute run–walk tests may also be appropriate. Evaluative norms for the 12-minute run are presented in Table 13.1.

Table 13.1 Fitness classifications based on distance covered (miles) in the 12-minute run–walk test.

Fitness Category		Distance Covered by Age (years)		
		13 – 19	20 – 29	30 – 39
Superior	males	≥ 1.93	≥ 1.78	≥ 1.71
	females	≥ 1.53	≥ 1.47	≥ 1.41
Excellent	males	1.74 – 1.87	1.66 – 1.77	1.58 – 1.71
	females	1.45 – 1.52	1.36 – 1.46	1.30 – 1.40
Good	males	1.58 – 1.73	1.51 – 1.66	1.47 – 1.57
	females	1.31 – 1.44	1.24 – 1.35	1.20 – 1.30
Fair	males	1.39 – 1.57	1.32 – 1.50	1.32 – 1.46
	females	1.20 – 1.30	1.12 – 1.23	1.07 – 1.19
Poor	males	1.31 – 1.38	1.22 – 1.32	1.19 – 1.31
	females	1.01 – 1.19	0.96 – 1.12	0.96 – 1.06
Very Poor	males	≤ 1.30	≤ 1.21	≤ 1.19
	females	≤ 1.00	≤ 0.96	≤ 0.95

1.5-Mile Endurance Run

Participants are encouraged to complete the 1.5 mile distance in the shortest possible time. They should be informed that they may walk or stop and rest at any time if necessary.

Several runners may be timed at the same time by one timer. The time is recorded for each participant to the nearest second. Evaluative norms are presented in Table 13.2.

YMCA 3-Minute Step Test

All that is required for this simple test is a bench that is 12 inches in height, a metronome set at 96 beats per minute, and a watch or timer. It is an ideal test for testing large groups of people, particularly for the initial testing of unfit subjects. The subject should first listen to the metronome to become accustomed to the rhythmic beat. After becoming familiar with the beat and practicing the steps, the subject then begins the test. He or she steps to a rhythm of 96 beats per minute following an "up–up, down–down" pattern, which results in 24 steps per minute. This continues for three minutes, after which time the subject steps down and sits down in order that a tester can record the heart rate over one minute. This one-minute recovery heart rate is the score for the test.

Table 13.2 Norms (min:sec) for the 1.5-mile run for boys and girls, 14 to 17 years old.

Percentile	Boys				Girls			
	14	15	16	17	14	15	16	17
95	9:57	9:38	9:18	9:29	12:02	12:17	11:58	11:14
90	10:21	9:59	9:49	9:45	12:43	12:57	12:24	12:24
85	10:43	10:23	10:08	10:08	13:28	13:31	12:38	12:45
80	11:00	10:39	10:25	10:21	13:51	14:01	13:09	13:06
75	11:09	10:50	10:42	10:32	14:16	14:19	13:22	13:31
70	11:22	11:02	10:50	10:42	14:34	14:36	13:41	13:57
65	11:34	11:15	11:03	10:50	14:49	14:56	14:21	14:11
60	11:50	11:25	11:10	11:02	15:05	15:17	14:47	14:28
55	12:08	11:36	11:21	11:05	15:30	15:38	15:15	14:50
50	12:16	11:51	11:32	11:16	15:51	16:02	15:44	15:13
45	12:29	12:04	11:50	11:29	16:07	16:10	16:02	15:39
40	12:40	12:23	12:02	11:52	16:32	16:37	16:26	15:58
35	13:03	12:36	12:20	12:07	16:50	16:55	16:44	16:20
30	13:25	12:51	12:36	12:26	17:07	17:21	17:06	16:45
25	13:51	13:16	13:05	12:40	17:32	17:31	17:37	17:31
20	14:11	14:03	13:15	13:06	17:59	18:20	17:56	18:05
15	14:40	14:46	14:08	13:33	18:51	18:58	18:37	18:53
10	15:26	15:45	14:57	14:27	19:22	19:58	19:33	19:39
5	16:38	17:03	16:10	16:40	20:41	21:29	21:15	22:15

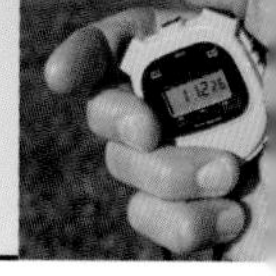

Queen's College Step Test

This test is satisfactory for males and females of college age or above. Bleachers or any stepping bench at a height of 16 to 17 inches is appropriate. A metronome and stopwatch are also needed to administer the test. Divide the group into pairs, with one partner being tested and the other counting the pulse rate. Before beginning, partners should familiarize themselves with pulse-counting procedures in order to perform properly (see Chapter 7).

Subjects step to a four-beat rhythm (up–up, down–down) for three minutes (Figure 13.4). Males step at 96 beats per minute (24 steps/min), while females step at 88 beats per minute (22 steps/min). After demonstrating and practicing at the required beat for about 15 seconds, begin testing. At the completion of the exercise, the subject remains standing and a heart rate is taken for a 15-second period (5 seconds after exercise). Recovery heart rates are converted into beats per minute (bpm) (15-second heart rate x 4). The following equations can then be used to predict $\dot{V}O_2max$ (ml/kg/min).

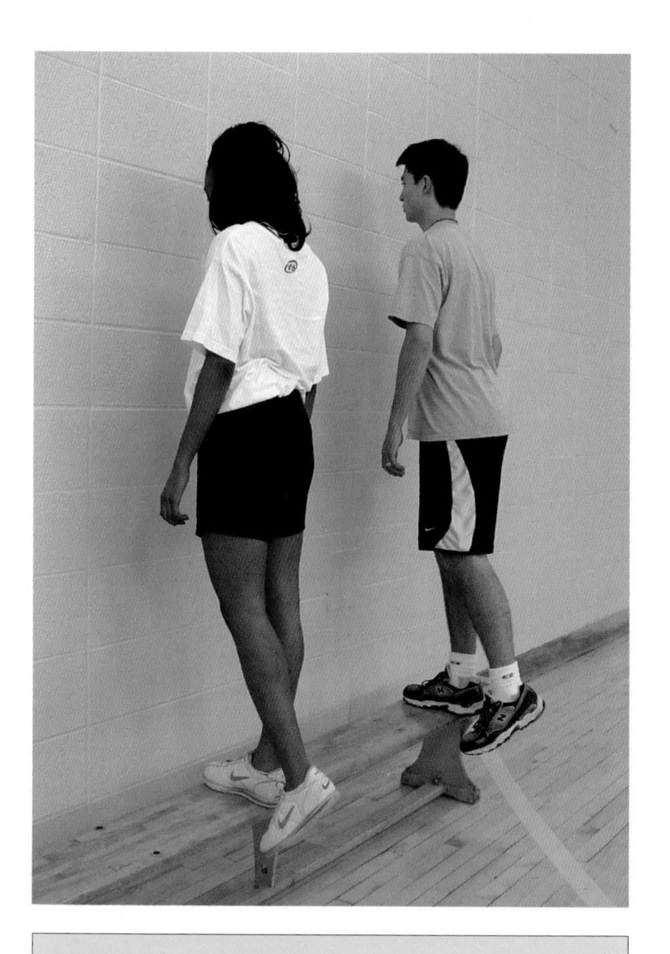

Figure 13.4 Participants follow an "up–up, down–down" stepping pattern for the step test.

$\dot{V}O_2max$ (males) = 111.33 – .42 (pulse rate in beats/min)

$\dot{V}O_2max$ (females) = 65.81 – .185 (pulse rate in beats/min)

In terms of accuracy of prediction, one can be 95 percent confident that the predicted value will be within 16 percent of the subject's true $\dot{V}O_2max$. Predicted $\dot{V}O_2max$ values can be obtained from Table 13.3.

Measuring Body Composition

Because obesity is a risk factor for various health conditions such as high blood pressure (hypertension), coronary heart disease (CHD), cancer, and type 2 (adult onset) diabetes, the accurate assessment of body composition is an important measurement goal. Many people today are concerned with their total body weight; however, the focus should be on losing excessive body fat rather than on total weight alone. Although numerous height–weight tables and indexes are used to assess body composition (e.g., BMI, see Chapter 15), you must be careful when interpreting information from such sources. An athlete who is well muscled, for example, may be considered overweight on a height–weight table even though he or she is actually quite lean. Indexes such as the BMI do not directly measure body fatness.

True measures of body composition (lean versus fat mass) involve the estimation of an individual's body fat percentage, requiring the determination of body density. A lean individual at a fixed body weight will have a higher body density (lower percent body fat) when compared to a fatter person

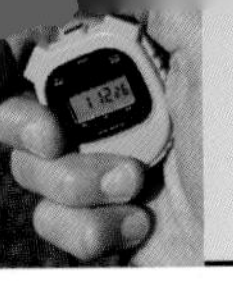

Table 13.3 Predicted maximal oxygen uptake ($\dot{V}O_2max$) for the step test (ml/kg/min).

15-Second Heart Rate	Heart Rate (bpm)	$\dot{V}O_2max$ – Females	$\dot{V}O_2max$ – Males
30	120	43.6	60.9
31	124	42.9	59.3
32	128	42.2	57.6
33	132	41.4	55.9
34	136	40.7	54.2
35	140	40.0	52.5
36	144	39.2	50.9
37	148	38.5	49.2
38	152	37.7	47.5
39	156	37.0	45.8
40	160	36.3	44.1
41	164	35.5	42.5
42	168	34.8	40.8
43	172	34.0	39.1
44	176	33.3	37.4
45	180	32.6	35.7
46	184	31.8	34.1
47	188	31.1	32.4
48	192	30.3	30.7
49	196	29.6	29.0
50	200	28.9	27.3

of the same weight. Many methods of measuring body density and body fat percentage exist, including chemical analysis of human cadavers, hydrostatic weighing, volumetry (body volume), total body water, total body electrical conductivity (TBEC), and radiographic (X-ray) analysis. Most of these methods are obviously not feasible for most schools or individuals for measuring body composition because they require special apparatus and/or complex procedures.

Skinfold measurements are one of the most feasible, reliable, valid, and popular methods used for estimating body composition. These tests involve measuring skinfolds (actually "fat folds") at particular sites on the body with special calipers (Figure 13.5). These measurements of

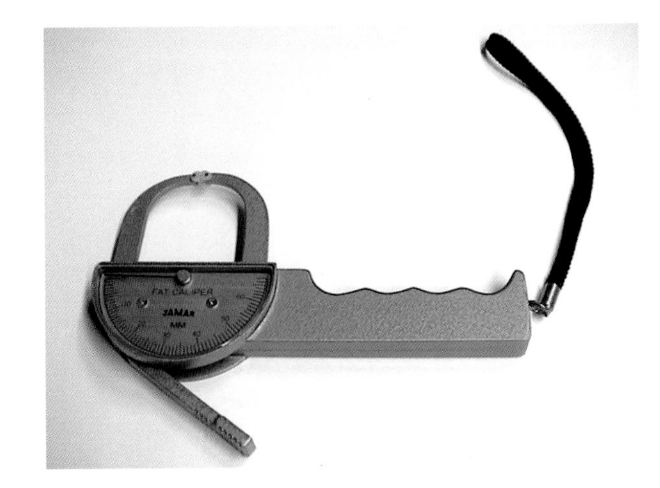

Figure 13.5 Skinfold calipers range in price, but more affordable plastic varieties are available for schools or organizations with limited budgets.

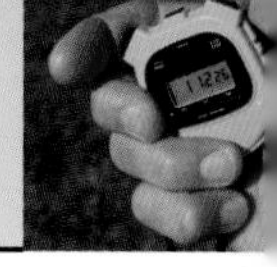

subcutaneous fat are based on the relationship that exists between fat located directly beneath the skin and internal fat and body density. The sum of a set of skinfolds can be used as an indication of the relative degree of fatness among individuals.

YMCA Skinfold Test

This test requires skinfold calipers. The process involves taking skinfolds at the abdomen, suprailium (crest of the hip bone), triceps (Figure 13.6), and thigh. The following steps should be followed when taking skinfold measurements:

(1) lift skinfolds two or three times before placing the calipers for a measurement;

(2) place the calipers below the thumb and fingers and perpendicular to the fold to allow easy reading of the measurement; completely release the caliper grip before reading the dial 1 to 2 seconds later;

(3) repeat this procedure three times; the measurements should not vary by more than 1 mm; use the median value, and allow at least 15 seconds between each measurement.

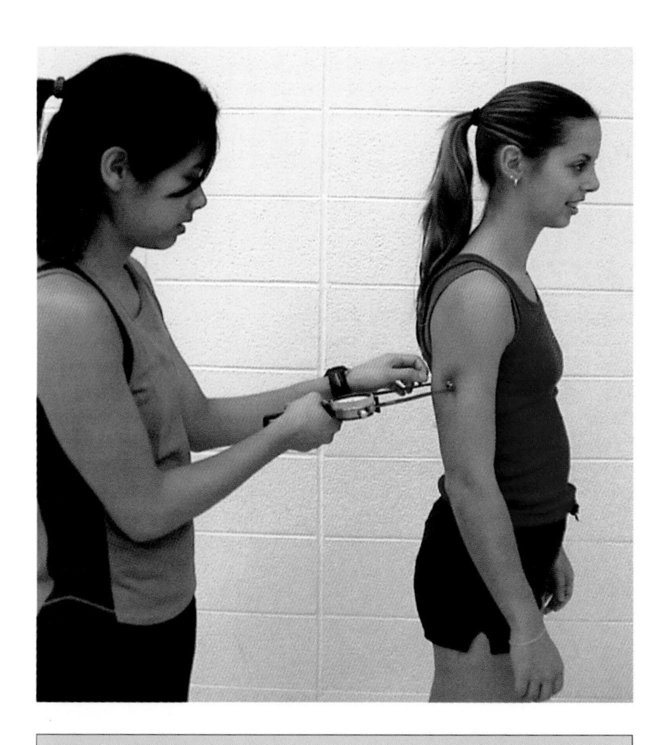

Figure 13.6 Caliper placement for measuring the triceps skinfold.

You must be aware that plenty of practice is required to obtain reliable and consistent results. You can convert the skinfold measures to percent body fat by using the following equations.

Four sites: abdomen, suprailium, triceps, and thigh:

Males

% fat = $.29288 \times (\text{sum of } 4) - .0005 \times (\text{sum of } 4)^2 + .15845 \times (\text{age}) - 5.76377$

Females

% fat = $.29669 \times (\text{sum of } 4) - .00043 \times (\text{sum of } 4)^2 + .02963 \times (\text{age}) + 1.4172$

Your body fat percentage can then be compared to norms for percent body fat (Table 13.4). However, in calculating your percent body fat, be aware that a standard error of estimate of up to 3.98 percent exists. Thus, a calculated percentage of 16 may actually range from 15.4 to 16.6.

Circumference (Girth) Measurements

The girth of various body segments can also be used to assess body composition. Using a cloth measuring tape, measurements must be made carefully at the correct sites and at right angles to the long axis of the body or specific body segment being measured (Figure 13.7). Plenty of practice is required to become an efficient tester.

Because obesity is characterized by large abdominal and hip girths in relation to chest circumference, these are particularly useful circumference measures to use. Some of the body sites most frequently measured include the:

- **neck** – immediately below the larynx;
- **chest** – in males, at nipple level; in females, measures are taken sometimes at the level of just above or just below the breasts (all measures of chest circumference should be taken at the end of an expiration);
- **hips** – from the maximal protrusion of the buttocks to the symphysis pubis;

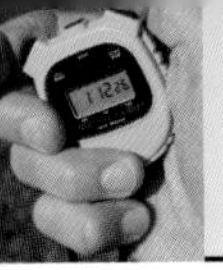

Table 13.4 Norms for percent body fat in males and females.

Rating	Males		Females	
	18 – 25	**26 – 35**	**18 – 25**	**26 – 35**
Very lean	4 – 7	8 – 12	13 – 17	13 – 18
Lean	8 – 10	13 – 15	18 – 20	19 – 21
Leaner than average	11 – 13	16 – 18	21 – 23	22 – 23
Average	14 – 16	19 – 21	24 – 25	24 – 26
Fatter than average	17 – 20	22 – 24	26 – 28	27 – 30
Fat	21 – 26	25 – 28	29 – 31	31 – 35
Overfat	27 – 37	29 – 37	32 – 43	36 – 48

- **thigh** – the point of maximal thigh girth;
- **calf** – the point of maximal calf girth;
- **biceps** – the point of maximal circumference when the arm is (1) fully flexed and muscles fully contracted, and (2) fully extended and muscles fully contracted; and
- **abdomen** – measurements have been taken at different sites:

(1) at the level of the umbilicus (belly button) and iliac crests;

(2) at the point of minimal girth, halfway between umbilicus and xiphoid process of sternum; and

(3) at the point of maximal abdominal girth; in women, about 2 inches (5 cm) below umbilicus.

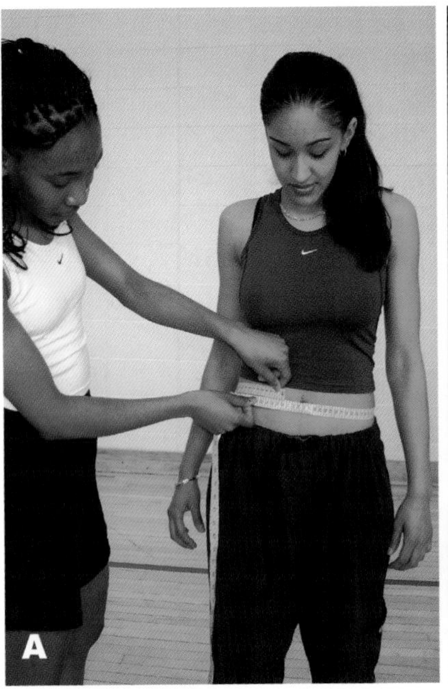

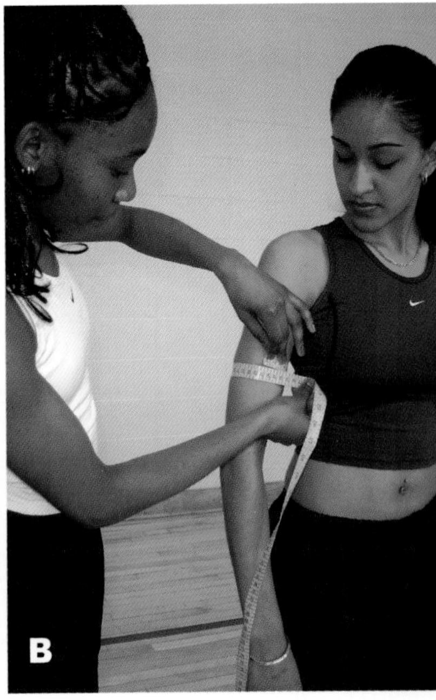

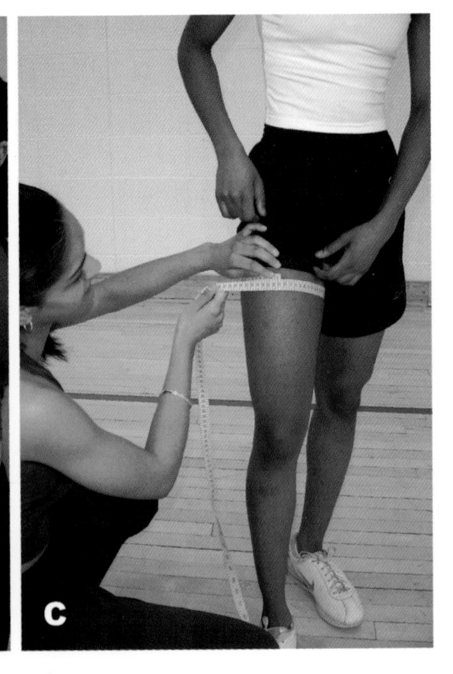

Figure 13.7 Common sites used for girth measurements. **A.** Abdomen. **B.** Biceps. **C.** Thigh.

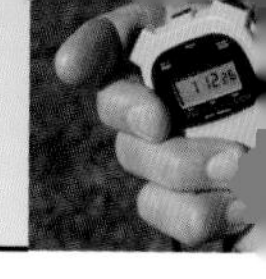

Measuring Muscular Strength

Strength is recognized as an important factor in human performance, particularly in the execution of physical skills. It can be defined as the maximum force that muscle can generate during a brief contraction against a single rigid resistance. Measures of strength involve tests that require one maximal effort for a given movement, often lifting an external weight or contracting against external resistance. An individual's body weight, however, has an impact on how "strong" he or she is deemed to be. For example, a 140-pound (64-kg) man who lifts 165 pounds (75 kg) (165/140 = 1.18) is stronger (relatively) than a 200-pound (91-kg) man who lifts 210 pounds (95 kg) (210/200 = 1.05). But the 200-pound (91-kg) man still possesses more **absolute strength** because he is able to lift a larger absolute weight.

Again, laboratory tests used to assess muscular strength require sophisticated equipment such as computerized dynamometers. Such an apparatus allows detailed measures of work, power, and so on but can be quite expensive. Although lab tests can be useful for physiotherapists, clinicians, athletic trainers, and rehabilitation centers, field methods are far more feasible for the average individual.

Grip Dynamometer

This is an isometric strength test that measures strength with a **grip dynamometer.** It is used to measure the grip strength of the hand but has correlated well with total body strength. It is adjustable to fit the size of any hand. A needle indicates scoring on the dial, which is marked off in pounds and/or kilograms – up to 220 pounds (100 kg). The subject simply takes in a breath, and while exhaling, squeezes the device maximally to obtain a reading. This is completed three times to calculate an average score for each hand. Evaluative norms are presented in Table 13.5.

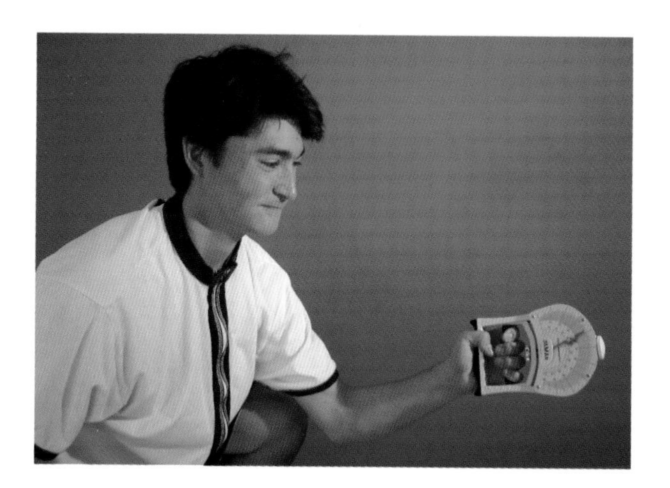

Table 13.5 Norms (lb) for grip strength of the dominant and non-dominant hands combined.

Performance Level	Grip Strength (Dominant and nondominant hands combined)	
	Males (15 – 19)	Females (15 – 19)
Excellent	247+	155+
Above Average	225 – 246	140 – 154
Average	208 – 224	129 – 139
Below Average	184 – 207	118 – 128
Needs Improvement	≤ 183	≤ 117

One Repetition Maximum (1RM)

One repetition maximum (1RM) refers to the maximum amount of weight an individual can lift just one time. 1RM tests can use values from the bench press or leg press. Dividing the 1RM values by the subjects' body weight allows you to make the strength measures equitable across weight classes. When testing for maximum strength, you must adhere to the following guidelines:

- have subjects warm up with stretching and light lifting;
- have subjects perform a lift below the maximum (a pretest session may be useful);
- have subjects rest at least two minutes between lifts to prevent fatigue;

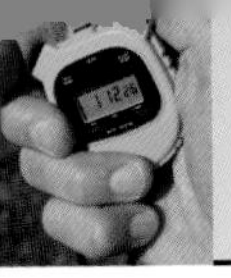

Maximal Strength – Muscular Endurance Relationship

It is neither necessary nor safe for an athlete or student to work against maximal resistance to calculate maximal strength capacity for a given exercise. Because of the close relationship between maximal strength and muscular endurance, determining an athlete's maximum number of repetitions against submaximal resistance will produce an accurate conclusion about maximal strength.

The relationship can be illustrated best with the following example. Student A is able to lift a 220-pound (100-kg) barbell, but partner B masters only 200 pounds (91) kg. If both students are challenged to clean and press a barbell of 190 pounds (86 kg) as often as possible, student A will perform 7 to 8 repetitions and B only 2 to 3 repetitions. Using a 175-pound (80-kg) barbell, student A can do 10 to 12 repetitions and athlete B only 5 to 6 repetitions. This comparison shows that the number of repetitions against high resistance is dependent on the maximal strength of the athlete. The table below shows the maximal number of repetitions possible for load levels of different resistance.

The maximal feasible number of repetitions of a particular load is referred to as the **repetition maximum (RM)**. If the RM of an exercise is 2 to 3, it can be deduced that an athlete can resist a force corresponding to approximately 95 percent of maximal strength capacity. If the athlete is able to perform maximally 7 to 8 repetitions with a particular weight, then this weight approximates 85 percent of his or her maximal strength capacity.

Maximum number of repetitions as a function of resistance.

Resistance Level	100%	95%	90%	85%	80%	75%
Repetition Maximum	1	2 – 3	5 – 6	7 – 8	approx. 10 – 12	approx. 12 – 16

- increase weight on subsequent lifts by small increments (5 or 10 pounds) (2.5 or 5 kg);
- continue procedure until subjects fail to lift a particular weight;
- record the last weight successfully lifted as the 1RM;
- divide the subjects' 1RM by their body weight.

If it takes more than five lifts to determine a subject's 1RM, consider retesting the subject the next day with a heavier starting weight.

Measuring Muscular Power

The term **power** is often (incorrectly) used as a synonym for the term strength. However, power specifically refers to the ability to release maximum force in the shortest possible time. Indeed time is the element that really distinguishes the two concepts. Activities that involve rapid muscular contractions such as the vertical jump, shot put, and standing broad jump require power to execute movements explosively. Many tests of power are easy to administer and are very practical in terms of time, effort, and equipment.

Standing Long Jump

This simple test can be used for both males and females from age six and up. All that is needed for the test is a floor or mat, a tape measure, and a marking material (chalk or tape) to indicate the distance jumped. Actually, it has never been easier to measure an athlete's explosive power in the legs using the standing long jump. Special standing long jump test mats have been made to make the test even simpler to administer (Figure 13.8). The special mat eliminates taping down measuring tapes to the gym floor and eyeballing the distance jumped since the measuring tape (in inches and cm) is printed directly on a thick, durable rubber material.

The goal of a two-footed long jump is to jump horizontally as far as possible from a standing

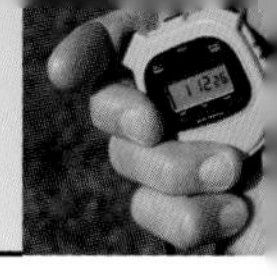

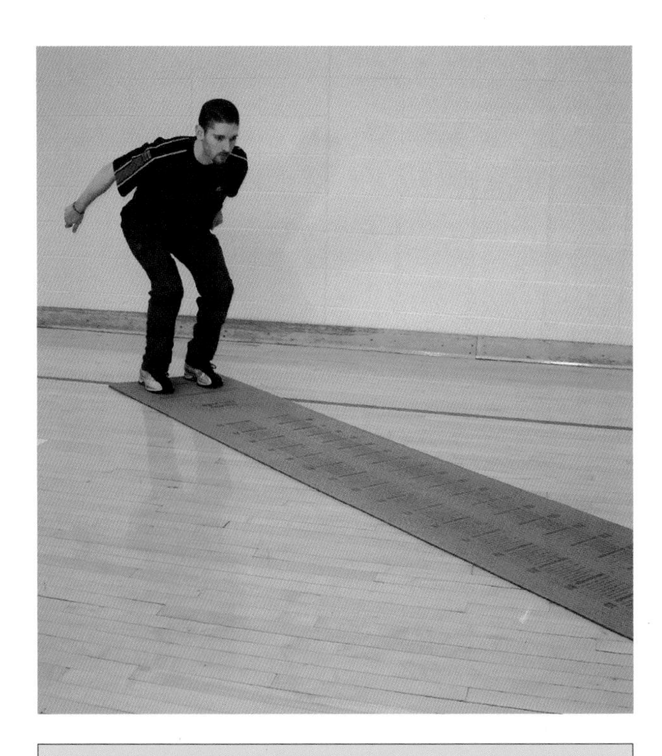

Figure 13.8 The rubber material of the mat provides excellent grip for takeoff and effectively cushions landings, eliminating the fear that students may slip on a wooden floor or other slick surface.

start. Begin by standing with the feet about shoulder-width apart, with the toes just behind the takeoff line. Then bend the knees and swing the arms backward and forward in preparation for the jump.

After attaining a feel for the jump, extend the hips, knees, and ankles from a crouch position as a unit while simultaneously swinging the arms forward for the jump. In addition, the trunk should be leaning slightly forward at the instant of takeoff and then upward as the arms swing in the direction of the jump. There should be no extra hop or step prior to the jump; it must be performed cleanly, with both feet entirely behind the takeoff line. The key to a successful jump is coordinating all parts of the body during the jump – ankles, knees, hips, arms, and trunk.

The measurement of the jump is the distance between the takeoff line and the heel touchdown (or other body part) closest to the takeoff line. Accurate readings are quick and easy with a specialized test mat. Allow each student at least three trials to obtain an average score. Evaluative norms are presented in Table 13.6.

Vertical Jump (Sargent Jump)

Another simple test used to measure power in the legs is the vertical jump, satisfactory for males and females age nine and up. A measuring tape or yardstick, chalk, and a smooth wall at least 12 feet (4 m) high is all that is required to complete the test. The subject simply stands sideways beside the wall,

Table 13.6 Norms (inches) for the standing long jump test.

Performance Level	Males			Females		
	Age (years)			Age (years)		
	15	16	17+	15	16	17+
Excellent	85.5 – 92.5	90.0 – 96.0	92.5 – 100.5	73.0 – 81.0	75.0 – 82.0	76.0 – 81.0
Above Average	81.0 – 85.0	85.5 – 90.0	88.0 – 92.5	68.0 – 73.0	69.5 – 75.0	70.0 – 75.5
Average	77.0 – 81.0	81.0 – 85.0	85.0 – 88.0	64.0 – 68.0	66.0 – 69.0	67.0 – 70.0
Below Average	69.5 – 76.5	77.0 – 81.0	79.0 – 85.0	59.0 – 64.0	61.0 – 65.0	62.0 – 66.5
Needs Improvement	51.5 – 69.0	66.5 – 76.5	66.5 – 79.0	49.0 – 59.0	48.0 – 60.0	50.5 – 61.5

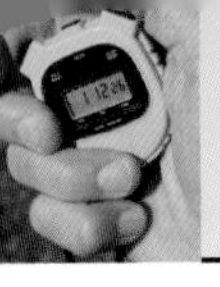

about an elbow's distance away (put the hand closest to the wall on your hip to determine this distance). Holding a small piece of chalk in the hand closest to the wall, the subject reaches up as high as possible with the heels on the floor and makes a mark on the wall (Figure 13.9 A). He or she then jumps as high as possible and makes another mark at the peak of the jump on the wall. It is important to bend the ankles, knees, and hips before explosively extending these joints from the crouch position for optimal power. Allow three trials of which the best score will count. The jump height is measured by subtracting the reach height from jump height.

Vertical Jump Test Mat Another special device has been developed to measure vertical jump height and power. The key feature in the design of this vertical jump test is a measuring tape feeder mounted on a rubber mat. This feeder allows the measuring tape to be fed through with minimal resistance as the athlete jumps, but stops the tape once the apex of the jump is reached (Figure 13.9 B). The length of measuring tape pulled through the feeder indicates the height of the jump, which is clearly displayed for recording. Evaluative norms are presented in Table 13.7.

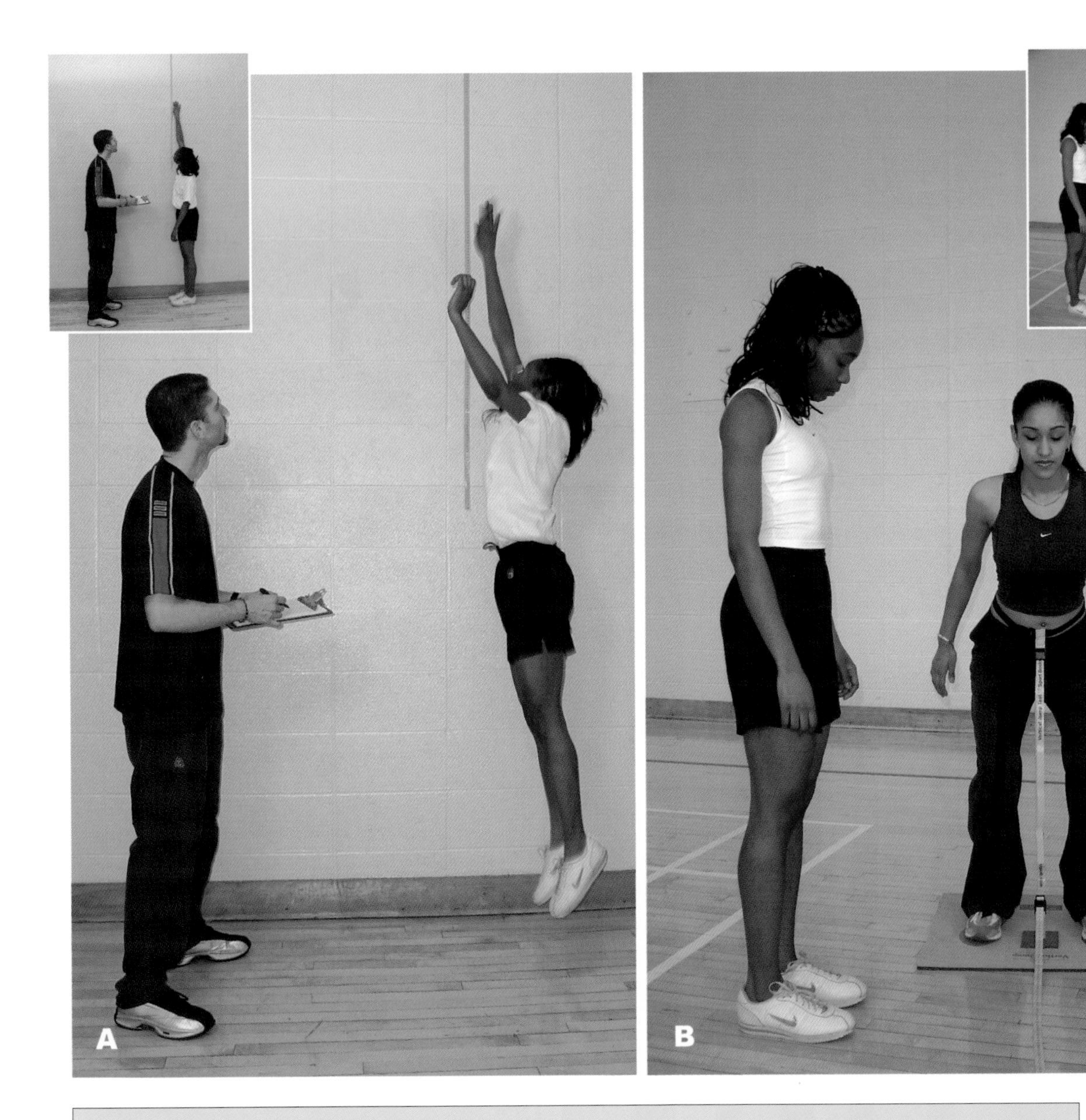

Figure 13.9 The vertical jump. **A.** Traditional Sargent jump. **B.** Using a vertical jump test mat.

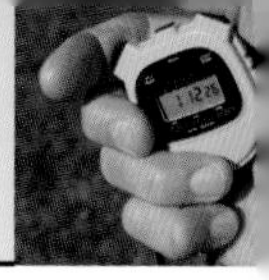

Table 13.7 Norms (inches) for the vertical jump test.

Performance Level	Males		Females	
	Age (years)		Age (years)	
	15 – 19	20 – 29	15 – 19	20 – 29
Excellent	≥ 20.0	≥ 22.0	≥ 14.5	≥ 15.5
Above Average	14.5 – 19.5	15.0 – 21.5	11.5 – 14.0	11.0 – 15.0
Average	10.5 – 14.0	12.0 – 14.5	8.5 – 11.0	8.0 – 10.5
Below Average	7.0 – 10.0	8.0 – 11.5	6.0 – 8.0	6.0 – 7.5
Needs Improvement	≤ 6.5	≤ 7.5	≤ 5.5	≤ 5.5

Measuring Muscular Endurance

Muscular endurance is characterized by the ability of muscle to maintain tension or to execute repeated movements versus submaximal resistance over time. Whether measures of endurance are static (e.g., flexed arm hang) or dynamic (e.g., pull-ups), most tests of muscular endurance are actually quite practical. The scoring for such tests usually involves recording the number of repetitions completed for a particular exercise or the length of time tension is maintained. Whether the test involves push-ups, sit-ups, bench presses, or squats, the ability to sustain muscular tension with repeated movements is what is being tested. It is important to note the difference between cardiorespiratory and muscular endurance. Muscular endurance, unlike cardiorespiratory endurance discussed earlier, refers to the endurance of skeletal muscle involved in activities, not the efficiency of the heart and lungs.

YMCA 1-Minute Sit-ups Test

This test is appropriate for males and females of most ages and requires subjects simply to perform the maximum number of sit-ups possible in one minute. The test is to be performed with bent knees, the feet flat on the ground shoulder-width apart, and the fingers behind the head (Figure 13.10). A partner holds the subject's feet during the test as he or she performs sit-ups to alternate sides (i.e., left elbow to right knee, right elbow to left knee). The total number of sit-ups performed in one minute is recorded to measure trunk endurance; repetitions are not to be counted if the fingers lose contact with the head. Evaluative norms are shown in Table 13.8.

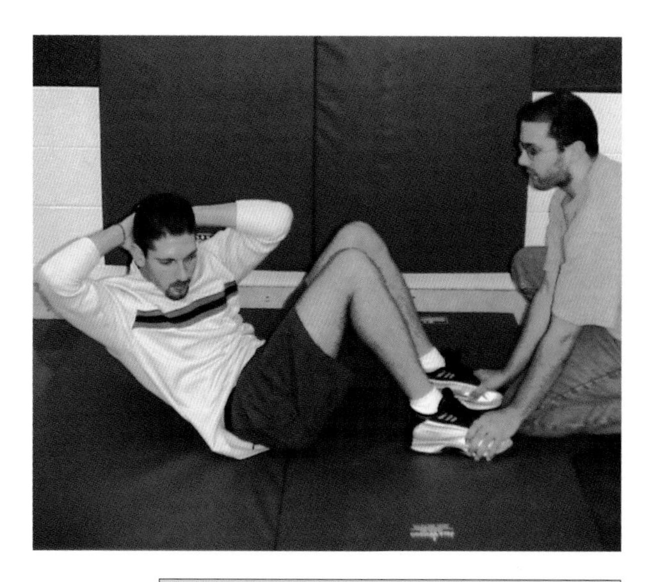

Figure 13.10 The YMCA sit-ups test.

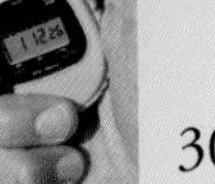

Table 13.8 Norms (number of repetitions) for the YMCA sit-ups test.

Performance Level	Age and Sex			
	Males		Females	
	16	17	16	17
Excellent	49+	47+	44+	45+
Above Average	43 – 48	42 – 46	38 – 43	40 – 44
Average	40 – 42	39 – 41	33 – 37	34 – 39
Below Average	34 – 39	34 – 38	26 – 32	28 – 33
Needs Improvement	≤ 33	≤ 33	≤ 25	≤ 27

Pull-ups and Flexed Arm Hang

Pull-up tests are popular for testing upper body muscular endurance. All that is required is a horizontal bar high enough from the ground that the tallest subject cannot reach the ground with his or her feet. An overhand grip (palms facing away) must be used. The test begins with the subject maintaining a straight arm hang (Figure 13.11 A). The subject's task is simply to pull himself or herself upward until the chin is above the bar (Figure 13.11 B); after each chin-up, the subject is to return to the starting position. This sequence is repeated as many times as possible to test muscular endurance of the arms and shoulder girdle. Evaluative norms are presented in Table 13.9.

The flexed arm hang is another effective test of muscular endurance, especially for participants who cannot pull their own body weight. In this test, two spotters assist the subject in attaining a flexed arm position (palms facing in) so the eyes are level with the bar (Figure 13.11 C). The subject is to hold this position as long as possible, and the

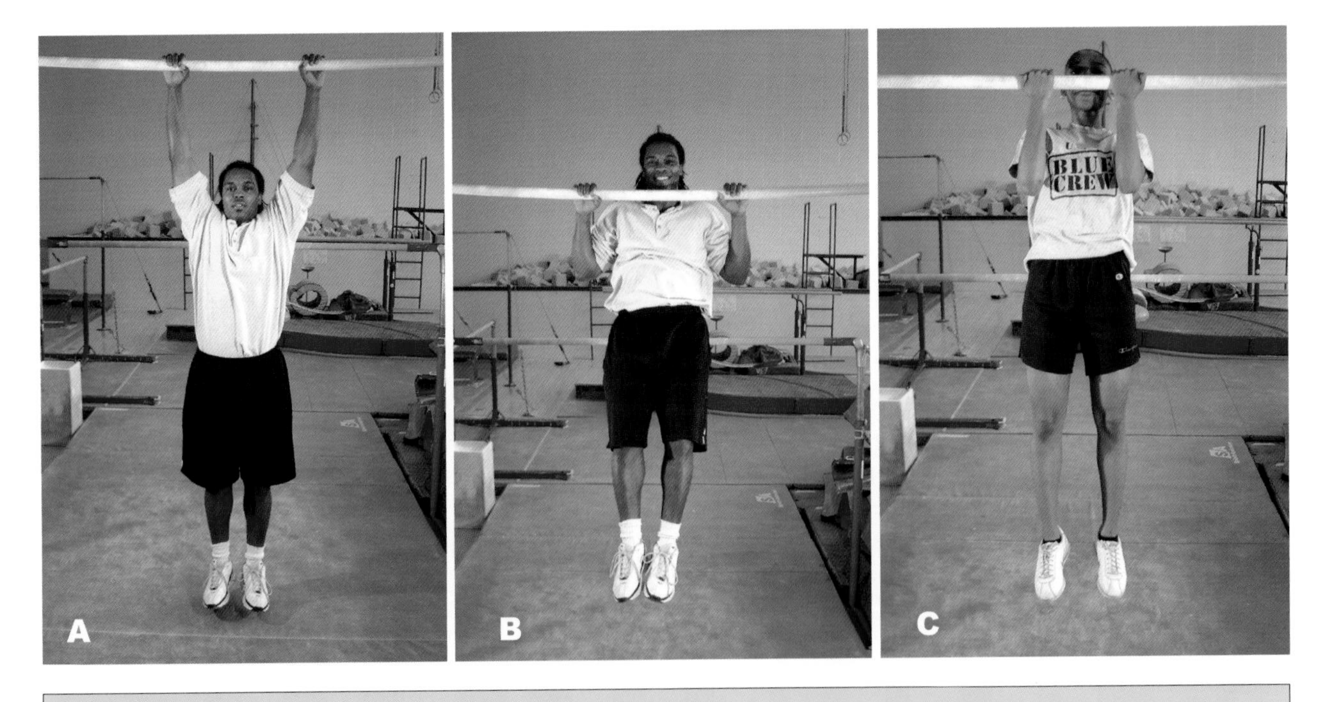

Figure 13.11 The pull-ups test. **A.** Starting position. **B.** Chin-up position. **C.** Flexed arm hang modification.

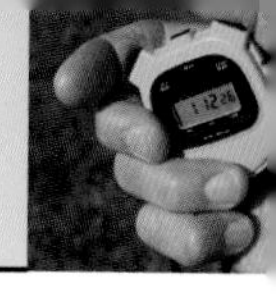

Table 13.9 Raw score norms (number of repetitions) for the pull-ups test for boys.

Percentile	Age				
	13	14	15	16	17+
95	10	12	15	14	15
75	5	7	9	10	10
50	3	4	6	7	7
25	1	2	3	4	4
5	0	0	0	1	0

number of seconds (to the nearest second) the subject maintains this position is the score that is recorded. Evaluative norms are presented in Table 13.10.

Push-ups Test

It doesn't get any easier for assessing upper body endurance – all you need is a mat. The goal of the test is to perform push-ups to exhaustion. The basic push-up position with hands under the shoulders and toes on the ground must be maintained throughout the test (no sagging or piking of the body) (Figure 13.12 A). The chest

Table 13.10 Norms (seconds) for the flexed arm hang, boys and girls 14 to 17 years old.

Percentile	Boys				Girls			
	14	15	16	17	14	15	16	17
95	80.8	84.0	92.0	80.8	58.0	53.0	52.0	55.0
90	72.5	72.5	80.5	73.1	46.5	45.3	46.1	47.5
85	66.9	67.3	74.3	69.5	41.8	40.5	41.4	43.0
80	63.1	64.2	68.8	66.7	36.3	36.0	39.2	40.1
75	61.1	62.4	65.8	65.2	31.9	31.3	35.8	37.1
70	59.6	60.9	63.0	63.9	29.4	28.8	32.8	34.1
65	56.8	59.7	61.8	62.5	26.5	25.1	30.2	32.5
60	54.0	57.1	60.8	60.9	24.2	23.4	27.1	30.8
55	51.6	53.8	59.8	58.3	22.6	21.5	24.6	28.7
50	48.7	51.6	57.0	56.0	20.3	20.0	21.4	25.4
45	45.8	50.1	53.7	52.3	18.5	18.5	19.2	24.0
40	42.7	47.4	51.0	49.8	16.6	15.8	16.7	21.3
35	39.9	44.8	48.7	46.7	14.1	14.2	15.1	19.1
30	36.3	42.3	45.3	43.7	12.0	12.4	12.8	16.9
25	33.8	38.3	42.0	41.5	10.2	10.6	10.6	14.8
20	31.0	34.5	39.8	38.9	8.8	8.6	9.0	12.0
15	26.8	29.1	35.1	34.8	6.9	7.1	7.8	9.1
10	21.8	24.1	29.8	30.7	5.2	5.8	5.8	6.2
5	12.5	15.5	18.3	24.5	3.5	3.3	3.9	4.5

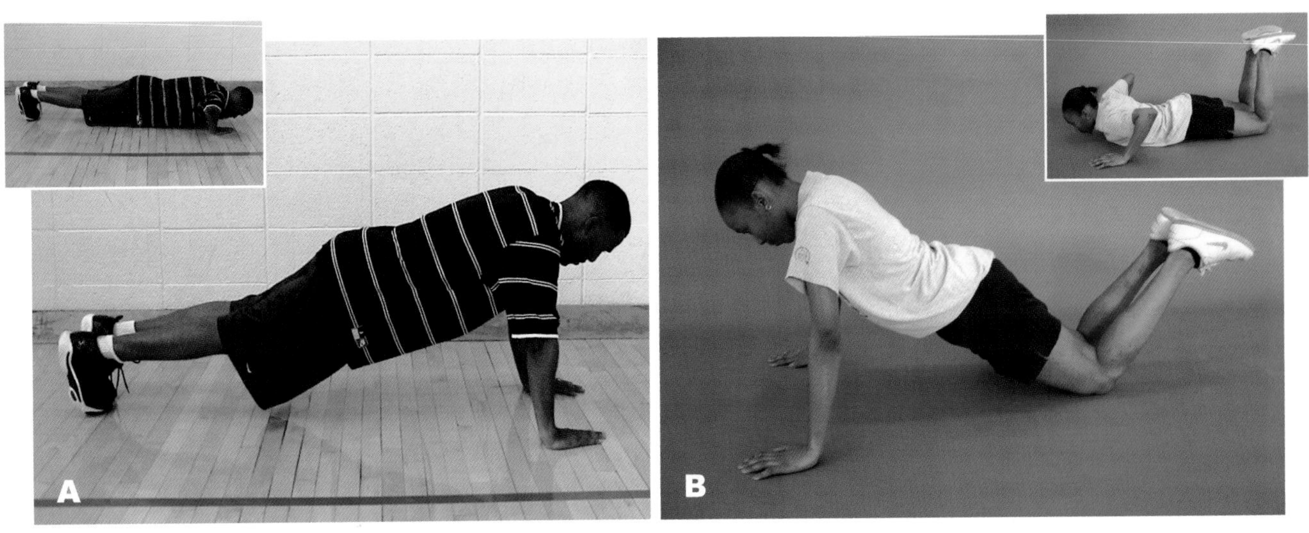

Figure 13.12 The push-ups test. **A.** Standard push-up. **B.** Modified push-up.

must touch the mat on each repetition to count in the score. Women may perform modified push-ups with the knees bent and touching the mat rather than the toes (Figure 13.12 B). The score is simply the number of push-ups successfully completed. Evaluative norms are presented in Table 13.11.

Continuous Burpee Test

This test measures the participant's general muscular endurance. Appropriate for both males and females, all that is required for this test is a stopwatch, wrist watch, or clock with a second hand. A burpee is performed in the following sequence: from standing, (1) the subject squats and places the hands on the floor in front of the feet; (2) propels the legs backward to a front-leaning rest position; (3) returns to the squat-rest position; and (4) rises back to a standing position (Figure 13.13). The test involves repeating this sequence as many times as possible after a "Go!" signal has been given. The subject's score is the total number of repetitions. Evaluative norms are presented in Table 13.12.

Table 13.11 Norms (number of repetitions) for the push-ups test (modified push-ups for females).

Performance Level	No. of Push-ups	
	Males (15 – 19)	Females (15 – 19)
Excellent	39+	33+
Above Average	29 – 38	25 – 32
Average	23 – 28	18 – 24
Below Average	18 – 22	12 – 17
Needs Improvement	≤ 17	≤ 11

Table 13.12 Norms (total number of burpees) for the continuous burpee test.

Performance Level	No. of Burpees	
	Males	Females
Excellent	94+	46+
Above Average	70 – 93	38 – 45
Average	39 – 69	20 – 37
Below Average	22 – 38	12 – 19
Needs Improvement	0 – 21	0 – 11

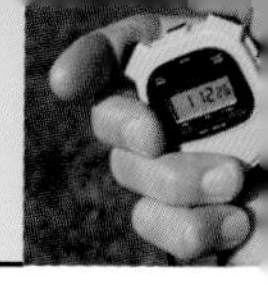

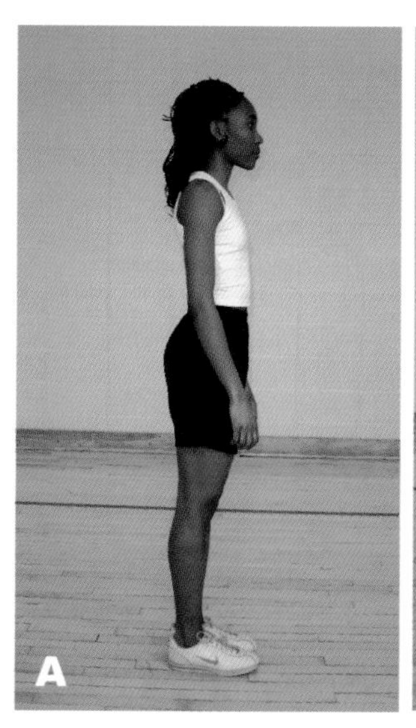

Starting position

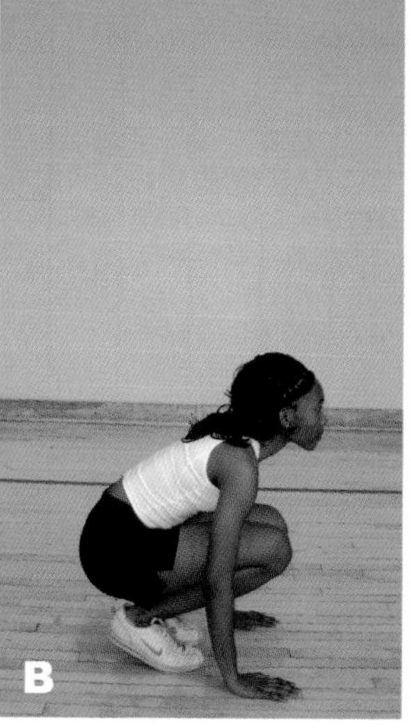

Squat or crouch position

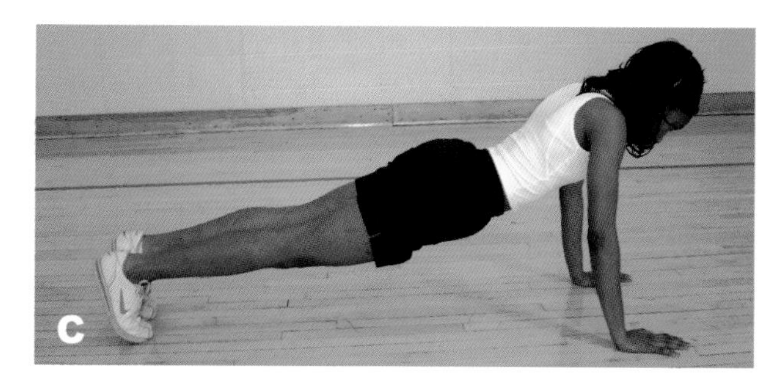

Front-leaning rest position

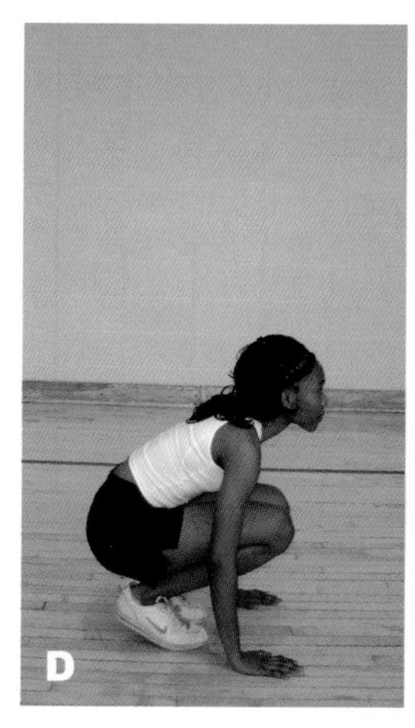

Return to squat position

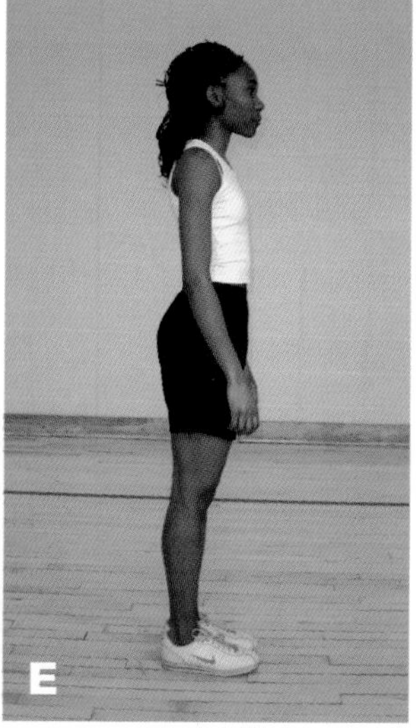

Return to standing

Figure 13.13 The sequence of a properly performed burpee.

Measuring Flexibility

Measuring **flexibility**, or joint range of motion, is an important measurement goal. Not only is flexibility important for performing physical skills, but it is also vital for performing daily tasks with comfort and ease. However, flexibility tends to be joint specific; therefore, a general test of flexibility really doesn't exist. Having flexible shoulders does not mean you will have flexible hamstrings. This creates a problem in measuring flexibility, unless the flexibility of a specific joint is being tested. Various laboratory methods exist that measure joint range of motion, including goniometry (manual, electric, and pendulum goniometers), radiography, photography, trigonometry, and linear measurements. While these methods are reliable and valid, many are not feasible for schools or average individuals. Other simple field tests exist that effectively measure flexibility.

Sit-and-Reach Test

This test assessing trunk and hamstring flexibility is satisfactory for both males and females from age five and above. Prior to testing, participants should warm up properly to stretch. These tests involve reaching as far forward as possible with the legs held straight. Some tests use a specially constructed box of specific dimensions with a measurement scale (Figure 13.14). However,

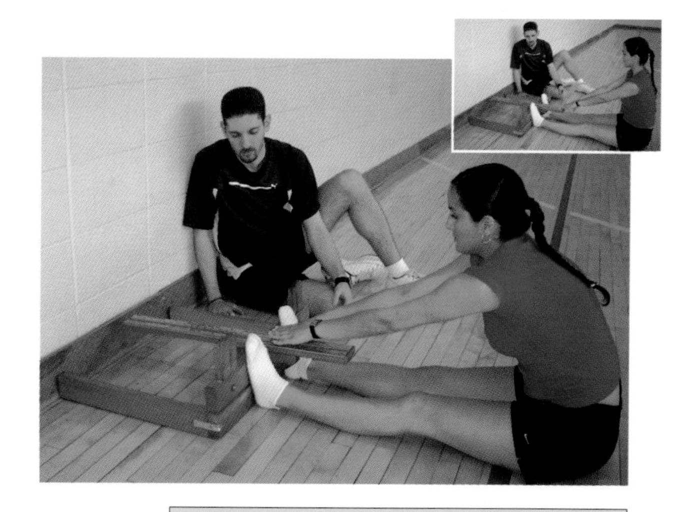

Figure 13.14 The sit-and-reach test.

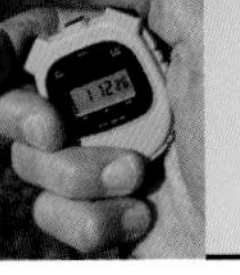

Table 13.13 Norms (inches) for the modified sit-and-reach test.

Males			Females		
Percentile Rank	Age Category		Percentile Rank	Age Category	
	Under 18	19 – 35		Under 18	19 – 35
99	21.0	20.0	99	22.5	21.0
95	20.0	19.0	95	20.0	19.0
90	18.0	17.0	90	18.5	17.5
80	17.5	16.5	80	17.5	16.5
70	16.0	15.5	70	16.5	16.0
60	15.5	15.0	60	16.0	15.5
50	14.5	14.5	50	15.5	15.0
40	14.0	13.5	40	14.5	14.5
30	13.5	13.0	30	14.0	14.0
20	12.0	11.5	20	12.5	12.5
10	9.5	9.0	10	11.5	10.0
05	8.0	8.0	05	9.5	9.0
01	7.0	7.0	01	8.0	7.5

the test may also be completed with a yardstick or measuring tape. For this modified test, the participant sits with one leg on either side of the yardstick or tape measure, with the feet and arms outstretched and the hips, back, and head against the wall (see background image in Table 13.13). The tape measure on the floor should be lined up with the edge of the participant's outstretched fingers. The participant's head and back can now come off the wall and gradually reach forward along the yardstick three times. On the third attempt, the participant stretches forward as far as possible and holds the final position for at least two seconds. The back of the participant's knees must remain flat on the floor. Each trial is scored to the nearest inch or centimeter. Two trials are allowed, and the final test score is calculated as the average of the two scores. Evaluative norms are presented in Table 13.13.

Bridge-up Test

Although little testing has been conducted on trunk extension, here is one test that is useful. It measures trunk extension and is particularly useful for assessing flexibility for sports such as the butterfly (swimming), high jump, modern dance and ballet, and the balance beam and floor exercise events in gymnastics. It is appropriate for both males and females, and all that is needed is a mat and a yardstick. Subjects begin in a supine position (on their backs) with their feet against a wall. Each

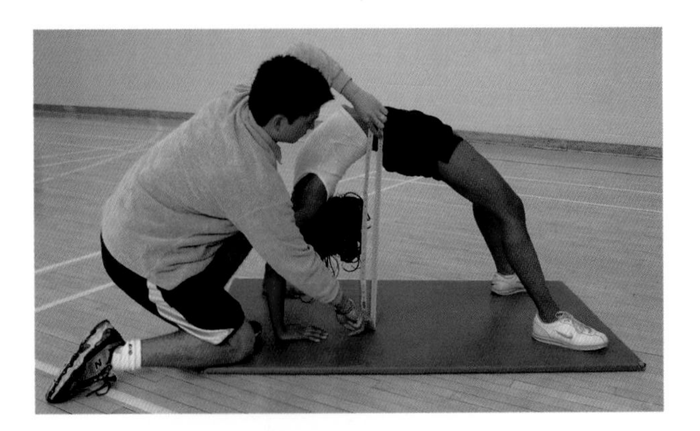

Figure 13.15 The bridge-up test.

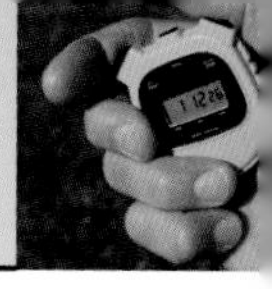

subject should tilt the head back, pushing upward and arching the back. The subjects then walk their hands and feet as close together as possible. A partner then measures the highest point of the arched back from the floor (Figure 13.15). Record the best score of three trials; this score is then subtracted from the subject's standing height (floor to navel). The smaller the difference, the better the performance.

Hamstring Looseness Test

This test is designed to assess hamstring looseness. Prior to testing, participants should be properly warmed up to stretch. The participant stands with the feet approximately hip-width apart. Keeping the knees straight, the participant bends over at the waist and lets the arms drop toward the ground, pushing the hands as far toward the floor as the hamstrings will allow. Refer to Figure 13.16 A-D and Table 13.14 to determine your performance level.

Table 13.14 Performance levels for the hamstring looseness test.

Performance Level	Position Reached
Excellent	Palms touch the floor (Figure 13.16 A)
Above Average	Knuckles touch the floor (Figure 13.16 B)
Average	Fingertips touch the floor (Figure 13.16 C)
Below Average	Fingertips touch the feet
Needs Improvement	Fingertips touch the ankles or higher (Figure 13.16 D)

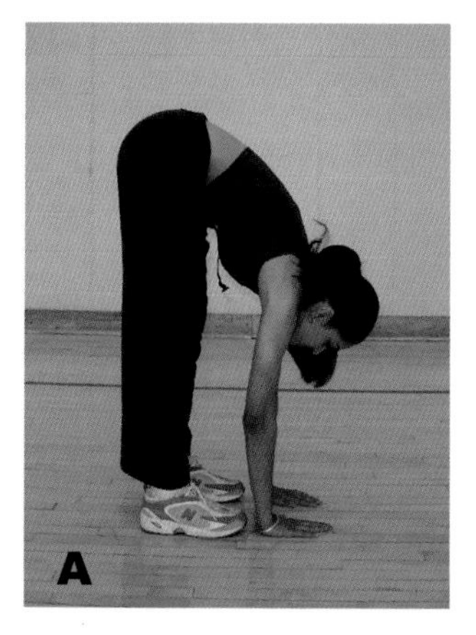

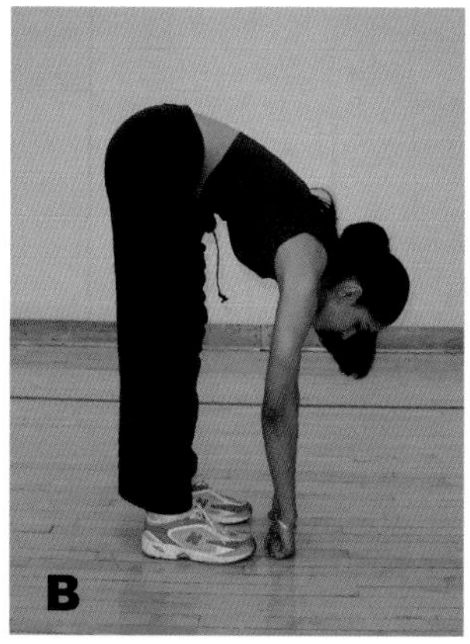

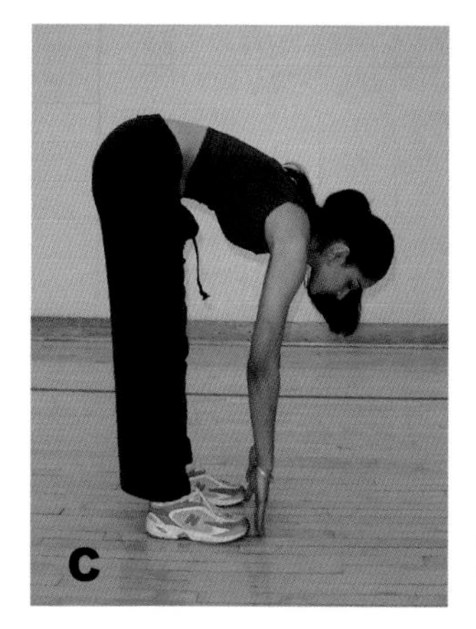

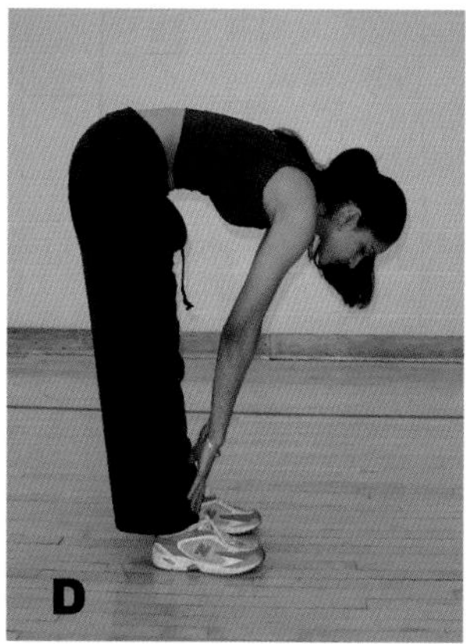

Figure 13.16 The hamstring looseness test. **A.** Palms touch the floor. **B.** Knuckles touch the floor. **C.** Fingertips touch the floor. **D.** Fingertips touch the ankles or higher.

Total Body Rotation Test

This simple test is designed to measure trunk flexibility. Begin by fastening a measuring tape on the wall at approximately shoulder height of the participant. At the 16-inch (40-cm) mark, draw a line with masking tape or chalk on the floor. Adjust the height of the measuring tape to each participant to ensure it is at shoulder height. Two stations are needed for testing both sides.

The participant should be properly warmed up to stretch. The participant stands sideways, an arm's length away from the wall. The toes must be lined up with the line on the floor, with the feet parallel and shoulder-width apart and the knees slightly bent. With the inside arm extended to the wall and

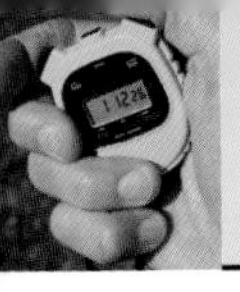

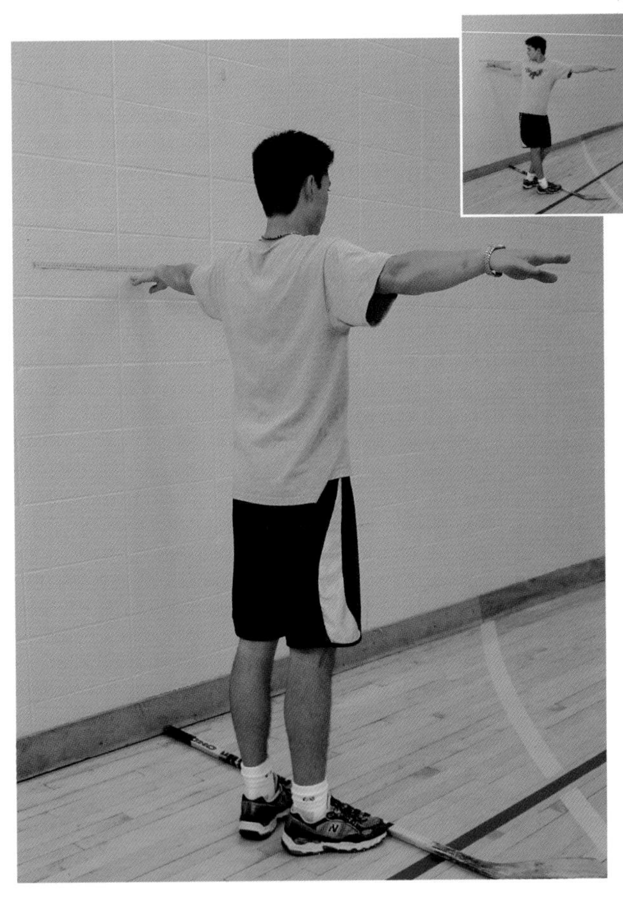

Figure 13.17 The total body rotation test.

the outside arm stretched out parallel to the floor, the knuckles must face the ceiling. Now rotate the trunk, the outside arm stretching backward until it touches the wall. Gradually slide the fist alongside the tape measure as far as possible. The final position must be held for a minimum of two seconds. The body must be kept as straight as possible, and the feet should always be pointing straight forward (Figure 13.17).

The test is conducted on either the right or left side of the body. Each participant is allowed two trials on the selected side. Each trial is scored to the nearest inch or centimeter at the knuckles and held for at least two seconds. The average of two trials is used as the final test score. Evaluative norms are presented in Table 13.15.

Measuring Agility

Agility, the physical ability that enables rapid and precise change of body position and direction, is important for many activities and sports. Athletes who participate in sports such as judo, wrestling, or badminton, which require quick maneuverability and agile reactions, undoubtedly possess a high degree of agility. Testing for agility may be accomplished in many ways, but only a few simple tests will be presented here.

Table 13.15 Percentile norms (inches) for the total body rotation test.

Percentile Rank	Left Rotation				Right Rotation			
	Under Age 18		Age 19 – 35		Under Age 18		Age 19 – 35	
	Male	Female	Male	Female	Male	Female	Male	Female
99	29.0	29.0	28.0	28.5	28.0	29.5	27.5	29.5
95	26.5	26.5	24.5	24.5	25.5	27.5	25.5	25.0
90	25.0	25.5	23.0	22.5	24.0	26.0	23.5	22.5
80	22.0	23.5	21.5	21.5	22.5	23.5	22.0	20.5
70	20.5	21.5	20.0	20.5	21.5	22.0	20.5	19.0
60	19.5	20.5	19.0	18.5	19.5	20.5	18.5	17.5
50	18.0	19.5	17.5	17.5	18.5	19.5	17.0	17.0
40	16.5	18.0	16.5	17.0	17.0	18.5	16.0	16.0
30	14.5	16.5	14.5	15.5	14.5	16.0	14.5	16.0
20	13.5	16.0	12.0	16.0	13.5	14.5	12.0	13.0
10	10.0	13.0	10.0	13.5	10.5	12.2	11.0	11.0
05	8.0	11.5	8.5	7.0	7.5	10.5	8.0	8.5

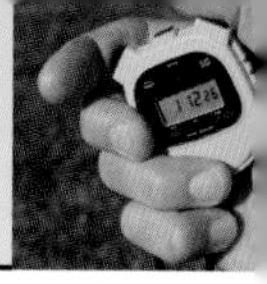

Table 13.16 Raw score norms (number of parts completed) for the burpee test.

Performance Level	College Men	High School and College Females	High School Boys
Excellent	≥ 34	≥ 30	≥ 32
Above Average	29 – 33	26 – 29	28 – 31
Average	17 – 28	14 – 25	16 – 27
Below Average	12 – 16	10 – 13	12 – 15
Needs Improvement	≤ 11	≤ 9	≤ 11

Burpee Test

This test, as described previously, can also be used for evaluating agility. It effectively measures how quickly participants can change their body position. The score represents simply the parts of the exercise sequence completed in 10 seconds. Squatting and placing the hands on the floor represents the first part (Figure 13.13 B); propelling the legs backward is the second (Figure 13.13 C); returning to the squat position is the third (Figure 13.13 D); and rising back to standing is the fourth (Figure 13.13 E). Scores are valid only if all parts of the exercise are performed properly as shown in Figure 13.13. Evaluative norms are presented in Table 13.16.

AAHPERD Shuttle Run

Shuttle runs are often used to measure the agility of individuals in running and changing direction. Both males and females age nine and up can complete this test. Marking tape, a stopwatch, and three beanbags (or three of any small object, e.g., blocks of wood) are all the equipment needed for the test.

One beanbag is placed beside the participant on the starting line and two beanbags are placed on a line 30 feet (10 meters) away. The participant stands behind the starting line. On the signal, the participant (1) runs 30 feet to the line; (2) picks up one beanbag (Figure 13.18); (3) returns to the start line; (4) sets the beanbag down across the line; (5) picks up another beanbag; (6) returns to the line 30 feet away; (7) exchanges the beanbag he or she is carrying for another; and (8) runs back across the finish line.

A "ready" warning signal should be given prior to the starting signal. Administer two trials,

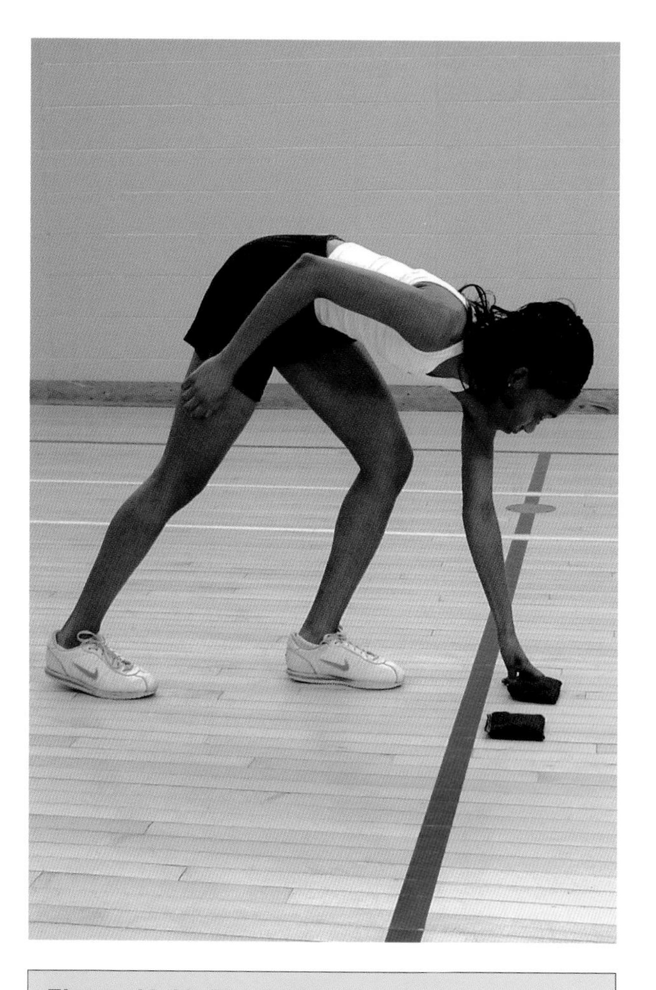

Figure 13.18 The shuttle run is a simple and easy way to test for agility.

Table 13.17 Norms (seconds) for the AAHPERD shuttle run, boys and girls 14 to 17 years old.

Percentile	Boys				Girls			
	14	15	16	17+	14	15	16	17+
95	8.9	8.9	8.6	8.6	9.7	9.9	10.0	9.6
75	9.6	9.4	9.3	9.2	10.3	10.4	10.6	10.4
50	10.1	9.9	9.9	9.8	11.0	11.0	11.2	11.1
25	10.7	10.4	10.5	10.4	12.0	11.8	12.0	12.0
5	11.9	11.7	11.9	11.7	13.1	13.3	13.7	14.0

with sufficient rest between them, and record the better of the two to the nearest tenth of a second. Evaluative norms are shown in Table 13.17.

Hexagonal Obstacle Test

This test is designed to assess agility, coordination, and balance. Begin by drawing or taping a hexagon on the floor (26 inches per side). To simplify the task, first draw a large circle with a radius of approximately 26 inches (66 cm); then insert the lines of the hexagon. Label the lines A to F (Figure 13.19 A).

Standing in the middle of the hexagon (Figure 13.19 B), the participant begins on signal to jump with both feet over side A and immediately back into the starting position within the hexagon. Then, without ever turning the body, the participant jumps over all sides to complete one round (Figure 13.19 C). The test continues until three full revolutions are completed. Time is recorded to the nearest tenth of a second. Time is stopped and recorded when the participant's feet enter the hexagon after jumping side F for the third time. The best time out of two trials is recorded (Table 13.18).

Summary

Physical fitness testing serves several important purposes, including diagnosis, placement, prediction, motivation, achievement, and program evaluation. When assessing physical fitness, it is important that reliable and valid fitness tests are selected. Reliability refers to the consistency of test scores, data, or

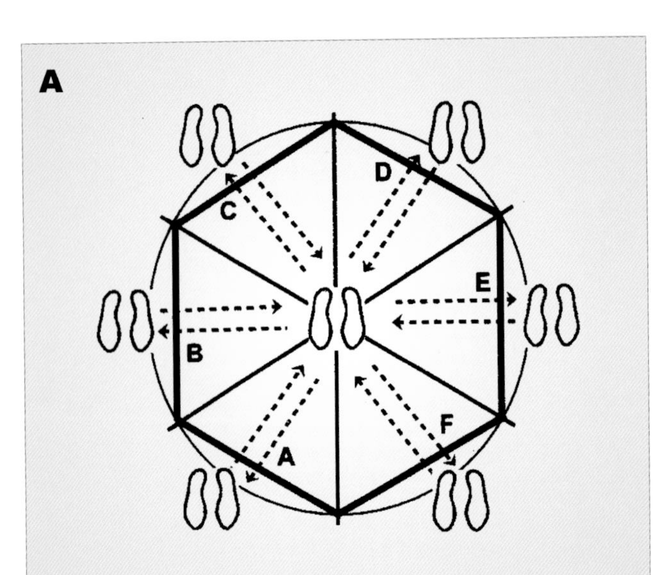

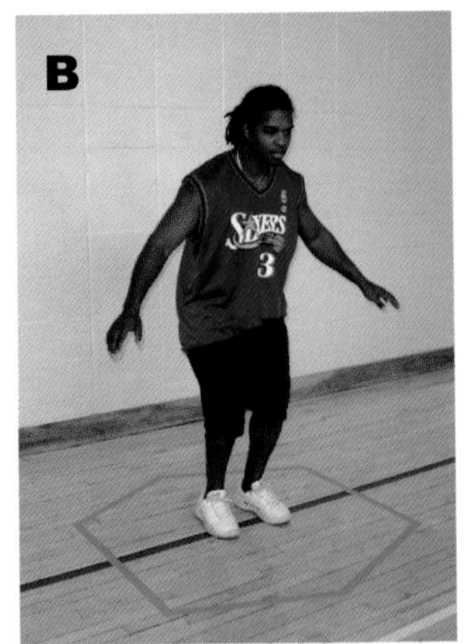

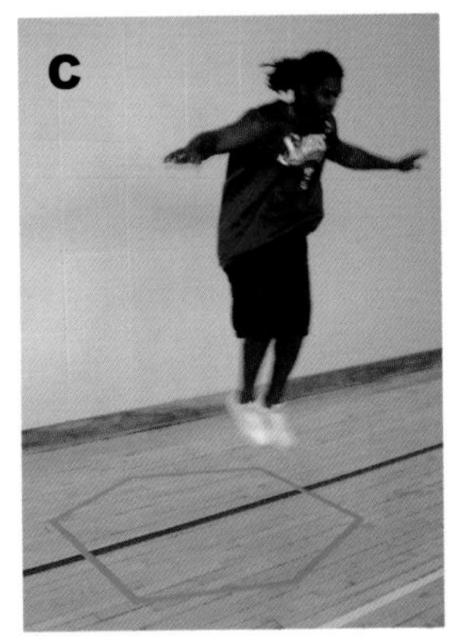

Figure 13.19 The hexagonal obstacle test. **A.** Schematic. **B.** Ready. **C.** Jump.

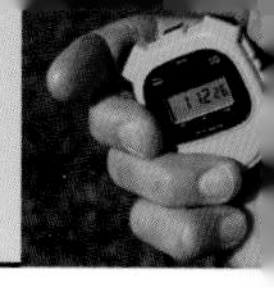

Table 13.18 Norms (seconds) for the hexagonal obstacle test.

Performance Level	Males	Females
Excellent	≤ 10.0	≤ 10.5
Above Average	10.1 – 12.5	10.6 – 14.5
Average	12.6 – 15.5	14.6 – 18.5
Below Average	15.6 – 18.5	18.6 – 21.5
Needs Improvement	≥ 18.6	≥ 21.6

observations, whereas validity refers to the extent to which a test measures what it proposes to measure. In addition, well-developed norms for all age categories help you compare and evaluate your personal test achievements relative to your peers.

Measures of physical fitness that are commonly assessed include aerobic capacity, body composition, muscular strength, muscular power, muscular endurance, flexibility, and agility. While more accurate test results can be obtained by using sophisticated laboratory equipment, many reliable and valid field tests (e.g., step tests, skinfold measurements, shuttle runs, and the sit-and-reach test) have proven to be useful in assessing the major components of fitness. However, you must realize that any assessment requires thorough preparation, practice trials, and attention to detail for sound measurement and evaluation of performance. Effective measurement and evaluation of your physical fitness should help you develop into a healthy and physically educated individual.

Key Terms

absolute strength
achievement
agility
diagnosis
field test
flexibility
grip dynamometer
laboratory test
maximal oxygen consumption ($\dot{V}O_2$max)
motivation
muscular endurance
muscular strength
norms
one repetition maximum (1RM)
placement
power
prediction
program evaluation
reliability
skinfold measurement
validity

Discussion Questions

1. List and briefly describe the six major purposes of testing and evaluation.

2. What are evaluative norms? Discuss their usefulness in interpreting test results.

3. Differentiate between the concepts of reliability and validity. Can a test have one without the other? Explain.

4. Discuss the advantages and disadvantages of laboratory versus field tests. Provide an example of each test.

5. List the most common sites used to measure skinfolds when estimating body composition. How do skinfold measurements differ from girth measurements?

6. Describe an alternative method of assessing maximal strength without performing a one repetition maximum (1RM) test.

7. Select one component of fitness and describe two field tests that can be used to assess it.

In This Chapter:

CHAPTER 14

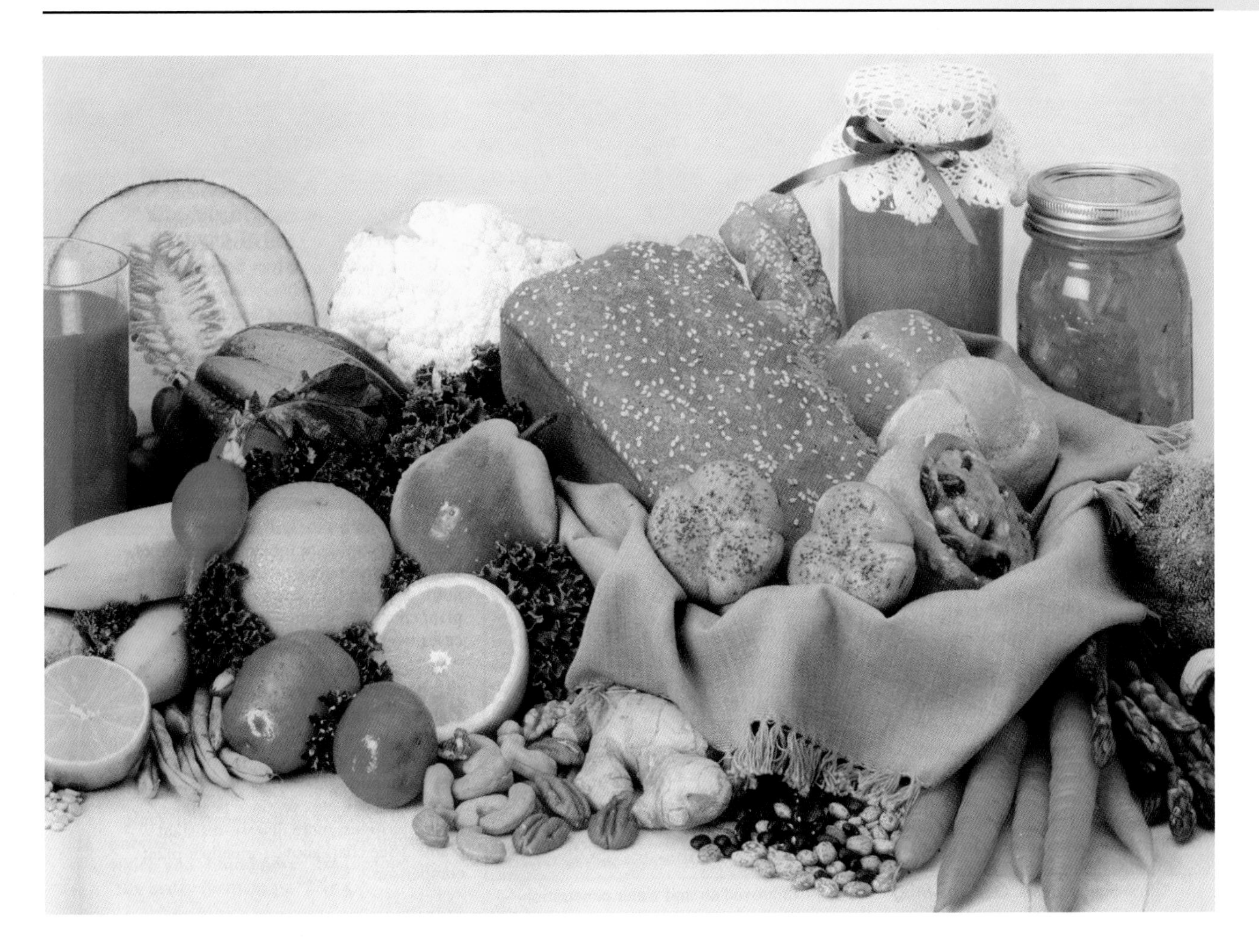

The Nutrition Connection

After completing this chapter you should be able to:

- describe the anatomy and physiology of the digestive system;
- identify the nutritional requirements and components of a healthy diet;
- outline the official nutritional advice provided for the United States;
- explain the unique nutritional needs of various populations;
- describe the effects of nutrition on athletic performance.

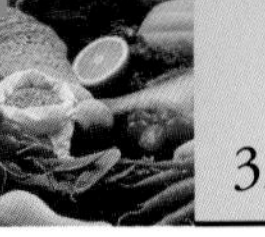

Not all the factors associated with health can be controlled, but your attitude and habits related to diet can influence your health in a positive way. The role of diet in overall health is significant and has profound effects on general well-being. Poor diets are often associated with disease and illness, but healthy diets can be sources of energy and vigor. Choosing foods that provide the necessary nutrients, while limiting those associated with disease, can therefore significantly affect the course your life and health will take. Furthermore, proper nutrition is essential for getting the competitive edge that athletes require to win, since it allows the body to perform at its best.

An understanding of what constitutes a healthy diet will allow you to make informed decisions about your nutrition-related concerns. While you should enjoy eating well and staying active, you must not assume that a healthy diet needs to be restricted to fat-free, low-sugar, and high-fiber foods all the time; in fact, the basics of a healthy diet are variety, balance, and moderation. And although you don't often hear that you should enjoy eating, this should also be part of a healthy diet. Too often, people are in such a rush to eat that they do not even realize they have eaten! Following these basic rules will effectively guide you to eating sensibly.

It is also important to understand that all foods are good – with one distinction: that some are good to have more often than others. There is nothing wrong with eating ice cream or a candy bar on occasion, just as long as it is *on occasion*. Labeling foods as good or bad sends a negative message about eating that should be avoided. (Note, too, that individuals with specific diseases or food allergies may not be able to eat certain foods.) An overall pattern of healthy eating should be your practical nutritional goal. We must not take for granted the remarkable ability of our bodies to deal with foods and substances over time, because it may catch up with us in the long run.

Students, for example, are faced with nutritional concerns on a daily basis over a simple matter such as what to eat for lunch. Bringing a lunch from home is always an option, but what kind of selection is there in school cafeterias (e.g., nutrition-wise, vegetarian dishes, and so on)? Many students settle for what is available to them, and fast foods (purchased within school cafeterias and from fast food restaurants, which are often conveniently located near schools) would not be considered ideal foods to eat on a daily basis.

A similar concern arises for the regular party-goer whose selection of foods and snacks is often limited to potato chips, cookies, and soft drinks (or alcohol) – all low nutrition-dense choices. It is up to the hosts of these parties, as well as those attending, to ensure that a variety of food is available for those who would prefer to eat on the lighter side. More often than not, however, individuals expect fattier foods at parties and may binge on these foods and beverages. It is important to note that healthier foods can also be very enjoyable, and if offered at a party, people will consume them. Providing different options helps make everyone feel at ease and keeps the occasion enjoyable for all.

Clearly, many issues are related to your nutritional habits, and their impact on your daily life is considerable. This chapter will attempt to outline the dietary recommendations made for the United States, helping you attain the tools necessary to incorporate a healthy diet in your own life.

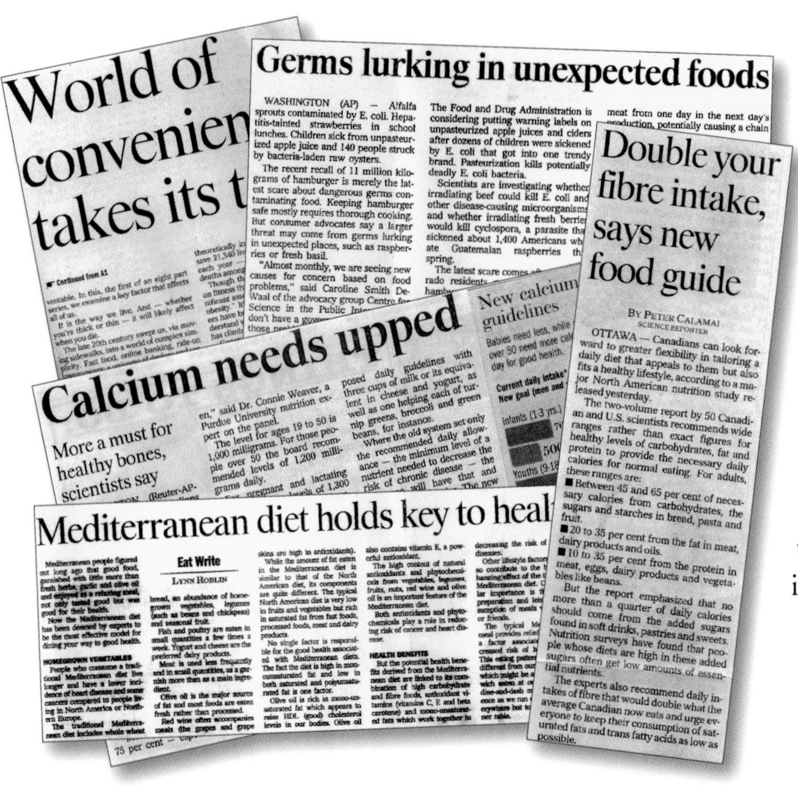

World of convenien[ce] takes its t[oll]

Continued from A1

ventable. In this, the first of an eight part series, we examine a key factor that affects all of us.

It is the way we live. And — whether you're thick or thin — it will likely affect when you die.

The late 20th century swept us, via moving sidewalks, into a world of complex simplicity. Fast food, online banking, ride-on

Germs lurking in unexpected foods

WASHINGTON (AP) — Alfalfa sprouts contaminated by E. coli. Hepatitis-tainted strawberries in school lunches. Children sick from unpasteurized apple juice and 140 people struck by bacteria-laden raw oysters.

The recent recall of 11 million kilograms of hamburger is merely the latest scare about dangerous germs contaminating food. Keeping hamburger safe mostly requires thorough cooking. But consumer advocates say a larger threat may come from germs lurking in unexpected places, such as raspberries or fresh basil.

"Almost monthly, we are seeing new causes for concern based on food problems," said Caroline Smith DeWaal of the advocacy group Centre for Science in the Public Int[erest] ...

The Food and Drug Administration is considering putting warning labels on unpasteurized apple juices and ciders after dozens of children were sickened by E. coli that got into one trendy brand. Pasteurization kills potentially deadly E. coli bacteria.

Scientists are investigating whether irradiating beef could kill E. coli and other disease-causing microorganisms and whether irradiating fresh berries would kill cyclospora, a parasite that sickened about 1,400 Americans wh[o] ate Guatemalan raspberries th[is] spring.

The latest scare comes ...

meat from one day in the next day's production, potentially causing a chain

Double your fibre intake, says new food guide

By Peter Calamai
Science Reporter

OTTAWA — Canadians can look forward to greater flexibility in tailoring a daily diet that appeals to them but also fits a healthy lifestyle, according to a major North American nutrition study released yesterday.

The two-volume report by 50 Canadian and U.S. scientists recommends wide ranges rather than exact figures for healthy levels of carbohydrates, fat and protein to provide the necessary daily calories for normal eating. For adults, these ranges are:

- Between 45 and 65 per cent of necessary calories from carbohydrates, the sugars and starches in bread, pasta and fruit.
- 20 to 35 per cent from the fat in meat, dairy products and oils.
- 10 to 35 per cent from the protein in meat, eggs, dairy products and vegetables like beans.

But the report emphasized that no more than a quarter of daily calories should come from the added sugars found in soft drinks, pastries and sweets. Nutrition surveys have found that people whose diets are high in these added sugars often get low amounts of essential nutrients.

The experts also recommend daily intakes of fibre that would double what the average Canadian now eats and urge everyone to keep their consumption of saturated fats and trans fatty acids as low as possible.

New calcium guidelines

Babies need less, while ... over 50 need more cal[cium] ... day for good health.

Current daily intake*
New goal (men and ...

Infants (1-3 yrs.)
Youths (9-18

Calcium needs upped

More a must for healthy bones, scientists say

(Reuter-AP-

en," said Dr. Connie Weaver, a Purdue University nutrition expert on the panel.

The level for ages 19 to 50 is 1,000 milligrams. For those people over 50 the board recommended levels of 1,200 milligrams daily.

posed daily guidelines with three cups of milk or its equivalent in cheese and yogurt, as well as one helping each of turnip greens, broccoli and green beans, for instance.

Where the old system set only the recommended daily allowance — the minimum level of a nutrient needed to decrease the risk of chronic disease — the

75 per cent —

Mediterranean diet holds key to heal[th]

Eat Write

Lynn Roblin

Mediterranean people figured out long ago that good food, garnished with little more than fresh herbs, garlic and olive oil and enjoyed as a relaxing meal, not only tasted good but was good for their health.

Now the Mediterranean diet has been deemed by experts to be the most effective model for dining your way to good health.

HOMEGROWN VEGETABLES

People who consume a traditional Mediterranean diet live longer and have a lower incidence of heart disease and some cancers compared to people living in North America or Northern Europe.

The traditional Mediterranean diet includes whole wheat bread, an abundance of home-grown vegetables, legumes (such as beans and chickpeas) and seasonal fruit.

Fish and poultry are eaten in small quantities a few times a week. Yogurt and cheese are the preferred dairy products.

Meat is used less frequently and in small quantities, as a garnish more than as a main ingredient.

Olive oil is the major source of fat and most foods are eaten fresh rather than processed.

Red wine often accompanies meals (the grapes and grape skins are high in antioxidants).

While the amount of fat eaten in the Mediterranean diet is similar to that of the North American diet, its components are quite different. The typical North American diet is very low in fruits and vegetables but rich in saturated fat from fast foods, processed foods, meat and dairy products.

No single factor is responsible for the good health associated with Mediterranean diets. The fact the diet is high in monounsaturated fat and low in both saturated and polyunsaturated fat is one factor.

Olive oil is rich in mono-unsaturated fat which appears to raise HDL (good) cholesterol levels in our bodies. Olive oil also contains vitamin E, a powerful antioxidant.

The high content of natural antioxidants and phytochemicals from vegetables, legumes, fruits, nuts, red wine and olive oil is an important feature of the Mediterranean diet.

Both antioxidants and phytochemicals play a role in reducing risk of cancer and heart disease.

HEALTH BENEFITS

But the potential health benefits derived from the Mediterranean diet are linked to its combination of high carbohydrate and fibre foods, antioxidant vitamins (vitamins C, E and beta carotene) and mono-unsaturated fats which work together in decreasing the risk of diseases.

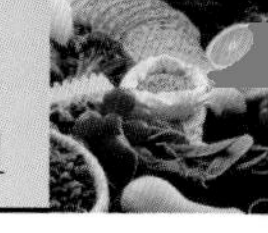

The Digestive System

You have probably wondered at one time or another how your body uses the food you eat to produce energy, and how energy-rich nutrients, water, and electrolytes are transferred into your body's internal environment. It is largely the role of the **digestive system**, composed of numerous structures and organs that work together, to accomplish this vital task. Although the components of the digestive tract are often discussed as separate structures according to the specialized functions they perform, the tract is actually continuous.

The **gastrointestinal tract** (digestive tract) portion of the system includes the mouth, pharynx, esophagus, stomach, small and large intestines, rectum, and anus; the **glandular organs** involved in the process include the salivary glands, liver, gallbladder, and pancreas (Figure 14.1). This effective organization allows food to be ingested and processed into forms that can be absorbed and used by the body. Keep in mind that the contents of the digestive tract actually remain part of the external environment until they have been absorbed across the gastrointestinal wall into the body.

The digestive system performs four basic digestive processes: digestion, secretion, absorption, and motility (Figure 14.2). Because the foods we eat contain nutrients that cannot cross the gastrointestinal wall (such as carbohydrates, proteins, and fats), the process of **digestion** is required to dissolve and break down these foods into molecules that can be absorbed by the body. Digestion works very closely with the **secretion** of numerous substances, including hydrochloric acid by the stomach, bile from the liver, and numerous other digestive enzymes. The **absorption** of the molecules produced by digestion occurs across a layer of epithelial cells lining the gastrointestinal wall to enter blood or lymph, where the circulatory system is able to distribute them to body cells. While foods are being digested, enzymes secreted, and digested molecules absorbed, the digestive tract is exercising **motility** through **peristalsis** – the muscular contractions that move the contents of the digestive tract forward. This process is important not only to propel the contents forward but also to mix food with digestive juices that promote digestion.

The Digestive Processes

The digestive system allows food to be ingested and processed into molecules that can be absorbed and used by the body by performing four basic digestive processes: *digestion, secretion, absorption,* and *motility*.

Although the purpose of the digestive system is to digest then absorb nutrients, some material is obviously excreted via the gastrointestinal tract as waste. This material is **feces**, consisting mainly of bacteria and ingested material that was not digested and absorbed (including fiber). Therefore, this system effectively allows us to absorb what we need and excrete what we don't need. Nonetheless, we do sometimes excrete what we need. Substances such as fiber, oxalates, and phytates can bind with minerals, for example, and prevent their absorption. This does not necessarily mean that you will be deficient in these nutrients, because the body will absorb more of a nutrient if it needs it; however, high consumption of substances that can decrease absorption *may* lead to a deficiency over time.

Functional Overview of the Gastrointestinal Organs

Thus far, we have discussed the functions and processes involved with the digestive system as a whole; but each portion of the system actually performs a specialized role. Digestion begins in the mouth, as chewing breaks food up into smaller pieces (bolus) that can be swallowed without choking. Further, **saliva** produced by three salivary glands in the head contains important mucus that moistens and lubricates food, as well as the enzyme **amylase**, which begins the digestion of carbohydrates.

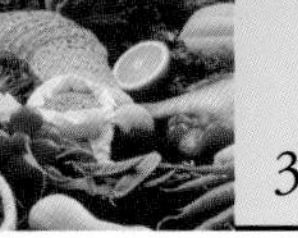

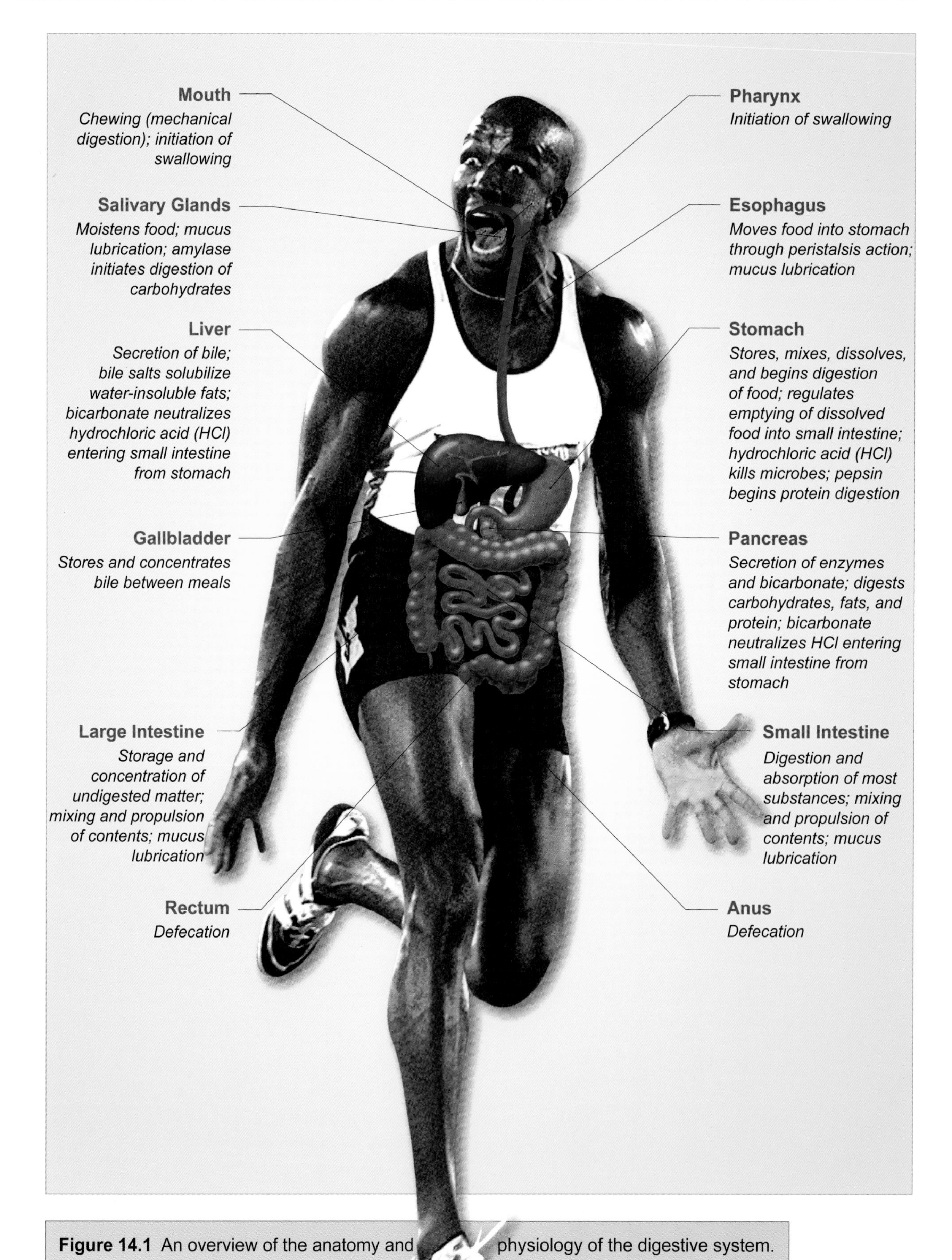

Figure 14.1 An overview of the anatomy and physiology of the digestive system.

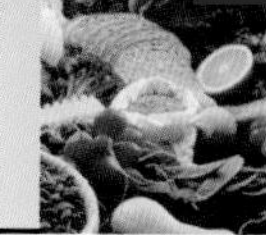

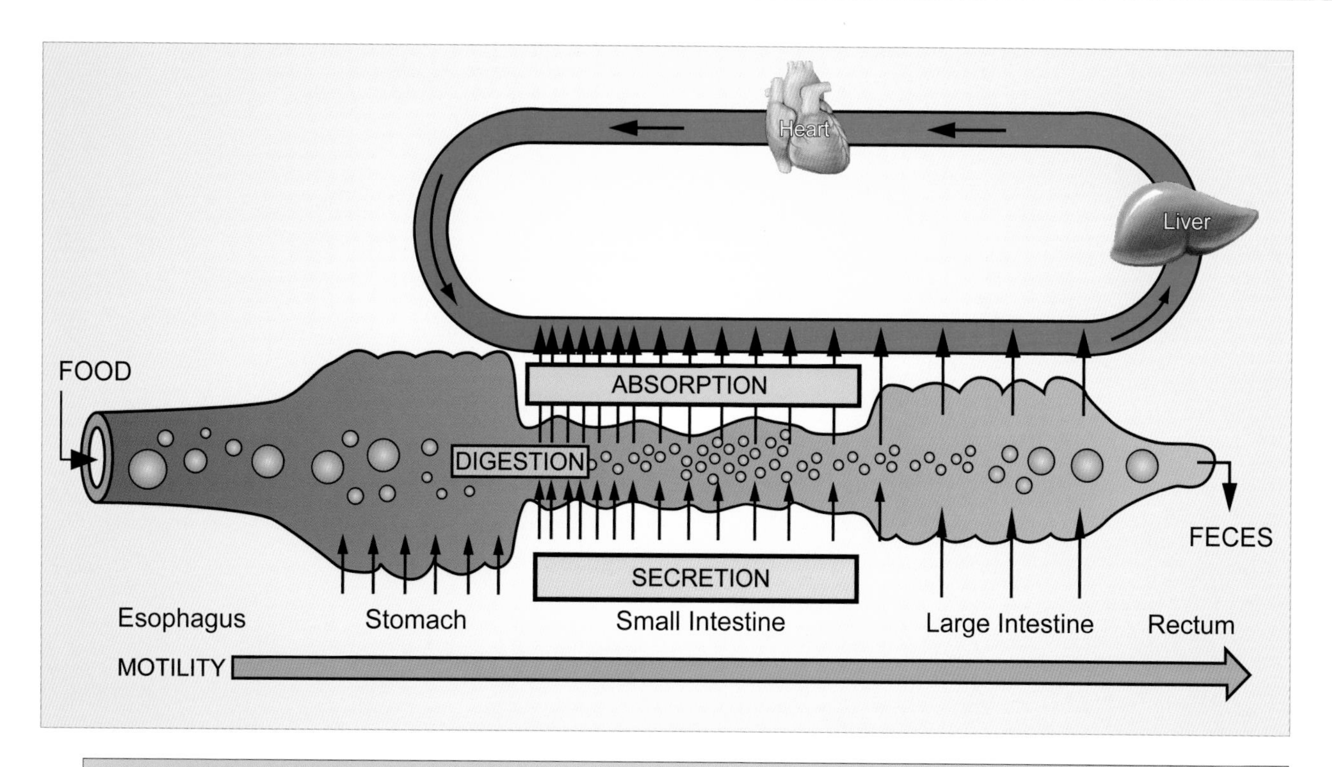

Figure 14.2 Schematic of the basic digestive processes: digestion, secretion, absorption, and motility.

The voluntary act of swallowing, initiated in the posterior mouth or **oropharynx**, results in movement of the food bolus into the **pharynx** and **esophagus**, where involuntary muscular contractions (peristalsis) take over and move the food down into the stomach. The **stomach** (a sac-like organ) serves as a storage site, dissolves and partially digests food, and prepares food for optimal digestion and absorption in the small intestine. Glands in the stomach's lining secrete a strong **hydrochloric acid** that serves to dissolve the particulate matter in food (except fat), and also kills bacteria that may have entered along with the food (though some do survive to flourish in the intestines). An enzyme called **pepsin** is also formed from the secreted precursor called **pepsinogen**. Pepsin begins protein digestion, and amylase (from the salivary glands) continues to break down carbohydrates into smaller fragments. However, despite the digestive actions that occur in the stomach, little absorption occurs across the stomach wall.

The next segment of the tract is the **small intestine**, where digestion is completed and most absorption occurs. The small intestine is approximately twenty feet in length and consists of three segments: the **duodenum**, **jejunum**, and **ileum**. Most absorption occurs in the duodenum and jejunum, including the absorption of vitamins, minerals, and water, which do not require enzymes to be digested. The existing molecules of carbohydrates, proteins, and fats are further broken down by hydrolytic enzymes into monosaccharides, amino acids, and fatty acids (absorbable units) respectively. While some of the necessary enzymes are located on the surface of the intestinal wall, others are provided by the pancreas and liver, which enter the duodenum of the small intestine via ducts.

The **pancreas** secretes both digestive enzymes, for each type of organic molecule, and an alkaline fluid consisting mainly of bicarbonate ions. The latter secretion serves to neutralize the acidic contents coming from the stomach to prevent damage to the small intestine wall and to provide an optimal pH for enzymes to function.

The **liver** also provides an important secretory product – **bile**. While the liver performs a myriad of functions, its exocrine functions related to the secretion of bile will be the focus here. Bile from the liver contains cholesterol, bicarbonate ions

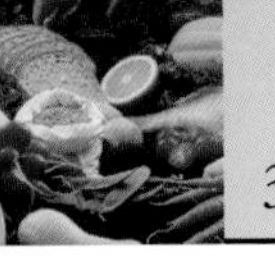

(like those from the pancreas), and **bile salts**. Bile salts are essential to the digestion and absorption of dietary fats, as they solubilize fats that are otherwise insoluble in water and convert large fat globules into smaller fat droplets (the process of homogenization). The **gallbladder** serves as a storage site for bile secreted from the liver; during a meal, the walls of the gallbladder contract to move the concentrated bile into the duodenum via ducts to exert its actions (mainly on fat).

In the small intestine, the molecules and ions are absorbed in a variety of ways, including diffusion (fatty acids), osmosis (water), active transport (mineral ions), and carrier-mediated transport (monosaccharides and amino acids). As the motility of the small intestine moves and mixes its contents, the material slowly moves toward the large intestine. By the time the contents reach the **large intestine**, which is approximately six feet in length, very little water, salts, and undigested material are left. It is the role of the large intestine to temporarily store these materials and concentrate them by reabsorbing salt and water. Once this is complete, the material (now feces) is moved to the **rectum** to be eliminated from the body through contractile activities, including associated sphincter muscles (the process is called **defecation**). This completes the long road that food must travel when providing us with the essential nutrients we need to lead a healthy life. The following sections will present the components of a healthy diet, what it means to eat well, and the importance of proper nutrition to healthy living.

Nutritional Requirements: Types and Sources of Nutrients

Nutrition, the science of food and how the body uses it in health and disease, encompasses a wide variety of topics and issues. When you consider what your diet is composed of, you probably think about the foods you eat. Really, what is important is what nutrients are contained in the foods you eat. Your body requires six categories of **essential nutrients**: proteins, fats, carbohydrates, vitamins, minerals, and water. The term "essential" refers to the fact that the body is unable to manufacture these substances (or not in adequate amounts to meet body needs), so they must be obtained from outside the body in the form of food or supplements. We rely on food to provide the nutrients we need to ensure proper growth and development (Figure 14.3). These nutrients are obtained when the foods we eat are digested (broken down) into compounds that can be absorbed and used by the body. It is vital to have a diet containing adequate amounts of all essential nutrients since they provide energy, as well as the ability to help build and maintain tissues and regulate body functions.

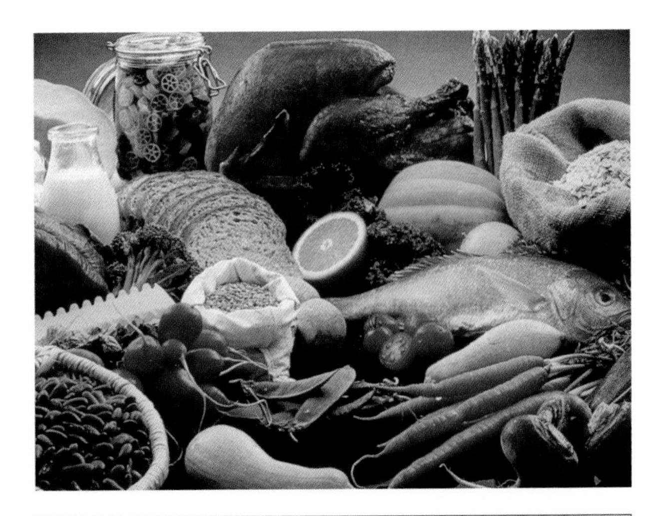

Figure 14.3 A balanced diet that includes all the essential nutrients is necessary to promote optimal growth and development.

There are three nutrients that provide your body with energy (**kilocalories**): proteins, fats, and carbohydrates. One kilocalorie (kcal) represents the amount of heat it takes to raise the temperature of 1 kg of water 1 degree Celsius. An average person needs approximately 2,000 kcal per day to meet his or her energy needs. Note that "energy" is the overarching term for kilocalories, calories, kilojoules, megajoules, and the like; different countries use different units to refer to energy. Therefore, "energy" will also be used in this chapter to represent kilocalories. Of the three classes of nutrients that supply energy, fats are the most energy dense, providing 9 kcal per gram.

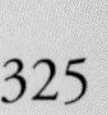

Kilocalories Versus Calories

In common usage, you will find that kilocalories are often referred to simply as **calories** (i.e., 1 kilocalorie contains 1,000 calories).

In contrast, proteins and carbohydrates each provide 4 kcal per gram. This difference is one reason why fats are recommended to be consumed in smaller amounts. Another source of energy (though not an essential nutrient) is alcohol, which provides 7 kcal per gram. Alcohol has no nutritional value, but its high energy content creates a problem with excess kilocalories being consumed (which often replace energy from nutritional sources).

Energy Densities of Various Energy Sources

Fats	9 kcal per gram
Alcohol	7 kcal per gram
Carbohydrates	4 kcal per gram
Proteins	4 kcal per gram

Energy needs are not our only concern. We also need a balanced intake of all the essential nutrients to achieve optimal growth and development. Just as the human body is largely composed of water (about 60 percent), the major component in foods is also water. Most foods, however, are composed of a mixture of nutrients, including vitamins and minerals, that perform special functions and fill unique roles. We take a closer look at each class of nutrient in the following section.

Proteins

Proteins may be found in every living cell, and they represent the basis of our body structure. Proteins not only provide important structural components or parts for muscles, bones, blood, enzymes, some hormones, and cell membranes but also function as an energy source. Proteins themselves are composed of chains of **amino acids**, the building blocks of life. There are 20 commonly recognized, naturally occurring amino acids; of these, the body can synthesize all but 9 – the so-called **essential amino acids** (*histidine, isoleucine, leucine, lysine, methionine, phenylalanine, threonine, tryptophan*, and *valine*).

Because amino acids are the building blocks of proteins, they are essential for our existence. But some sources of proteins are better than others in providing these essential amino acids. Individual protein sources are "complete" if they supply all 9 essential amino acids. Such **complete protein** sources are animal products, such as meat, fish, poultry, eggs, milk, and cheese. Sources of food that do not contain all the essential amino acids are called **incomplete protein** foods. These usually come from plant sources such as grains, beans, peas, and nuts. Although these sources are usually low in 1 or 2 amino acids, they are still good sources of essential amino acids.

Although incomplete protein sources on their own will not provide the appropriate complement of amino acids, various sources may be combined to achieve the full range to make a meal complete (Figure 14.4). This can be particularly important for vegetarians who must prepare meals consisting of plant foods, combining foods that account for the essential amino acids missing in some foods. Some common combinations include peanut butter and bread, rice and beans, milk and cereal, and macaroni and cheese. It used to be thought that protein complementation had to be conducted in the same meal; however, research has shown that as long as people consume different sources of protein

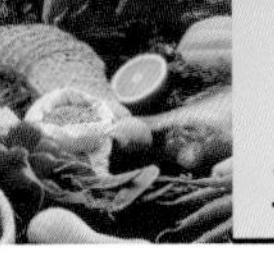

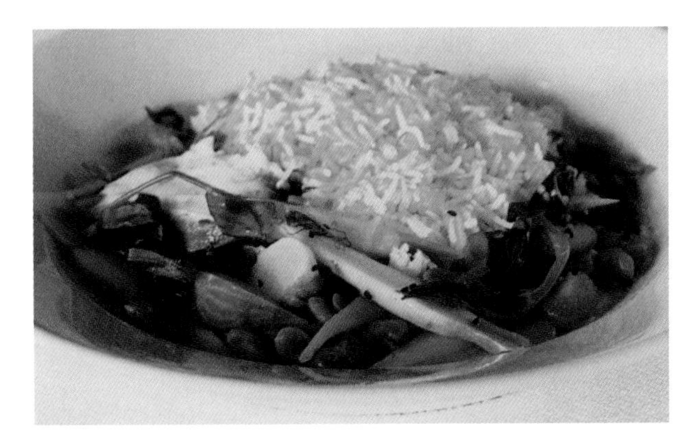

Figure 14.4 Rice and beans are examples of complementary protein sources.

throughout the day, not necessarily within the same meal, they will meet their needs. Nonetheless, most individuals will naturally combine, for example, milk and cereal in the same meal because these foods go well together.

Protein is essential for promoting growth and the maintenance of body tissues; but eaten in excess, protein can pose a problem. Any protein consumed beyond the body's needs is synthesized into fat for storage or used as a source of energy. The **dietary reference intake (DRI)** for protein for adults is 0.8 grams per kilogram of body weight. On average, this equals about 10 to 15 percent of your total daily energy intake; however, the DRI states that the **acceptable macronutrient distribution range (AMDR)** for protein is from 10 to 35 percent for individuals 19 years of age and older. On the other end of the spectrum, a drop in energy intake below your needs can lead to protein being selectively broken down to provide glucose for the body, which can hamper the growth and repair of body tissues. In *extreme* situations where your diet lacks an adequate amount of proteins and carbohydrates, the body turns to its own proteins, which causes damaging muscle wasting. Thus, an intermediate range of kilocalories must be consumed for optimal development. Therefore, starving yourself, even for short periods of time, can lead to muscle being used for energy, which is not a good thing. It is a myth that fat is burned first – protein is used first so your body can protect itself with the fat that surrounds your organs.

Fats

Negative associations around the word "fat" would appear to be general and widespread. Anything in excess can be detrimental to your health, but fat in moderation is essential.

Fat (also known as **lipids**) is an important nutrient in our diets for many reasons. It represents a source of usable energy, serves to insulate our bodies, cushions our organs, is involved in the synthesis of many hormones, and aids in the absorption of the fat-soluble vitamins (which would otherwise pass through our bodies). Further, the presence of fats in foods adds important flavor and texture (palatability), which is one reason why many people find it difficult to cut down on some of their favorite foods (which happen to contain fat). Still, being the most concentrated source of energy, the consumption of fat should be closely monitored. The DRI for fat ranges from 20 to 35 percent of total energy for individuals 19 years of age and older.

The fats in food are mostly in the form of **triglycerides**, composed of groupings of a glycerol (an alcohol) and three fatty acid molecules. Fats can be classified as saturated, monounsaturated, and polyunsaturated, based on the degree of saturation (the number of double bonds contained between the carbon atoms) of the fatty acid molecules. If no double bonds exist, these are **saturated fats**. When one double bond exists, the fatty acids are called **monounsaturated fats**, while those with two or

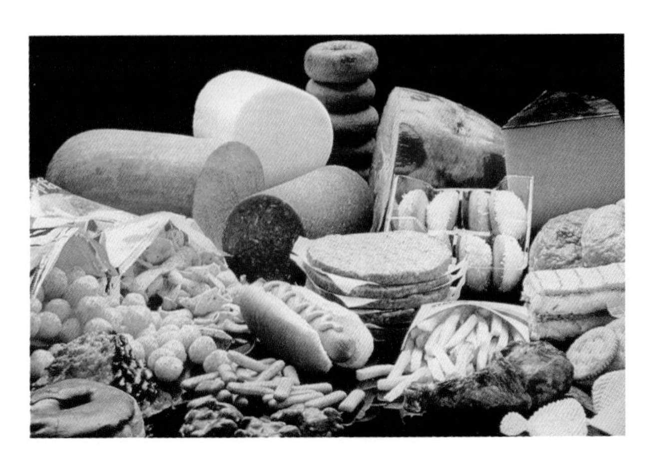

Figure 14.5 Foods containing high levels of saturated fat have been linked to heart disease.

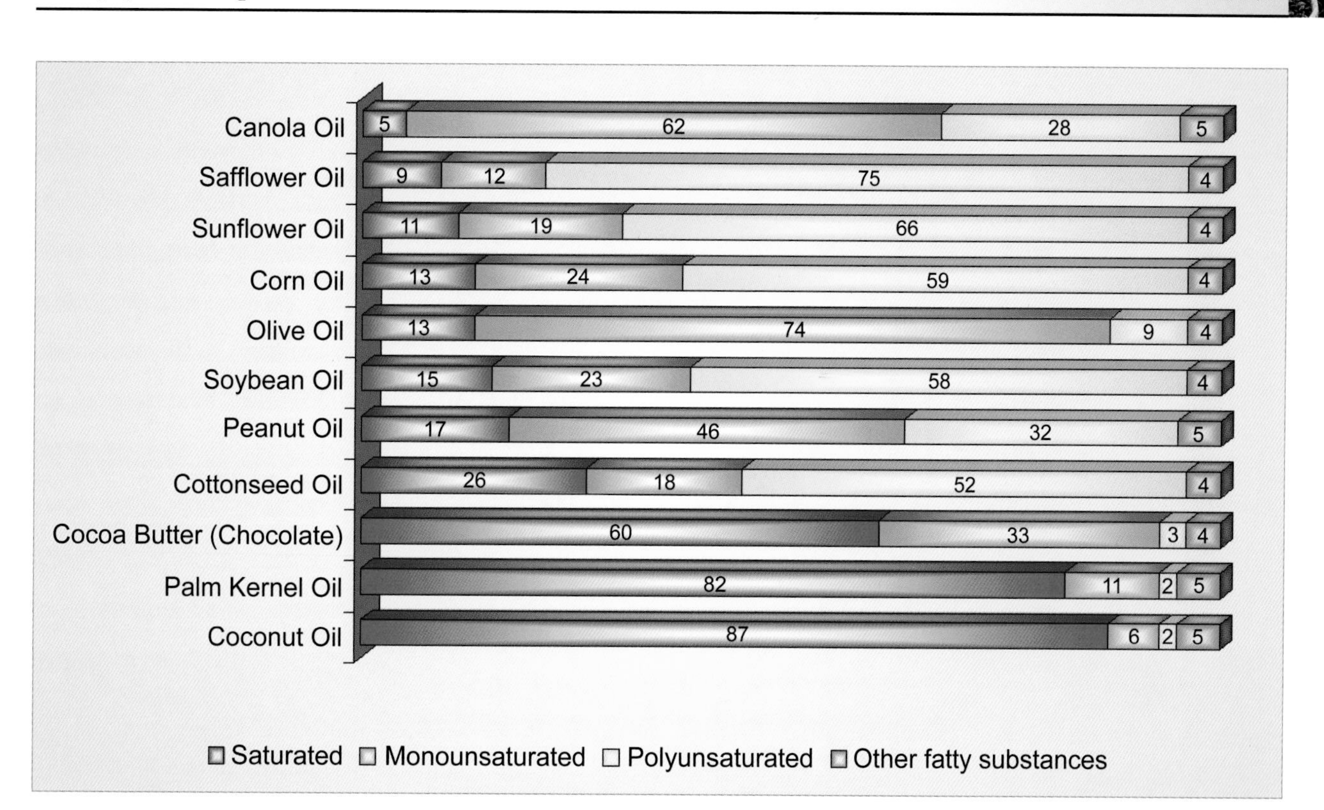

Figure 14.6 Percentages of saturated, monounsaturated, and polyunsaturated fats in common oils.

more double bonds are called **polyunsaturated fats.**

While most foods contain some combination of these fats, the dominant type of fatty acid determines the characteristics of the fat. Foods that contain an abundance of saturated fat are usually solid at room temperature – commonly found in animal products such as meats, dairy products, eggs, and many baked products. This is the type of fat most closely associated with numerous cardiovascular diseases such as heart disease and should be eaten less often (Figure 14.5).

Those foods that contain large amounts of unsaturated fats usually come from plant sources and are liquid at room temperature (so-called "oils"). These unsaturated fats come in two forms, mono- and polyunsaturated fats. These fats are deemed more desirable, as they are not linked to cardiovascular disease as are saturated fats; in fact, monounsaturated and polyunsaturated fats may lower blood cholesterol levels and reduce the risk of heart disease. Monounsaturated fats are found in large amounts in olive, canola, sesame, and peanut oils. Sunflower, safflower, and corn oils contain mostly polyunsaturated fats (Figure 14.6).

Unfortunately, not all fats from plant sources are low in saturated fats. Palm oil and coconut oil (tropical oils often used in processed foods) contain a high quantity of saturated fat. Furthermore, the process of **hydrogenation** turns what were double bonds in unsaturated fats to single bonds, yielding a more solid fat from an oil. This process is often used for three main reasons: (1) to extend the shelf life of fat (preventing its breakdown or its turning rancid), (2) to add the desired texture of pastry and cake products, and (3) because it is less expensive than using butter. Hydrogenated oils and fats should be used sparingly, and it is important to read labels in order to identify those products that use the process of hydrogenation.

The issue of serum (blood) cholesterol levels as it relates to the intake of dietary cholesterol and saturated fats is an important issue to consider in attempting to control your blood cholesterol levels. While **cholesterol** is synthesized by our own bodies and is an important constituent of all animal tissue, high levels of cholesterol and triglycerides

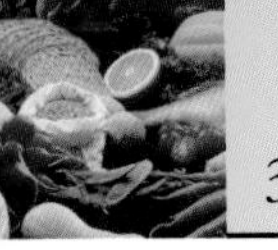

"Good" vs. "Bad" Cholesterol

Excess amounts of cholesterol in the body can accumulate on the inner walls of arteries, leading to a host of health implications, including atherosclerosis and heart disease. The actual amount of circulating cholesterol itself, however, appears not to be as important as the ratio of total cholesterol to a group of compounds called **lipoproteins**.

Lipoproteins serve as transport facilitators for cholesterol in the blood and come in two basic forms: **high-density lipoproteins (HDLs)** (so-called "good" cholesterol) and **low-density lipoproteins (LDLs)** (so-called "bad" cholesterol). HDLs transport circulating cholesterol to the liver for metabolism and elimination, while LDLs transport cholesterol to the body's cells. Therefore, individuals with higher levels of HDLs have been shown to be at lower risk for developing plaque in the arteries and subsequent heart disease.

Participation in regular physical activity, consumption of monounsaturated fats such as olive oil, maintaining a healthy body weight, and not smoking appear to play a role in reducing cholesterol levels by increasing levels of HDLs.

have also been implicated with the development of cardiovascular disease. There is evidence to show that an elevated intake of saturated fats may increase the levels of cholesterol in the blood. However, the relationship between the intake of dietary cholesterol (from sources such as egg yolk and animal fat) and blood cholesterol levels is uncertain. The process of hydrogenation mentioned earlier has another downside – it produces **trans fatty acids**, which are thought to increase blood cholesterol levels as well. Simply put, in the normal chemistry of a fat, the hydrogen atoms on a double bond form a "cis" configuration, meaning the hydrogen atoms for each double bond are on the same "side." When hydrogenation occurs (i.e., when hydrogen atoms are added to a fat to make it more saturated), the process actually impacts the double bonds and forces the hydrogen atoms to opposite sides, referred to as the "trans" configuration. The body does not react well to trans fatty acids, and they have been deemed worse than saturated fatty acids when it comes to cardiovascular disease. Trans fatty acids also occur naturally in some animal products, but not to the extent that results from hydrogenation of the many processed foods in our society.

Carbohydrates

When we are looking for food to give us a boost of energy, the foods containing high amounts of carbohydrates should be the ones we reach for (Figure 14.7). **Carbohydrates** are the primary source of energy in our diet. Based on the DRI, we should consume about 130 grams of carbohydrate per day, or it should make up 45 to 65 percent of our total daily energy needs. Carbohydrates are themselves composed of a number of glucose units, or saccharides, and can be divided into three groups based on the number of saccharides that form the molecule: monosaccharides contain one, disaccharides two, and polysaccharides more than two glucose units respectively. As a group,

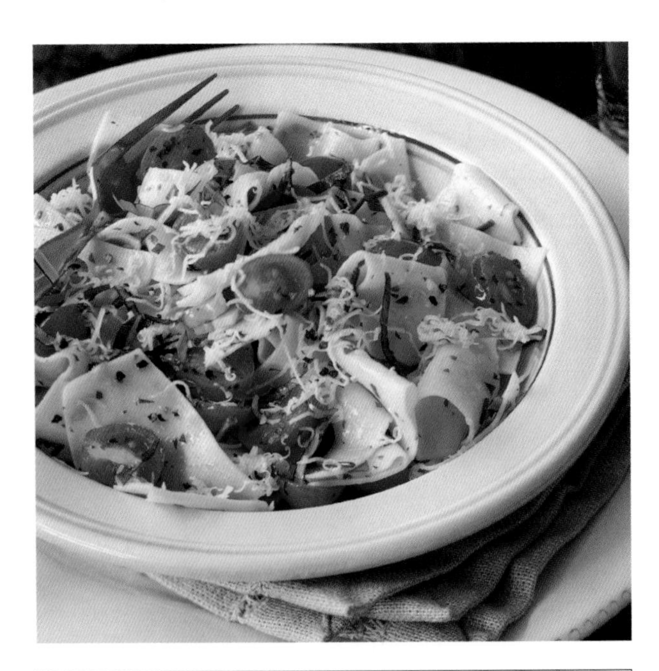

Figure 14.7 Pasta is an example of a food high in carbohydrates.

the mono- and disaccharides are considered sugars, while polysaccharides are commonly called starches. Note that the best sources of carbohydrates are those that come from whole grains (e.g., whole wheat bread); more processed carbohydrates (e.g., white bread) do not provide as many nutrients or as much fiber.

Monosaccharides

Monosaccharides are the simplest of sugars. These would include glucose (also known as dextrose), fructose (also called levulose), and galactose. Because glucose makes up the blood sugar as the body's primary source of energy, it is the most important monosaccharide; in fact, the brain and nervous system use glucose for fuel almost exclusively. Glucose tends to be found in foods such as fruits, vegetables, and honey, whereas fructose is often found in fruits and berries.

Disaccharides

When you think of sugar you probably think of table sugar. Table sugar, as it is commonly known, is actually a disaccharide – sucrose (a combination of glucose and fructose). As stated earlier, **disaccharides** are made up of two monosaccharides, of which one is always a glucose molecule. Other familiar examples of disaccharides include lactose, a combination of glucose and galactose (found in milk), and maltose, a combination of two glucose molecules (derived from germinating cereals). Along with the monosaccharides, the disaccharides provide much of the sweetness in the foods we eat. Sugar is abundant in our diets, although it is often hidden. We do not associate foods such as ketchup, salad dressings, or canned fruits and vegetables as containing significant amounts of sugar, but they do. The primary concern related to sugar consumption is dental caries (cavities), which can be combated by regular brushing and flossing.

Polysaccharides

Polysaccharides are commonly found in vegetables, fruits, and grains (e.g., pasta, bread, and rice). These are complex carbohydrates composed of extended chains of many sugar units (better known as *starches*). Aside from their role in providing a source of energy, starches often contain numerous vitamins, minerals, water, and protein. Dietary fiber is also a very important complex carbohydrate (see next section).

Before starches and double sugars can be taken up and used for energy, your body must digest them (break them down) into single sugar molecules (such as glucose) for absorption. Once in the bloodstream, glucose is able to provide cells with an energy source. The liver and muscles also store glucose in the form of **glycogen**. When such glycogen stores are full, any carbohydrates consumed above the body's needs are synthesized into fat and stored. Consuming large amounts of complex carbohydrates is beneficial to athletes since it enhances the amount of stored energy in the liver and muscles, providing an extended source of fuel for events of long duration. This does not mean that athletes should go above the DRI recommendations. It does mean that, in general, athletes should consume approximately 65 percent of their total energy needs from carbohydrates (especially complex carbohydrates in the form of whole grains).

Recommended Percentage of Total Daily Energy Supplied by the Three Major Nutrients (Based on the Dietary Reference Intakes)

Proteins	10 to 35 percent
Fats	20 to 35 percent
Carbohydrates	45 to 65 percent

Fiber

Fiber is not a nutrient by definition, but it is still an important component of our diets. For the most part, fiber includes plant substances that cannot be digested by humans; as a result, they pass through the digestive tract relatively unchanged, adding bulk for feces to facilitate elimination. Because some fiber can be metabolized by bacteria in the large intestine (producing acids and gases as by-products), a large

Types of Fiber

Fiber can be classified generally as soluble or insoluble. While sources of *soluble fiber* (such as fruit, legumes, oats, and barley) have been shown to help reduce blood cholesterol levels and maintain glucose balance, sources of *insoluble fiber* (such as vegetables, wheat, grains, and cereals) assist in bulking and softening feces, improving elimination, and preventing colorectal cancer.

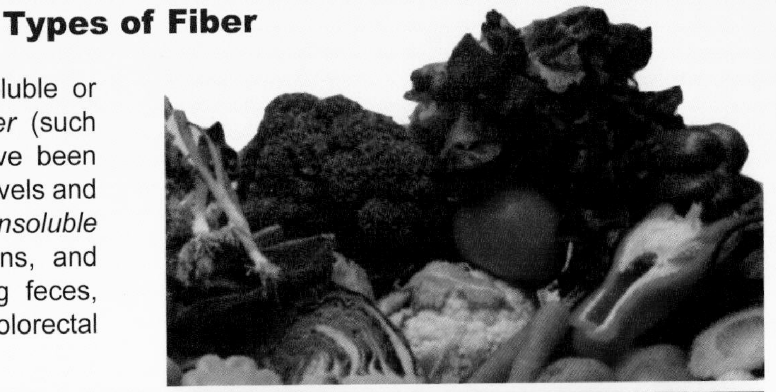

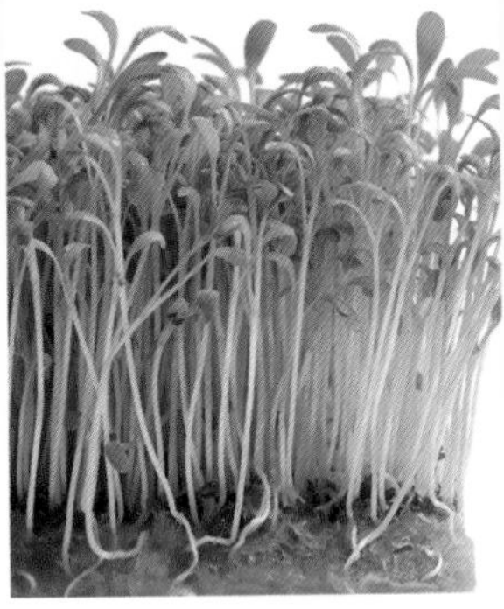

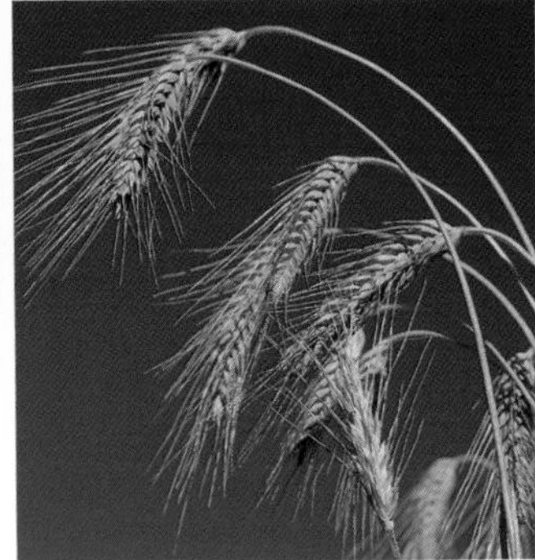

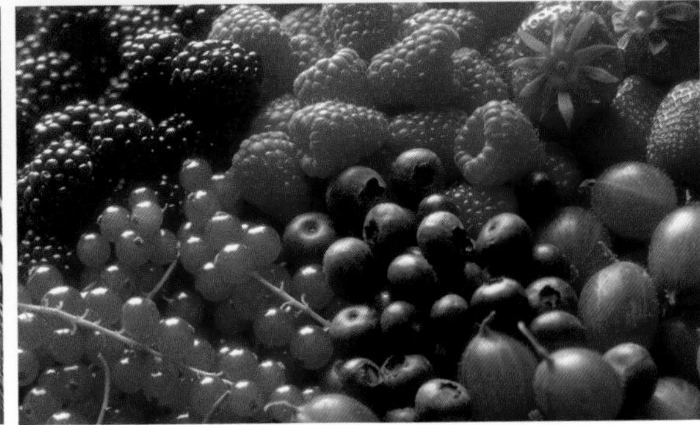

intake of fiber can lead to intestinal gas. The DRI for fiber ranges from 19 to 38 grams per day, depending on age and gender.

Fiber can be classified as soluble or insoluble, and each has significant physiological effects on your body. **Soluble fiber** has the ability to bind cholesterol-containing compounds in the intestines, thus lowering blood cholesterol levels by clearing cholesterol from the intestinal tract. Soluble fiber has also been known to slow your body's absorption of glucose, having potential implications for the treatment of diabetes.

Fiber that is classified as insoluble also offers important benefits for good health. Its main function is to absorb water from the intestinal tract, thereby aiding in making feces softer and bulkier to improve elimination. A diet with adequate amounts of **insoluble fiber** can effectively prevent a variety of health concerns such as constipation and some forms of cancer of the lower intestinal tract.

It is important to note that all plant foods contain some dietary fiber, though some more than others. Some rich sources of soluble fiber include fruits, legumes (e.g., beans, peas, lentils), oats, and barley. Other sources of dietary fiber such as wheat, grains, vegetables, and some cereals are classified as insoluble sources. It is always a good idea to eat fresh fruits and vegetables and whole-grain foods, since the processing of foods can remove some of their valuable fiber content. Try eating a variety of fiber-rich foods, but do so gradually so as to avoid upsetting your digestive system. In addition, make an attempt to choose alternatives – try whole wheat bread instead of white bread, or oranges in the place of orange juice. These types of habits can offer benefits that last a lifetime. When increasing fiber intake, be sure to increase your fluid intake as well. Though it is thought that too much fiber can lead to diarrhea, if you consume a lot of fiber and not enough fluids (e.g., water), constipation can actually occur.

Vitamins

Unlike the nutrients discussed thus far, vitamins do not provide energy; instead, they serve as **coenzymes**, facilitating the action of enzymes in a variety of responses and chemical reactions. Thus, vitamins are often part of energy reactions within the body, but they themselves do not provide energy (kilocalories).

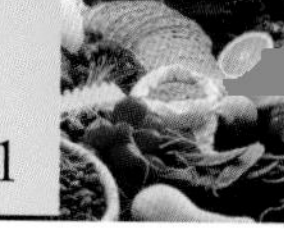

Table 14.1 The major water-soluble vitamins.

Vitamin	Physiological Functions	Vitamin Food Sources	Deficiency Effects
Thiamine (B_1)	Glucose metabolism; nervous system synaptic functioning	Enriched breads and cereals; pork, kidney; peas; pecans	Constipation; nausea; depression, fatigue, irritability; loss of hand-eye coordination; gait changes; often seen in anorexia nervosa
Riboflavin (B_2)	Red blood cell formation; glycogen synthesis; energy release from glucose and fatty acids; growth; adrenal cortex activity	Beef, liver, heart; yogurt, milk, cheese; almonds, broccoli, asparagus; produced by intestinal flora	Personality shifts, depression; cracked mouth and lips; purplish-red tongue; dry skin; fetal development effects
Niacin (B_3)	Protein and fat synthesis; energy release from all nutrient forms	Meat, poultry, liver; peanut butter	Diarrhea; depression, irritability, headaches; sleeplessness; personality disorientation; pellagra-dermatitis; death
Pyridoxine (B_6)	Protein, lipid, and carbohydrate metabolism; neurotransmitter synthesis; hemoglobin synthesis; antibody production; fetal nervous system function; synthesis/ breakdown of amino acids	Chicken, fish; egg yolk; bananas, avocados; whole-grain cereal	No known deficiency in adults; poor growth; anemia; skin lesions; decreased niacin production, convulsions; decreased antibody production
Cobalamin (B_{12})	Red blood cell formation; metabolism of folate; growth and function of nervous system	Meat, liver, kidney; eggs; dairy products	Pernicious anemia in adults; however, not caused by lack of B_{12}, but a lack of intrinsic factor influencing absorption
Folate (folic acid)	Red blood cell formation; fetal development; DNA synthesis required for rapid cell division	Bread; oranges and orange juice; meat, poultry, fish, eggs; broccoli, lima beans, asparagus, spinach	Megaloblastic anemia; infections; rheumatoid arthritis; chronic alcohol use leads to inadequate absorption; toxemia of pregnancy
Ascorbic acid (vitamin C)	Tooth development; maintenance of scar tissue; folic acid formation; absorption of iron and calcium; neurotransmitter synthesis	Peppers, broccoli, kale, cauliflower, strawberries, lemons, papayas, spinach, asparagus; liver	Scurvy; fatigue, shortness of breath, muscle cramps, skeletal pain; dry skin; anorexia; bleeding gums; depressed glucose tolerance; personality disorders

Vitamins are organic (carbon-containing) substances that are required in small amounts for normal growth, reproduction, and maintenance of health.

A distinction can be made between two broad classifications of vitamins: **water-soluble** (able to dissolve in water) and **fat-soluble** (able to dissolve in fat or lipid tissue). The water-soluble vitamins are not readily stored, so any excess is usually eliminated from the body during urination. Nonetheless, some water-soluble vitamins can be stored in some form, so overconsumption of any one vitamin is not good practice or good for health. Water-soluble vitamins include vitamin C and the B-complex vitamins (Table 14.1). On the other hand, the fat-soluble vitamins (A, D, E, and K), taken in excess, are able to be stored in fat (adipose) tissue in the body (Table 14.2). As a result there is a concern that consuming and retaining too many of these particular vitamins (especially vitamin A) may lead to toxicity. Obviously, a diet lacking a particular vitamin (adequate amounts) will lead to characteristic symptoms of a deficiency (Tables 14.1 and 14.2). In general, we return to the basics of balance, variety, and moderation. Consuming too much of one vitamin can be harmful, yet not consuming enough can also be harmful. A varied

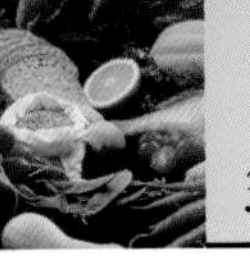

Table 14.2 The major fat-soluble vitamins.

Vitamin	Physiological Functions	Vitamin Food Sources	Deficiency Effects
A	Bone growth; night vision; sperm production; growth of epithelial cells; estrogen synthesis; mucus gland secretion	Eggs, cheese, liver, milk; yellow, orange, and dark green vegetables; broccoli, carrots, cantaloupe, spinach	Night blindness, corneal deterioration; skin changes; enamel alteration; diarrhea; respiratory infections
D	Bone growth; calcium and phosphorus absorption; kidney resorption of calcium and phosphorus; neuromuscular activity	Egg yolk; fortified milk; fish-liver oil, tuna; sunlight stimulates the body's production of the vitamin	Osteomalacia; osteoporosis; tooth malformation; rickets
E	Vitamin A absorption; prevents lipid peroxidation (antioxidant function); heme synthesis for red blood cell function	Wheat germ, whole-grain cereal; vegetable oils; liver; leafy green vegetables	Deficiency rarely seen in humans; destruction of red blood cell membrane
K	Synthesis of clotting factors in the liver; involved in bone metabolism	Dark green leafy vegetables, cabbage, cauliflower, tomatoes; eggs; liver; produced by intestinal flora	Prolonged coagulation time, bleeding, bruising

diet will help maintain balance.

Another fact to consider concerning water-soluble vitamins is that they will dissolve fairly quickly in water. It is therefore important not to overcook fresh fruits and vegetables because the longer they remain cooking, the more vitamins will be lost (unless you also plan to use the water in which the food was cooked). Steaming vegetables rather than boiling them is the best way to retain their nutritional content.

Some vitamins form substances that act as **antioxidants**. These aid in preserving healthy cells in the body. As the body breaks down fats or uses oxygen, compounds called **free radicals** are formed. These free radicals require electrons, so they react with fats, proteins, and DNA, damaging cell membranes and mutating genes along the way. Antioxidants serve to react with these free radicals (donating electrons) making them harmless to you. Such antioxidants in our diet include vitamins E, C, and beta-carotene (the vitamin A derivative). A regular intake of these nutrients goes a long way in maintaining a healthy body over time.

Minerals

Minerals are inorganic (non-carbon-containing) materials that are needed in small amounts to perform numerous functions in the body. Minerals function as structural elements (e.g., in teeth, muscles, hormones), regulate body functions (e.g., muscle contraction, blood clotting, heart function), aid in the growth and maintenance of body tissues, and act as catalysts in the release of energy. There are approximately 17 to 21 identified essential minerals for human health; the major minerals found in relatively large amounts in our bodies include calcium, phosphorus, magnesium, sulfur, sodium, and potassium (Table 14.3).

Other minerals (also known as **trace elements**) that are needed in relatively small amounts include zinc, iron, copper, fluoride, iodine, and selenium (Table 14.4). Although needed only in small quantities, trace elements are nonetheless essential to good health. Minerals are also involved in antioxidant activity. Such examples include iron, copper, and zinc.

Mineral intake is like the intake of vitamins. Any essential mineral taken in an amount that is either too small or too large can lead to deleterious symptoms. Calcium and iron are two minerals that are commonly lacking in our diets, leading to the potential conditions of **osteoporosis** and iron-deficiency **anemia**, respectively. The best way

Table 14.3 Major minerals and their roles.

Mineral	Physiological Functions	Mineral Food Sources	Deficiency Effects
Calcium	Bone ossification; tooth formation; general body growth; cell membrane maintenance; neuromuscular function	Milk and milk products; turnip greens, collards; broccoli; shellfish; soy products; molasses	Osteoporosis; osteomalacia; tetany
Phosphorus	Tooth and bone development; energy release (ADP/ATP); fat transport; acid–base balance; synthesis of proteins, enzymes, and DNA/RNA	Meat, poultry, fish; eggs; cereal products; peanuts; cheddar cheese; carbonated soft drinks	Fatigue; demineralization of bone occurs in people taking high doses of antacids; often seen in anorexia nervosa
Potassium	Protein synthesis; fluid balance; acid–base balance; nerve transmission; energy release	Potatoes; bananas; liver; milk; apricots, cantaloupe, avocados; lima beans	Abdominal bloating; muscle weakness; heart abnormalities; respiratory distress; most often seen in infants with vomiting and diarrhea
Sulfur	Metabolism; blood clotting; collagen synthesis; detoxification of body fluids	Protein foods	Not clearly established
Sodium	Nerve transmission; acid–base balance; formation of digestive secretions	Bacon; olives; table salt; processed cheese; sauerkraut	Unlikely to occur; vomiting or extreme sweating in children could reduce sodium
Chloride	Acid–base balance; carbon dioxide transport; acidity of stomach	Table salt	Unlikely to occur; may be lost as a result of vomiting
Magnesium	Protein, lipid, and carbohydrate metabolism; energy production; protein synthesis; nerve transmission; tooth enamel stability	Nuts; soy beans; whole grains; spinach; green leafy vegetables; clams; cocoa	Uncertain effects; nervousness, irritability, convulsions; skin changes; vasodilation; related to vomiting

to ensure that you consume adequate amounts of essential minerals is by eating a balanced diet with variety.

Water

Why do athletes consistently drink water before, during, and after periods of exercise? Water is a vital nutrient that is often ignored, but it is perhaps the most essential nutrient to life. Water composes such a large percentage of our bodies and the food we eat that its importance cannot be overstated. How can we overlook a substance that provides the medium for nutrient and waste transport, aids digestion and absorption, helps regulate our body temperature, forms the base of fluids that serve as lubricants (e.g., synovial fluid within joints), and plays a key role in the majority of the chemical reactions that take place within our bodies?

Water is an essential part of our diet. You can live without food for several weeks (up to 50 days), but only a few days without water. Yet many of us still underestimate the importance of an adequate daily intake of water. Each day, you experience a loss of body fluids through urine, feces, sweat, and evaporation in your lungs. In order to maintain a balance between the water you consume and the water that is lost each day, you need to consume about 1 ml of water for each kilocalorie you burn. It is important to note that you can hydrate yourself through other forms of beverages. For example, 100 percent fruit juices, milk, and yes, even coffee, do count toward your hydration needs. It used to be thought that a person would need to drink an

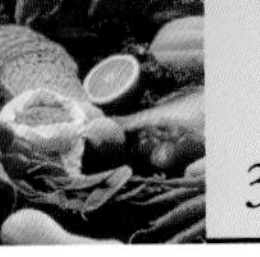

Table 14.4 Trace minerals and their roles.

Mineral	Physiological Functions	Mineral Food Sources	Deficiency Effects
Iron	Oxygen and carbon dioxide transport; red blood cell formation; vitamin A synthesis; antibody production; collagen synthesis; removal of lipids from the blood	Spinach, peas, greens, asparagus; liver; enriched breads and cereals; clams; beans	Iron-deficiency anemia; fatigue
Zinc	DNA/RNA synthesis; enzyme formation; acid–base balance; collagen production; fetal development; wound healing; HCl production; enhanced appetite and taste	Meats, seafood (especially oysters); whole-grain bread, whole wheat; cashew nuts	Immune function problems; depressed growth; skeletal problems; impaired wound healing; reproductive problems
Copper	Hemoglobin, protein, and cholesterol synthesis; energy release; enzyme formation; myelin sheath development	Liver; oysters; cherries; mushrooms; whole-grain cereal; nuts; cocoa	Anemia; skeletal, dermal, and vascular defects; central nervous system defects
Iodine	Protein, thyroxine, cholesterol, and vitamin A synthesis; cell metabolism	Water supply (depending on location); seafood; dairy products; iodized salt; spinach	Goiter (mainly in developing nations)
Fluoride	Skeletal stability; prevention of osteoporosis, dental caries, and periodontal disease	Water supply; tea; rice; spinach; soy beans; mackerel, salmon	N/A
Selenium	Antioxidation; energy release; heart muscle function	Meats, organ meats; cereal; milk and dairy products; fruits; plant sources depend on soil concentrations	Cardiomyopathy; osteoarthritis; hair loss; growth retardation

extra cup of water for every cup of coffee consumed, but this is not true because coffee still provides a person with fluids. The DRI for water is 2.7 liters per day for women 19 years of age and older, and 3.7 liters per day for men 19 years of age and older, and these needs can be met by foods (usually about 20 percent of the diet) and fluids (about 80 percent of the diet). Of course, people living in a warmer climate or exercising may have greater water requirements.

Dehydration is more of a problem than many acknowledge. Although thirst alerts us to consume more water, it is not always a reliable indicator of dehydration. For example, during an illness or during intense exercise, you may not feel the urge to drink, but that does not mean that your body is fully hydrated. On days that we feel uncharacteristically weak or fatigued, it just may be that we are slightly dehydrated and need to take in more fluids. An extreme bout of dehydration can cause severe weakness and land you in the hospital or even lead to death.

The opposite of dehydration is overhydration, which can manifest itself as *hyponatremia* (or below normal levels of blood sodium). Though not a common occurrence, hyponatremia can lead to dizziness, nausea, vomiting, and even death. This

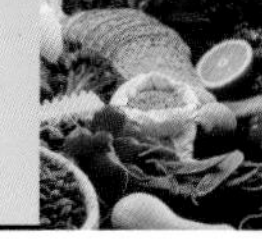

condition has been in the news a bit more lately because some marathon competitors have died from hyponatremia. These runners overconsumed water during the course of the race while also insufficiently replacing their sodium losses with carbohydrate–electrolyte drinks. Thus, just like other nutrients, it is important to consume the proper balance of water. The average person with normal kidney function who consumes too much water need not worry about hyponatremia.

Nutrition Guidelines and Recommendations

Most of us know what kinds of foods are good for us, and which we should perhaps eat less often, but where do we get this information? Various groups have established nutrition guidelines that help us plan a diet that is healthy and balanced. Based on current research, these authorities on nutrition recommend nutrient requirements according to age, sex, body size, and activity level. These **dietary reference intakes (DRIs)**, or **recommended nutrient intakes (RNIs)** in Canada, are designed to meet the needs of virtually the entire healthy population; as a result, the recommended intake of any nutrient will exceed the requirements of most people. DRIs and RNIs allow for a margin of safety, taking into account the vast individual variation that exists.

An easy way to understand these concepts is to think of them as doorways. If all doorways were made the height of the average person, that would leave all those above the average height hitting their heads. But if the doorways were made higher than average height, this would allow just about every individual to pass safely. It is important to note that although DRIs and RNIs are expressed on a daily basis, they should be regarded as an average recommended intake over a period of time (days or even weeks).

Dietary Guidelines for Americans

One set of guidelines for the United States is the Dietary Guidelines for Americans. These guidelines are revised about every 5 years, most recently in 2005 (visit the following website for more information: www.healthierus.gov/dietaryguidelines). The Dietary Guidelines for Americans promote overall healthier eating and increased physical activity. The key recommendations of the Dietary Guidelines for Americans 2005 are as follows:

- ***Adequate nutrients within energy needs***
  - Choose a variety of nutrient-dense foods and beverages from the basic food groups.
  - Limit the intake of saturated and trans fats, cholesterol, added sugars, salt, and alcohol.
  - Adopt a balanced eating pattern, such as the U.S. Department of Agriculture (USDA) Food Guide or the Dietary Approaches to Stop Hypertension (DASH) eating plan.
- ***Weight management***
  - To maintain a healthy body weight, balance kilocalories from foods and beverages with kilocalories expended.
  - To prevent gradual weight gain, make small decreases in kilocalorie intake and increase physical activity.
- ***Physical activity***
  - Reduce sedentary activities.
  - Engage in regular physical activity to promote health, psychological well-being, and a healthy body weight.
    - To reduce the risk of chronic disease, perform at least 30 minutes of moderate-intensity physical activity (above usual activity) on most days of the week.
    - Most people can obtain greater health benefits by engaging in physical activity of more vigorous intensity or of longer duration.
    - To prevent gradual weight gain in adulthood, engage in approximately 60 minutes of moderate to vigorous activity on most days of the week while not exceeding energy intake needs.
    - To sustain weight loss in adulthood, participate daily in at least 60 and up to 90 minutes of moderate-intensity physical activity while not exceeding energy intake

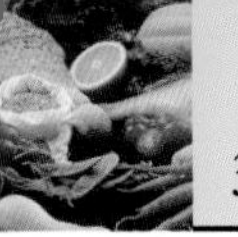

needs. Consult a health care provider before participating in this level of activity.

- Include cardiovascular conditioning, stretching exercises for flexibility, and resistance exercises or calisthenics for muscle strength and endurance.

▪ ***Food groups to encourage***

- Eat a sufficient amount of fruits and vegetables while staying within energy requirements. For a 2,000-kcal intake, two cups of fruit and 2.5 cups of vegetables are recommended per day.
- Enjoy a variety of fruits and vegetables each day. Select from all five vegetable subgroups (dark green, orange, legumes, starchy vegetables, and other vegetables) several times a week.
- Consume three or more ounce-equivalents of whole-grain products per day. The remaining recommended grains should come from enriched or whole-grain products. In general, at least half your grain choices should be whole grains.
- Consume 3 cups of fat-free or low-fat milk or equivalent milk products daily.

▪ ***Fats***

- Consume less than 10 percent of energy from saturated fatty acids and less than 300 mg of cholesterol each day. Keep trans fatty acid consumption as low as possible.
- Keep total fat intake between 20 and 35 percent of total energy. Most fats should come from polyunsaturated and monounsaturated fatty acids, such as fish, nuts, and vegetable oils.
- Choose lean, low-fat, or fat-free meat, poultry, dry beans, and milk or milk products.
- Limit intake of fats and oils high in saturated or trans fatty acids.

▪ ***Carbohydrates***

- Choose fiber-rich fruits, vegetables, and whole grains often.
- Select and prepare foods and beverages with little added sugars or caloric sweeteners. See the USDA Food Guide and the DASH eating plan for recommended limits.
- Reduce dental caries by practicing good oral hygiene and consuming sugar- and starch-containing foods and beverages less frequently.

▪ ***Sodium and potassium***

- Consume less than 2,300 mg of sodium (approximately 1 teaspoon of salt) per day.
- Select and prepare foods with little salt. Consume potassium-rich foods, such as fruits and vegetables.

▪ ***Alcoholic beverages***

- If you choose to drink alcoholic beverages, do so sensibly and in moderation – up to one drink per day for women and up to two drinks per day for men.
- Some people should not consume alcoholic beverages, including those who cannot restrict their alcohol intake, women of childbearing age who may become pregnant, pregnant and lactating women, children and adolescents, individuals taking medications that can interact with alcohol, and those with specific medical conditions.
- Individuals engaging in activities that require attention, skill, or coordination, such as driving or operating machinery, should avoid alcoholic beverages.

MyPyramid

The United States Department of Agriculture (USDA) revised the original Food Guide Pyramid in 2005 to a new pyramid system called **MyPyramid** – Steps to a Healthier You (Figure 14.8). The website to access this information is http://mypyramid.gov. The idea behind MyPyramid is that everyone's nutritional needs are specific, and thus more individualized pyramids may help people better understand what their bodies need. The USDA basically states that "one size doesn't fit all." The website is fairly interactive and allows individuals to insert their approximate energy expenditure to estimate total energy needs. For more specific nutrition information, a registered dietitian should be consulted.

MyPyramid
STEPS TO A HEALTHIER YOU
MyPyramid.gov
PEACHES
RAISINS
FAT-FREE MILK
1% MILK
TUNA
GRAINS
VEGETABLES
FRUITS
MILK
MEAT & BEANS
Eat at least 3 oz. of whole-grain cereals, breads, crackers, rice, or pasta every day
1 oz. is about 1 slice of bread, about 1 cup of breakfast cereal, or 1/2 cup of cooked rice, cereal, or pasta
Eat more dark-green veggies like broccoli, spinach, and other dark leafy greens
Eat more orange vegetables like carrots and sweetpotatoes
Eat more dry beans and peas like pinto beans, kidney beans, and lentils
Eat a variety of fruit
Choose fresh, frozen, canned, or dried fruit
Go easy on fruit juices
Go low-fat or fat-free when you choose milk, yogurt, and other milk products
If you don't or can't consume milk, choose lactose-free products or other calcium sources such as fortified foods and beverages
Choose low-fat or lean meats and poultry
Bake it, broil it, or grill it
Vary your protein routine – choose more fish, beans, peas, nuts, and seeds
For a 2,000-calorie diet, you need the amounts below from each food group. To find the amounts that are right for you, go to MyPyramid.gov.
Eat 6 oz. every day
Eat 2 1/2 cups every day
Eat 2 cups every day
Get 3 cups every day; for kids aged 2 to 8, it's 2
Eat 5 1/2 oz. every day
Find your balance between food and physical activity
Be sure to stay within your daily calorie needs.
Be physically active for at least 30 minutes most days of the week.
About 60 minutes a day of physical activity may be needed to prevent weight gain.
For sustaining weight loss, at least 60 to 90 minutes a day of physical activity may be required.
Children and teenagers should be physically active for 60 minutes every day, or most days.
Know the limits on fats, sugars, and salt (sodium)
Make most of your fat sources from fish, nuts, and vegetable oils.
Limit solid fats like butter, stick margarine, shortening, and lard, as well as foods that contain these.
Check the Nutrition Facts label to keep saturated fats, trans fats, and sodium low.
Choose food and beverages low in added sugars. Added sugars contribute calories with few, if any, nutrients.

MyPyramid.gov
STEPS TO A HEALTHIER YOU

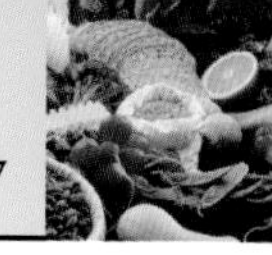

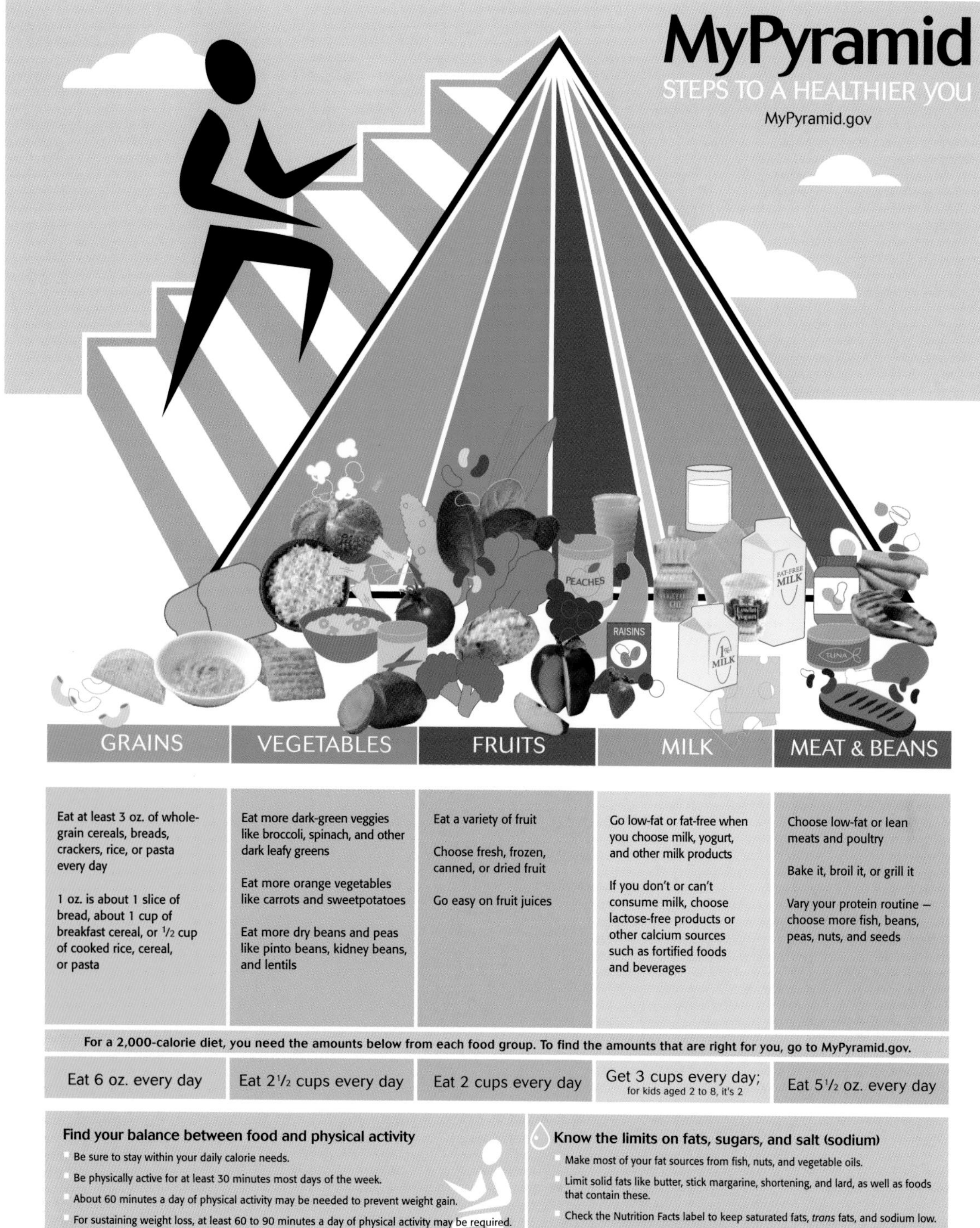

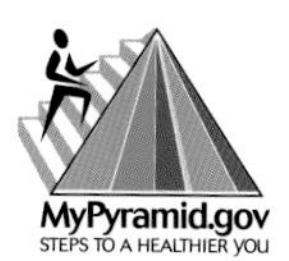

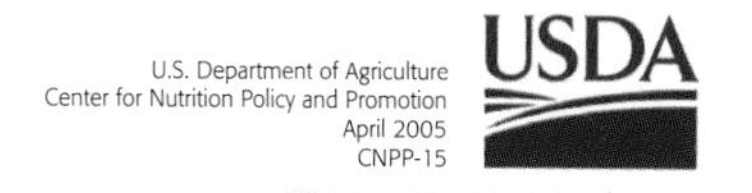

Figure 14.8 The original Food Guide Pyramid was revised to a new pyramid system called *MyPyramid – Steps to a Healthier You* to reflect the diversity of the American population.

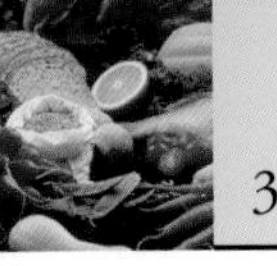

The Food Groups

Though we do not discuss the food groups as we used to years ago, MyPyramid does display six colors, representing, in essence, six food groups. The size of each of these "mini" pyramids reflects the emphasis you should place on consuming specific foods each day.

The orange triangle represents grains, of which we should strive to consume 6 ounces per day, with at least half coming from whole grains. The green triangle corresponds to vegetables, of which 2.5 cups should be consumed per day, with emphasis on varying the types of vegetables we eat, as well as on choosing deep green and orange vegetables for antioxidants. Red is the next color on MyPyramid, and it signifies fruits, of which we should consume 2 cups each day, again varying the type. The next mini pyramid is yellow. It is the thinnest because it represents fats, sugars, and salt, all of which we should consume sparingly. The emphasis is on "good" fats, such as fats from oils, nuts, and fish. The blue triangle represents milk, and 3 cups per day of skim or low-fat dairy (e.g., milk, yogurt) are recommended to ensure proper calcium intake. The final triangle, which is purple, corresponds to meat and beans, of which 5.5 ounces per day are recommended in the form of lean meats, poultry, fish, nuts, beans, peas, and seeds. The USDA also recommends that we broil, bake, or grill meat, poultry, and fish as much as possible to keep the fat content even lower.

Dietary Guidelines for Canadians

The established RNIs form the basis of eight recommendations presented by Health Canada, defining the desirable characteristics of the Canadian diet based on a review of the scientific literature. These recommendations provide a technical look at nutrition, targeting mainly educators and health professionals (see box *Nutrition Recommendations for Canadians*). The nutrition recommendations are reviewed regularly and act as the foundation for all healthy eating and nutrition programs in the country.

Nutrition Recommendations for Canadians

The Canadian diet should:

- provide energy consistent with the maintenance of body weight within the recommended range
- include essential nutrients in amounts recommended
- include no more than 30 percent of energy as fat (33 g/1,000 kcal or 39 g/5,000 kJ) and no more than 10 percent as saturated fat (11 g/1,000 kcal or 13 g/5,000 kJ)
- provide 55 percent of energy as carbohydrate (138 g/1,000 kcal or 165 g/5,000 kJ) from a variety of sources
- have a reduced sodium content
- include no more than 5 percent of total energy as alcohol, or two drinks daily, whichever is less
- contain no more caffeine than the equivalent of four regular cups of coffee per day

The nutrition recommendations are made more user-friendly in a report called *Action Towards Healthy Eating*, which outlines five general statements to keep in mind when choosing what foods to eat. These constitute *Canada's Guidelines for Healthy Eating*. The language used is simple, is easy to understand, and is aimed at all Canadians. The guidelines are as follows:

- ***Enjoy a variety of foods.***
- ***Emphasize cereals, breads, other grain products, vegetables, and fruits.***
- ***Choose lower-fat dairy products, leaner meats, and foods prepared with little or no fat.***
- ***Achieve and maintain a healthy body weight by enjoying regular physical activity and healthy eating.***
- ***Limit salt, alcohol, and caffeine.***

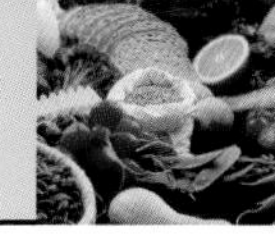

Canada's Food Guide to Healthy Eating

Nutrition recommendations are intended to provide guidance in the selection of a general dietary pattern that will supply recommended amounts of all essential nutrients. However, we eat food, not nutrients. That's where **Canada's Food Guide** comes in. The six-page handbook on healthy eating effectively translates nutrient recommendations or RNIs into a food group plan that provides a guide to ensuring a balanced intake of essential nutrients. *Eating Well with Canada's Food Guide* (Figure 14.9) takes Canada's Guidelines for Healthy Eating one step further by helping you plan healthy meals through a daily selection of food and allowing you to evaluate your eating habits in a general way.

A new version of Canada's Food Guide was released in early 2007 – the first revision of the Guide in 15 years. For the first time, the Food Guide is gender- and age-specific for Canadians over the age of two, offering tailored dietary advice for three different age groups of children, teens, and two different age groups of adults. And also for the first time, a national food guide for First Nations, Inuit, and Métis – *Eating Well with Canada's Food Guide: First Nations, Inuit and Métis* – has been developed to reflect the unique values, traditions, and food choices of aboriginal populations.

Just as no two people are exactly alike in appearance, personality, or interests, the same holds true when it comes to food and nutritional needs – different people need different amounts and types of food. The amount of food you need each day from the various food groups differs according to your age (e.g., teenagers have higher energy needs), body size (e.g., nutrient and energy needs are greater for those with a larger body size), sex (e.g., men generally have higher nutrient and energy needs), activity level (e.g., the greater the activity, the higher the energy and nutrient needs), and whether you are pregnant or breast-feeding. The Food Guide accounts for these differences and makes daily planning easier for all individuals.

The Food Groups

Most of us have heard and learned about food groups. These groups are created to help us choose foods that will lead to a healthy diet, emphasizing the ideas of balance, variety, and moderation. Choosing foods from each group in appropriate amounts will improve your chances of having a healthy diet. The Guide presents a recommended number of servings from four food groups: vegetables and fruit; grain products; milk and alternatives; and meat and alternatives. A small amount (30 to 45 ml) of healthy unsaturated oils or fats is also recommended daily for optimal health. All foods can be a part of a healthy eating pattern.

Although all the food groups in Canada's Food Guide are vital to a healthy diet, you will notice that the amounts required from each group vary – the rainbow design depicting the food groups provides a visual representation of this idea. The vegetables and fruit arc occupies the largest (outer) portion of the rainbow, while the meat and alternatives arc occupies the smallest (inner) portion of the rainbow. Notice also the directional statements that offer key points for choosing appropriate foods within each food group.

Vegetables and Fruit:

- ***Eat at least one dark green and one orange vegetable each day.***
- ***Choose vegetables and fruit prepared with little or no added fat, sugar, or salt.***
- ***Have vegetables and fruit more often than juice.***

Grain Products:

- ***Make at least half of your grain products whole grain each day.***
- ***Choose grain products that are lower in fat, sugar, or salt.***

Milk and Alternatives:

- ***Drink skim, 1%, or 2% milk each day.***
- ***Select lower-fat milk alternatives.***

Health Canada Santé Canada
Your health and safety… our priority. Votre santé et votre sécurité… notre priorité.

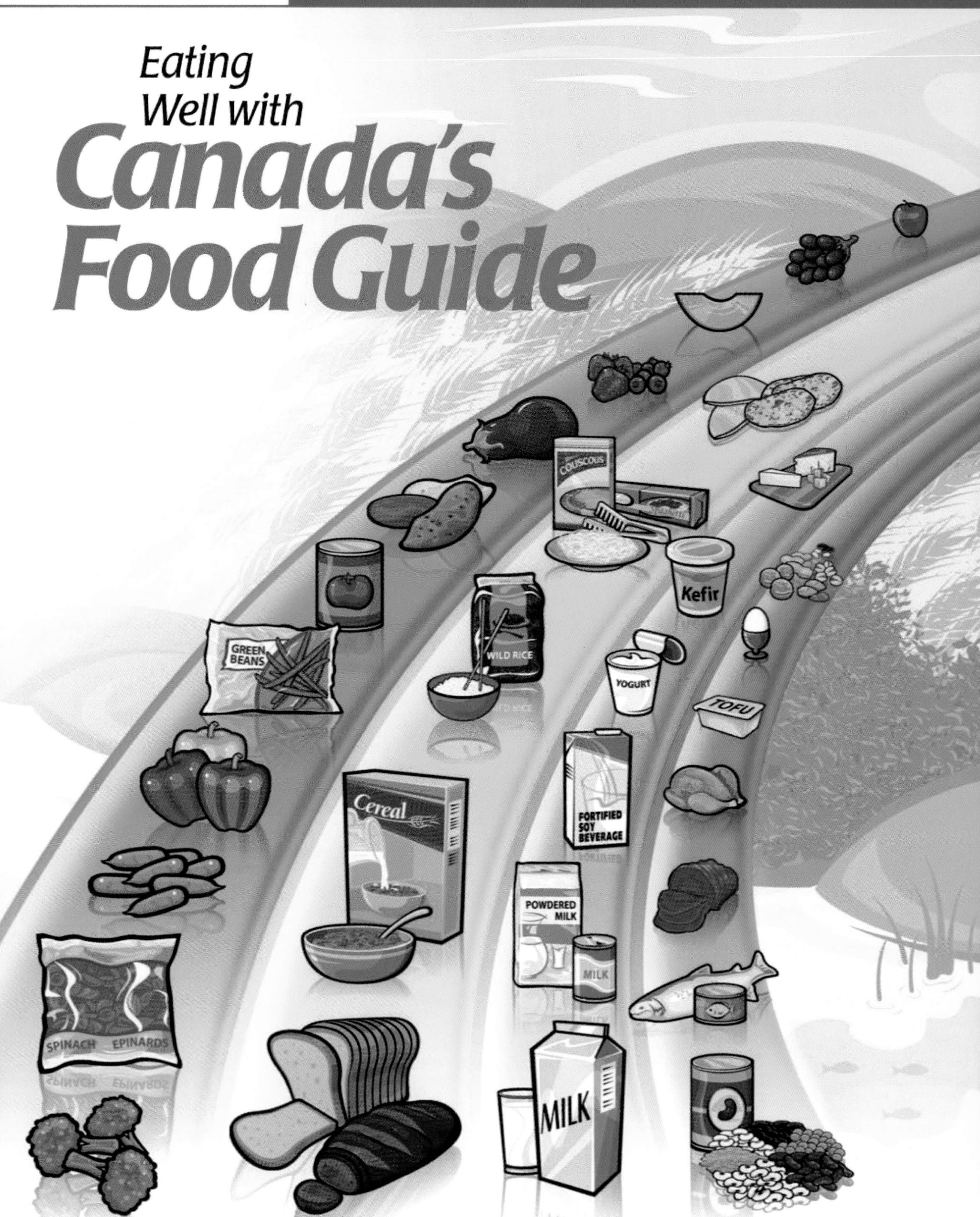

Canada

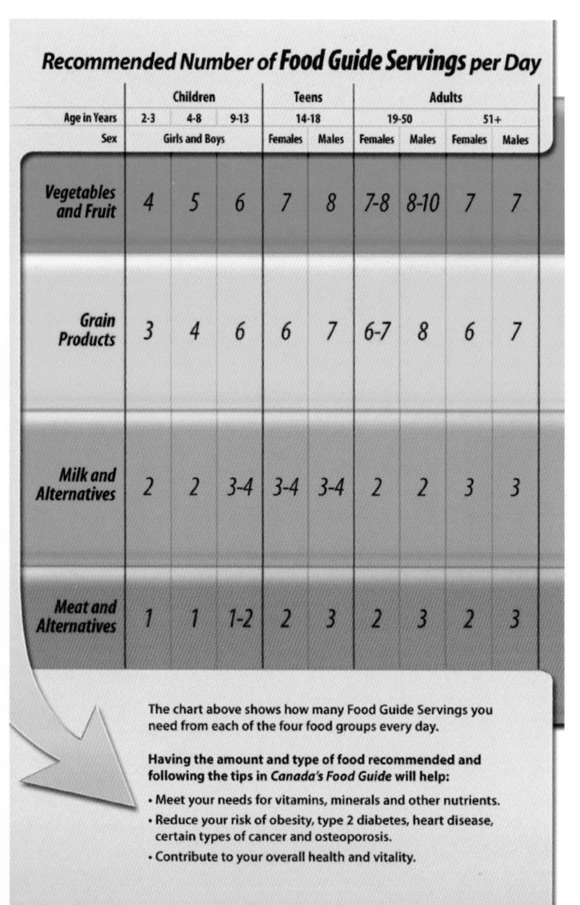

Recommended Number of Food Guide Servings per Day

	Children			Teens		Adults			
Age in Years	2-3	4-8	9-13	14-18		19-50		51+	
Sex	Girls and Boys			Females	Males	Females	Males	Females	Males
Vegetables and Fruit	4	5	6	7	8	7-8	8-10	7	7
Grain Products	3	4	6	6	7	6-7	8	6	7
Milk and Alternatives	2	2	3-4	3-4	3-4	2	2	3	3
Meat and Alternatives	1	1	1-2	2	3	2	3	2	3

The chart above shows how many Food Guide Servings you need from each of the four food groups every day.

Having the amount and type of food recommended and following the tips in *Canada's Food Guide* will help:

- Meet your needs for vitamins, minerals and other nutrients.
- Reduce your risk of obesity, type 2 diabetes, heart disease, certain types of cancer and osteoporosis.
- Contribute to your overall health and vitality.

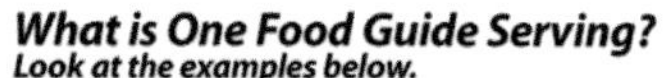

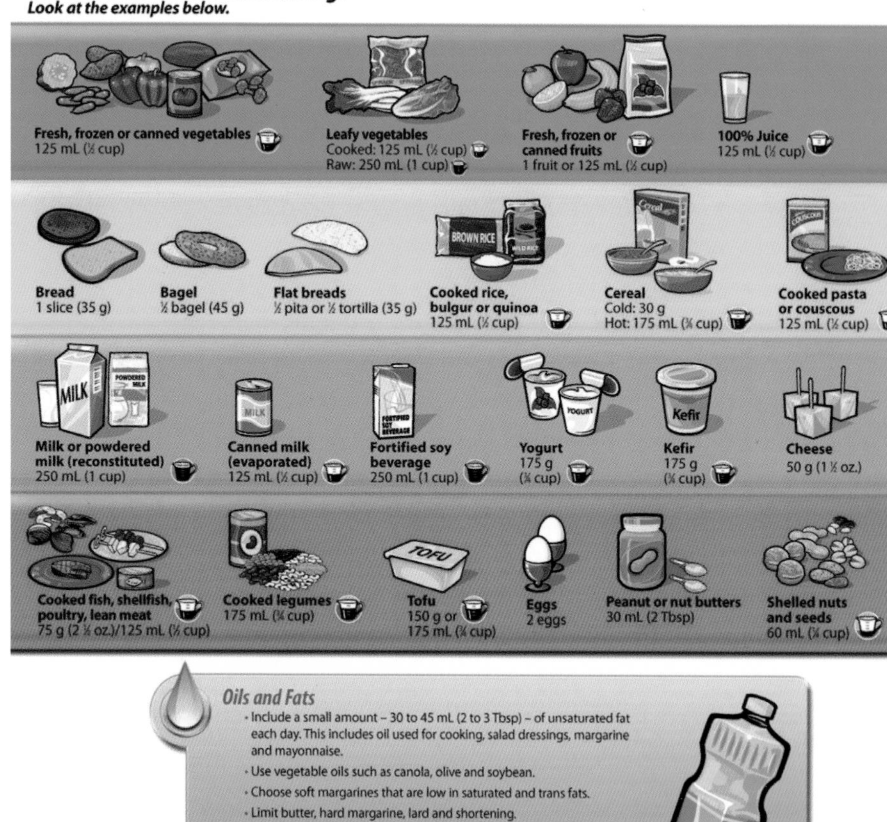

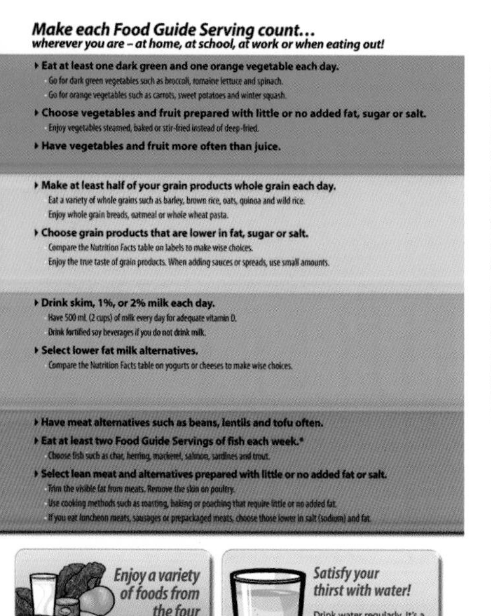

* Health Canada provides advice for limiting exposure to mercury from certain types of fish. Refer to www.healthcanada.gc.ca for the latest information.

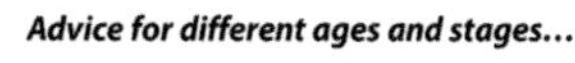

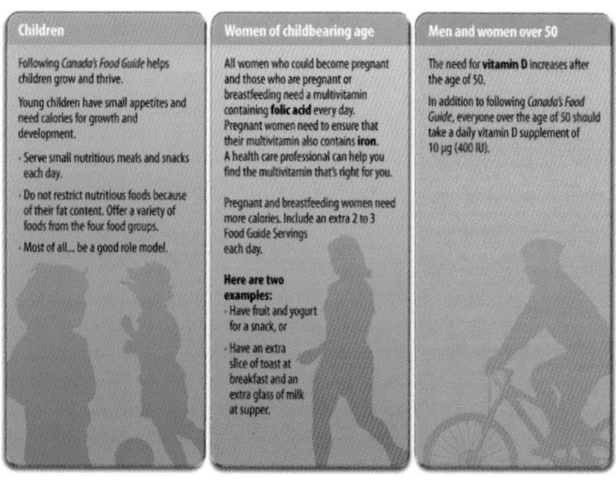

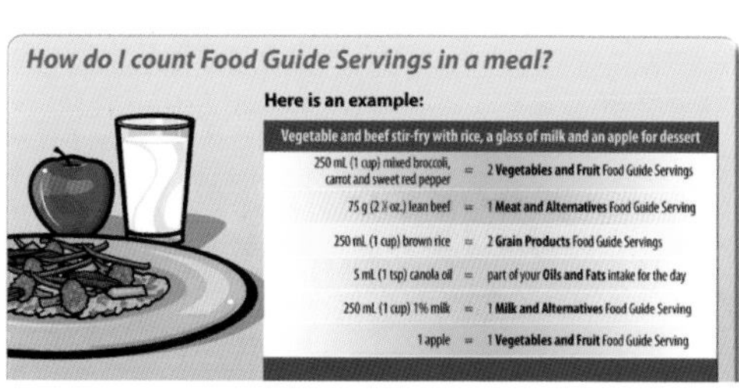

Eat well and be active today and every day!

The benefits of eating well and being active include:

- Better overall health.
- Lower risk of disease.
- A healthy body weight.
- Feeling and looking better.
- More energy.
- Stronger muscles and bones.

Be active

To be active every day is a step towards better health and a healthy body weight.

Canada's Physical Activity Guide recommends building 30 to 60 minutes of moderate physical activity into daily life for adults and at least 90 minutes a day for children and youth. You don't have to do it all at once. Add it up in periods of at least 10 minutes at a time for adults and five minutes at a time for children and youth.

Start slowly and build up.

Eat well

Another important step towards better health and a healthy body weight is to follow *Canada's Food Guide* by:

- Eating the recommended amount and type of food each day.
- Limiting foods and beverages high in calories, fat, sugar or salt (sodium) such as cakes and pastries, chocolate and candies, cookies and granola bars, doughnuts and muffins, ice cream and frozen desserts, french fries, potato chips, nachos and other salty snacks, alcohol, fruit flavoured drinks, soft drinks, sports and energy drinks, and sweetened hot or cold drinks.

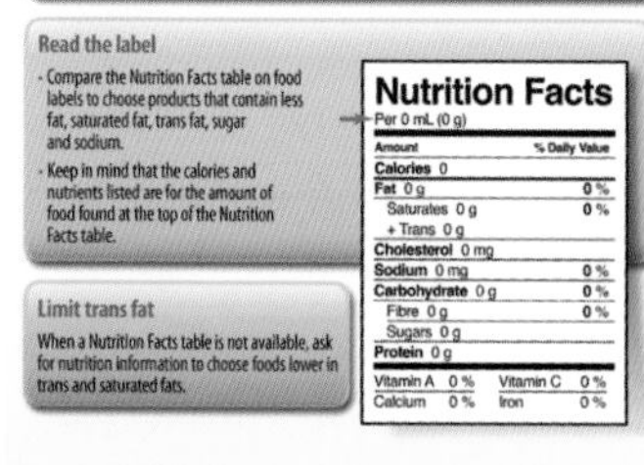

Take a step today…

- ✓ Have breakfast every day. It may help control your hunger later in the day.
- ✓ Walk wherever you can – get off the bus early, use the stairs.
- ✓ Benefit from eating vegetables and fruit at all meals and as snacks.
- ✓ Spend less time being inactive such as watching TV or playing computer games.
- ✓ Request nutrition information about menu items when eating out to help you make healthier choices.
- ✓ Enjoy eating with family and friends!
- ✓ Take time to eat and savour every bite!

For more information, interactive tools, or additional copies visit Canada's Food Guide on-line at:
www.healthcanada.gc.ca/foodguide

or contact:

Publications
Health Canada
Ottawa, Ontario K1A 0K9
E-Mail: publications@hc-sc.gc.ca
Tel.: 1-866-225-0709
Fax: (613) 941-5366
TTY: 1-800-267-1245

Également disponible en français sous le titre : Bien manger avec le Guide alimentaire canadien

This publication can be made available on request on diskette, large print, audio-cassette and braille.

 HC Pub.: 4651 Cat.: H164-38/1-2007E ISBN: 0-662-44467-1

Figure 14.9 Eating Well with Canada's Food Guide. For more information, visit the Food & Nutrition section of Health Canada's website at www.hc-sc.gc.ca/fn-an/food-guide-aliment/index_e.html.

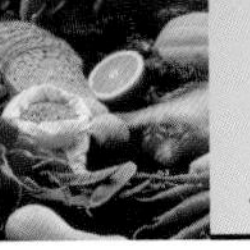

Meat and Alternatives:

- ***Have meat alternatives such as beans, lentils, and tofu often.***
- ***Eat at least two Food Guide servings of fish each week.***
- ***Select lean meat and alternatives prepared with little or no added fat or salt.***

The revamped Guide provides more details than ever on how to choose foods within the four food groups, and a wider variety of foods (e.g., couscous, flatbreads, tofu, and bok choy) are included to reflect the ethnic and cultural diversity of the population. To help you understand how much food from a specific food group makes up a Food Guide serving, more detailed information is also provided on serving sizes and food portions. For example, one slice of whole wheat bread, half a bagel, and half a cup of cooked pasta are each considered one serving from the Grain Products food group.

Canada's Food Guide also puts a spotlight on the importance of physical activity in maintaining a healthy body and mind. Eating well and being active work together to help you achieve better overall health, including a healthy body weight, stronger muscles and bones, and a reduced risk of various cardiovascular and other diseases. The Guide not only tells you to eat well and be active but also offers practical tips and guidelines on how to get there.

Nutrition Questions and Answers

There are several issues in choosing which diet to follow and in making decisions that apply to your own nutritional needs. This section will attempt to highlight some of these issues, now that you understand the basis of good nutrition and a healthy diet.

How bad is fast food, really?

The term "fast food" is synonymous with greasy, high-fat foods that have little or no nutritional value. But unlike junk foods, the nutritional value of fast foods prepared in walk-in or drive-through restaurants can vary immensely (Table 14.5). Still, the amount of fat (particularly saturated fat) and cholesterol found in most fast foods (especially those that are fried) makes consumption of these foods a poor nutritional choice. The limited variety of foods containing sources of dietary fiber available at most fast food establishments also represents a concern.

The picture is not all bad, however. Fast food restaurants have recently made an attempt to offer a wider variety of foods to meet the nutritional needs of the population. Menus have been extended to include salad bars, lower-fat meats, whole wheat breads, and lower-fat milk products. Nutritional information is also provided by the larger restaurants, and some fast foods can offer some real nutritional value. Although an excess of fast food consumption as a primary source of nutrition is undoubtedly unwise (and expensive), it can offer variety in a meal, which is the key to preventing most nutrient deficiencies. Still, fast foods are high in energy, fat, and salt, so you must be cautious when it comes to eating out. If you find yourself going to fast food restaurants often, then be wise in your choices – vary what you eat, and minimize the number of times you consume fried foods. For example, choose a salad instead of French fries and a grilled chicken sandwich instead of a fried one. Your body will thank you for it.

Why should I read food labels? What do they tell me?

If you are to make intelligent choices about what you eat, it is important to know how to read and understand food labels. Establishing healthy eating patterns begins at the grocery store where you choose your food. Increasingly, food

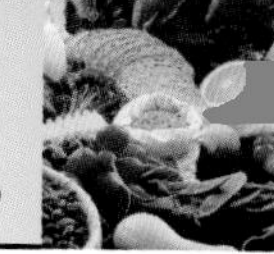

Table 14.5 Selected fast food facts.

Food	Energy (kcal)	Protein (g)	Carbohydrate (g)	Fat (g)	Energy from Fat (%)	Cholesterol (mg)	Sodium (mg)
Hamburgers							
McDonald's hamburger	263	12.4	28.3	11.3	38.6	29.1	506
McDonald's Big Mac	570	24.6	39.2	35	55.2	83	979
Dairy Queen single hamburger with cheese	410	24	33	20	43.9	50	790
Wendy's double hamburger (white bun)	560	41	24	34	54.6	125	575
Burger King Whopper	640	27	42	41	57.6	94	842
Chicken							
Arby's chicken breast sandwich	592	28	56	27	41	57	1340
Burger King chicken sandwich	688	26	56	40	52.3	82	1423
Dairy Queen chicken sandwich	670	29	46	41	55	75	870
KFC Nuggets (one)	46	2.82	2.2	2.9	56.7	11.9	140
Others							
McDonald's Filet-O-Fish	435	14.7	35.9	25.7	53.1	45.2	799
Arby's roast beef sandwich	350	22	32	15	38.5	39	590
McDonald's french fries (regular)	220	3	26.1	11.5	47	8.6	109
Wendy's french fries (regular)	280	4	35	14	45	15	95
Drinks							
Dairy Queen shake	710	14	120	19	24	50	260
McDonald's vanilla shake	352	9.3	59.6	8.4	21.4	30.6	201
Coca-Cola	154	—	40	—	—	—	6
Diet Coke	0.9	—	0.3	—	—	—	16
Sprite	142	—	36	—	—	—	45
Diet Sprite	3	—	0	—	—	—	9

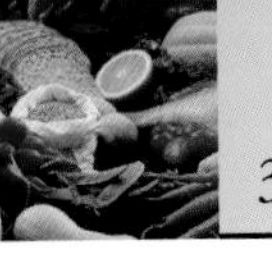

labels are providing more information relevant to nutrition.

Nutrition labels are standardized presentations of the nutrient content of food, designed to aid your choices as a consumer (Figure 14.10). The Nutrition Labeling and Education Act (NLEA) of 1990 requires nutrition labeling for most foods (except meat and poultry) and allows for the use of nutrient content claims and proper Food and Drug Administration (FDA)-endorsed health claims. For more information on nutrition labels, visit the following website: www.fda.gov/opacom/backgrounders/foodlabel/newlabel.html#daily.

Each label consists of a heading, a serving size, and values for energy, protein, fat, and carbohydrate based on the serving size. Some labels may also include the breakdown of fat into fatty acids (i.e., saturated, monounsaturated, and polyunsaturated, as well as trans) and cholesterol; the breakdown of carbohydrates into sugars, starch, and dietary fiber; as well as the sodium, potassium, and vitamins and minerals contained. The nutrients are expressed as a percentage of the **daily values**, which are label reference values based on a 2,000 kcal per day diet. Always check the serving size carefully, as all subsequent values on the label are calculated based on this amount of the product.

Serving Size

Are you eating the serving size indicated on the label? If not, you must adjust the nutrient and energy values accordingly.

Total Fat

It's a good idea to cut back on fat (especially saturated and trans fats) for heart health and general well-being. Look for products with low-fat alternatives.

Sodium

You know it better as salt. High sodium consumption is associated with high blood pressure in some individuals, so keep your intake low. If you are an athlete, however, and you do not have a reason to lower your salt intake, it is beneficial for you to consume more salt in your diet to keep you well hydrated.

Protein

Where are you getting your protein? Animal proteins are usually higher in fat and cholesterol. Emphasize low-fat or skim milk, yogurt, and cheeses, and try vegetable proteins such as beans and cereals as well as nuts and seeds.

Nutrition Facts

Serving Size: 3/4 Cup (30g)
Servings Per Package: About 7

Amount Per Serving	Cereal	Cereal With 1/2 Cup Skim Milk
Calories	120	160
Calories from Fat	15	15
	% Daily Value**	
Total Fat 1.5g*	**2%**	**2%**
Saturated Fat 0g	**0%**	**0%**
Trans Fat 0g		
Polyunsaturated Fat 0g		
Monounsaturated Fat 0.5g		
Cholesterol 0mg	**0%**	**1%**
Sodium 220mg	**9%**	**12%**
Total Carbohydrate 26g	**9%**	**11%**
Dietary Fiber less than 1g	**2%**	**2%**
Sugars 13g		
Other Carbohydrate 12g		
Protein 1g		
Vitamin A	0%	6%
Vitamin C	0%	2%
Calcium	0%	15%
Iron	25%	25%
Thiamin	25%	30%
Riboflavin	25%	35%
Niacin	25%	25%
Vitamin B6	25%	25%
Folate (Folic Acid)	25%	25%
Zinc	25%	30%

* Amount in cereal. One-half cup skim milk contributes an additional 65mg sodium, 6g total carbohydrate (6g sugars) and 4g protein.
**Percent Daily Values are based on a 2,000 calorie diet. Your daily values may be higher or lower depending on your calorie needs:

	Calories:	2,000	2,500
Total Fat	Less than	65g	80g
Saturated Fat	Less than	20g	25g
Cholesterol	Less than	300mg	300mg
Sodium	Less than	2,400mg	2,400mg
Total Carbohydrate		300g	375g
Dietary Fiber		25g	30g

Calories (Energy)

Are you watching your weight? This value tells you how many kilocalories are contained in a single serving of the product.

Daily Value (Daily Intake)

What percentage of your DRI or RNI does a serving of this product give you? Use these numbers as a guide.

Total Carbohydrate

Need a boost of energy? Carbohydrates provide a major source of energy and are found in foods such as breads, cereals, and fruit. But watch out for foods high in simple sugars. Consume at least half of your carbohydrates as whole grains.

Dietary Fiber

Soluble and insoluble sources of fiber help prevent heart disease and cancer, respectively, as well as keep you regular.

Vitamins and Minerals

Eat a variety of foods daily to ensure an adequate intake of vitamins and minerals needed for vital body functions.

Figure 14.10 Sample nutrition label.

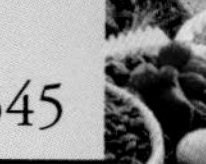

Nutrition Claims and What They Mean

Often presented in a bold, banner format on the product package, nutrition claims highlight a nutritional feature of a product. Since the U.S. government requires that these claims must always be backed up by detailed facts relating to the claim, look for more information on the label.

- ***Free.*** The product contains no amount of, or only trivial amounts of, one or more of the following components: fat, saturated fat, cholesterol, sodium, sugars, and kilocalories.
- ***Low.*** (Also "little," "few," "low source of," and "contains a small amount of") Applies to foods that can be eaten frequently without exceeding dietary guidelines for one or more of the following components: fat, saturated fat, cholesterol, sodium, and kilocalories.
  - ***low fat***: 3 g or less per serving
  - ***low saturated fat***: 1 g or less per serving
  - ***low sodium***: 140 mg or less per serving
  - ***very low sodium***: 35 mg or less per serving
  - ***low cholesterol***: 20 mg or less and 2 g or less of saturated fat per serving
  - ***low calorie***: 40 calories or fewer per serving
- ***Lean and extra lean.*** Used to describe the fat content of meat, poultry, and seafood.
  - ***lean***: less than 10 g fat, less than 4.5 g saturated fat, and less than 95 mg cholesterol per serving and per 100 g
  - ***extra lean***: less than 5 g fat, less than 2 g saturated fat, and less than 95 mg cholesterol per serving and per 100 g
- ***High.*** One serving of the food contains 20 percent or more of the daily value for a particular nutrient.
- ***Good source.*** One serving of the food contains 10 to 19 percent of the daily value for a particular nutrient.
- ***Reduced.*** Applies if a nutritionally altered product contains at least 25 percent less of a nutrient or of calories than the regular, or reference, food. A reduced claim cannot be made if the reference product already meets the requirement for a "low" claim.
- ***Less.*** (Also "fewer") The food, whether altered or not, contains 25 percent less of a nutrient or of calories than the food to which it is compared.
- ***Light.*** There are two possible meanings:
  - A nutritionally altered product contains one-third fewer calories or half the fat of the reference product. If the food derives at least 50 percent of its calories from fat, the reduction must be 50 percent of the fat.
  - The sodium content of a low-calorie, low-fat product has been reduced by 50 percent. Food in which the sodium content has been reduced by at least 50 percent may be labeled "light in sodium."

  The term "light" can still be used to describe properties such as texture and color as long as the label explains the intended meaning (e.g., "light brown sugar").
- ***More.*** A serving of food, whether altered or not, contains at least 10 percent more of the daily value of a specific nutrient than the reference food. The 10 percent of daily value also applies to "fortified," "enriched," "added," "extra," and "plus" claims, but in these cases, the food must be altered.

In Canada, **recommended daily intakes (RDIs)** serve as a reference standard for nutrition labeling purposes only. Based on the RNIs, RDIs represent the highest RNI that exists for a nutrient for that age group and are expressed on labels as a percentage of the nutrient's RDI (not mg, etc.). Two sets of RDIs exist – one for infants (<2 years) and one for children (>2 years) and adults.

Food labels not only make comparing products easier but also enable you to choose foods for healthy eating that reflect the nutrition recommendations. You must be careful about reading nutrition claims, however. These claims (often appearing in a clear, bold format) highlight a specific nutritional feature of a product, trying to influence your buying habits (see box *Nutrition Claims and What They Mean*). Because the words used in claims are government-defined (e.g., *low,*

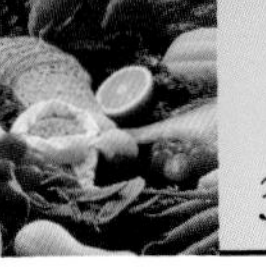

less, light), their meaning is standardized. The term "less," for example, is used to compare one product with another. A package of bacon that claims to have "50 percent less salt" may have half the amount of salt found in the product to which it is being compared, but it does not necessarily mean the product is itself low in salt (half the amount may still be a lot of salt) – you should check the label for more information.

How safe is the food supply?

We rarely inquire about what is actually in the food we eat especially if it is already prepared. But the quality and safety of the food we eat are important factors. There are in fact many concerns pertaining to environmental contaminants present in foods (e.g., pesticides), the presence of potentially dangerous additives, and the threat of bacteria and microorganisms that cause food-borne illness. Unfortunately, the occurrence of various food-borne illnesses is fairly prevalent; in fact, the last time you thought you had the flu, you may have actually been suffering from the effects of a food-borne illness. This mistake can be made because the symptoms are so similar – diarrhea, vomiting, weakness, and fever. Although the effects of most food-borne illnesses are usually not serious, elderly people and children are at higher risk.

The source of most food-borne illnesses is bacteria and the toxins they produce; they are caused by a variety of factors and can largely be prevented. Food can become contaminated by bacteria if it is not prepared or stored properly. This is especially true of eggs, meat, milk, and poultry (which can lead to **Salmonella** poisoning, the most common type of food-borne illness). Another type of bacteria is **Staphylococcus aureus**, which lives primarily in nasal passages and skin sores; it manages to spread to food when you handle food, or sneeze or cough over it. Ham, cheese, eggs, and seafood are common sources of this bacteria. More dangerous types of bacteria also exist including **Clostridium botulinum** (causing botulism) and **Escherichia coli** (*E. coli* for short), which arise mainly from improperly canned foods (particularly meats and vegetables) and are found in the intestinal tract of humans and other animals respectively. Therefore, it is important to handle food with extreme care and be vigilant about what you eat in restaurants when you eat out (Table 14.6). A simple way to prevent the spread of bacteria in foods is to wash your hands before and after handling food.

The multitude of substances added to processed foods can also be an issue of concern. While most are added for good reason (e.g., to improve nutritional quality, taste, and appearance, or to maintain freshness), additives can lead to allergic reactions in some individuals. Sulfites, for example, which protect vegetables from turning brown, have been known to cause wheezing, hives, diarrhea, vomiting, and dizziness in some individuals. The use of coloring agents (e.g., yellow No. 5) and flavor enhancers such as MSG (monosodium glutamate) can also lead to reactions – another reason to pay attention to labels. Yellow No. 5 can cause hives, itching, a runny nose, and even asthma in some, while MSG may lead to bouts of high blood pressure and sweating in those who are sensitive. Therefore, if you are sensitive to any substance or are concerned about what is in the food you eat, check the labels carefully to avoid any potential reaction or illness. When you go out to eat, it is important to ask how foods are prepared and with what ingredients.

Is vegetarianism a healthy alternative?

Some people choose to eliminate or restrict meat and other animal-derived foods from their diets for various reasons (philosophical, health, environmental). A **vegetarian** diet can provide the necessary nutrients required by the body if a few rules are followed (children and pregnant women require special individual guidance). In fact, a well-planned vegetarian diet can offer immense benefits to adults and can lead to better health than an omnivorous diet.

Vegetarians are often placed under one broad heading, but there are several types. **Vegans** restrict

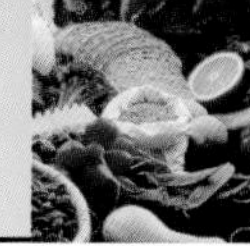

Table 14.6 Tips on food safety.

Food can become contaminated by bacteria if it is not handled, prepared, or stored properly. Keep the following tips in mind to avoid the potentially serious effects of food-borne illnesses.

- Thoroughly clean dishes, cutting boards, counters, and other utensils with soap and warm water after use, particularly if used with raw foods such as meat, fish, or eggs.
- Wash hands thoroughly with warm water and soap before and after handling all foods.
- Pesticide residues tend to concentrate in animal fat; therefore, trim excess fat from meats or remove skin, which contains most of the fat. Remove fats and oils from soups and pan drippings.
- When handling food, cover any cuts on your hands, and avoid sneezing or coughing over the food.
- When preparing foods to be eaten raw (such as vegetables), use a different cutting board than one used for meats. The relative worth of plastic over wooden cutting boards remains contentious. Whichever you use, have separate cutting boards for vegetables and fruits versus meats, and wash all thoroughly with soap and warm water after each use.
- Do not leave groceries in the car for extended periods of time – bacteria thrive in warm temperatures. Purchase products that require refrigeration last to keep them as cool as possible.
- When cooking with poultry, cook stuffing separately, or wash poultry well and stuff immediately before cooking; transfer to a separate dish immediately after cooking.
- Wash and scrub produce thoroughly under running water to help loosen any trapped dirt.
- Cook all foods thoroughly (especially meats and eggs), which will kill most microorganisms. Avoid eating raw animal products.
- To avoid the deadly botulism toxin, do not buy prepackaged foods in containers that leak, are dented, or bulge.
- The outer leaves of leafy vegetables should be removed. Wash and scrub other fruits and vegetables well (with a brush if possible) or peel them if necessary (even though some nutrients may be lost).
- Use only pasteurized milk and juices.
- Avoid leaving cooked or refrigerated foods at room temperature for more than two hours. Foods should be stored below 40 degrees Fahrenheit (4 degrees Celsius).
- When fishing, throw back the big ones – smaller fish tend to have lower concentrations of pesticides and other harmful residues.
- Do not barbecue more than three times per week to avoid ingestion of cancer-causing compounds. Avoid overcooking (burning) foods for the same reason.
- Do not eat eggs with runny yolks or batter made with raw eggs; over 80 percent of Salmonella outbreaks can be linked to eggs. Assume that all eggs have salmonella.

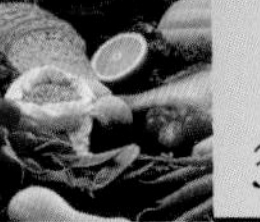

Vegetarian Styles

Although they are often categorized as one large, homogeneous group, vegetarians are actually quite a diverse population. Here are the various vegetarian diets, ranging from strict to lax:

- **Sproutarianism:** A diet based around sprouted seeds, such as bean sprouts, wheat sprouts, and broccoli sprouts. Usually supplemented with additional raw foods. This is not a varied and healthy diet; it is not recommended because it is too strict with food allowances.
- **Fruitarianism:** A diet consisting of raw or dried fruits as well as grains, nuts, seeds, legumes, honey, and vegetable or olive oil. Basically, includes any part a plant can easily replace. This is not a varied and healthy diet; it is not recommended because it is too strict with food allowances.
- **Raw Foodism:** A diet built primarily on raw foods, excluding anything cooked past 48 degrees Fahrenheit (9 degrees Celsius). This is not a varied and healthy diet; it is not recommended because it is too strict with food allowances.
- **Veganism:** An all-vegetable diet, excluding meat, milk products, eggs, and any other animal products – including honey. This can be a healthy diet, but you need to ensure it is varied; supplementation with B_{12} is usually required.
- **Ovo-vegetarianism:** A diet including vegetables as well as eggs. This can be a healthy diet, but you need to ensure it is varied.
- **Lacto-vegetarianism:** An all-vegetable diet plus dairy products – no eggs. This can be a healthy diet, but you need to ensure it is varied.
- **Lacto-ovo-vegetarianism:** An all-vegetable diet plus dairy products and eggs. This can be a healthy diet, but you need to ensure it is varied.
- **Pesco-, Pollo-, and Semi-vegetarianism:** A diet including vegetables plus some group(s) of animal products such as fish (pesco) or chicken (pollo). Semi-vegetarians who frequently, but not systematically, avoid meat and dairy products are not considered true vegetarians. This is typically the most varied diet, and therefore it can be healthy, depending on food choices.

their diet to plant foods; **lacto-vegetarians** also eat plant foods but include dairy products; **lacto-ovo-vegetarians** choose to eat plant foods and dairy products as well as eggs; finally, **semi-vegetarians** eat plant foods, dairy products, eggs, and usually a small selection of poultry, fish, or other seafood (see box *Vegetarian Styles* for a complete summary of all the various vegetarian diets). Those vegetarian diets that offer a wider variety make it easier to meet nutritional requirements. While there is relatively little risk associated with the others, a vegan diet requires a higher degree of nutritional understanding to avoid malnourishment.

One potential concern is whether a vegan diet includes sources of all the essential amino acids because no single plant source contains all of them. However, a careful combination of nonmeat, high-quality **complementary proteins** (proteins that supply the essential amino acids missing in each other) can prevent amino acid deficiencies. Some examples include black beans and rice, peanut butter and wheat bread, and tofu and stir-fried vegetables with rice. Other potential difficulties include maintaining adequate intakes of vitamin B_{12}, calcium, iron, and zinc, as well as a concern with satiation (satisfaction of hunger). Early satiation as a result of large amounts of fiber in the diet may lead to a decrease in carbohydrate intake. Many vegans consume smaller meals throughout the day, which is also a healthier practice, and this allows them to obtain the needed nutrients and energy without feeling quickly satiated.

It takes planning and common sense to put together a vegetarian diet that works. Thus, if you are a vegetarian or are considering becoming one, think carefully about eating a variety of foods, and plan ahead to ensure that your nutritional needs are adequately met. In addition, the number of vegetarian options in supermarkets has greatly increased, providing more variety and allowing

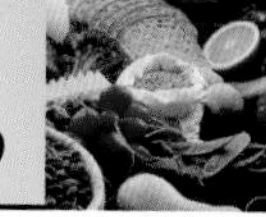

vegetarians of all types to more easily obtain their nutrient and energy requirements.

Do I need vitamin or mineral supplements?

You may wonder whether you could benefit from taking a vitamin or mineral supplement. Promotional tactics often try to convince consumers that supplements are essential to health. The question you need to ask yourself is whether you are following the Dietary Guidelines for Americans or Canada's Food Guide. If you enjoy a balanced diet that has adequate variety, most nutritionists would agree that the need for supplements is low or nonexistent; in fact, megadoses (very high doses of any one or more than one vitamin or mineral) may even lead to toxicity. Many people use supplements as nutritional insurance, making sure they get all the nutrients they need, but there is no reason why most people can't obtain the vitamins and minerals they need from a healthy, balanced diet.

That being said, there are several special cases where vitamin and mineral supplementation should be considered (Figure 14.11):

- women with excessive bleeding during menstruation may need to supplement with iron;
- pregnant or breast-feeding mothers may require iron, folate (also known as folic acid), and calcium (inadequate amounts of folate during pregnancy have been linked to birth defects called neural tube defects – typically, women who are pregnant or breast-feeding take prenatal vitamins prescribed by their physicians);
- individuals with low energy intakes (e.g., people who live alone and often eat by themselves, elderly, heavy drinkers/alcoholics, cigarette smokers);
- some vegetarians (typically vegans) may need calcium, iron, zinc, and vitamin B_{12};
- exclusively breast-fed infants and shut-in elderly may need vitamin D (lacking in human milk and in an environment lacking sunlight); and
- people with certain illnesses or on medication may need supplements.

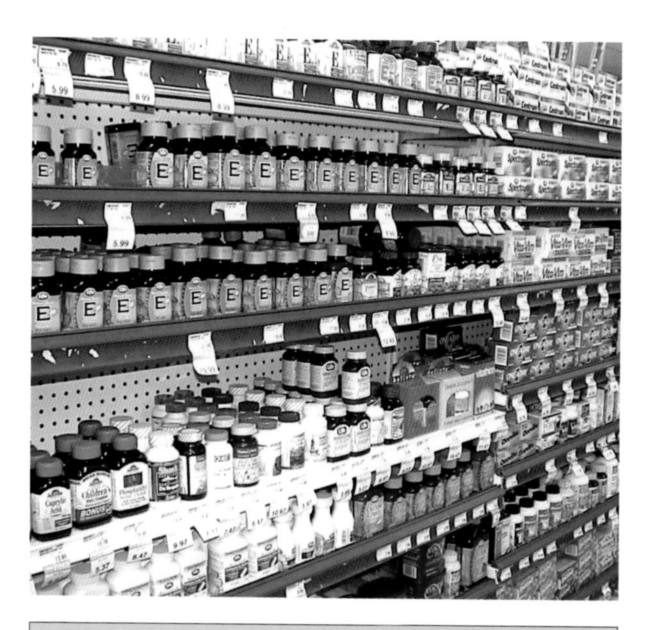

Figure 14.11 Vitamin and mineral supplementation may be necessary for some individuals.

Although most of us can rely on a healthy diet to provide us with the nutrients we need, if you choose to use nutrient supplements, do so only after consulting with a public health nutritionist or registered dietitian. Whether you require supplements due to one of the aforementioned conditions or not, always remember that they are "supplements" (i.e., they are not meant to *be* your diet but to *supplement* your diet). For healthy individuals who eat well but want to have the "insurance" of supplements, taking a multivitamin/mineral supplement every other day may be more than adequate – and will also save some money.

What's the scoop on sugar?

Many of us crave sugar but believe it is detrimental to good health. Sugar is often linked with fatness, despite research showing that obese individuals do not consume more sugar than normal-weight people. Nonetheless, sugar can create a unique dilemma – while sugar itself does not make you overweight, sugary foods in our diets also tend to be high in fat

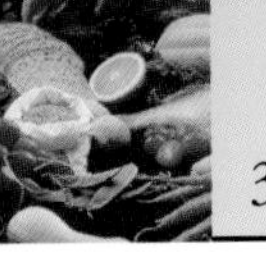

and kilocalories, which *can* make you gain weight (i.e., consuming more energy than your body needs will result in weight gain). Any kilocalories consumed beyond body needs that are not burned off during activity are inevitably stored as fat.

How about the effects of sugar on children's behavior? Does sugar consumption increase hyperactivity, delinquency, or learning disorders in children? Although these are popular beliefs held by many, there is no evidence that clearly validates these claims. Nonetheless, children (and adults) *do* acquire a taste for high-sugar (and high-salt) foods, and thus they should still be consumed in moderation.

The primary health problem linked to sugar is tooth decay (dental caries). For many years, sugar has been known to cause tooth decay (leading to fluoridated drinking water) – a problem that can be effectively combated by regular brushing, flossing, and dental checkups. It is also worth noting that eating *sweets* with other foods is less damaging to your teeth, as a result of increased saliva and foods that buffer the acid effect in your mouth.

Sugar has also been linked to type 2 **diabetes mellitus**. This disease, typically a result of obesity, affects the insulin receptors within the body, altering normal metabolism. When we eat food, our blood sugar rises. Individuals with type 2 diabetes mellitus produce enough insulin in the pancreas; however, many of the receptors for insulin at the cells do not recognize this insulin, leading to an elevated blood sugar level. While high sugar consumption will not cause diabetes, those who are genetically susceptible to the condition may want to limit the amount of sugar they eat. The indirect link still remains, however. A high-energy diet can lead to obesity, which is a risk factor for developing type 2 diabetes mellitus.

How do nutritional needs change as we grow older?

It should come as no surprise that nutritional needs change as we age (Figure 14.12). The main factors that account for this are the physiological changes that accompany the aging process, diseases that may develop affecting nutrition (directly or indirectly),

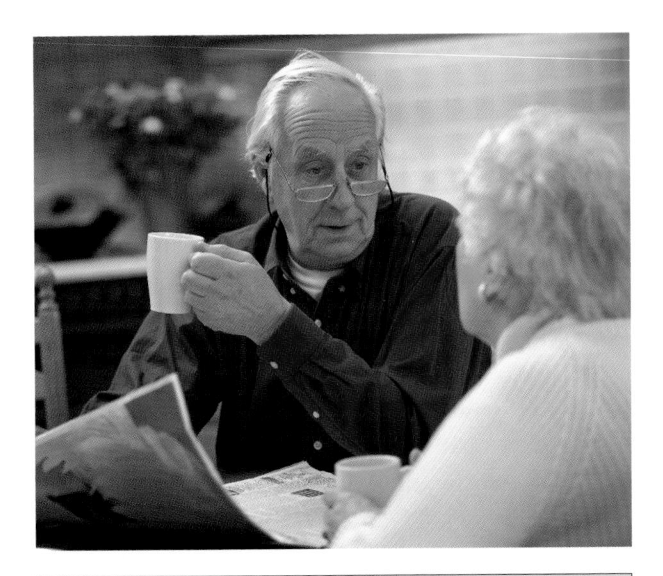

Figure 14.12 Age-related physiological changes alter the nutritional needs of older adults.

as well as psychosocial factors. We will now look at these individually.

Aging may (but does not always!) lead to a decrease in physical activity, which may lead to a lower metabolic rate and a lower total energy requirement. This, in turn, often leads to less food intake among the elderly. Still, while the need for energy declines, the need for vitamins and minerals still remains vital. Not only do many elderly people sense the need for less food, but changes in teeth, salivary glands, taste buds, oral muscles, gastric acid production, and peristalsis make it more difficult to chew and make eating less pleasurable. Other changes that may occur, such as an increased occurrence of constipation, further add to a declining interest in food.

In addition, a variety of diseases and disorders can significantly affect the nutrition of the older adult. Dental problems, swallowing disorders, mood disorders (e.g., depression), and gastrointestinal disorders are commonplace. But elderly individuals also suffer from chronic infections more regularly, and many must deal with musculoskeletal problems such as osteoporosis and arthritis, which indirectly affect nutrition (for example, eating with arthritic hands can be a real challenge) and may directly affect physical activity.

Perhaps psychological factors are the most overlooked influence on nutrition in the older adult.

Social isolation, poverty, transportation limitations, and institutionalization (nursing homes) are all factors that figure into the lifestyle of the elderly. These factors may change the enjoyment and ease with which foods may be prepared and consumed, affecting nutrition greatly.

Nonetheless, it is important that the elderly not be stereotyped. Many older individuals are still very active, even competing in athletic events. This is what we, as a society, should strive for – to expect that as we age, we will continue to be active, whether or not we compete, and to allow ourselves the best quality of life that we can through healthy eating and daily physical activity. Our older population is growing, and soon one in every five individuals will be over the age of 65; thus, it is important that public health messages be directed to everyone, at all life stages, so that every person strives for the best quality of life he or she can achieve.

Can diet improve athletic performance?

Athletes are always searching for the formula for success in maximizing their potential; sound nutrition is certainly part of it. Eating particular types of foods before participating in athletic events can be more beneficial than others. But what specific nutritional concerns do athletes face? How can an athlete prepare a diet that will maximize performance?

Ergogenic Aids and Supplements

Research and experience have shown that athletes have a greater need for energy, proteins, and amino acids than moderately active or inactive people (see box *Training and Competition Make a Difference*). However, the North American diet seems to be adequate to meet the protein needs of most individuals, including athletes, as long as energy requirements are met. Further, amino acid supplementation cannot be scientifically justified. Because all athletes have higher energy needs in general, a diet that aims to provide 15 percent of total energy intake as protein should be adequate for athletes as well (some athletes may need higher amounts; however, there is no need for athletes to go above the DRI-established AMDR for protein of between 10 and 35 percent). Even in the presence of extra protein, the body can only build muscle so fast, and excess protein is broken down to be eliminated as waste. So athletes should focus on maintaining a balanced diet with adequate energy rather than look to supplements. It is especially important to note here that athletes should not supplement with single amino acids because this can lead to competition of different amino acids

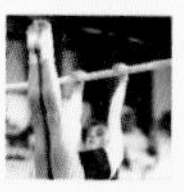

Training and Competition Make a Difference

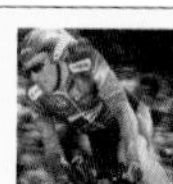

Individuals who are engaged in intense physical activity experience increased daily energy needs to match their higher level of daily energy expenditure. Their daily food intake contains the essential and many nonessential nutrients in amounts that are two or more times greater than the amounts eaten by nonathletes. Furthermore, depending on the activity, energy needs of athletes can range from a low of 1,700 to a high of 8,000 kcal (or higher) to meet the special requirements of an athlete. Energy requirements vary according to age, activity, and metabolism. For example, the average daily nutrient intake of a 14-year-old, 110 pound (50-kg) gymnast is drastically different from the nutrient requirement of a 28-year-old, 165 pound (75-kg) road cyclist.

The practice of eating specific amounts of protein, carbohydrates, and fats is essential for the enhancement of athletic performance. Additionally, meal timing and frequency are important. While nonathletes can maintain their health by consuming three moderately sized, well-balanced meals per day, athletes must utilize a diet that is much more complex. For example, to facilitate muscle recovery athletes need to consume high-quality protein several times a day. To ensure an adequate supply of energy, athletes must consume specific amounts of high-quality carbohydrates several times a day. Overall, the main goal is to consume the proper amount of energy; athletes must consider their protein, carbohydrate, and fat requirements, both within the DRIs and within their needs as active individuals.

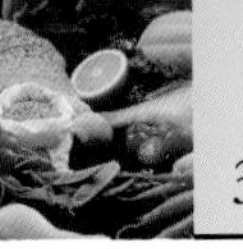

within the body, which would be more detrimental than helpful.

There is widespread interest in the effects of carbohydrates on endurance performance. Carbohydrates are recognized as the major fuel for most athletic performance, and its depletion from muscle stores (as glycogen) is associated with fatigue in endurance exercise. The practice of **carbohydrate loading** can increase muscle glycogen stores by gradually reducing the duration of training sessions during the week before an important competition and progressively increasing the consumption of dietary carbohydrates. This technique has been shown to be effective before endurance-type competition (over 60 minutes), although some drawbacks can be identified. Some individuals feel gastrointestinal discomfort and sluggishness as a result of the increased carbohydrate intake. Carbohydrate loading is not recommended for athletes with diabetes or heart irregularities, and the long-term effects of this practice on muscles have not been studied yet. Any such program should be done under the supervision of a qualified coach, trainer, or sport nutritionist who is also a registered dietitian. It is also important to note that true carbohydrate loading should be saved for very big events, and athletes, in general, should consume more carbohydrates (within the AMDR established by the DRI) to restore glycogen stores.

What Are Ergogenic Aids?

Ergogenic (*work producing*) refers to the application of a nutritional, physical, mechanical, psychological, or pharmacological procedure or aid to improve physical work capacity, athletic performance, and responsiveness to exercise training.

Other substances such as caffeine, sodium bicarbonate, and various vitamins and minerals have been shown to have an effect on athletic performance. Caffeine, for example, found in coffee, tea, and colas, has been identified as a possible **ergogenic aid**. It is believed to enhance the release and use of free fatty acids, conserving glycogen and prolonging endurance when taken before exercising. Although some studies have shown positive results, some individuals react negatively to caffeine (usually those who are caffeine-naïve). Its use should be controlled and introduced on a trial basis only. The International Olympic Committee used to ban caffeine, but it has been taken off the banned substance list. It is wise not to consume too much caffeine before an event, especially if you are caffeine-naïve, as it may result in nervousness and tachycardia (a heart rate greater than 120 beats per minute).

Pre-event Meals

Before an athlete is fully ready to compete, there are certain nutritional guidelines that should be followed. First, meals before a competition should be high in carbohydrates and low in fat because carbohydrate-containing foods leave the stomach more quickly than other foods (fats are slowest)

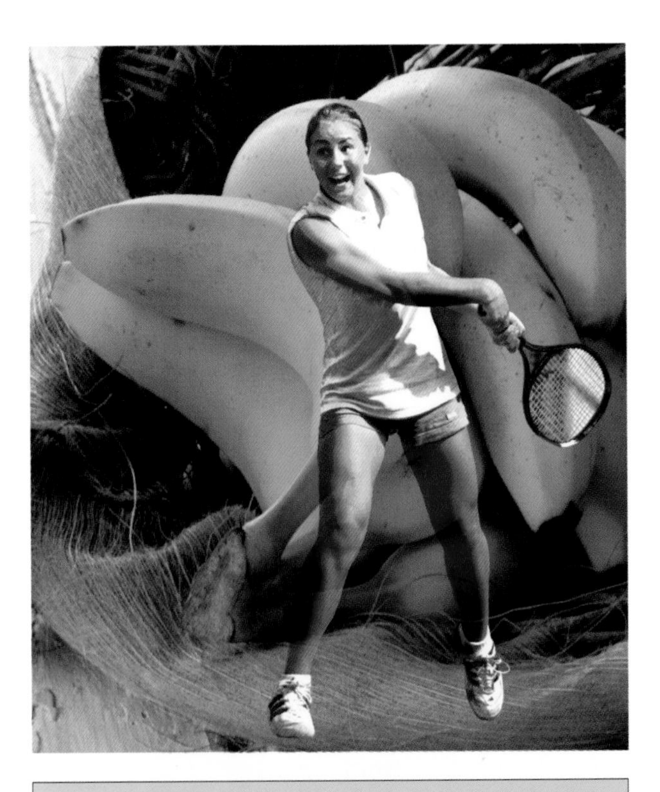

Figure 14.13 Packed with an assortment of vitamins and minerals, bananas make a great snack to boost energy before, during, and after a bout of exercise.

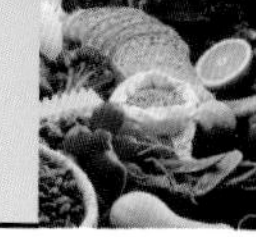

(Figure 14.13). Food in the digestive system makes a demand on the circulatory system, so it is beneficial to have food move quickly through the system to allow needed oxygen to be supplied to the working muscles. In stressful competitive conditions, muscle damage can occur if muscles are deprived of energy-yielding oxygen. Second, only familiar foods should be eaten before an event to avoid any strange or surprising reactions.

Hydration

We have already stressed the importance of water as a nutrient. The need for water is increased during exercise because of increased losses through the lungs and sweat losses. Fluid losses can be dramatic, especially in warm and humid environments, so keeping hydrated by drinking fluids is essential (Figure 14.14). It is important to drink early (prior to exercise), often (during exercise), and also after exercise. Cool drinks also make your performance more effective by cooling your body. Waiting until you "feel" thirsty is not recommended because your body may not feel the need for fluids even when it is there. An adequate supply of water is therefore a key to performing your best. As previously discussed in this chapter, sports drinks may be needed if you compete in events longer than one hour or if you compete in multiple events in one day or in tournaments. Sports drinks provide the energy (carbohydrate) and electrolytes (sodium) you need for longer events.

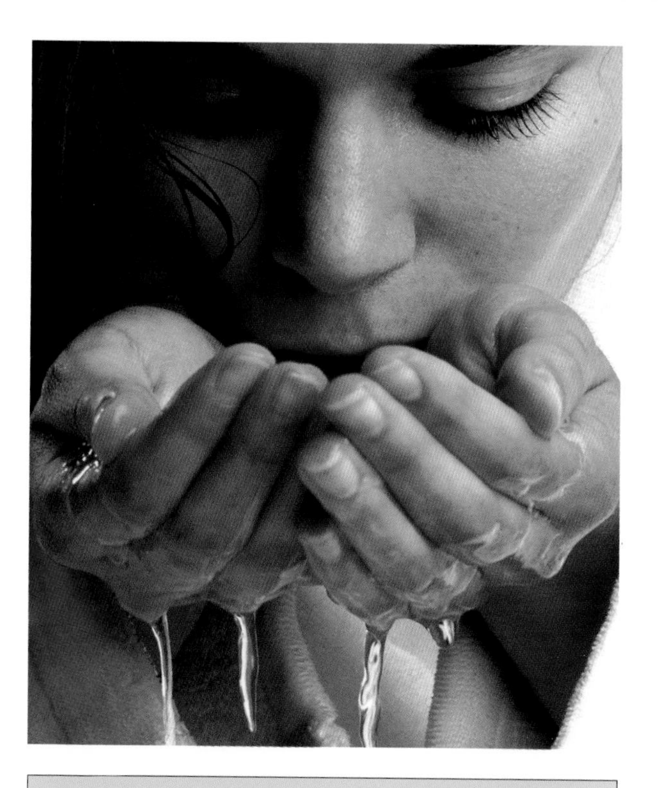

Figure 14.14 Although often taken for granted, water is perhaps the most essential nutrient.

Summary

Nutrition is an important science concerned with food and how our bodies use it in health and disease. Our attitudes about nutrition and diet can influence our health in a positive way. Because some diets are associated with disease, while others protect us from them, we must choose foods that provide us with the essential nutrients. This means understanding the essential nutrients (carbohydrates, proteins, fats, vitamins, minerals, and water) and what foods contain them. This is where DRIs, RNIs, the Dietary Guidelines for Americans, MyPyramid, and Canada's Food Guide can help you establish sound eating patterns and vitality. While all foods are good to eat, some are good to eat more often than others.

Of course, individuals have different needs, and these needs change as we age. Understanding the nutritional needs of various populations (e.g., children, the elderly, athletes, individuals with diabetes mellitus) is important if we are to assist those around us as well as adapt our own nutritional habits as we change over the years. Then, there's always the issue of weight and maintaining a healthy body image, which all comes down to balancing your energy intake and following a lifestyle that includes regular exercise (see Chapter 15). Other relevant information concerning food labels, nutrient supplements, the safety of the food supply, or the risks associated with vegetarianism are important in formulating a nutritional program that is right for you. Any way you put it, nutrition has profound effects on your general health and well-being.

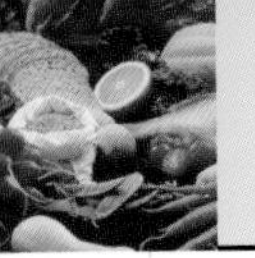

Food for Thought

GARFIELD—By Jim Davis

THERE ARE MANY WAYS TO MAKE A DIET MORE APPEALING

SOME SAY IT HELPS TO DRESS YOUR FOOD UP
© 1987 United Feature Syndicate, Inc.

I SAY IT STILL LOOKS LIKE CELERY
JIM DAVIS 5-19

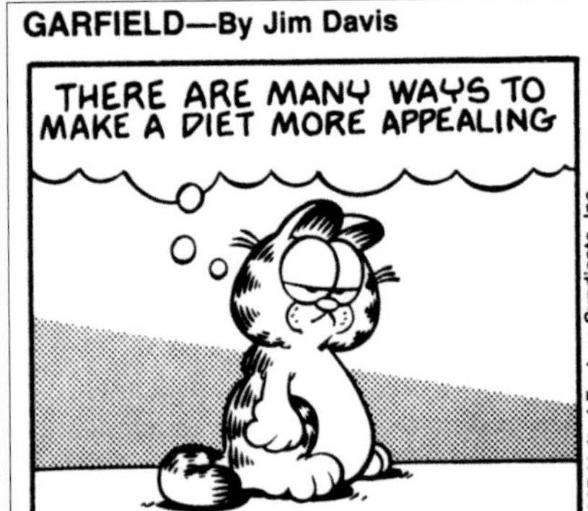

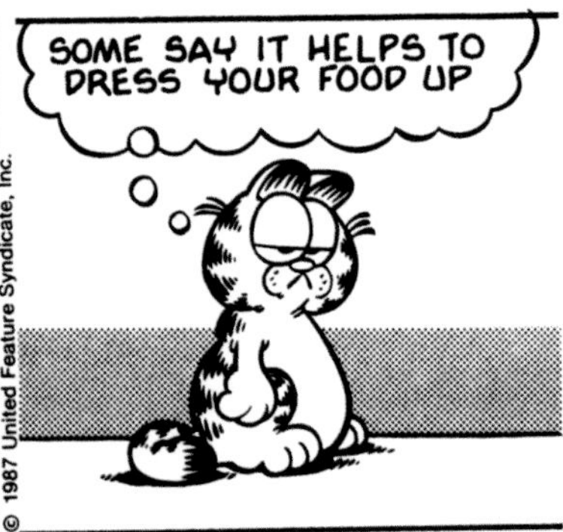

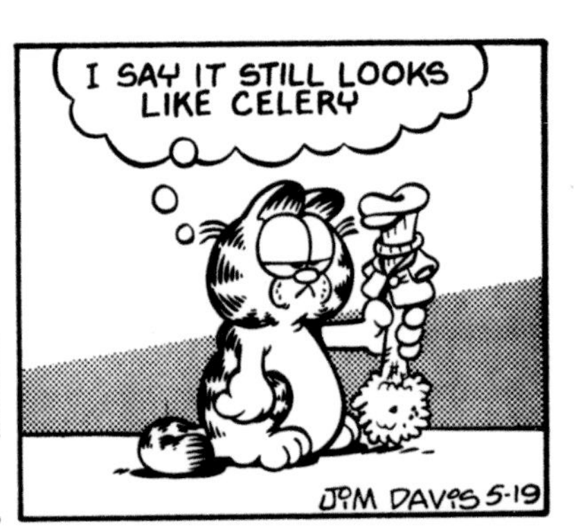

You can make your eating experience nutritious and fun. Remember, what pleases the eye pleases the palate.

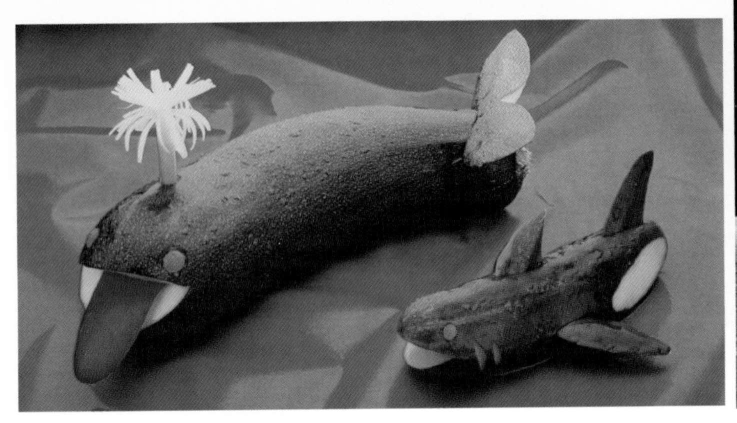

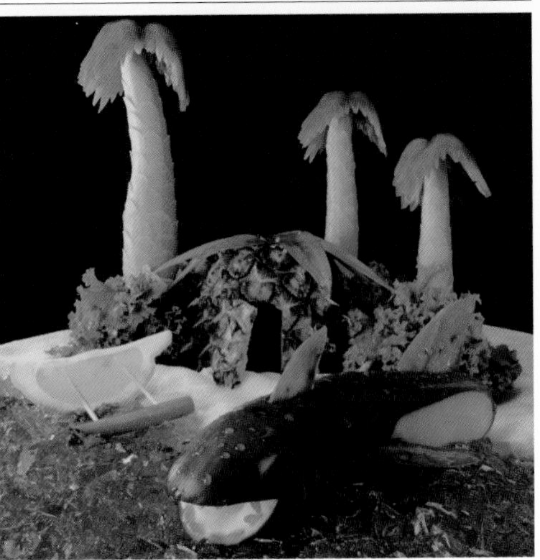

Key Terms

absorption
acceptable macronutrient distribution range (AMDR)
amino acid
amylase
antioxidant
bile
bile salts
carbohydrate
carbohydrate loading
cholesterol
complementary proteins
complete protein
daily value
dietary reference intake (DRI)
digestion
digestive system
disaccharide
ergogenic aid
esophagus
essential amino acids
essential nutrients
fat-soluble vitamins
free radicals
gallbladder
gastrointestinal tract
glycogen
hydrochloric acid
hydrogenation
incomplete protein
insoluble fiber
kilocalorie
large intestine
lipid
lipoprotein
liver
minerals
monosaccharide
monounsaturated fat
motility
MyPyramid
nutrition
pepsin
peristalsis
polysaccharide
polyunsaturated fat
protein
recommended daily intake (RDI)
recommended nutrient intake (RNI)

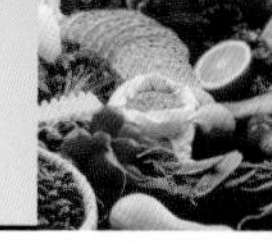

saliva
saturated fat
secretion
small intestine
soluble fiber
stomach
trans fatty acid
triglyceride
vegetarian
vitamins
water-soluble vitamins

Discussion Questions

1. List the four basic digestive functions. What is the role of the small intestine?

2. What is a nutrient? Identify the six essential nutrients and explain their contribution to growth and development.

3. List the energy densities of the three classes of nutrients that supply energy. Which nutrient is the most energy dense?

4. Identify the two major classifications of dietary fiber and provide two examples of each type.

5. Distinguish between the DRIs and the Dietary Guidelines for Americans and the RNIs and Canada's Guidelines for Healthy Eating. What are the DRIs and RNIs used for?

6. How many food groups are included in MyPyramid and in Canada's Food Guide? Give an example of three foods and sample serving sizes from each group.

7. Describe the different vegetarian diets. If not followed correctly, which type may put you at the most risk for nutrient deficiencies?

8. Are vitamin and mineral supplements necessary for health? Explain.

9. What is carbohydrate loading? Can all athletes benefit from it?

10. What factors affect the nutrition of the older adult?

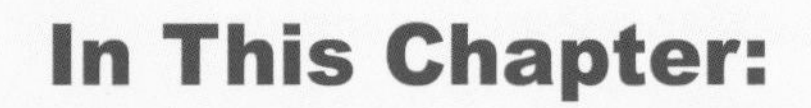

In This Chapter:

CHAPTER 15

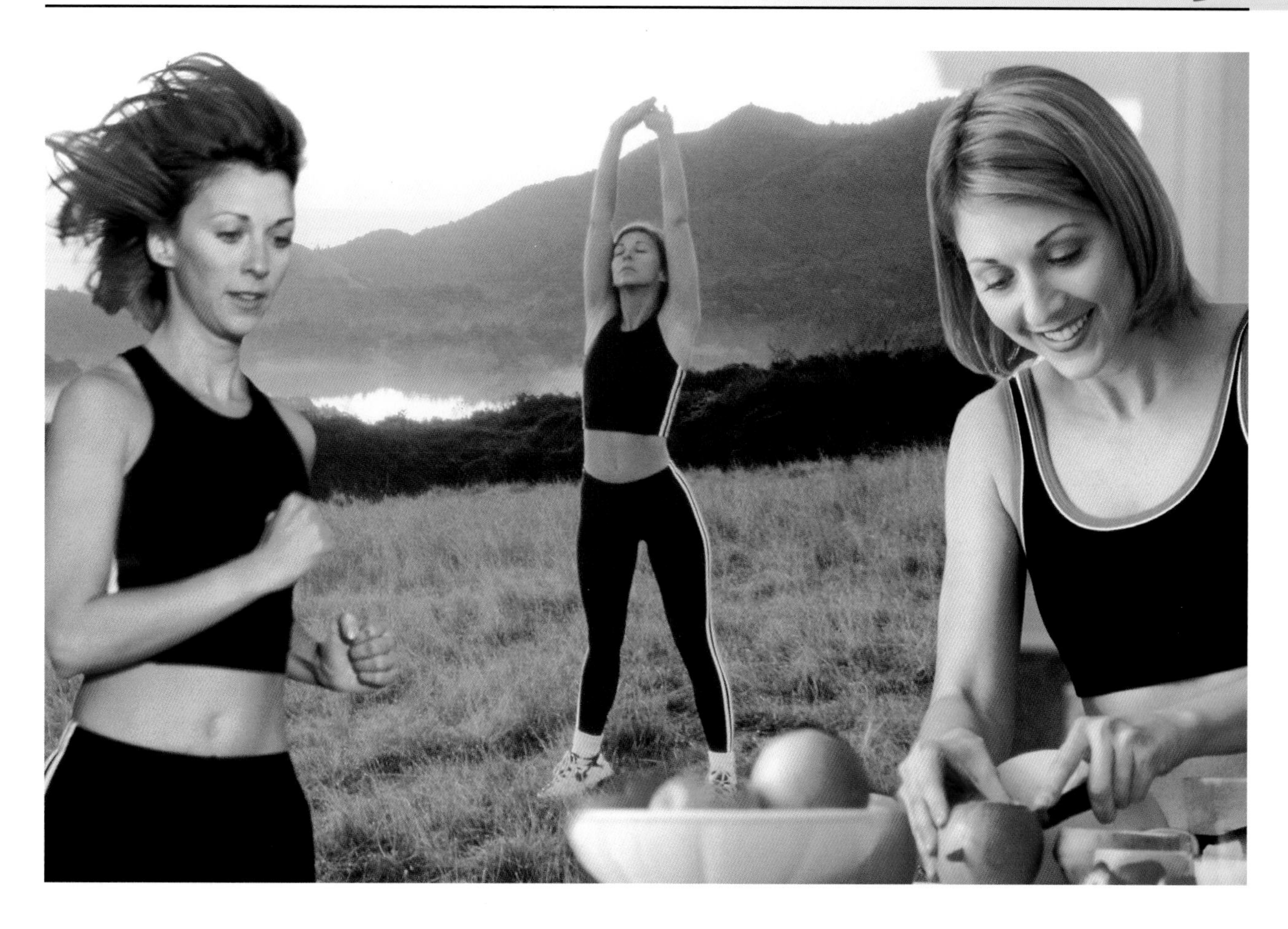

Weight Management: Finding a Healthy Balance

After completing this chapter you should be able to:

- discuss the differences between overweight and obese and their implications for health;
- explain the concept of energy balance in weight management;
- describe the role of exercise and lifestyle modification in maintaining a healthy body weight;
- discuss the consequences of dieting and eating disorders;
- set and evaluate personal goals for maintaining a healthy body weight.

Weight is an issue for all of us. Many people feel obliged to buy diet books, try fad diets and supplements, attempt special programs, and even consider medical procedures, all in the pursuit of attaining an "ideal" body weight. The key to weight management lies not in some vague ideal or perfection but in sensible dietary practices and adequate levels of physical activity.

Despite the efforts of many people, the United States is clearly in a state of nutritional crisis and in need of sound remedies. The statistics are sobering. Collectively, we have grown fatter over the years. Today, more than 50 percent of adults and 30 percent of children are considered overweight or obese, and these statistics continue to increase. Too many children and young adults are facing an epidemic of numerous obesity-related diseases that were unheard of just a generation ago.

We live in an environment where physical activity has been engineered out of day-to-day life, and the food environment has become more "toxic" by the day (Figure 15.1). Eating disorders have also emerged in greater numbers as the social pressure to be thin has increased, especially among adolescents and young adults.

Energy Balance Equation

Human beings come into the world well equipped to regulate what scientists call the **energy balance equation** (Figure 15.2). On one side of the equation is the energy we burn through exercise and other bodily processes (such as digestion and absorption). Kilocalories (kcal) consumed beyond the body's needs are stored as fat. In short, one gains weight when energy input exceeds energy output (Figure 15.2 B) and loses weight when the opposite occurs (Figure 15.2 C). One's weight will remain constant if energy input and output are the same, and one's body is said to be in **energy balance** (Figure 15.2 A).

Although it is more common to hear about people who want to lose weight, there are those who have the desire to put on a few pounds to look better or to "bulk up" for athletic events. Just as weight loss is based on energy balance, so is weight gain. This can be achieved by increasing your food intake while participating in an activity program aimed at developing muscular strength. This increase in mass is due to an increase in functional muscle tissue, not fat.

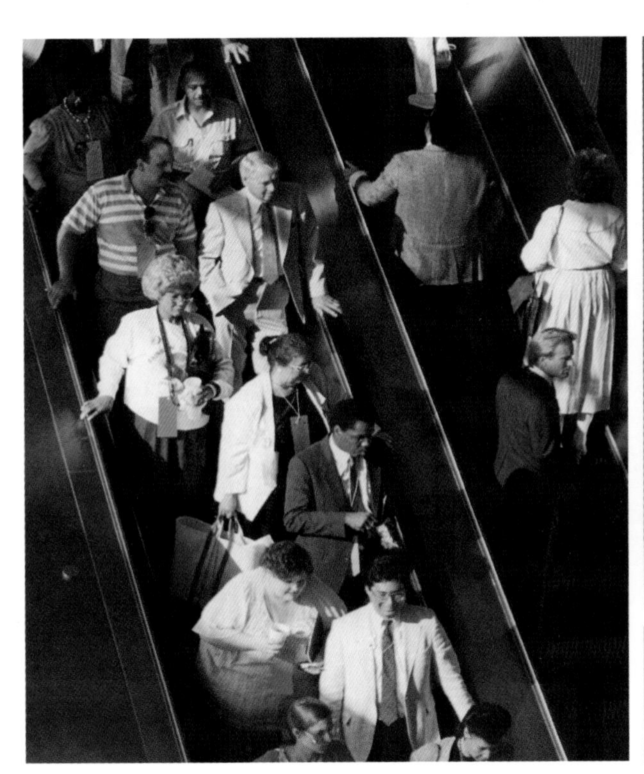

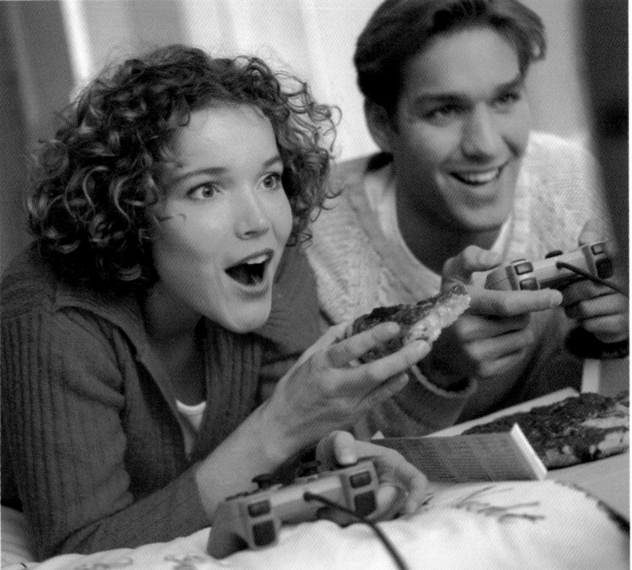

Figure 15.1 Modern conveniences, lower levels of activity, and poor nutritional choices contribute to a myriad of weight and health issues.

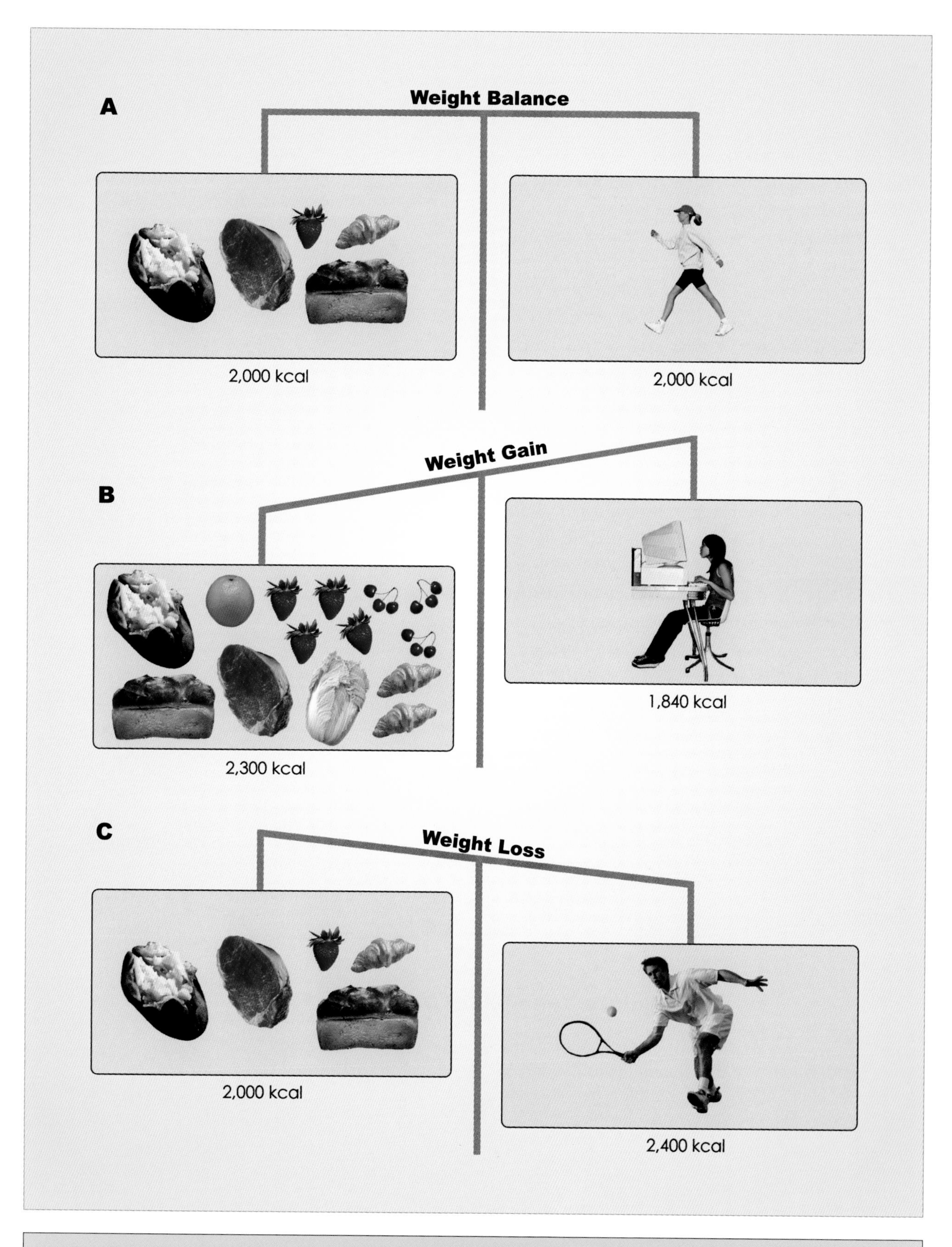

Figure 15.2 The energy balance equation. **A.** Energy input equals energy output. **B.** Energy input exceeds energy output. **C.** Energy output exceeds energy input.

Energy Needs of the Body

Of the total energy you require on a daily basis, the highest proportion is used for basal metabolism. Your basal metabolism, or **basal metabolic rate (BMR),** is defined as the minimum amount of energy the body requires to carry on all vital functions at rest (including blood circulation, respiration, and brain activity). Thus, your basal metabolism will vary throughout your life. As a general rule, your BMR is relatively high at birth and continues to increase until the age of two, after which it will gradually decline as your life progresses (except for a rise at puberty). Other variables also affect your BMR, such as body composition (muscular bodies have higher BMRs), physical fitness (fit people have higher BMRs), sex (the BMRs of men are approximately 5 percent higher than those of women), sleep (BMRs are 10 percent lower during sleep), pregnancy (a 20 percent increase in BMR), and body temperature (a one degree rise in body temperature – for example, when you have a fever – increases BMR about 7 percent). Among all these factors, age is probably the most significant because many people fail to recognize their changing metabolic needs, and do not adjust their food intake to reflect these changes. Many people put on extra pounds as they grow older for this very reason.

To calculate your BMR, use the formula presented in the box below (*Calculate Your Basal Metabolic Rate*).

Total Energy Expenditure

Total energy expenditure (TEE) (kcal/day) = BMR (~60 percent of TEE) + the thermic effect of food (TEF) (energy used in digestion and absorption after a meal) + the thermic effect of activity (energy used during physical activity) + nonexercise activity thermogenesis (NEAT) (energy used when someone is fidgeting, for example).

Exercise and Weight Management

When you exercise, the body's needs for energy increase significantly beyond basal metabolic needs. The amount of extra energy or kilocalories required depends upon the volume of exercise (how long you exercise or the quantity of exercise performed), the intensity of exercise (the rate of exercise per unit of time), and the type of exercise performed (Table 15.1). It must be stressed, however, that exercise on its own can be a slow way to lose weight. For example, if you are a woman weighing 121 pounds (55 kg), you would have to walk over two hours or cross-country ski for over one hour to burn off the kilocalories consumed in a single vanilla milkshake (Figure 15.3, Table 15.1). But combined with controlled eating patterns involving energy reduction, your chances for success are greatly enhanced. Exercise is a great

Calculate Your Basal Metabolic Rate

Your basal metabolic rate (BMR) reflects the amount of energy in kilocalories (kcal) needed to maintain basic body functions such as breathing and blood circulation. Use the simple equation below to help you determine your approximate BMR. NOTE: a woman's BMR is approximately 5 percent lower than that of a man the same age.

BMR per day = 1 kcal x body weight (kg) x 24

Example: 70-kg man

BMR per day = 1 kcal x 70 x 24
= 1,680 kcal

This individual needs approximately 1,680 kcal to maintain his body at rest. Of course, any additional activity above this level raises energy requirements accordingly.

[NOTE: 1 kg = 2.2 lb]

Walk 3.5 miles (5.6 km)
Cross-country ski briskly for 1 hr
Cycle 7.5 miles (12 km)
Tennis at an easy pace for 90 min
Housework for 120 min
1 Vanilla Milkshake
700+ kcal

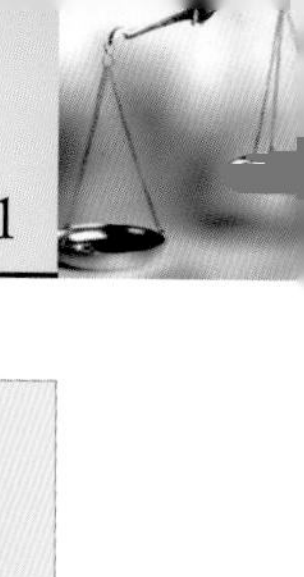

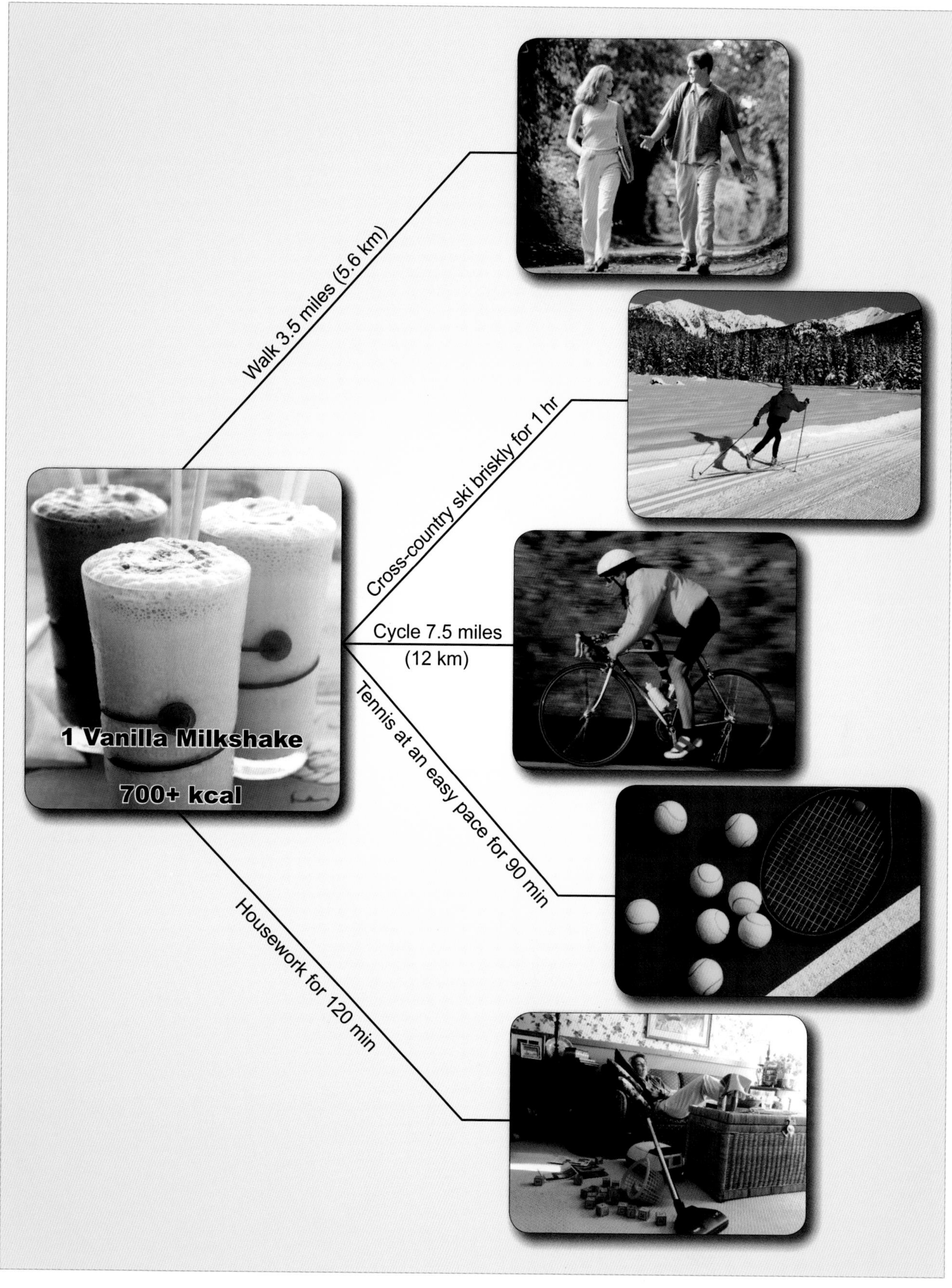

Figure 15.3 Using food energy. How much activity would it take to burn off the kilocalories from a single shake?

Table 15.1 Approximate kilocalories expended for male (154 lb) and female (121 lb) participants in sporting and recreational activities lasting an hour.

Activity	Male (154 lb)	Female (121 lb)	Kcal/hour/lb
Sporting Activity			
Basketball	581.0	456.5	3.8
Cycling (racing)	714.0	561.0	4.6
Ice hockey	875.0	687.5	5.7
Running 8 min/mile	868.0	682.0	5.6
7 min/mile	959.0	753.5	6.2
6 min/mile	1050.0	825.0	6.8
Cross-country skiing	679.0	533.5	4.4
Soccer	546.0	429.0	3.5
Squash	889.0	698.5	5.8
Swimming breaststroke	686.0	539.0	4.5
Tennis (singles)	462.0	363.0	3.0
Weight training	294.0	231.0	1.9
Leisure Activity			
Cycling 6 miles/hour	266.0	209.0	1.7
10 miles/hour	413.0	324.5	2.7
Canoeing	182.0	143.0	1.2
Dancing	350.0	275.0	2.3
Golfing	357.0	280.5	2.3
Hiking	385.0	302.5	2.5
Jogging (11 min/mile)	553.0	434.5	3.6
Rowing ergometer	735.0	577.5	4.8
Walking	329.0	258.5	2.1

way to maintain the weight that is lost, and it also helps keep metabolism higher.

If you doubt the importance of exercise to such a program geared at weight loss, consider this. Not only does regular exercise (especially endurance type) strengthen the heart, improve endurance, provide a means of managing stress, and help prevent osteoporosis, it also burns energy and keeps your metabolism using food for energy rather than storing kilocalories.

As described earlier, a higher amount of fat-free mass (muscle) and a higher level of physical fitness are associated with higher metabolism. These can both be achieved by engaging in regular physical exercise. Individuals with elevated or normal metabolic rates are less likely to become overweight. When your metabolism is more active, you can eat more without necessarily gaining weight, and your body will burn more energy even when you are not exercising. Weight management becomes much easier with a lifestyle that includes regular exercise.

Body Composition

The human physique includes three interrelated aspects of the body: size, structure, and composition. **Size** refers to the volume, mass, length, and surface area of the body, while body **structure** refers to how certain aspects such as the skeleton, muscle, and fat are arranged or distributed throughout the body. **Body composition** refers to the amount of body constituents, such as fat, muscle, bone, and organs, and is regarded as one of the major components of physical fitness.

The composition of the human body can be divided into many components. However, a two-component model dividing the body into lean body mass and fat mass, or total body fat, is the most common.

Lean Body Mass

Perhaps the most important component of the body is **lean body mass (LBM)**. It refers to the "nonfat" or "fat-free" component of the human body and generally consists of skeletal muscle, bone, and water. LBM can be calculated by using the following simple formula:

$$LBM = TBM - TBF$$

By subtracting the **total body fat (TBF)** from **total body mass (TBM)** we arrive at lean body mass. TBF is calculated by multiplying TBM, or weight, by percent body fat (see calculation in next section) divided by 100. For example, if a subject weighs 150 pounds and has 10 percent body fat, he has 15 pounds (150 pounds x 10/100 = 15 pounds) of TBF. If TBF is known, LBM can be calculated. In our example, this works out to an LBM of 135 pounds (150 pounds – 15 pounds). Individuals with high amounts of lean body mass normally have higher rates of metabolism.

Note that the terms "lean body mass" and "fat-free mass" are often used interchangeably; however, they are not exactly the same thing. Lean body mass refers to all the lean mass in the body, as described previously; it is measured indirectly, by such instruments as skinfold calipers and underwater weighing. Fat-free mass can really only be measured on a cadaver – that is, when all the fat-free mass can be separated from any fat mass.

Lean body mass may represent a biological lower limit beyond which a person's body mass cannot be reduced without impairing health. In women, excessive leanness may increase the chances of developing amenorrhea (absent menstruation). Amenorrhea should be viewed as a red flag, and women with amenorrhea should discuss their condition with a knowledgeable sports physician.

The reproductive system can be compromised in situations where an athlete does not consume enough energy to support her body's metabolism and exercise needs, leading to a decrease in estrogen production. The body will try to conserve kilocalories and shift metabolism down, which in turn shuts down the reproductive system's production of estrogen. Estrogen plays an important role in maintaining bone health, and thus females with low levels of estrogen are at a greater risk of developing osteoporosis. Both amenorrhea and disordered eating can lead to osteoporosis. This trio of complications, known as the female athlete triad, will be discussed in more detail later in this chapter.

Fat Mass

Fat mass, or **total body fat**, can be divided further into two types of fat. **Storage fat (SF)** is fat that accumulates as adipose tissue (fat cells). This fat serves as an energy reserve (should the body be subjected to starvation) and also serves to protect internal organs by cushioning them. The main storage site for SF is beneath the skin surface; this fat is thus often referred to as subcutaneous fat. The average man has about 12 percent of body weight as SF, while the average woman has about 15 percent of body weight as SF. Individuals require some fat to exist; however, excess fat is associated with numerous health problems.

The second type of fat is **essential fat (EF)**, which is the fat that is required for normal physiological functioning. Some of this fat is present in the bone marrow, heart, lungs, liver, spleen, kidneys, intestines, muscle, and the lipid-rich tissues of the central nervous system. To maintain normal health and metabolism, men require a minimum essential body fat of 3 percent, while the minimum essential body fat for women is 12 percent. Not surprisingly, this sex-specific essential fat is located in the mammary glands and pelvic region and is involved in hormone-related functions and pregnancy.

Measuring Body Fat

There are many ways to assess total body fat, and most involve an *indirect* method. The *direct* method is simply to grind tissue and measure the amount of fat through **chemical analysis**. Obviously, this is impractical for living organisms, and this method is generally used only on cadavers.

The most common indirect method involves measuring skinfold thickness with **skinfold calipers**. This indirect method requires some technical expertise but is relatively inexpensive (see Chapter 13). The measurements obtained can be used to predict or estimate total body fat based on the assumption that subcutaneous fat is directly related to total body fat. To perform this technique, the skin is pulled away from muscle and pinched between two flattened prongs of the fat calipers, which exert a constant tension. The accuracy of skinfold measurement is about ±3.98 percent when performed correctly by an experienced individual. By measuring skinfolds at a number of sites and comparing results to tables or using mathematical formulas, a percentage of body fat can be predicted.

A second indirect method of determining percent body fat is to use **hydrostatic weighing**, or underwater weighing (Figure 15.4 A). This is a more accurate means of measuring body composition and the standard for other indirect techniques. It is based on Archimedes' principle of water displacement. According to this principle, when an object is submerged in water, there is a buoyant force equal to the weight of the water displaced. Since bone and muscle have a greater density than water, an individual with a high percentage of fat-free mass will weigh more in the water than an individual with a high percentage of body fat. To use hydrostatic weighing, one must first determine body density by measuring (a) body weight on land, (b) underwater body weight, (c) water density at the temperature used for the test, and (d) residual lung volume (the amount of air left in the lungs after a forceful expiration). It is important to measure residual lung volume because if it is not accounted for, body fat will be overestimated. Once body density has been determined, equations (e.g., the Siri equation) can be used to calculate **percent body fat**.

Another method of measuring body fat is the **Bod Pod** (also known as air-displacement plethysmography), a somewhat expensive but

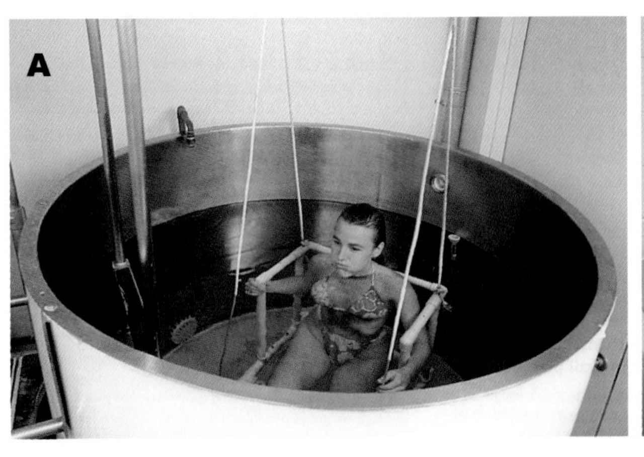

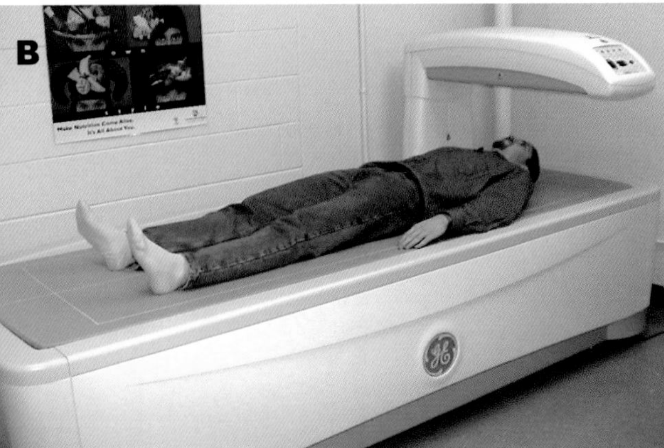

Figure 15.4 Research methods for establishing percent body fat. **A.** Hydrostatic weighing. **B.** Dual energy x-ray absorptiometry (DEXA).

accurate method that does not require underwater submersion and may facilitate measuring very heavy or large individuals. **Bioelectrical impedance analysis (BIA)** is yet another method based on differences in electrical conductivity between fat-free mass and fat mass. By passing an electrical current through the body, a change in voltage is detected, which allows body density, and hence percent body fat, to be calculated. One disadvantage of BIA is the extent to which measurements are influenced by the hydration level of the subject. Other indirect methods of measuring body fat are also available such as **dual energy x-ray absorptiometry (DEXA)**, which is also used to determine bone mineral content and bone mineral density (Figure 15.4 B). DEXA often "competes" with underwater weighing as the gold standard for measuring body composition. Furthermore, the fact that it can also measure bone mineral density means that a three-component model of body composition can be obtained.

Body Mass Index

Except for skinfold calipers, the measurement of body mass can be expensive and time consuming. It is largely limited to research labs and hospitals. Therefore, **body mass index (BMI)** can be used as an easy alternative to assess healthy body weight using an individual's weight (kg) and height (m) measurements. BMI is calculated by dividing total body weight (kg) by body height (m) squared:

$$\text{BMI} = \text{weight (kg)} / \text{height (m)}^2$$

For example, a person who is 167 cm (1.67 m) tall and weighs 70 kg would have a BMI of 25.1 kg/m^2 [$70/(1.67)^2 = 70/2.79 = 25.1$ kg/m^2]. Once the BMI has been obtained, its relationship to desirable body mass indexes can be determined using Table 15.2 A and B.

BMI can also be calculated using pounds and inches by multiplying weight (in pounds) by 703 and dividing this number by height (in inches) squared. A person who is 63 inches tall and weighs 110 pounds would have a BMI of 19.5 [$(110 \times 703)/(63)^2 = 77{,}330/3{,}969 = 19.5$].

BMI has three general ranges: an underweight range, a healthy or acceptable weight range, and an overweight range. The overweight range may be further subdivided. BMI scores above 30 are classified as obese, and scores in this range or above increase one's risk of developing health problems. Use of the BMI is generally intended for men and women aged 20 to 65; it is not useful for babies, children, teenagers, pregnant women, or very muscular people, such as athletes, who may have a high BMI due to their muscle mass. Nonetheless, for the average population, BMI correlates well with body composition.

Table 15.2 A. BMI values in relation to sex. **B.** Desirable BMIs in relation to age.

A

Weight Status	Men	Women
Underweight	< 20.7	< 19.1
Acceptable weight	20.7 – 27.8	19.1 – 27.3
Overweight	27.8	27.3
Severely overweight	31.1	32.3
Morbid obesity	45.4	44.8

B

Age Group (years)	BMI
19 – 24	19 – 24
25 – 34	20 – 25
35 – 44	21 – 26
45 – 54	22 – 27
55 – 65	23 – 28
> 65	24 – 29

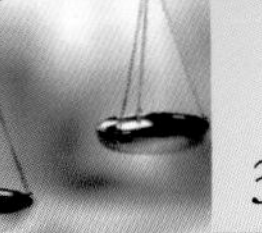

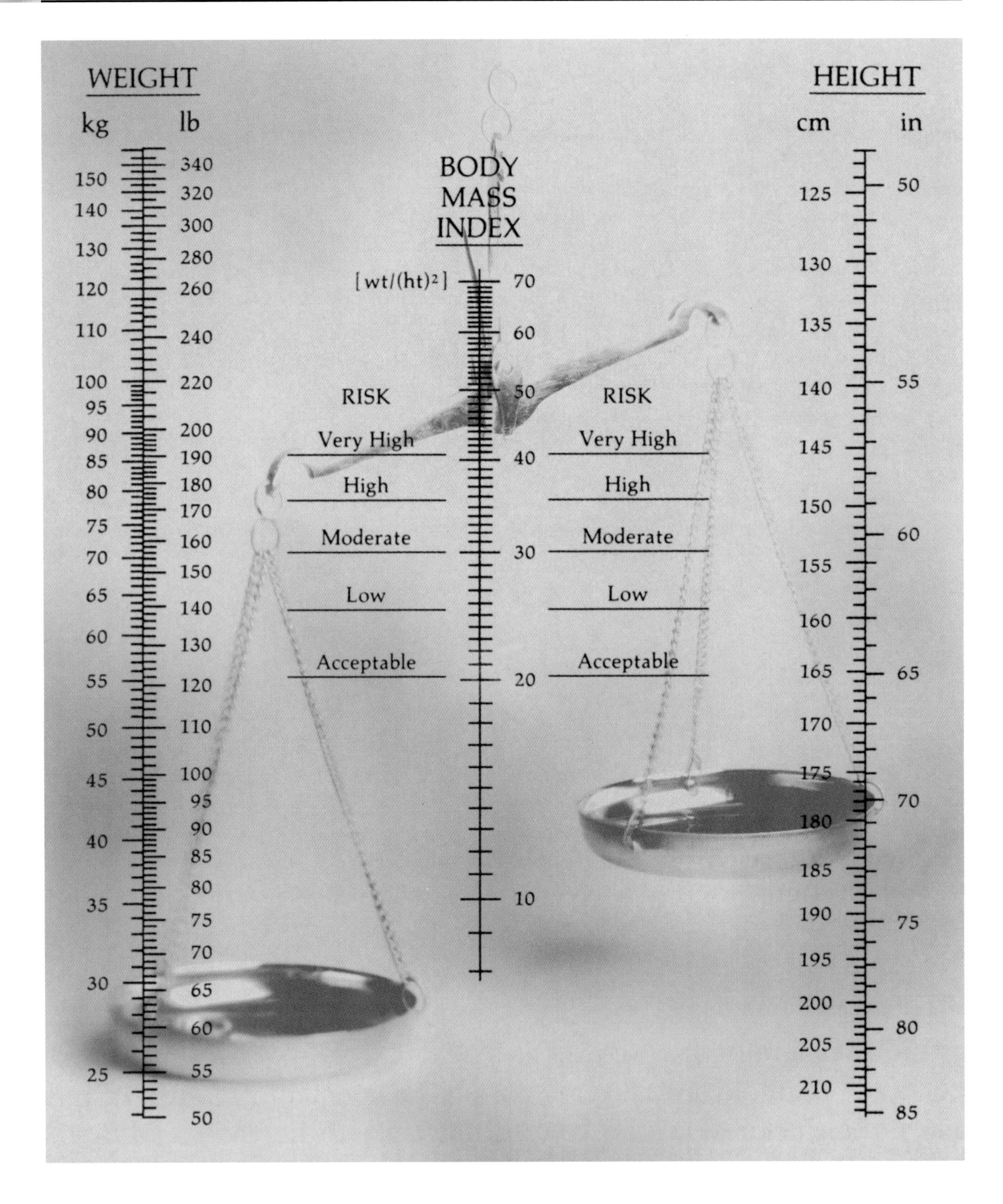

Figure 15.5 Use the nomogram above to determine your BMI. First, find and mark your body weight (kg or lb) on the scale to the left and your height (cm or in) on the scale to the right. Then simply place a straight edge connecting the two values. Your BMI is read where the line intersects the scale in the center. The degree of risk associated with your BMI is also indicated to the left or right of the scale.

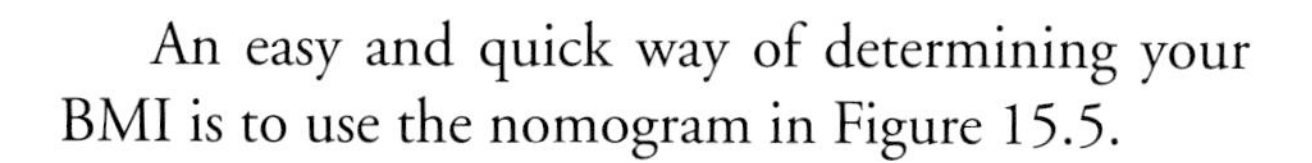

An easy and quick way of determining your BMI is to use the nomogram in Figure 15.5.

Misleading Norms

Weight norms must be interpreted with caution. Being overweight according to norms does not necessarily mean that one is obese. Consider two individuals who are both 71 inches (180 cm) tall and weigh approximately the same weight. One 154-pound (70-kg) person might be very fit and have only 7 percent (10.8 lb, or 4.9 kg) body fat, while another 154-pound (70-kg) person might have 30 percent (46.2 lb, or 21 kg) body fat. Clearly, both individuals have the same mass, but their body composition differs drastically. Thus, although an excess of muscle and other lean body mass can render an individual overweight by normative standards, it does not render him or her obese, since he or she may not have an excess of body fat.

Somatotyping

The human body is composed of **roundness**, **muscularity**, and **linearity**. Based on these three components, individuals can be classified into three major body types. **Endomorphs** exhibit a predominance of the gut and visceral organs, giving them a round appearance. **Mesomorphs** exhibit a predominance of muscle, while **ectomorphs** exhibit a predominance of linearity, tending to be tall and thin.

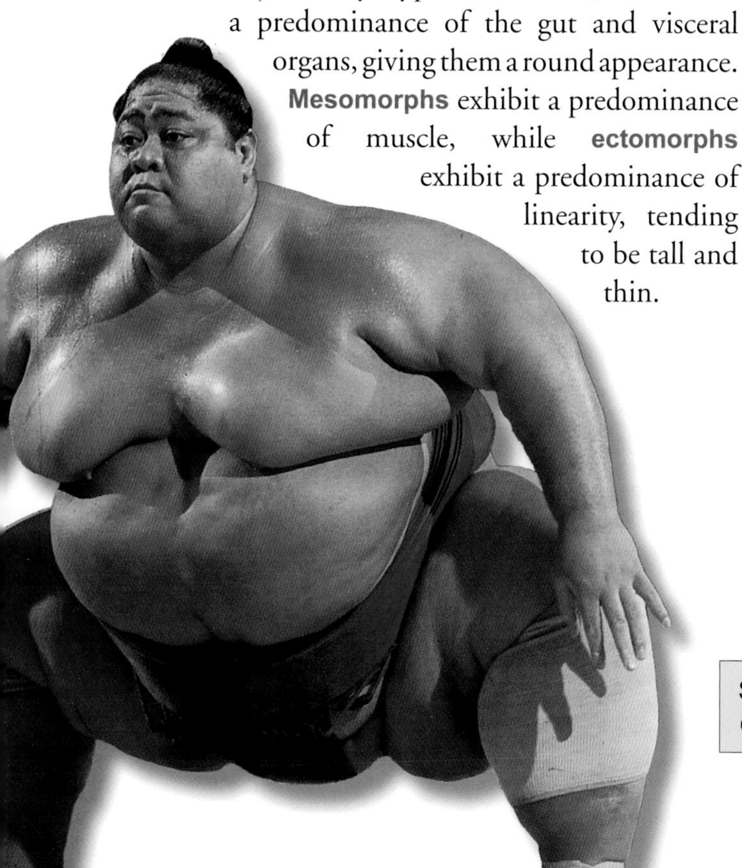

Typically, various sporting activities require sport-specific body types for achieving optimal performance. Therefore, it is not surprising that athletes from different sports demonstrate different somatotypes (Figure 15.6).

An example of a predominantly endomorphic individual would be an obese person or athlete participating in sports like sumo wrestling (Figure 15.6 A). A body builder, a gymnast, and a running back in football (Figure 15.6 B) are examples of mainly mesomorphic individuals. An example of a predominantly ectomorphic individual would be a basketball player, a long-distance runner, or a high jumper (Figure 15.6 C).

Obesity

Obesity is defined as having an excess of body fat beyond some particular standard that is usually based on age and sex (i.e., norms derived from a large number of people). To be classified as obese, men and women between the ages of 17 and 50 require a body fat percentage of greater than 20 and 30 percent, respectively. Older individuals are granted more leeway, although it is not clear why body fat should increase with age.

Obesity has become an epidemic in the Western world, and 30 percent of all adults in Western countries can be considered obese. Unfortunately these numbers seem to be getting worse, not better.

Obesity is a complex condition that may involve environmental, social, psychological, and genetic factors, although only a small percentage of people are genetically predisposed to be obese (Figure 15.7). Research has shown that obesity poses serious health problems, increasing the risk of coronary heart disease, stroke, hypertension, type 2 diabetes mellitus, osteoarthritis, some forms of cancer, and other diseases. On the bright side, obesity can be prevented and by itself is perhaps less harmful than the many health complications that are associated with the condition.

Sumo wrestlers represent an extreme example of endomorphy and obesity.

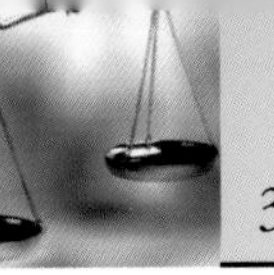

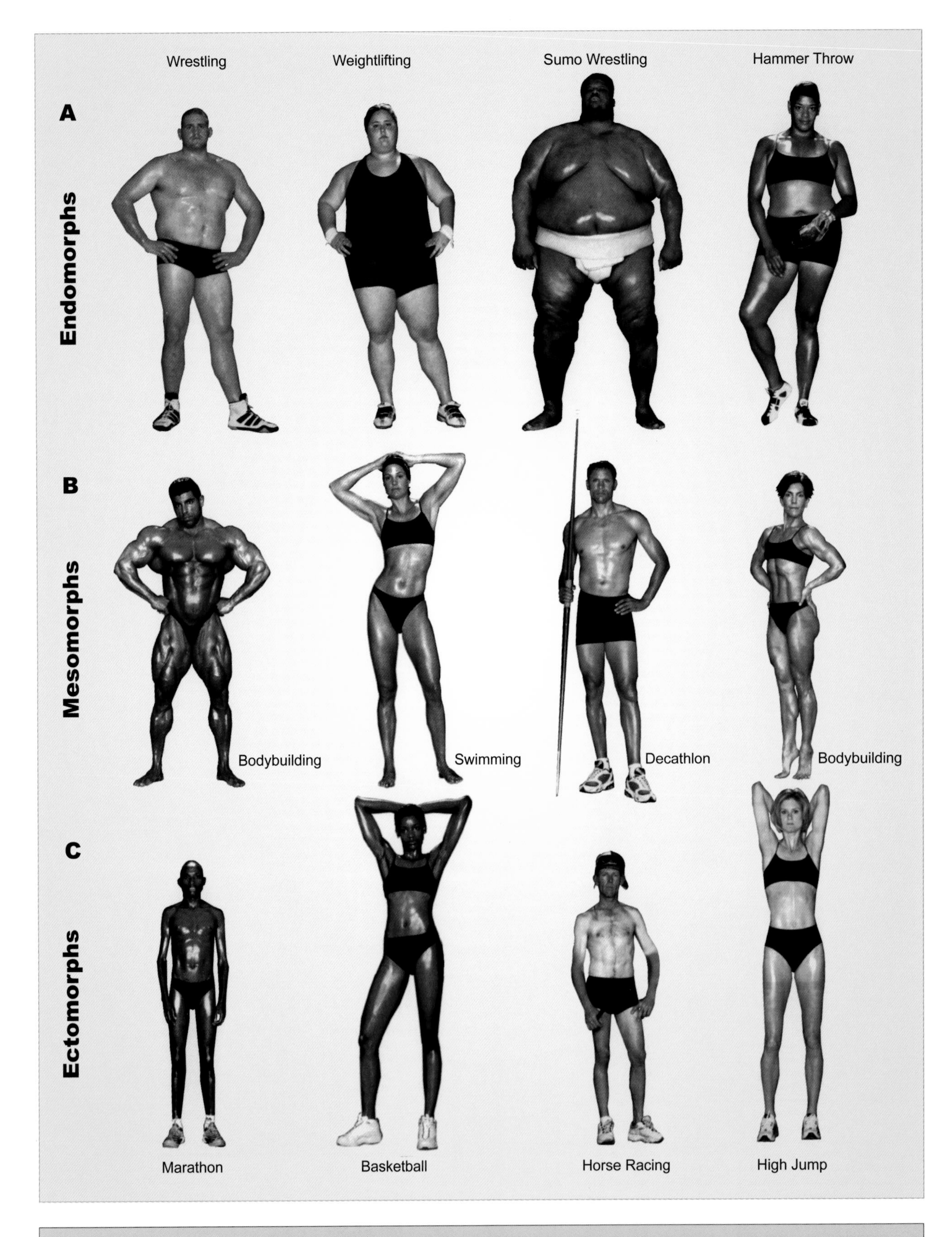

Figure 15.6 Typical body types across a variety of sporting activities. **A.** Endomorphs. **B.** Mesomorphs. **C.** Ectomorphs.

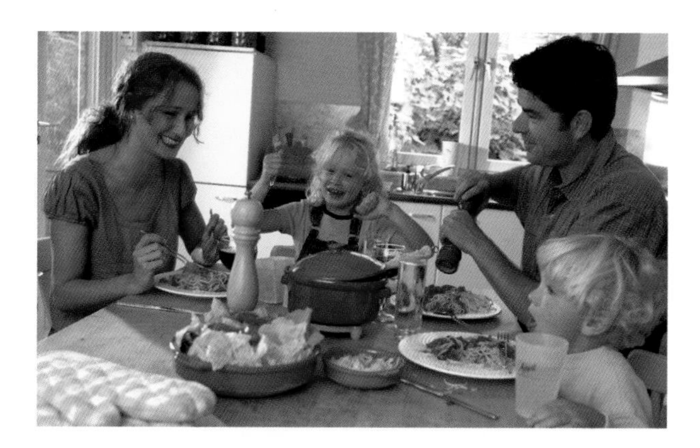

Figure 15.7 Good eating habits are developed early and may help prevent obesity in the long run.

Creeping Obesity

Although obese individuals are often viewed as gluttonous, they generally do not consume large amounts of kilocalories. In fact, physically active individuals have been shown to consume more kilocalories than do obese individuals. Thus, obesity is often the result of too little activity rather than overeating, bringing about **creeping obesity**: a slight change in the energy balance occurring over a period of time causes a gradual increase in fat mass each year. As people age, their metabolic rates and physical activity patterns often decline. If their energy intake is not reduced to rebalance with energy expenditure (according to the energy balance equation in Figure 15.2), then body mass will increase because of excess kilocalories stored as fat.

Consider This

If you consume only one potato chip per day (roughly 10 kilocalories) in excess of energy expenditure, then over a year (365 days) you will have accumulated 3,650 extra kilocalories, equivalent to approximately 1 pound (0.5 kg) of body fat. In view of this, it is easy to understand how one can gradually become obese.

Creeping obesity is often experienced by individuals who were active in their teens and twenties but for various reasons (work, family, and so on) reduced their physical activity levels later in life, only to realize years later that they have an excess amount of body fat.

Weight-loss Industry

There are a variety of fad diets that people use in an attempt to achieve weight loss. The weight-loss industry has become a billion-dollar industry as more and more people battling obesity seek help from food-industry experts and nutritionists. High-protein, low-carbohydrate diets; high-carbohydrate, low-protein diets; fasting–starvation diets; high-fiber, low-energy diets; and limited food choice diets are just a few of the many possibilities available. In most cases, these approaches are ineffective and potentially harmful. Following the dietary guidelines and recommendations presented in Chapter 14, coupled with an active lifestyle that includes regular exercise, seems to be the best approach to weight management (Figure 15.8 B).

Stuck on Soda?

After water, carbonated beverages are the most popular drinks in North America. And there is no shortage of choices. From Cherry or Vanilla Coke to Pepsi Twist or Blue, new flavors, colors, and labels are constantly being developed to entice consumers – especially young consumers (12- to 24-year-olds) who comprise the majority of high-consumption soda drinkers. According to statistics, Americans guzzle more than 50 gallons (200 liters) per person per year.

Our love for these carbonated beverages, which often come full of empty kilocalories, has contributed to the overweight epidemic facing individuals in the United States, both young and old. Next time you consider reaching for a can of soda, consider the impact it can have on your health. And remember, even small changes can make big differences; for example, not drinking one soda a day may lead to approximately 12 pounds of weight loss in a single year.

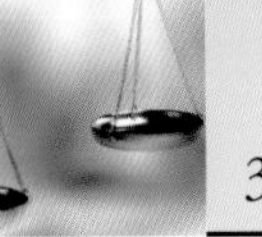

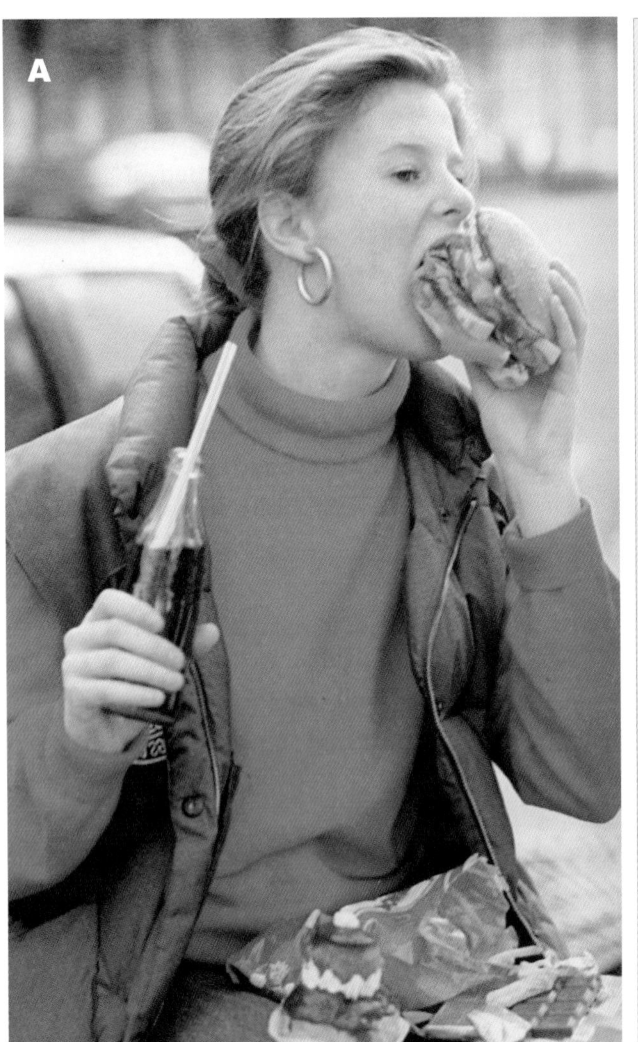

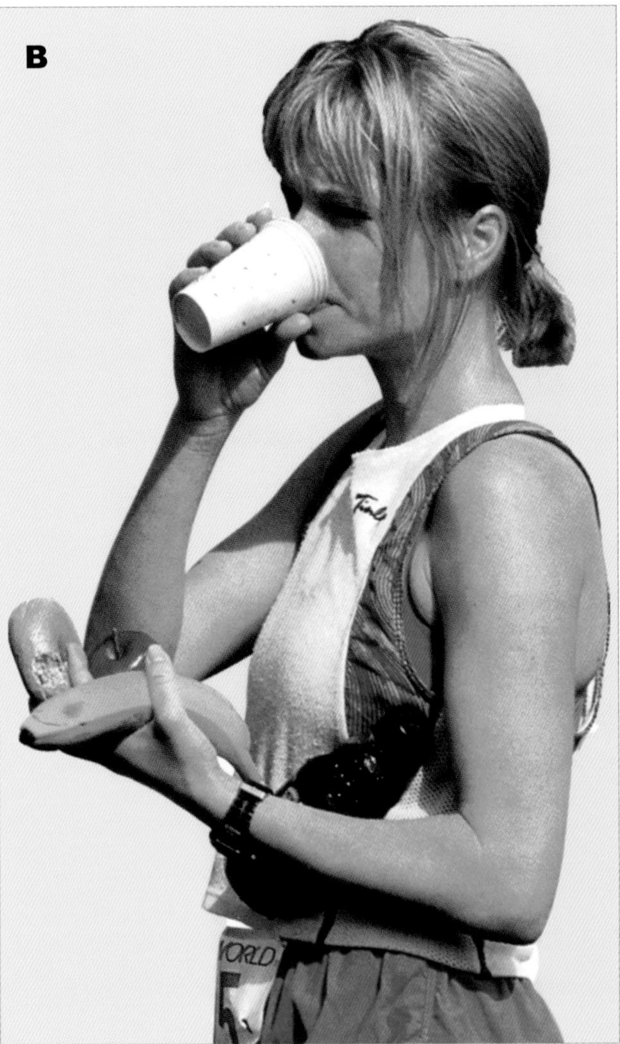

Figure 15.8 It is your choice when it comes to making sensible eating decisions.

Consequences of Dieting

Dieting for the purposes of improving health, working capacity, or athletic performance can be positive if you follow the recommended guidelines for healthy eating. Unfortunately, cultural pressures to be thin (especially among girls and young women) and the stigma of being overweight have pushed many weight-conscious youths to dieting and abnormal eating patterns lacking nutritional balance. Dieting for these reasons not only is distressing but also sets you up for failure in the long run. Although obesity can be a real health concern, your weight needs to be managed in an atmosphere that is both positive and realistic – not under conditions in which eating itself seems like a crime.

Should we be preoccupied with the issue of weight if it does not pose a major health risk? This is a question young people especially should ask themselves. At one time or another, you have probably questioned your weight or the way you look because of cultural pressures to be "thin and attractive." But chronic dieting, especially among teenagers, can be a serious concern because it can lead to retardation of physical growth, menstrual irregularities in women, a lowering of metabolic rate, and the development of eating disorders.

Self-esteem and Body Image

Many of today's adolescent girls have an appallingly low sense of self-worth, poor views of their value to society, and often less confidence than boys of similar age. To combat this trend, the notion that self-esteem should be based less on outward appearance and body shape and more on other assets – musical, athletic, creative, and scholastic abilities or other talents – must be reinforced for all adolescents. It is also important that overweight children of all ages not be condemned for their body weight because this will lead to poor self-esteem.

Eating Disorders

The term "eating disorders" does not reveal the true seriousness of these conditions. Problems with weight management are not just problems of avoiding excess body fat. In fact, these disorders have increased in frequency and pose specific public health risks among athletes, dancers, models, and others who become preoccupied with body weight and shape. Disorders of this nature also put women at risk of developing the female athlete triad, a deadly combination of eating disorders, amenorrhea, and osteoporosis.

The two major eating disorders characterized by abnormal eating behaviors are *anorexia nervosa* and *bulimia nervosa*. These disorders develop as a result of many factors, including dissatisfaction with body image, which stems from distorted thinking, unrealistic expectations, and excessive self-criticism. A fear of being overweight, excessive dieting, and a preoccupation with food become obsessive. Related issues are *binge eating* and *subclinical eating disorders* among athletes. Another problem is *cognitive restraint*, a psychological means of intentionally restraining intake to lower dietary intake.

Anorexia Nervosa

Individuals with **anorexia nervosa** fail to eat an adequate amount of food to maintain a reasonable body weight – to the point of starvation. Anorectics have an intense fear of gaining weight or becoming fat, so they often avoid eating and may use compulsive exercise to reduce body weight. They begin by restricting their intake of high-energy foods, which eventually leads to a restriction of virtually all foods from their diet. Typically, anorectics weigh less than 85 percent of normal body weight for their age and height (Figure 15.9). Some of the physical

Knowledge Check

For each of the following statements below, indicate whether it applies to *anorexia nervosa* (**AN**), *bulimia nervosa* (**BN**), or both (**AB**) eating disorders. After you have finished reading this chapter, take the test again.

1. Need or desire for perfection. ( )
2. Recurrent episodes of binge eating. ( )
3. Low self-esteem and sense of self-worth. ( )
4. Extreme concern about appearance. ( )
5. Evidence of purging (through vomiting or use of laxatives, diuretics, or excessive exercise). ( )
6. Amenorrhea (loss of menstrual periods). ( )
7. Signs of starvation (thinning of hair, yellow appearance of palms or soles). ( )
8. Refusal to maintain body weight at or above normal weight for age and height. ( )
9. Frequent, unusual dental problems. ( )
10. Frequent weight fluctuations. ( )

(Answers: 1. AB; 2. BN; 3. AB; 4. AB; 5. BN; 6. AN; 7. AN; 8. AN; 9. BN; 10. BN) symptoms include dry skin, amenorrhea, reduced bone mass, brittle nails, and carotene pigmentation (yellowish appearance of the palms and soles of the feet).

The psychological problems associated with anorexia nervosa, such as depression and other clinical disorders, can be even more serious than the physical ones. It has been reported that between 5 and 18 percent of anorectics commit suicide or develop serious, irreversible medical problems.

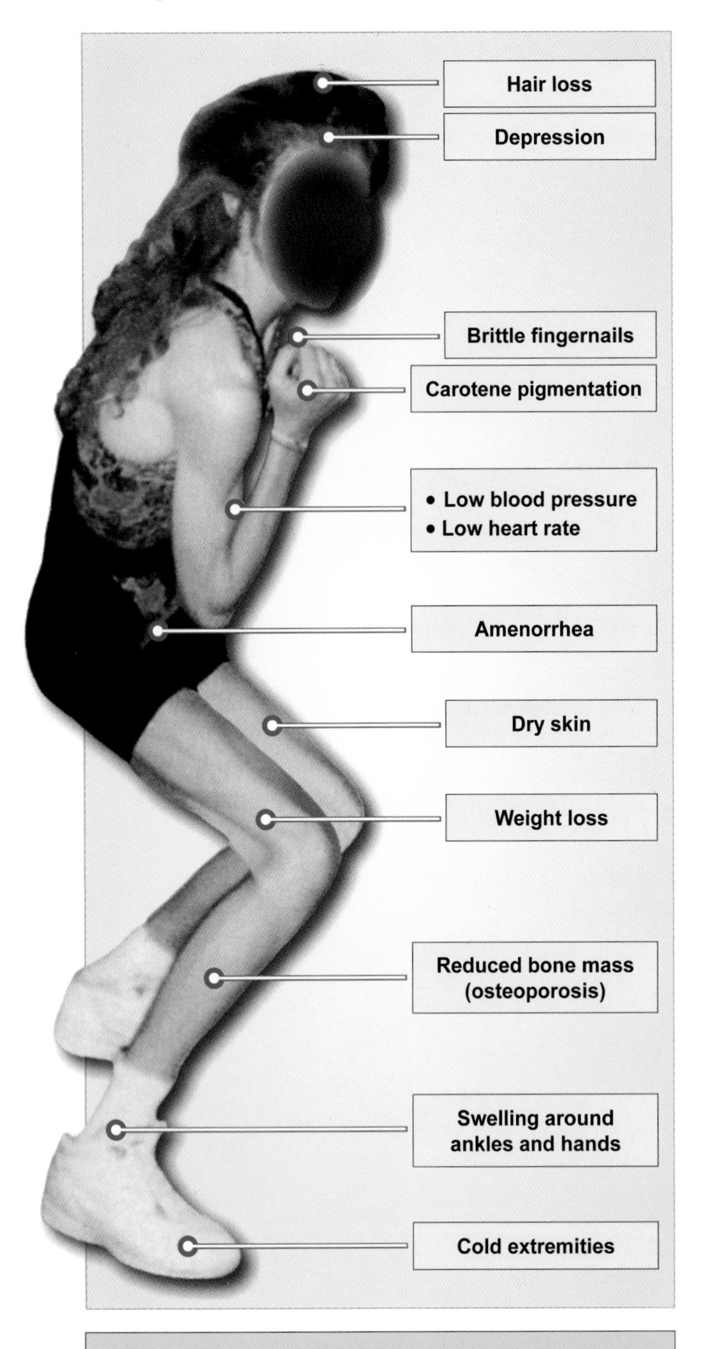

Figure 15.9 The effects of anorexia nervosa.

Bulimia Nervosa

Bulimia nervosa is characterized by recurring episodes of binge eating (large amounts of food consumed in a discrete period) followed by purging. Bulimics feel a lack of control when they binge, unable to stop what and how much they eat. After a binge, bulimics compensate by vomiting or using laxatives or diuretics to rid the body of the food they just ate. Frequent vomiting often leads to dental problems, as the acid reflux from the stomach damages the teeth and gums in the mouth. Bulimics may also engage in vigorous exercise to compensate for the increased energy consumed during a binge.

Bulimics are more difficult to identify because their body weight is often normal, and they usually conceal their eating habits well (Figure 15.10). However, look for warning signs such as secretive eating patterns, repeated isolation soon after a meal, disappearance of large amounts of food, nervous or agitated behavior immediately after eating, or the loss or gain of extreme amounts of weight. Bulimics may experience weight fluctuations exceeding 10 pounds (4.5 kg) during periods of binge eating.

Bulimia nervosa is generally considered to be less serious than anorexia nervosa, since treatment is effective in the majority of cases and most individuals experience a full and lasting recovery. All eating disorders should be taken seriously, however, and managed promptly.

Binge Eating Disorder

A syndrome related to eating disorders, and obesity in particular, is **binge eating disorder (BED)**, which involves ingesting large amounts of food without the purging behavior characteristic of bulimia nervosa. Although this is considered to be a hazardous health behavior, it is actually encouraged in such sports as sumo wrestling and football (linemen), where gaining greater mass is an asset. It is worth noting, however, that binge eating leads to obesity in most cases.

Female Athlete Triad

Modern society and the media place enormous

Recognizing Binge Eating Disorder

Presented below are a few signs and symptoms characteristic of *binge eating disorder (BED)*.

1. Recurrent episodes of binge eating. An episode of binge eating is characterized by both:

- eating an amount of food during a discrete period that is larger than most people would eat during the same time and in similar circumstances; and
- a sense of lack of control over eating (what or how much) during the episode.

2. During most binge episodes, *at least* three of the following behavioral indicators of loss of control are present:

- eating much more rapidly than usual;
- eating until feeling uncomfortably full;
- eating large amounts of food even when not feeling physically hungry;
- eating alone because of being embarrassed by how much one is eating; or
- feeling disgusted with oneself, depressed, or very guilty after overeating.

3. The binge eating causes episodes of considerable distress.

4. Binge eating occurs, on average, at least two days a week over a six-month period.

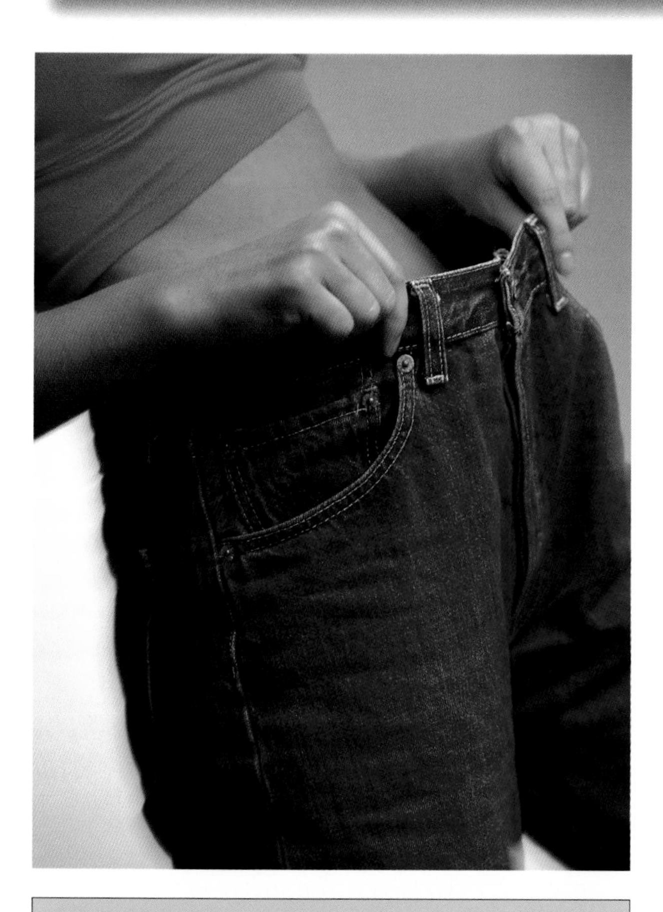

Figure 15.10 Distorted thinking and excessive self-criticism lead many bulimics to constantly monitor their weight and appearance in the pursuit of an ideal figure.

pressure on individuals, and especially on young women, to maintain a thin body image. Such goals are unrealistic, but many athletes pursue them through extreme dieting and overtraining. They thereby risk developing a medical syndrome known as the **female athlete triad**. Although athletes from all types of sports run this risk, those who participate in gymnastics, dance, figure skating, ballet, lightweight rowing and sculling, and cross-country running are the most susceptible because these sports demand an unrealistic stereotypical body shape or weight.

Three distinct interrelated problems form the female athlete triad condition: disordered eating, amenorrhea, and osteoporosis (Figure 15.11).

Disordered Eating The term **disordered eating** refers to a spectrum of poor and unhealthy nutritional behaviors that can be as extreme as anorexia nervosa and bulimia nervosa or as subtle as consciously restricting food intake.

Amenorrhea The occurrence of irregular or absent menstrual periods for at least three months is referred to as **amenorrhea**. When an athlete stops having a menstrual period or menstrual periods become irregular, it should not be viewed

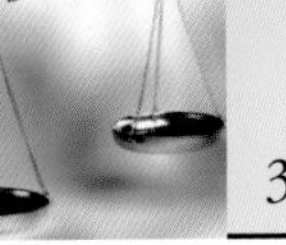

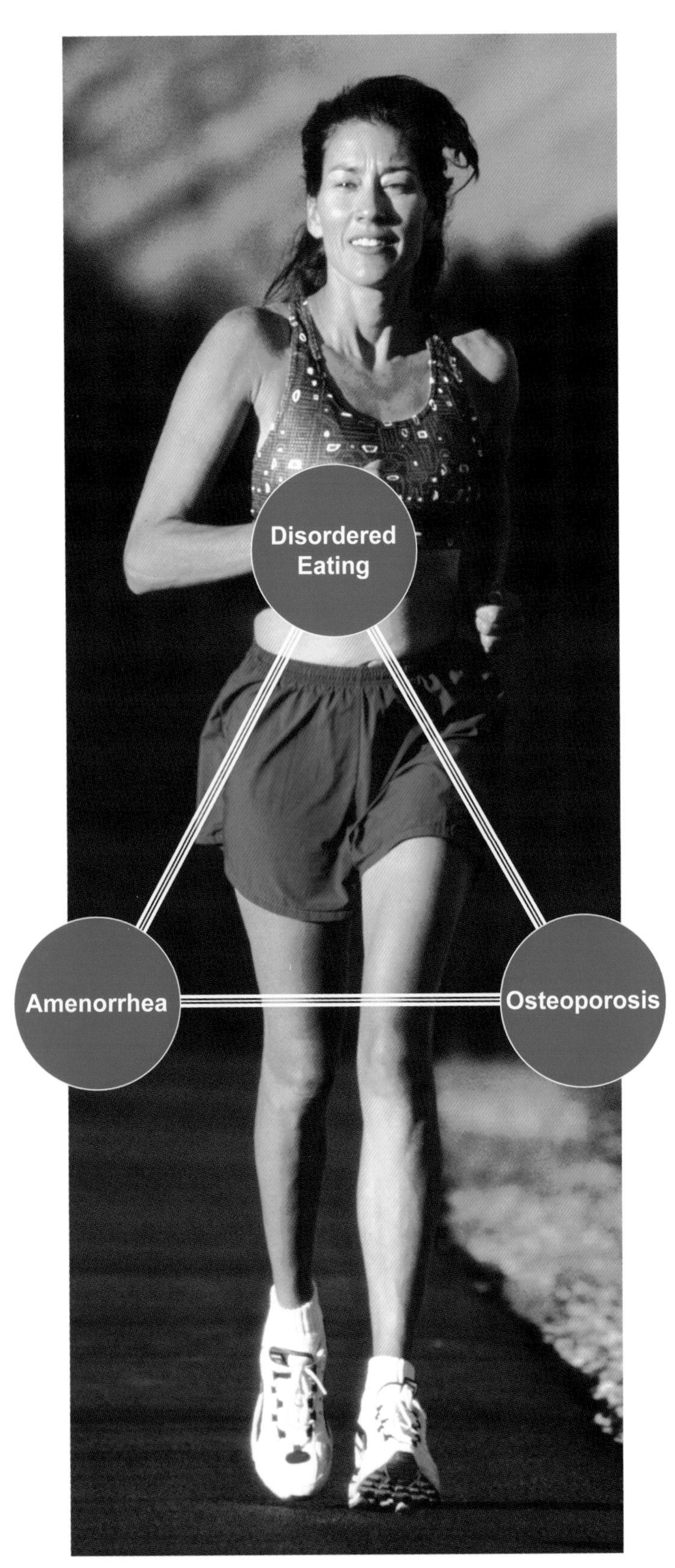

Figure 15.11 The female athlete triad represents a series of three progressive conditions that should be taken seriously.

as a normal adaptation to exercise training. It is actually a classic sign of the triad, and medical intervention should be initiated.

Osteoporosis If amenorrhea persists over long periods, it leads to **osteoporosis**, or a weakening of the bones, which unfortunately is not entirely reversible. Osteoporosis refers to low bone mass; bones become weak and brittle, which in turn increases the risk of fracture. An athlete who suffers a stress fracture may also be struggling with the female athlete triad; in fact, a stress fracture should be considered by coaches and athletes as a possible indicator of an unhealthy approach to training.

Take the Female Athlete Triad Seriously

The *female athlete triad* is a serious medical condition that can be fatal in some cases. An athlete who has any symptoms of the triad (disordered eating, osteoporosis, menstrual dysfunction) should seek medical counsel. Early intervention is more likely to result in successful treatment.

How to Prevent the Female Athlete Triad The single best strategy to prevent the female athlete triad is to consume more kilocalories, especially during intense or increased exercise training. Eating a healthy and balanced diet is very important for maintaining bone and muscle mass. Female athletes should also ensure they get enough calcium in their diets. Young women require 1,300 mg of calcium a day to maintain strong and healthy bones, since the years before and after puberty are the most important bone building years.

Eating Disorders Among Athletes

Although eating disorders are an issue faced predominantly by girls and women concerned with body image, many athletes rely on extreme dieting measures to achieve or maintain a desired

Case Study

Anthropometric Data:

Height: 5 ft, 8 in
Weight: 119 lb
LBW: 102 lb
Her goal was to be 108 to 110 lb.
She had amenorrhea.

Present Dietary Pattern:

Breakfast: Nil
On the way to dance class a power bar, various flavors

Lunch: Nil
Diet Coke during the day

Dinner: Steamed vegetables and fruit

An intelligent 16-year-old dancer wanted to reduce her body weight prior to her final examination to help her make the national junior squad, which was to travel abroad to compete at an international tournament (see data on the left).

After following this pattern for some time, the problem began: binge eating on anything that was in the house (bread – dry or with peanut butter or jam, biscuits and cheese, breakfast cereal, ice cream, and so on), followed by discomfort and guilt and finally induced vomiting before bedtime. The pattern would be repeated the next day.

Solution

The instructor, with the professional help of a registered dietitian, was able to explain to the dancer the negative effects of her nutrition practice on performance. Furthermore, the instructor suggested nutrition counseling. The registered dietitian was able to persuade the dancer that it is possible to eat normally and still lose weight. A low-energy diet was planned, with emphasis on a high percentage of carbohydrate intake. A multivitamin/mineral was recommended to supplement the low-energy diet.

Result

At the review visit six weeks later, the dancer's weight had decreased by 3.3 pounds. She felt well, was able to follow the nutritional regimen, and had achieved her goals. She continued to lose weight and was selected to the squad.

body weight. Many athletes competing in sports with weight classes often strive to make weight in lower weight classes (e.g., wrestling, boxing, weightlifting) or maintain the minimum weight allowed (e.g., jockey in horse racing, coxswain or lightweight crew in rowing) to gain a competitive advantage. For these athletes, the issue of body weight is secondary to the objective of performing well. Dieting issues are only temporary in most cases for these individuals. Contrast this with the more prolonged issues faced by individuals battling the eating disorders described previously, which stem from issues of self-esteem, self-evaluation, and self-identity. Nonetheless, these short-term but frequent dieting episodes can still be harmful to health and could lead to a true eating disorder.

Summary

The human body is made up of components that are arranged and distributed in different ways. Individuals may exhibit different amounts of roundness (endomorphs), linearity (ectomorphs), or muscle (mesomorphs) and thus have different body types. Various sporting activities require sport-specific body types for achieving optimal performance.

Basal metabolic rate (BMR) is defined as the minimum amount of energy the body requires to carry out all vital functions. Energy requirements increase with any additional activity above this level. Weight management is a matter of balancing the kilocalories consumed with the energy expended; body weight will remain constant if energy input and output are the same.

Lean body mass (LBM) refers to the "nonfat" components of the human body (i.e., muscle, bone, and water). LBM can be calculated by subtracting total body fat from total body mass. One way of indirectly measuring body fat is through skinfold measurements. This method uses calipers to measure skinfold thicknesses at various sites on the body, and the results are then used to predict total body fat. An easy way of assessing healthy weight is to divide body weight (kg) by body height (m) squared to arrive at a measure known as body mass index (BMI).

Obesity is defined as having excess body fat beyond some particular standard, usually based on age and sex. The proportion of muscle and fat you have greatly influences your risk of disease, and obesity poses serious health problems including coronary heart disease, stroke, hypertension, and type 2 diabetes mellitus. At the other extreme, cultural pressures to be thin and the stigma of being overweight have led some individuals along the dangerous path of extreme dieting and abnormal eating patterns. Examples of common eating disorders include anorexia nervosa, bulimia nervosa, and binge eating.

Fortunately, body weight is one body component that we do have control over. By coupling an awareness of sufficient energy intake with adequate amounts of physical activity, a healthy body weight can usually be achieved.

Key Terms

amenorrhea
anorexia nervosa
basal metabolic rate (BMR)
binge eating disorder (BED)
bioelectrical impedance analysis (BIA)
Bod Pod
body composition
body mass index (BMI)
bulimia nervosa
creeping obesity
disordered eating
dual energy x-ray absorptiometry (DEXA)
ectomorph
endomorph
energy balance
energy balance equation

essential fat (EF)
female athlete triad
fat mass (FM)
hydrostatic weighing
lean body mass (LBM)
mesomorph
obesity
osteoporosis
percent body fat
skinfold calipers
storage fat (SF)
total body fat (TBF)
total body mass (TBM)

Discussion Questions

1. Briefly describe the energy balance equation. What situation would need to exist for someone to lose weight? To gain weight?

2. What is a basal metabolic rate? How does exercise influence it?

3. What is the two-component model? Discuss each component of the model and how it relates to overall body composition.

4. Identify and define the two major types of body fat. How do levels of each type differ in males and females?

5. List four indirect methods used to measure body fat. Which methods are most accurate? Least accurate?

6. What does BMI stand for? How is it used to assess body weight? What is a healthy BMI value?

7. Individuals can be classified into three main body types. List them and briefly describe each one.

8. Define creeping obesity.

9. Body weight norms can be misleading. Discuss the implications of this statement.

10. Distinguish between the two major types of eating disorders. How do these differ from binge eating disorder and eating disorders among athletes?

A Career in Nutrition

NAME: Stella Lucia Volpe
OCCUPATION: Associate Professor and Miriam Stirl Term Endowed Chair of Nutrition
EDUCATION: BSc Exercise Physiology, University of Pittsburgh
MSc Exercise Physiology, Virginia Tech
PhD Human Nutrition, Virginia Tech

What do you do?

I am a professor at the University of Pennsylvania. My primary responsibility is to conduct research. My research focuses primarily on obesity prevention through exercise and nutrition, especially in changing the environment to require people to become more active and eat more healthily. I also conduct research in mineral metabolism and diabetes, as well as mineral metabolism and exercise, and in body composition. I teach classes in sports nutrition and basic nutrition. I am also a registered dietitian and certified as an exercise specialist by the American College of Sports Medicine.

What is unique about your job?

My job is always diverse! I write a lot – grants, manuscripts, book chapters, books. I travel to present my research, I teach, I mentor graduate students, I review manuscripts, I am on a number of committees on campus. I enjoy that I get to be around so many diverse people, too, because I learn a lot from them and their respective disciplines. It is also helpful to have such diversity on a university campus because it allows for a great deal of collaboration on research.

Why did you choose a career in nutrition? What was your motivation for pursuing this field?

I always enjoyed learning from my professors, both in the classroom and through their research. I like the challenge of thinking about research questions, then writing grants and learning from others. I enjoy writing, and my field requires a lot of writing.

How did studies in kinesiology benefit your career choice?

The combination of exercise physiology and nutrition has been excellent for me. They are two fields that I really enjoy, having been an athlete my entire life, and I am still a competitive athlete; so they bridge together two very linked disciplines.

What do you enjoy most about your profession?

I really enjoy being on a university campus. I also enjoy the fact that I have freedom to pursue my research interests and that I have wonderful colleagues with whom to collaborate.

What career advice would you give to students interested in entering this field?

Keep open as many options as possible. Try to bridge together two fields that you enjoy because this will open more doors for you. Keep an open mind, and don't be afraid to pursue an area of research you are passionate about.

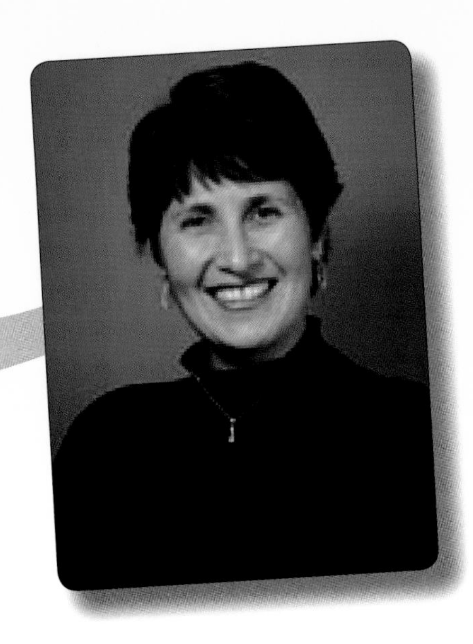

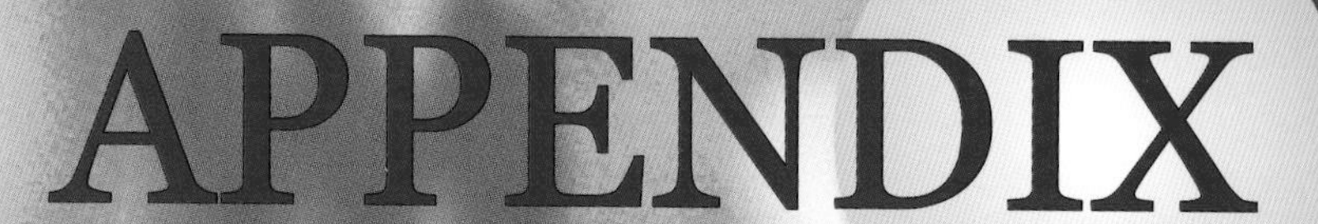

Career Opportunities in Kinesiology

- Career Opportunities in Kinesiology

In This Chapter:

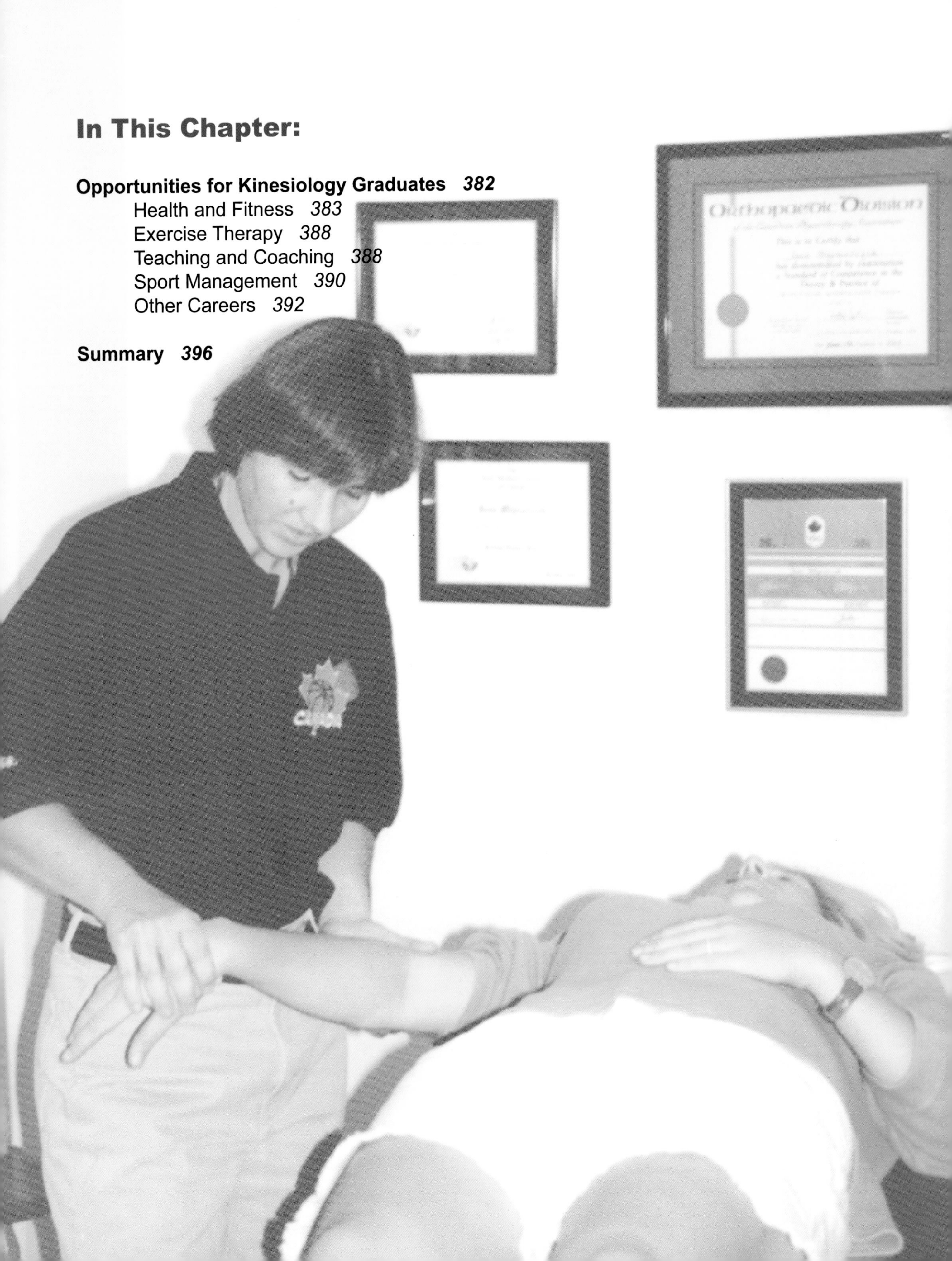

APPENDIX

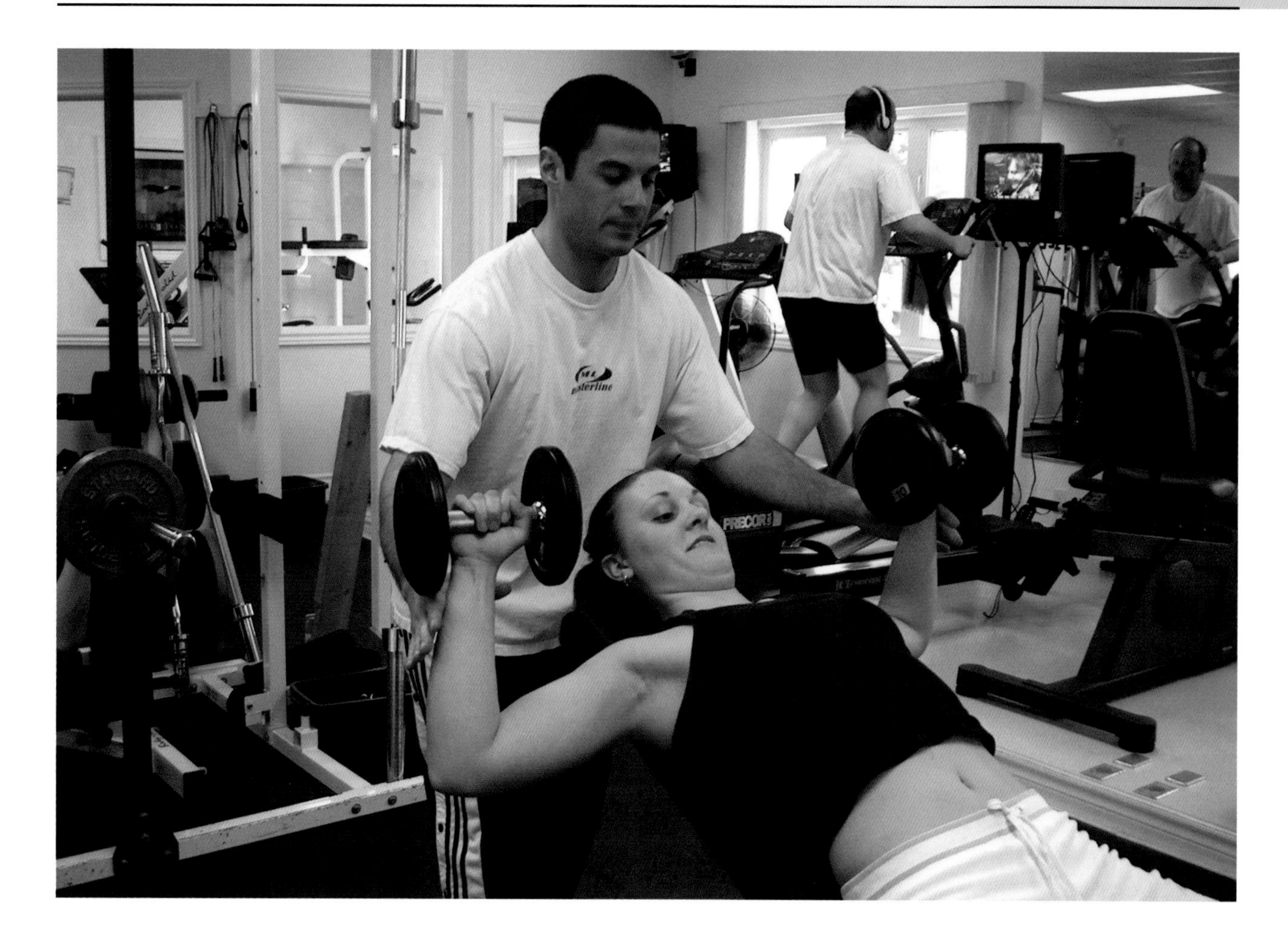

Career Opportunities in Kinesiology

After completing this chapter you should be able to:

- describe the diversity of college and university programs in physical education;
- identify career opportunities available to kinesiology graduates;
- describe the role of kinesiology in today's society.

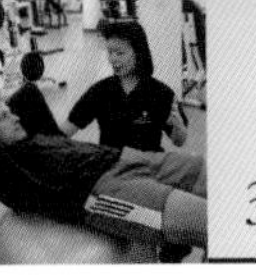

Notions based on outdated stereotypes sometimes make physical education out to be a field for "dumb jocks." So it is not surprising that when people think about careers in health and fitness, visions of their high school physical education teachers often come to mind. However, secondary school teaching represents but one of many opportunities available to graduates in physical and health education. The increased emphasis on physical activity in today's society as a means to better health as well as improved business productivity has meant a corresponding expansion of career possibilities in a variety of fields. The diverse positions filled by physical and health education graduates is a continuing reminder that the old stereotypes and caricatures are fast disappearing.

At one time, "physical education" was the name given to all health and fitness programs because they were initially formed to train elementary and secondary school physical education teachers. Since then a huge evolution has occurred in the diversity of knowledge and its application in the field. This includes major developments in areas such as exercise physiology and biochemistry; sports medicine and exercise rehabilitation; fitness, nutrition, and health; sports psychology; biomechanics and applied ergonomics; sports and recreation administration; and fitness for elderly, disabled, or very young populations, as well as advanced training and coaching techniques for elite athletes. This vast expansion of the scope of the discipline has also resulted in the growth of new and exciting areas of employment for graduates.

With the evolution of this expansion has come diversification and partial fragmentation of college and university physical and health education programs. To avoid a narrow association of physical education with training for the school system, many university programs have changed their names. Some of the names that physical and health education has evolved into include kinesiology, human kinetics, kinanthropology, and exercise science.

Whether university programs are called physical and health education, kinesiology, or some other related term, most deal primarily with various aspects of the study of human movement. Some programs specialize in the more scientific or quantitative aspects of this study, others more in health and fitness areas, and still others in recreation and leisure. However, most programs are diverse and comprehensive enough to allow for study in many of these areas along with the development of various student interests. This chapter will survey the diverse learning and career opportunities available in the field of fitness and health.

Opportunities for Kinesiology Graduates

"So what are you going to do with that?" is the question many students face when they first tell their parents about their choice of major. The real question is, can you earn a living with that background? The answer for kinesiology students is an unequivocal "Yes!"

Kinesiology is a field that attracts many people with athletic backgrounds. Some are varsity athletes who juggle higher education and athletics. Others are former high school athletes who, for a variety of reasons, do not compete at the collegiate level but retain deep interest in sport. And while kinesiology graduates used to be relegated to narrowly defined careers as athletic coaches and trainers, today societal changes have opened the door to a wide variety of career opportunities.

Back in the late 1800s, when the first professional athletic competitions arose, few people would have predicted that sport would become a multibillion dollar industry in North America. That growth, coupled with an explosion of amateur and club sports, on top of concerns about health, fitness, and weight management, all contribute to robust career opportunities for kinesiology students.

Concerns about obesity, establishment of new guidelines for healthy eating, and the aging of the "baby boom" generation are all contributing to the need for the knowledge, skills, and capabilities of kinesiology graduates. The health and fitness

Figure 16.1 Percent change in wage and salary employment, service-providing industry divisions, 1994 to 2004 and projected 2004 to 2014.

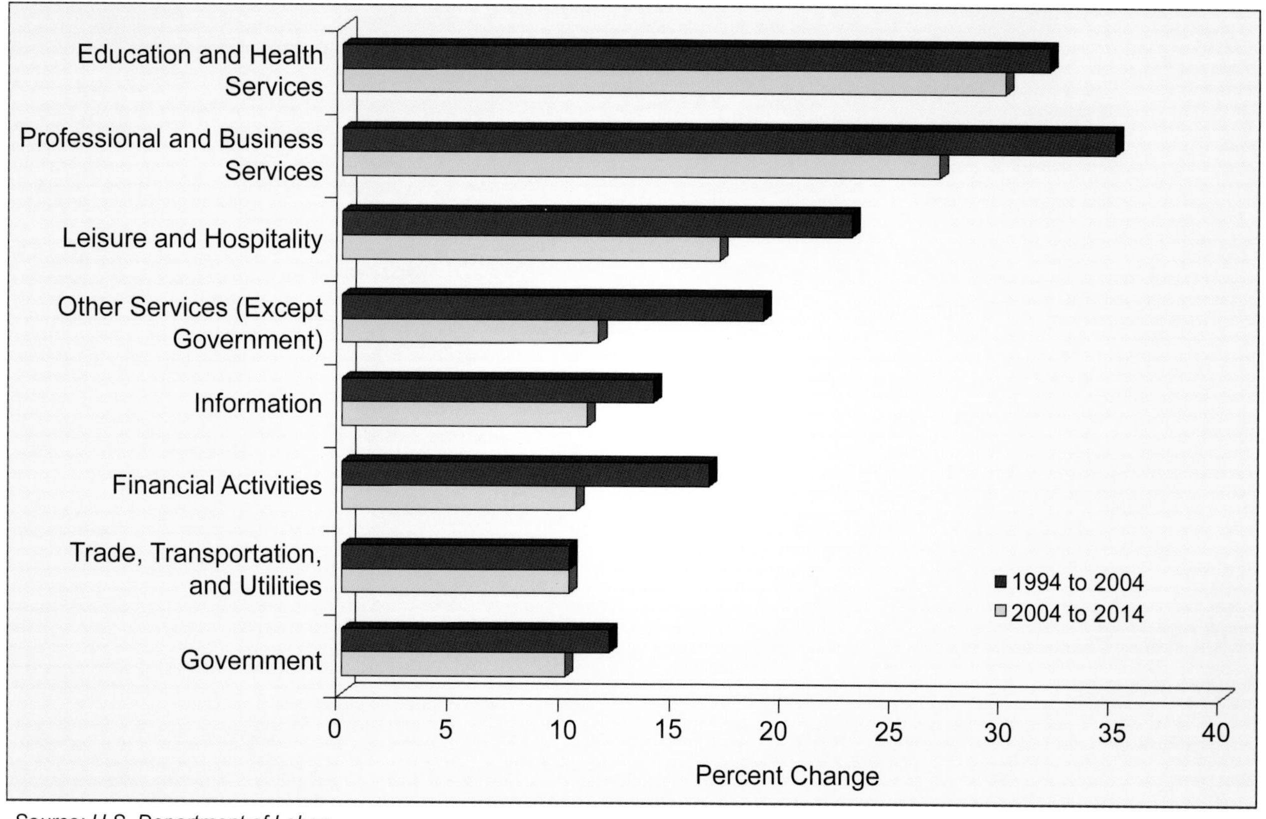

Source: U.S. Department of Labor

industry integrates exercise, personal responsibility, and prevention in ways that meet the needs of popular North American culture. Decades of research and reports by the U.S. Surgeon General, Centers for Disease Control, U.S. Food and Drug Administration, Public Health Agency of Canada, and Health Canada all point to the need for physical activity to promote health.

The U.S. Department of Labor is forecasting that the health services and leisure and hospitality industries will continue to be among the highest-demand positions in the country (Figure 16.1). When it comes to prospects for kinesiology students, Figure 16.2 provides an insight to where the opportunities may be greatest.

Health and fitness careers fall into several fields, each with its own subcategories:

- Health and fitness
- Exercise therapy
- Teaching and coaching
- Sport management
- Other careers

Health and Fitness

The **health and fitness industry** is a phenomenon of the late 20th century – and the explosion of career opportunities for kinesiology graduates has matched its evolution. For example, Life Time Fitness was founded by Bahram Akradi in 1992 after cofounding and working for U.S. Swim & Fitness in the 1980s. (And Mr. Akradi's 2005 compensation is listed as more than $40 million!) Today, Life Time Fitness has 48 large fitness centers in nine states, with plans to open 6 to 10 each year. Each requires a full staff, ranging from personal trainers to physiotherapists and nutritionists – from entry-level positions to

Figure 16.2 Percent change in employment in occupations projected to grow fastest, 2004 to 2014.

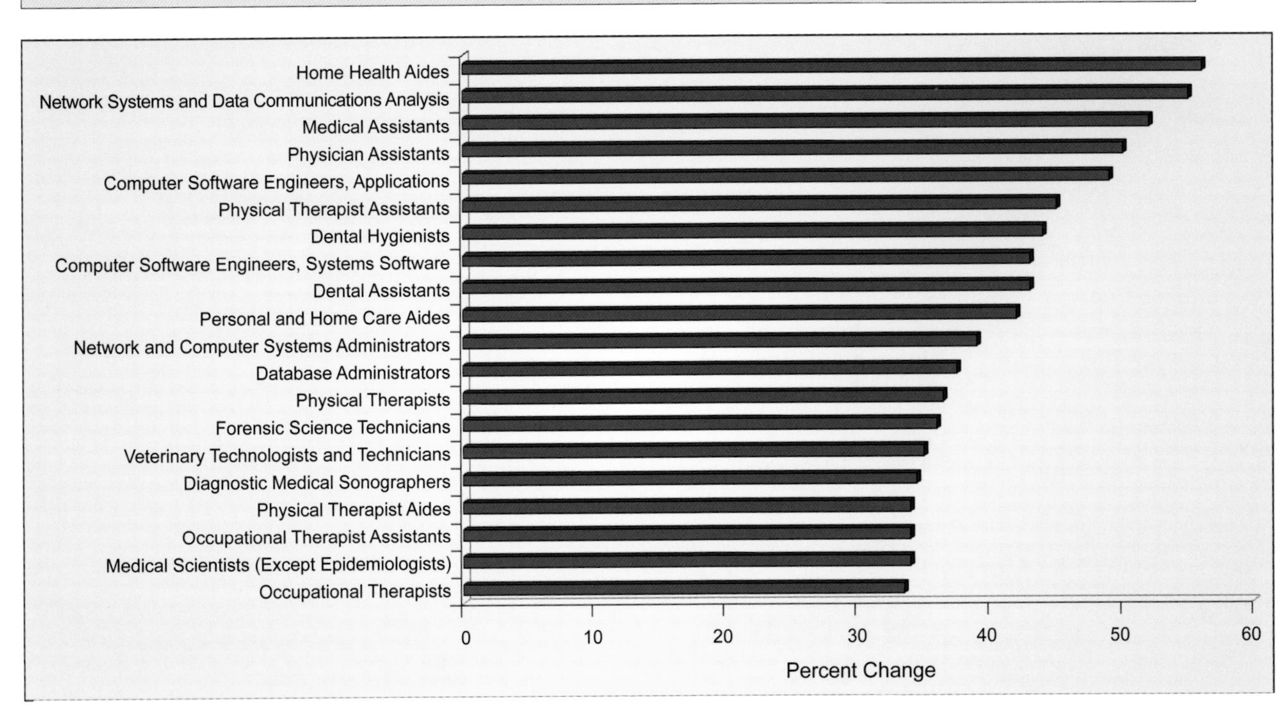

Source: U.S. Department of Labor

experienced professionals with highly specific training.

But this is just one type of development in the health and fitness category. Typically this field involves four principal programs – worksite, commercial, clinical, and community – in varying stages of development or service delivery. For example, at the University of Minnesota, worksite programs entail self-managed and self-directed activity encouraged by employee communications. There are on-site fitness facilities for students, faculty, and staff, but the delivery of fitness programs for employees is at the personal level at each person's worksite.

Worksite Programs

Health care costs are skyrocketing, and companies are reaching out via employee health and fitness programs in an effort to manage the expense. The side benefits of improved health are improved worker productivity and reduced absenteeism.

Worksite programs first appeared in the early 1980s, exploded in the 1990s, and extended to include health education classes, health risk appraisals, and lifestyle change initiatives. In the boom economy of the late 1990s, the quality of worksite programs was a hiring differentiator for some companies – especially in fields where competition for key skills was most intense. Many companies with worksite fitness facilities contract out the staffing and management of the facilities, recognizing that it requires specialized skills and knowledge. Many kinesiology students find themselves employed as these "consultants" in a wide variety of corporations and institutions.

Commercial Programs

Many different types of health and fitness activities can be classified as commercial programs. They all have one thing in common – their objective is to generate a profit for their owners or shareholders. Some are large franchised or corporate-owned chains such as Bally Total Fitness, GoodLife Fitness Clubs, and Gold's Gym. Others are independent, locally owned and managed operations, such as the Southview Athletic Club in St. Paul, Minnesota; gender-specific facilities, such as Curves for women; or focus-specific facilities, such as L.A.

A Career in Personal Training

NAME: Kelby James Klosterman
OCCUPATION: Owner/Director Personal Training Company (TrailRipped™ LLC)
Spa and Fitness Manager at a Private Country Club (Superstition Mountain Golf and Country Club)
BACKGROUND/EDUCATION: BSc Exercise Science, University of North Dakota
Minor: Psychology
MSc Exercise and Wellness, Arizona State University
Emphasis/Thesis: Strength and Conditioning, Testosterone
Certified Strength and Conditioning Specialist (CSCS) (NSCA)
CPR/AED/First Aid

What do you do?

I currently own and direct a seasonal outdoor personal training company called TrailRipped located in Phoenix, Arizona. Along with myself, there are two other trainers who lead resistance training and heart rate-based sessions throughout the valley's trails. As an addition to the trail sessions, TrailRipped also offers year-round sport-specific performance training and in-home personal training. TrailRipped also provides individualized exercise protocols, body fat analysis, nutritional analysis, and monthly newsletters, as well as professional exercise consulting.

I also manage a spa and fitness center at a private country club where I oversee daily operations and budgeting as well as spa services, group fitness, and personal training personnel. I also lead group fitness classes; conduct personal training; and create health/fitness seminars, fitness incentives, and newsletters.

What is unique about your job?

Being the director of TrailRipped is unique because it allows me to be creative in exercise design and with each individual and group on the trail. It is an intense workout that combines resistance, flexibility, and cardiovascular-monitored training unlike any other exercise program. TrailRipped was designed as a way to improve overall health issues such as weight loss, muscular development, aerobic conditioning, and nutritional habits outside of the health club environment. TrailRipped has been shown to be one of the most intense and personally satisfying workouts available anywhere. TrailRipped provides a *real* step on the path to healthy living. It is especially appealing to outdoor enthusiasts because we embrace the outdoors as nature helps us achieve our health and fitness goals. TrailRipped can be tailored to meet any fitness level, from beginner to advanced.

Why did you choose a career in exercise science? What was your motivation for pursuing this field?

I chose a career in exercise science because of my passion for athletics and the opportunity to affect others' levels of health and fitness. Originally I was motivated to pursue a career in sport performance and held strength and conditioning positions with college and professional teams. However, I soon decided to operate TrailRipped as well as pursue a career with the general population in the country club setting because I felt there was less resistance for the rate of promotion. I suppose you could say I was motivated by the opportunity to manage myself and others as well as the opportunity for rapid salary advancement. Because of this choice to manage early, many different options are now available within the health and fitness field.

What do you enjoy most about your profession?

My profession allows for daily interaction with others who are interested in increasing their health and fitness levels and constantly seeking reliable knowledge. The exercise science field is very gratifying in the fact that as a reputable source you can affect others' quality of life while creating mutually rewarding relationships.

What other career options are available to students interested in this area?

Many career options are available to aspiring students in the exercise science field. Viable options include doctor of philosophy (professor/researcher), strength and conditioning, personal training, cardiac rehabilitation, fitness and spa management, sport nutrition, sport psychology, massage therapy, physical therapy, coaching, and many more.

What career advice would you give to students interested in entering this field?

Pursuing a master's degree was the one stepping stone that allowed me the opportunity to begin my career at my desired level. It provided me with the knowledge and respect from others to design and operate TrailRipped. As well, without a master's degree I believe I would be years behind in acquiring the corporate position of where I started. Without any hesitation, I would recommend pursuing a master's degree as a minimum to any entrepreneur in the exercise science field.

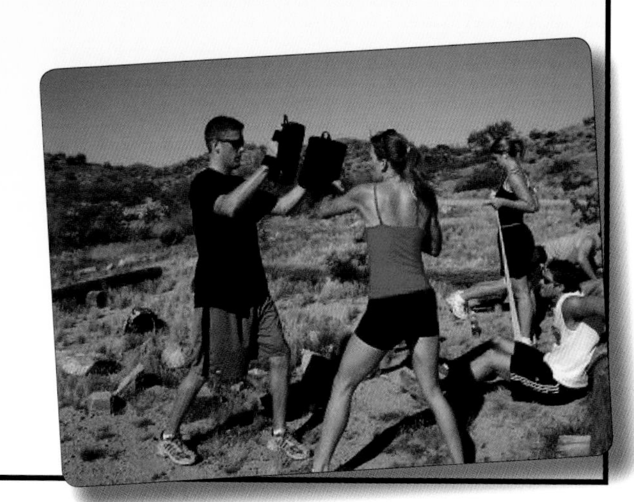

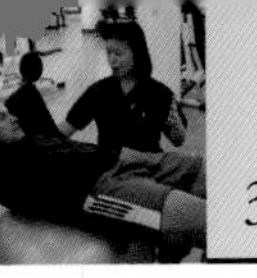

Weight Loss centers. YMCAs sell health club memberships to offset the cost of other programs offered by the nonprofit organization. Should YMCA health and fitness programs be included in the commercial sector? You decide.

Membership sales are the major focus of these facilities, supported by retail sales of clothing and equipment, restaurant and entertainment facilities, special events such as tennis tournaments, fees for consulting and training, and fees for weight-loss programs and accompanying specialized meals. Health and fitness is *big* business in sales-based facilities across North America today.

Some commercial facilities focus more on member retention by meeting the long-term needs of their clients. Market research shows that it costs far more to attract a new member than to retain an existing member, so facilities that follow the retention business model tend to advertise and promote less than sales-based facilities.

Clinical Programs

Hospitals, general medical clinics, and specialized clinics such as physiotherapy facilities represent one of the largest segments – though often hidden – in the health and fitness field. The services offered in clinical programs are often more specific than in commercial programs. Health screenings, health risk identification, cardiac rehabilitation, nutrition and weight management consulting, water exercise therapy, and even childbirth and parenting education are all found in clinical health and fitness programs.

Some clinical programs are leaning toward the commercial model in that they are extending services to local employers to manage worksite programs for a fee. So the overall trend in the field is a blurring of boundaries between types of programs, with many areas of overlap and competition.

Community Programs

The city of Minnetonka, Minnesota, competes head to head with local and national fitness facilities with its city-owned and managed Williston Fitness Center. It also operates the Lindbergh Center, a multisport fitness and training facility shared with an area high school. The Lindbergh Center is a multicourt basketball facility featuring an indoor running track, weight training rooms, exercise facilities, and a swimming pool.

Although community recreation facilities are nothing new, the expensive multidimensional complexes built in recent years as nonprofit municipal facilities are a relatively new phenomenon. For example, Chaska, Minnesota, owns and operates a large recreational water park, and neighboring Hennepin County operates a large outdoor water park open only in the summer months, cross-country running and ski trails, downhill ski parks, and water sport facilities. Every dimension of community programs employs a wide range of skill sets.

Common jobs in all four of these programs include group exercise instructors, often focusing on aerobic programs; fitness instructors focusing on specific strength development; health and fitness counselors who work one on one with clients to help them develop personalized programs and achieve their goals, often involving changes in lifestyle; personal trainers who typically cater to clients in upper-income sectors; and specialists in a variety of settings (e.g., nutritionists, dietitians, physical and occupational therapists) (Table 16.1).

Many people with this type of experience go on to become directors of facilities – which requires training in health and fitness disciplines as well as management training such as accounting, sales management, and organizational development. These individuals require a multidisciplinary educational background and a strong foundation in kinesiology. Often they are called on to conduct market research, identify emerging trends in our society, and help develop plans for new facilities or equipment.

Today's health and fitness professionals, more than ever, need to obtain a broad education across a core scientific, behavioral science, and liberal arts curriculum. Students should strive to achieve a combined degree – perhaps a kinesiology major

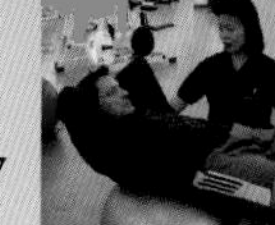

Table 16.1 Job descriptions chart.

Job Title	Evolution	Job Duties	Skills and Competencies
Group Exercise Instructor	This position has transitioned away from exclusively teaching aerobic dance classes. This position now involves teaching a broad range of classes to a diverse population.	Lead group exercise classes for various population groups including seniors, children, pre- and postnatal women, and medically based clients.	Bachelor's degree in kinesiology or another health and fitness related discipline preferred. Certification by a nationally recognized organization required. Additional certifications in a specialized area may also be required in order to teach specific types of classes. Strong teaching skills are a must.
Health/Fitness Counselor	This position has evolved from the more traditional fitness instructor position. The health/fitness counselor provides counseling on a broad range of health topics in addition to conducting fitness assessments and designing exercise programs.	Provide guidance to a diverse population in areas such as behavior change, stress management, smoking cessation, social participation, weight management, and exercise programming.	Bachelor's or graduate-level degree in kinesiology or another health and fitness related discipline required. Certification by a nationally recognized organization required. Additional skills in counseling, behavior change, cultural diversity, and teaching are a must. Marketing and promotional skills are also essential.
Personal Trainer	This position has transitioned from exclusively providing individualized exercise programs to providing individualized services on a broad range of health topics.	Provide ongoing support and guidance to a diverse population of clients on topics such as physical fitness, weight management, stress management, and sport conditioning.	Bachelor's degree in kinesiology or another health and fitness related discipline preferred. Certification by a nationally recognized organization required. Background in exercise programming is a must. Counseling and teaching skills are a must. Business, marketing, sales, and promotion training are also essential.
Specialist Positions	Examples include physical therapists, registered dietitians, clinical exercise specialists, and health educators.	Provide specialized health and fitness services to clients with special needs.	Graduate-level degree required. Additional certifications and licensure may be required in order to practice in specific states or provinces. Other specific experiences and skills are required for each type of specialist position.
Health/Fitness Director	Programming all health and fitness programs that are delivered in a facility. Responsibilities include delivery of programs to address all dimensions of health.	Manage all aspects of a health and fitness department. Responsibilities include departmental leadership, staff management, programming, and all aspects of business administration.	Bachelor's or graduate-level degree in kinesiology or another health and fitness related discipline required. Additional skills in business administration, management, marketing, and promotion are required. Previous experience in an entry-level health and fitness position required.

From S.L. Hoffman and J.C. Harris, Introduction to Kinesiology: Studying Physical Activity, table 14.2, page 472.

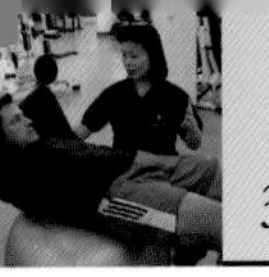

with a business or sociology minor, for example. Some students find it beneficial to have a business major with a kinesiology minor. The choice of curriculum is highly individual, dependent on a student's interests and strengths.

Exercise Therapy

Exercise therapy aims to develop or restore specific physical capabilities – it can be directed at capabilities such as strength or endurance, or at specific muscle groups or neuromuscular coordination of specific portions of the body. Typically, exercise therapy is viewed as either rehabilitative, which involves restoring skills or functions that have been lost, or habilitative, which aims to help an individual acquire skills and functions. In both cases, permanent disabilities or impairments need to be considered as factors in establishing goals for the individual. For example, a paraplegic may have significant upper-body strength but less than needed for daily routines. Habilitative therapy can be used to improve the person's lifestyle.

Exercise therapy can be used effectively to rehabilitate athletic injuries, workplace accidents, injuries caused by repeated physical stress of one part of the body, postsurgical effects, or cardiopulmonary conditions. Most people are familiar with neuromuscular injuries caused by accidents, in which an individual's muscles and nervous system may no longer function properly. Therapeutic exercise is an important part of the treatment process. A long period of immobilization, perhaps while recovering from a severe car accident, can manifest itself in widespread physical problems. Not only may specific limbs degrade in physical capacity, but the entire cardiovascular system may degrade as well. Exercise therapy can help the individual return to his or her previous level of functioning – and even beyond.

Rehabilitation directed at older populations can lead to both physical and emotional improvements. The psychological benefits of exercise (e.g., reducing stress and improving sleep function) cannot be overlooked as part of the rehabilitation portfolio.

Habilitative exercise therapy helps people who have developmental deficiencies or a personal desire to improve some aspect of their capacity. For example, specialized sports training such as power skating camps can be considered habilitative. Similarly, the nation's concern about obesity has led to a plethora of weight-loss and exercise or nutritional enterprises that can all be considered habilitative therapy.

Individuals with physical abnormalities or physical limitations can often benefit from a scientific and systematic habilitative therapy program. Teaching children with disabilities how to use equipment, how to strengthen specific muscle groups, or how to use a prosthetic device all fall under the realm of habilitative therapy.

Professionals practicing both rehabilitative and habilitative exercise therapy can be found in hospitals, outpatient clinics, sports settings, or even private individual practices. Many kinesiology students interested in this aspect of the field go on to obtain specialized training as occupational therapists, as physiotherapists, or as cardiac rehabilitation specialists. These specialized professions have varying accreditation and licensure requirements, usually involving rigorous academic study and intensive field experience. Many of these professions require a master's degree or doctoral-level degree accompanied by professional certification. Details on requirements are available from universities and colleges, state and provincial governments, and national professional associations such as the American Physical Therapy Association or the Canadian Physiotherapy Association. Requirements and standards change frequently, so it is advisable to obtain current information pertaining to your area of interest – much of it is readily available on the Internet.

Teaching and Coaching

Many kinesiology students pursue their passion for sport and exercise by finding rewarding careers as teachers or sports coaches. There is an extremely

A Career in Physical Therapy

NAME: Peter Bzdusek
OCCUPATION: Physical Therapist/Athletic Trainer
EDUCATION: BSc Kinesiology/Exercise Science, University of Wisconsin-Madison
MSc Physical Therapy, University of Wisconsin-Madison

What do you do?

I work as a physical therapist in an orthopedic clinic in Minneapolis, Minnesota. I have worked at this location for the last four months and see patients with orthopedic injuries and/or postoperative conditions (ACL reconstructions, rotator cuff repairs, and so on). There are five other physical therapists at the clinic, as well as a hand clinic with four occupational therapists.

What is unique about your job?

Every patient is unique. Patients are seen from a variety of races and socioeconomic backgrounds (Somalian, Russian, Hmong, Korean, American, Mexican). Also, because we work closely with university physicians, we see the most current surgical procedures that are supported by research, and I see surgical revisions (surgeries that have failed elsewhere).

Why did you choose a career in physical therapy? What was your motivation for pursuing this field?

During my sophomore year in college, I realized I wanted a career in health care. My background in athletic training drove me toward that field. During my senior year I decided I wanted an advanced degree and a broader area of study, which led me to physical therapy. I toyed with the idea of medical school but did not want to commit that much additional time to school. I am very pleased with my decision.

As for my motivation, during one of my athletic training affiliations, I worked closely with a physical therapist and learned a great deal from this person. The field also gives me the opportunity to work with non-sport-related conditions or pathologies (e.g., CVAs, Parkinson's disease).

How did studies in kinesiology benefit your career choice?

Kinesiology gave me the backbone on which to build my career. The studies provided me with the knowledge to pursue and succeed in my career choices.

How competitive is the field?

Physical therapy is a growing and evolving field. Currently the physical therapy market is favorable for the employee. The market is not saturated. There is competition depending on the setting one desires. For example, it is very easy to find a position in a nursing home or home health care setting.

What are the future job prospects in the field?

The future shows more private practices evolving, as well as PTs in the emergency department. The vision of the profession is for all therapists to have a doctorate degree by 2020. Most programs currently are doctorate programs, and many are providing classes for practicing therapists to complete the necessary coursework to obtain a doctorate. Direct access is another hot topic. This involves seeing patients directly, prior to a physician visit. For example, a patient suffers an ankle sprain and instead of seeing the doctor and being referred to a PT, the patient sees the PT first. Screening is critical here, and the importance of the doctorate in providing the necessary education is key. A PT must be able to know when to treat, when to treat and refer to an MD, or when to simply refer to the MD.

What do you enjoy most about your profession?

I love the daily interaction with individuals. It is rewarding to guide patients through therapy and see them return to the activities they enjoy and were unable to perform. People are interesting, and I learn a great deal from my patients. Mechanics have given me tips on car maintenance. Fishermen have revealed their secret spots. But I'm still waiting for someone I'm treating to predict the winning lottery numbers!

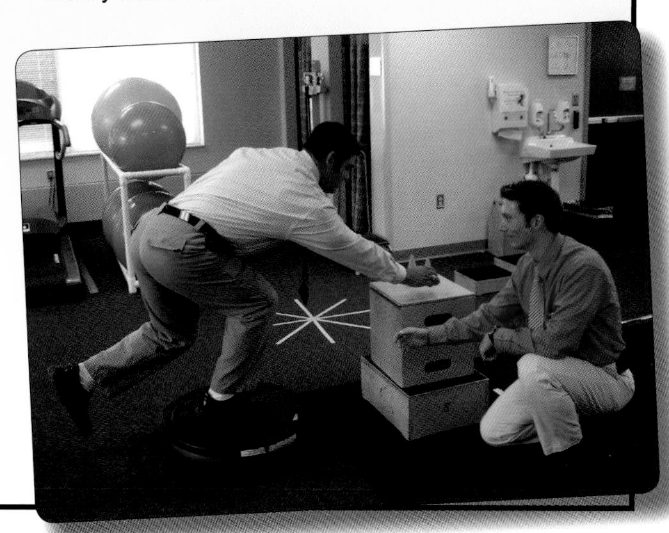

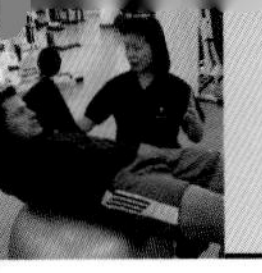

wide diversity of roles and settings involving **teaching and coaching** – from preschool play time to intercollegiate sports, and from local sandlot games to professional sports. Coaches and teachers find roles in nonprofit organizations and corporations, often leading to management responsibilities.

The roles of teachers and coaches are so closely intertwined that they often cannot be easily differentiated. Both professions are concerned with developing and maintaining fitness and motor skill performance in various settings. One possible difference is that teachers often deal with base audiences – those with no natural selection process involved. Consequently, a wide range of capabilities and interest levels is evident in any given group. Coaches, on the other hand, often deal with a highly selective audience, one in which skill levels are more developed and where the individuals have a high degree of interest and aspiration. Which would you rather be?

Although the actions and methods of teaching and coaching are very similar, some aspects of teaching and coaching are quite different – different workdays, different audiences, and different accreditation requirements. Each professional group has its own subcultural attributes, with some members actively involved in both roles.

Many people find themselves coaching at the community level. Tee-ball, mites soccer, and tennis leagues exist for very young participants, and all require large numbers of people to coordinate, manage, and coach activities. Similarly, sport-specific clubs exist in almost every activity, all requiring coaches for various levels. National sport governing bodies have long recognized that the diversity of coaching capabilities within their sports is a serious problem, so most have developed coaching training and certification programs to help ensure adequate coaching standards – with the side benefit of making the sport more enjoyable for participants and leading to the growth of the sport. Time after time, sport after sport across the country, we can see that participation thrives when coaching excels. Coaches are the catalyst for growth in virtually every sport.

Teacher-coaches can be found in K–12 settings, both private and public, and in junior colleges and some universities. And all these settings also provide opportunities for people to teach various aspects of exercise science without any formal coaching responsibility. So when it comes to career selection in the teaching/coaching field, there are many different possibilities and combinations. Finding the right one for yourself is usually a matter of personal preference – there is no "right" or "wrong" role or function; they are simply different. Some settings combine teaching with coaching, others separate the two functions. Some revolve around elite athletes, some specialize in specific sports, and others place emphasis on adapted sports to ensure opportunity for all to participate in physical activity and competitive sport.

When asked the philosophy of the school district relative to sport – is it to provide activity and develop skills, or is it to develop elite athletes? – most school districts do not have a ready answer. It's not a topic that has been addressed frequently in the past, but as budget constraints continue and cocurricular programs dwindle, it's a question that will probably be raised more frequently because it will be ever more difficult to fund both areas. It's similar to the debate about eliminating men's athletic programs to make room for new women's programs. There is no easy answer.

Sport Management

There are a myriad of potential careers in **sport management** – in athlete representation (professional agents); in event management (think of what it takes to plan the Super Bowl each year); and in sporting goods, promotional materials, and clothing. Sport is big business, and every aspect of that business requires people with management skills.

Sport represents one of the largest segments of the North American economy. And with a background in physical activity, supplemented with strong communication skills, kinesiology

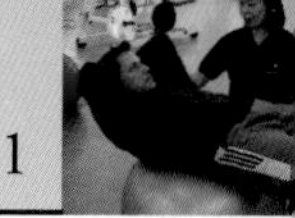

A Career in Coaching

NAME: Mark Temple
OCCUPATION: Director of Swimming and Head Coach, Mississauga Aquatic Club; Canadian and Olympic Coach
EDUCATION: BPHE, University of Toronto
MBA, MSBA, University of Southern California

What does the coach of a community-based swimming club do?

My role function has three key aspects. First, I use my leadership skills and knowledge experience to articulate and implement the vision and mission of the swimming club on behalf of a volunteer board of directors and the general membership. Second, within the business operations I must recruit and develop a skilled coaching staff for all competitive levels of community swimmers. Third, I design the training programs that, over time, will allow the community's competitive swimmers to develop as student athletes to a world top-50 level. For the most successful student athletes, I coach them to the world championships and Olympic Games.

What skills are required to be a professional coach?

First and foremost you must have a passion and enthusiasm for pursuing goals. The pursuit of excellence is in the process. The coach's primary task is to develop favorable situations so the athletes experience success in graded levels of stress. You must demonstrate a successful combination of leadership style and knowledge of human motivations. The successful coach is a great communicator and possesses extensive knowledge of skill acquisition, sport science, and program design.

How did your studies in physical and health education benefit your career?

I was already coaching when I entered the BPHE program at the University of Toronto. From my previous engineering studies and continued coaching, I developed a fascination for human physiology and performance so I enrolled in every physiology course I could, read every medical school text book, and delved into the psychology of the impossible. I did a master's level study in leadership theory in one of my electives. This eclectic education prepared me to ask good questions and be mentored by some of the world's finest coaches and sport scientists. I now prepare training programs for Olympic hopefuls. If you have the will to succeed, then continual learning and advanced education can greatly benefit your career.

What do you enjoy most about your profession?

I enjoy watching student athletes strive to master difficult skills and fitness challenges in their pursuit of being the best they can be in a highly competitive environment. Their individual performances are an inspiration to everyone about dreaming the goal and mastering the psychology of the impossible.

What career advice would you give to students interested in amateur club coaching?

Mentoring is key. Learn from the most successful leaders within your area. Visit them. Interview them. Coaching swimming and being a teacher is a terrific combination of professional balance until your success allows you to take on a full-time position as a coach. Being a teacher would refine your teaching skills by working with the appropriate age groups involved in club sports.

What advice would you give to students entering this field?

Coaching is about a portfolio of lifelong success. Your product is the student-athlete. In many respects the profession is akin to farming. One cannot cram for a successful harvest. There is a time to plant, to measure and nurture, and then, only then, the harvest. Then, each year, you begin the process again – one eye on the horizon and one eye on the next step.

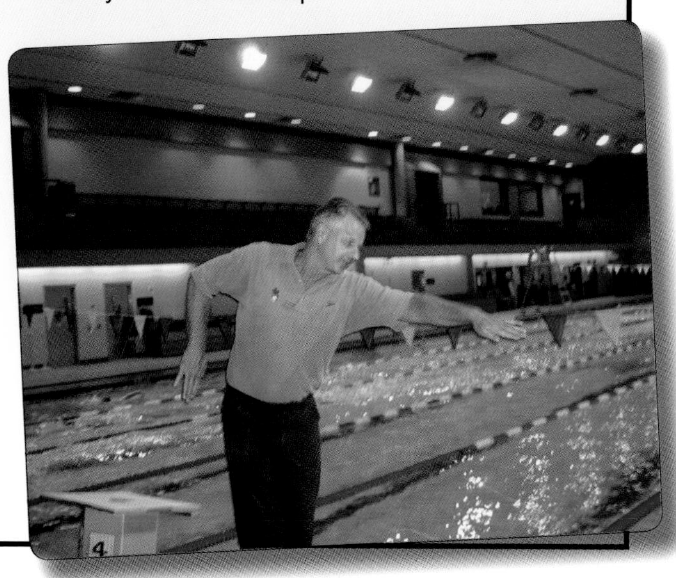

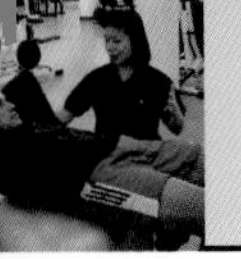

graduates often make ideal managers – especially if they round out their education with supporting courses in finance, human resource management, or marketing.

Sport management roles can be found at all levels of the sport industry – professional, local amateur, for-profit companies, and nonprofit organizations. At the same time, sport management is part of the entertainment industry, and many people who start careers in sport management find themselves transitioning into other aspects of the entertainment industry, such as music, television, and even Hollywood.

And while mainstream sport management careers are abundant, there are also many supporting careers and part-time positions as well. These supporting functions, called sport services, may include insurance company representatives specializing in sport coverage, talent scouts who work within major-league "farm" organizations, writers for various publications that deal with the subject of sport management, and promoters of licensed products. The list of career possibilities in sport management is almost limitless.

Some kinesiology students who aspire to work in a highly specialized segment of sport management often find it advantageous to obtain an advanced degree – perhaps an MBA, law degree, or master's degree in industrial relations. Some sports managers focus on the issue of risk management (i.e., risks to players, spectators, and organizers, all of which carry the potential for significant litigation when calamity strikes). The well-prepared sport management candidate develops knowledge in the area of risk management. The range of topics goes from understanding potential physical injuries and financial losses to the risks posed by not complying with rules of governing bodies or regulatory agencies.

Not everyone wants to focus his or her career on things that can potentially go wrong; many want to focus efforts on things that can go right, such as marketing programs to make sport organizations more successful. Some people think sports marketing is almost as much fun as participating in the sport being promoted! Part of the reason is that the potential specialties in sports marketing range from public relations and advertising to on-air or in-stadium public address announcing; research on sports fans' attitudes; and creating, producing, and promoting sports memorabilia.

Other Careers

Many students are puzzled about where or how to start their career investigation. One good idea is to identify and establish a relationship with someone already working in the field. Ask to "job shadow" that person for a day. Most professionals will be honored by a student's request. There is no better way to determine if you will like a career than to observe the work firsthand and possibly participate in it. Many organizations offer both paid and unpaid internships so that students can learn about the job function and make informed career decisions for themselves.

When asked what skill sets or capabilities they want in employees, most CEOs respond that they want people who can communicate effectively, both verbally and in writing. That has been true for many years, and the rush into the Internet age has only intensified the need for strong communication capabilities. Kinesiology students typically have strong interpersonal and verbal communication skills developed through the nature of the research and curriculum they undertake. As a result, many find careers that have these capabilities as prerequisites (e.g., sales and customer service). Kinesiology students typically are found in the sales forces of pharmaceutical and medical equipment manufacturers such as Pfizer and Stryker.

Others use their knowledge and experience in strength training to enter fields where personal strength and endurance are assets – firefighting and police work, nursing, and a variety of skilled positions in construction. And of course, advanced education offers kinesiology graduates opportunities in other fields – both related and unrelated.

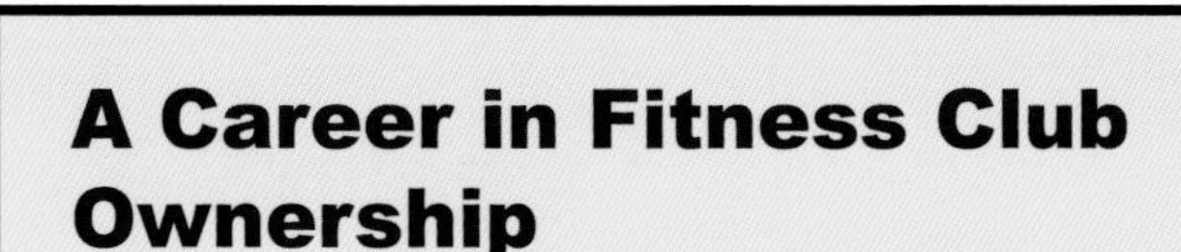

A Career in Fitness Club Ownership

NAME: David Patchell-Evans
OCCUPATION: Founder and CEO, GoodLife Fitness Clubs
EDUCATION: BA, Honors (Physical Education), University of Western Ontario

What do you do?

I am the founder and CEO of the largest group of fitness clubs in the world owned by a single individual. By December 2007, GoodLife Fitness will have over 150 clubs stretching across Canada from Newfoundland to British Columbia and servicing in excess of 400,000 members. My job is to lead our strategic planning team with a clear vision that demonstrates caring for our members and staff with a simple goal of making all Canadians fit and healthy.

What is unique about your job?

Fitness club ownership has almost unlimited growth opportunity globally. The world's population for the most part is informed about the need to exercise and the health benefits of doing so, yet only an estimated 9 to 13 percent of people belong to a fitness facility. In Canada, that figure is 15 percent of the population. That means there is a huge population of unfit people who would benefit from a fitness membership. The other side, I would caution though, is that this is also a highly competitive and risky field. To survive and grow a thriving business, you must have a smart plan, know your ROI [return on investment] margins, and deftly adapt your business to any shifts in the market.

Why did you choose a career in fitness club ownership?

While attending university, I had a very serious motorcycle accident at age 19 that put me in rehabilitation for six months at a sports injury clinic on campus. I had come to university to do a business degree, but this time spent working out alongside athletes created a new-found interest for me in exercise physiology and biomechanics. This experience not only crystallized my interests in a physical education degree but also focused my motivation as to what I wanted to do with my life. I wanted to change lives by helping people lead their best lives through fitness.

What are the future job prospects in the field? Where is it heading?

The profession is growing by leaps and bounds! Prospects for a career in fitness have never been brighter, and this trend will continue to outperform many other careers for decades to come. From 2000 to 2004, the fitness industry in Canada experienced a 27 percent growth. GoodLife Fitness offers a range of exciting, dynamic, and challenging careers. As a company, we believe in promotions from within and rewarding top performers with rapid advancement and management/leadership opportunities as we increase our number of clubs across Canada to 200 by 2009.

A career as a manager at a club could include a defined career path as a fitness manager, personal training regional manager, general manager, cluster manager, or divisional manager. Our management trainee program provides employees with training in fitness, leadership, business, sales, and service in order to successfully run their own multi-million-dollar world-class businesses.

What other career options are available?

There are four primary types of health and fitness clubs: commercial clubs (e.g., GoodLife), nonprofits (e.g., community centers), miscellaneous clubs (e.g., corporate clubs), and other types of clubs (including those attached to hospitals and universities).

In addition there will be jobs in related areas of teaching, group exercise instructors, sports attorneys, government (including research and writing), lifestyle coaching, sports trainers, consulting, corporate wellness, and sports medicine to name a few. Large companies will have an infrastructure of positions including marketing, public relations, operations, and human resources.

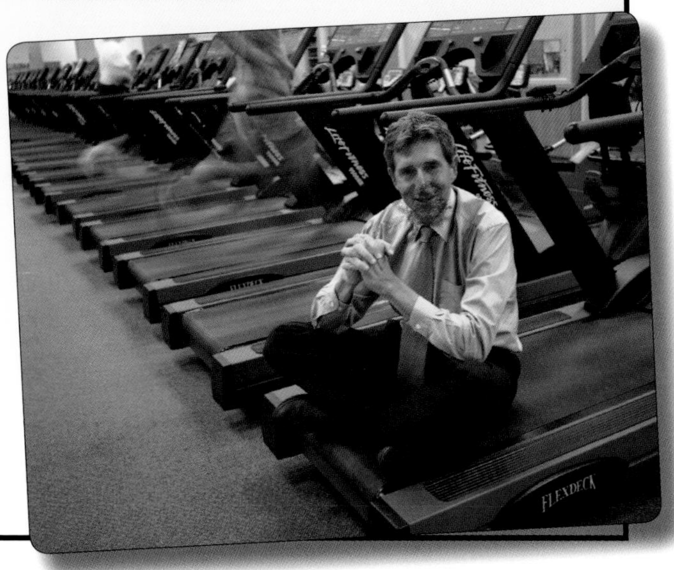

Figure 16.3 An overview of occupations in kinesiology and the related educational requirements.

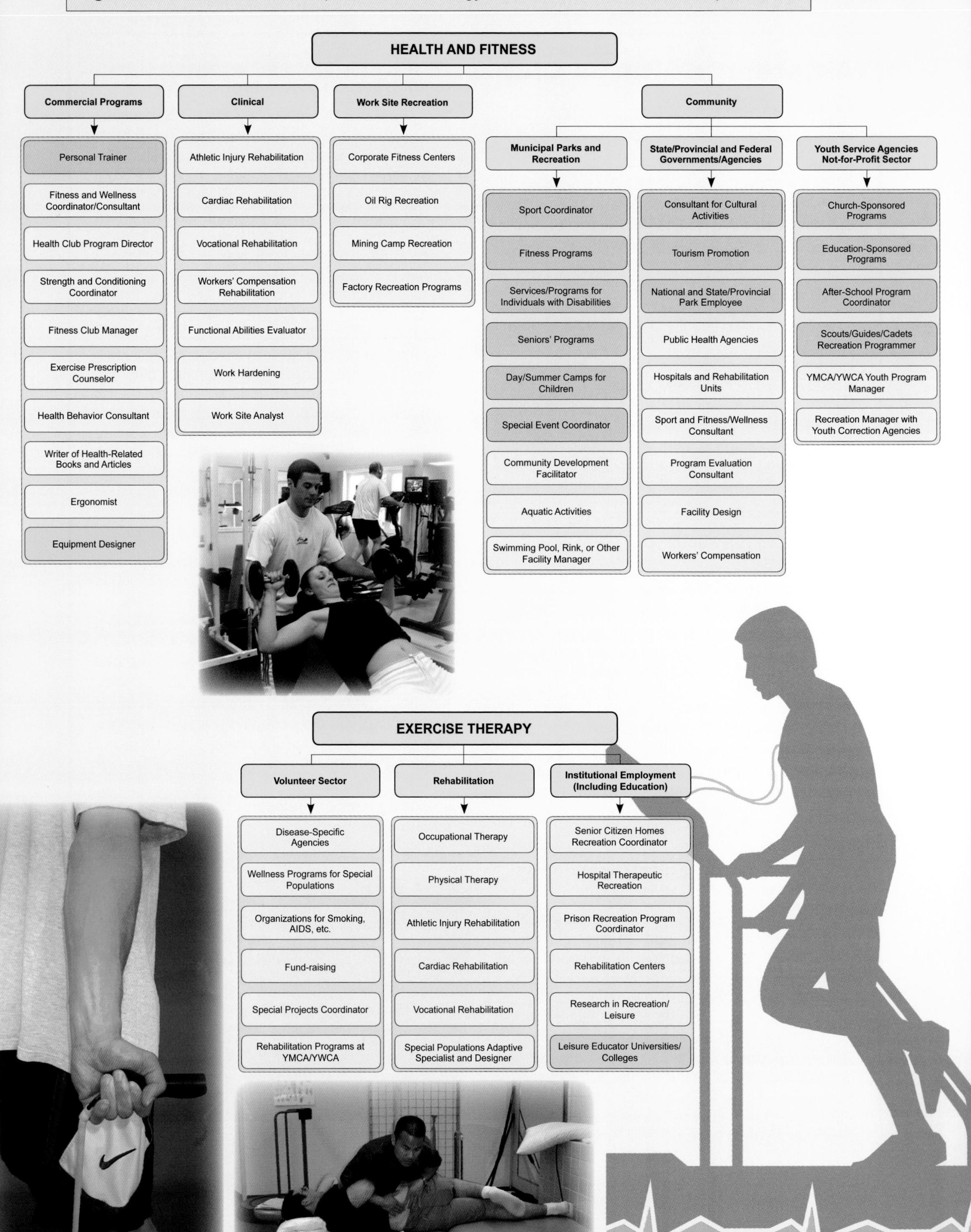

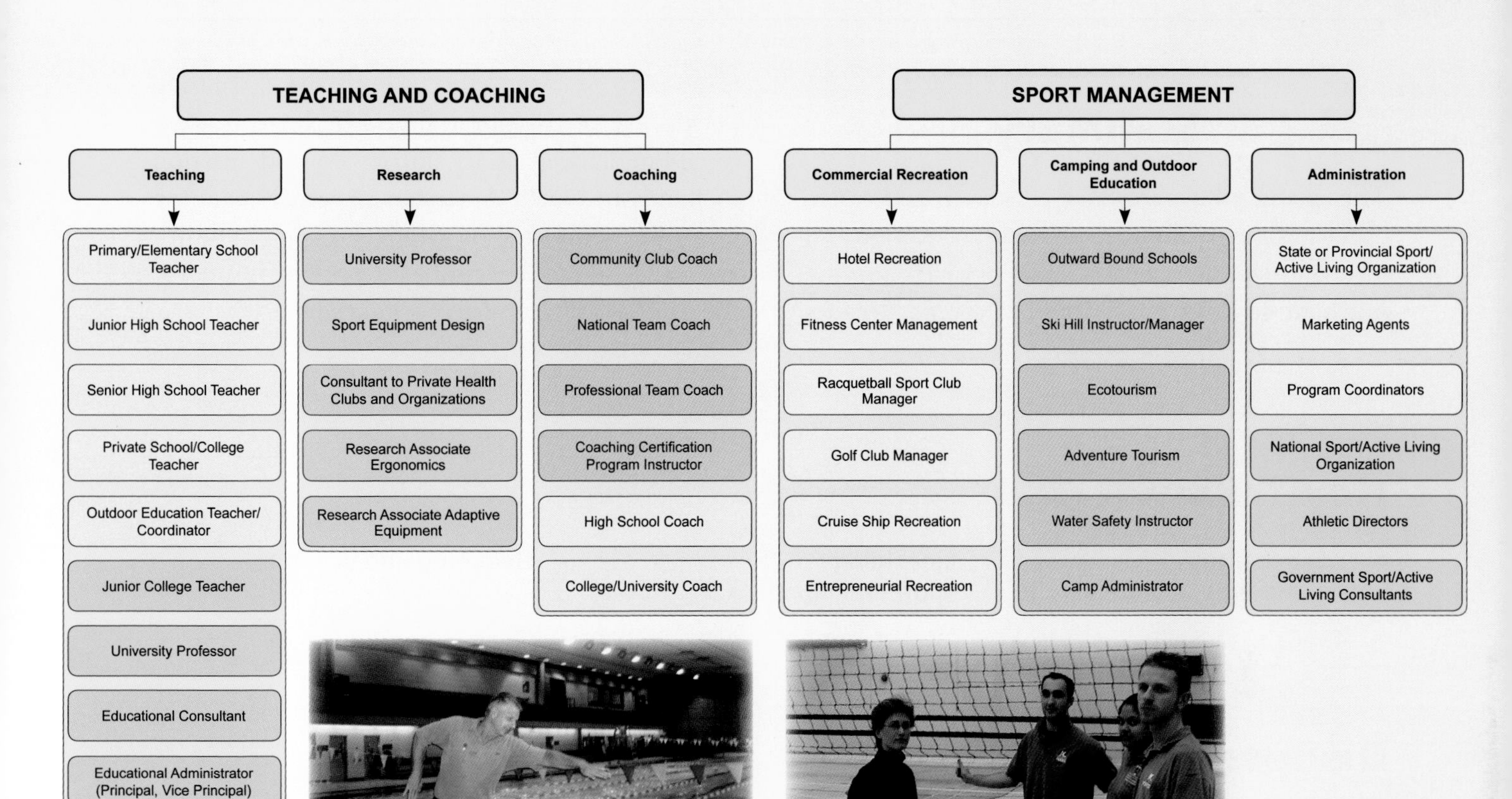

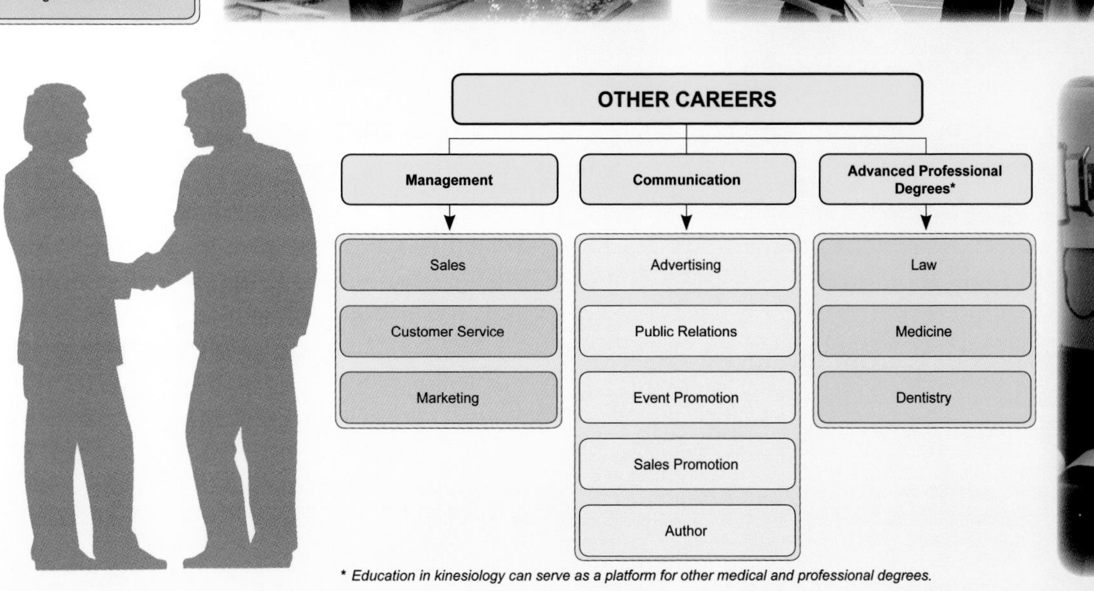

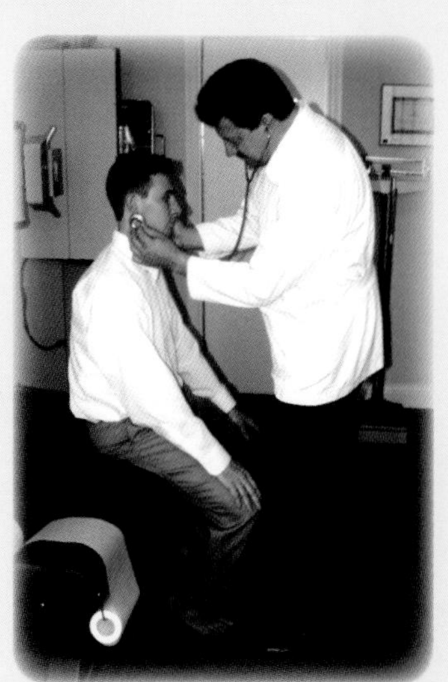

* *Education in kinesiology can serve as a platform for other medical and professional degrees.*

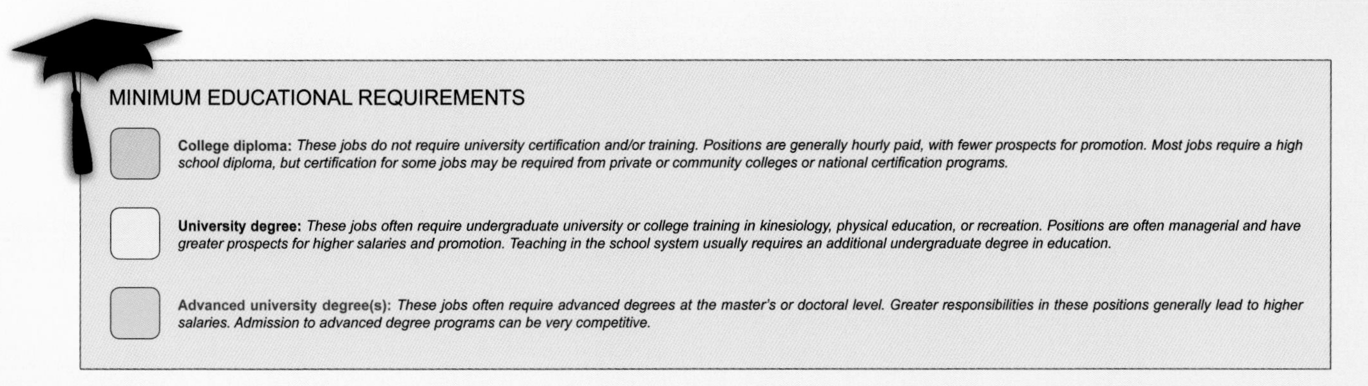

MINIMUM EDUCATIONAL REQUIREMENTS

College diploma: *These jobs do not require university certification and/or training. Positions are generally hourly paid, with fewer prospects for promotion. Most jobs require a high school diploma, but certification for some jobs may be required from private or community colleges or national certification programs.*

University degree: *These jobs often require undergraduate university or college training in kinesiology, physical education, or recreation. Positions are often managerial and have greater prospects for higher salaries and promotion. Teaching in the school system usually requires an additional undergraduate degree in education.*

Advanced university degree(s): *These jobs often require advanced degrees at the master's or doctoral level. Greater responsibilities in these positions generally lead to higher salaries. Admission to advanced degree programs can be very competitive.*

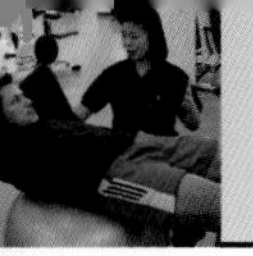

Summary

This chapter illustrates how education and career opportunities in physical and health education and related disciplines such as kinesiology have become much more diverse over the last several decades (Figure 16.3). This reflects both the expanding perspective of the physical and health education discipline as well as its impact on and reaction to trends in North American society. Expanding career opportunities for students trained in health and fitness disciplines indicate a bright future for the field and those pursuing its study.

Key Terms

exercise therapy
health and fitness industry
kinesiology
sport management
teaching and coaching

Discussion Questions

1. How has the field of physical education changed in recent years? What brought about these changes?
2. Which physical and health education career areas appear to be growing at present?
3. Identify and briefly describe the four program areas of the health and fitness industry.
4. What are the two kinds of exercise therapy? Give examples of each.
5. Name one area in which teaching and coaching are similar and one area in which they are different.
6. Why are business skills important for some careers in sport management?
7. How do the diverse employment prospects for kinesiology graduates reflect trends in North American society?

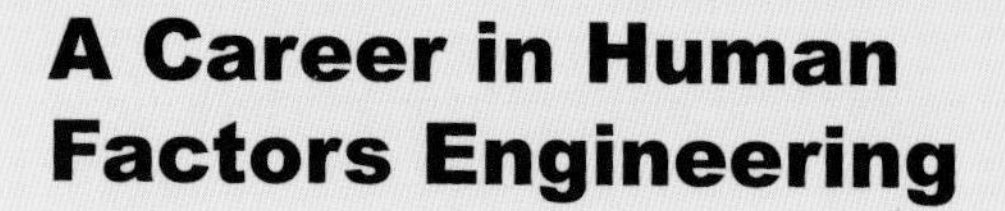

A Career in Human Factors Engineering

NAME: Paul Cassidy
OCCUPATION: Human Factors Engineer
EDUCATION: BA Psychology, University of Connecticut
MA and PhD Kinesiology, University of Minnesota

What do you do?

I am a human factors engineer. I work at Exponent Failure Analysis Associates, Inc. in Natick, Massachusetts, as a managing scientist. I was previously employed at the 3M Company in St. Paul, Minnesota, as a human factors specialist. At Exponent, I provide expert consulting services to clients in two general areas: product development and litigation support. I currently help clients design consumer products and medical devices, as well as help attorneys address human factors issues pertaining to matters of personal injury and vehicle accidents. At 3M, I also had two different job roles. As a member of the 3M Software, Electronics, and Mechanical Systems Technology Center, I worked with multidisciplinary engineering and design teams to develop dozens of different consumer, industrial, and medical products and systems. I also founded and ran the 3M Human Performance Research Lab, where I led several research efforts investigating the safety and performance enhancement effects of various 3M products (e.g., respirators, retro-reflective safety garment materials, anti-fatigue mats) on human performance and behavior.

What is unique about your job?

At both Exponent and 3M, there are very few human factors engineers (but far more than at most companies). Therefore, in one way, the uniqueness of my job is that I provide human factors expertise! Another unique aspect of my work at Exponent is that I get to apply visual perception, motor coordination, cognitive psychology, and biomechanics principles toward designing and developing medical devices and forensic investigations of matters such as jet ski collisions and slips and falls down stairwells. At 3M, as the first kinesiologist in its more than 100 years of existence, I was able to provide empirical evidence of product safety and performance benefits to product developers and marketers; such efforts had either never been at 3M or had always been outsourced.

Why did you choose a career in human factors engineering? What was your motivation for pursuing this field?

I chose the field of human factors engineering after being inspired during my graduate studies at the University of Minnesota, where I worked as a research assistant at the Human Factors Research Laboratory. My mentors, Drs. Michael Wade, Peter Hancock, Allen Burton, and Thomas Smith, all fostered in me an appreciation and passion for understanding how to optimize the relationship between people and machines, particularly by applying principles of ecological psychology and dynamic systems theory in the context of motor coordination. After completion of my graduate studies, I found employment at 3M, where I was able to apply my human factors skills toward developing advanced technology products and systems.

How did studies in kinesiology benefit your career choice?

As a human factors engineer trained in kinesiology, I have always been able to provide unique, complementary insights and services to clients regarding physical aspects of product design or litigation matters. Because the majority of human factors engineers are trained in psychology, they traditionally address cognitive, perceptual, and social or organizational factors that affect human performance, but they often do not have expertise in traditional ergonomic areas. I can offer expertise on physical, or ergonomic, factors while also addressing many of the other areas (my undergraduate studies were in psychology).

How competitive is the field?

There are many different career options, but very few jobs are available annually. The field of human factors engineering is small compared with other engineering disciplines such as mechanical engineering, but awareness of our field is continuing to grow along with demand, fortunately. Most positions require a PhD in psychology, industrial engineering, biomedical engineering, kinesiology, or another related discipline. I would recommend that a kinesiology student interested in human factors become a student member of the Human Factors and Ergonomics Society (www.hfes.org) and take full advantage of the many services offered to student members. Also, discuss with other students, professors, and professionals in the industry how your unique skills in kinesiology can give you a strong self-marketing advantage during your job search.

What career advice would you give to students interested in entering this field?

During your undergraduate or graduate studies in kinesiology, focus heavily on the areas of biomechanics and motor learning and control. So much human factors engineering work pertains to issues of human physical interaction with systems, objects, and products, and the overwhelming majority of human factors engineers are trained in cognitive, perceptual, and experimental psychology. As a human factors engineer with kinesiology training, you will be able to provide an extremely valuable complementary perspective toward the design and testing of products or offer unique expert forensic opinions as to how accidents occurred or products failed. Bear in mind, though, that depending on the size of the human factors group and the number of other kinesiologists you work with at a company, you may be expected to also know almost *anything* about exercise physiology. This can be daunting – but stimulating, challenging, and rewarding at the same time. Furthermore, if you pursue your graduate degree in motor learning and control, regardless of your persuasion toward direct or indirect perception issues, learn as much as you can about both theories. If you are a kinesiology student, this will mean pursuing elective courses in related disciplines such as cognitive psychology, perceptual psychology, neuroscience, and child development.

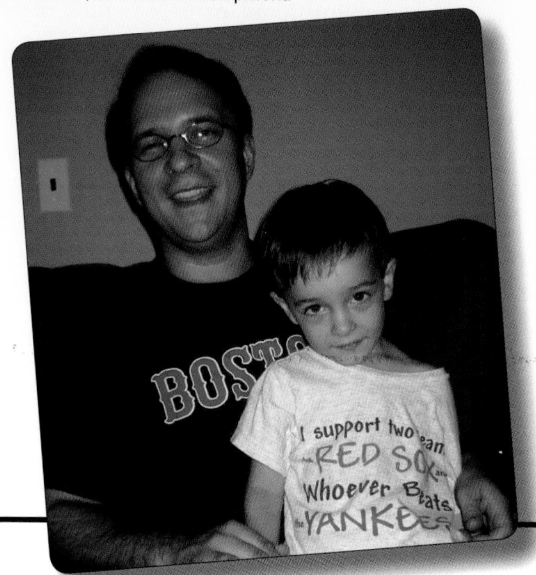

Glossary

A

abduction: Movement away from the midline of the body.
absolute refractory period: A period (about a millisecond) in which a second action potential is not possible.
absolute strength: A measure of strength independent of a person's body mass.
absolute $\dot{V}O_2max$: An aerobic power measurement that is related to mass, especially muscle mass, and is expressed in liters per minute (L/min).
absorption: Movement of molecules, produced by digestion, across a layer of epithelial cells lining the gastrointestinal wall into the blood or lymph, where the circulatory system distributes them to body cells.
acceleration: The rate of change of velocity.
acceptable macronutrient distribution range (AMDR): Range for acceptable daily energy intake for nutrients.
achievement: How an individual has fared at a particular task, determined through a measurement or evaluation process.
actin: The thin myofilament that makes up the sarcomere.
action potential: An electrical impulse generated by the sinus node.
action–reaction principle: See Newton's third law.
active flexibility: The range of movement generated by individual effort.
activity cross training: Type of training that involves participating in several different physical activities to provide variety.
acute mountain sickness: A variety of symptoms caused by the body's inability to adapt to a sudden or large change in altitude.
adduction: Movement toward the midline of the body.
adenosine diphosphate: By-product of the chemical reaction during which the chemical bond between ATP and its phosphate subgroup is broken.
adenosine triphosphate: Provides the energy for all biochemical processes of the body (i.e., it is the energy currency of the body).
aerobic cross training: Type of training that involves performing different aerobic activities to provide variety.
aerobic metabolism: Energy or ATP production in the presence of oxygen.
aerobic power: The maximal rate at which the body can take up, transport, and utilize oxygen; expressed as maximal oxygen uptake, or $\dot{V}O_2max$.
aerodynamics: The study of objects moving relative to a fluid, such as air.
afferent neurons: Neurons that carry signals to the brain or spinal cord.
agility: The physical ability that enables rapid and precise change of body position and direction.
agonist: The muscle or group of muscles producing a desired effect.
agonist–antagonist training: Approach to strength training that includes exercises for a joint's agonist and antagonist muscles, achieving balanced development of strength.
air (wind) resistance: A force that air exerts on objects moving through it.
all-around athlete: Individuals who perform well in several sports; these athletes differ from average individuals in the number of abilities in which they are superior.
all-or-none law: A synaptic transmission will cause an action potential in the postsynaptic cell as long as its strength is above a minimum threshold level.
all-or-none principle: An impulse of a certain magnitude is required to cause the innervated fiber to contract.
altitude: Above sea level.
alveoli: Tiny air sacs that make up and are the functional units of the lungs.
amenorrhea: Occurrence of irregular or absent menstrual periods for at least three months; one of the three conditions of the FAT.
amino acid: The building block of proteins.
amylase: Digestive enzyme found in saliva that begins the digestion of carbohydrates.
anaerobic alactic system: One of two divisions of anaerobic energy systems; it does not result in the production of lactic acid (i.e., the high energy phosphate system).
anaerobic glycolysis: A stepwise breakdown of glucose or glycogen without the presence of oxygen into pyruvic acid and ATP.
anaerobic lactic system: One of two divisions of anaerobic energy systems; it results in the production of lactic acid (i.e., the lactic acid system).
anaerobic metabolism: Energy or ATP production in the absence of oxygen.
anaerobic threshold: The exercise intensity at which lactic acid begins to accumulate within the blood,

associated with the feeling of discomfort and a burning sensation in the muscles.
anatomical position: The position of the human body that is used as a point of reference in anatomy.
angle of attack: The tilt of an object relative to the flow velocity.
angular acceleration: The measure of change in angular velocity per unit of time.
angular displacement: The direction and smallest angular change between a rotating body's initial and final position.
angular kinetics: Study concerned with the generation of rotation about an axis of rotation and the control of these rotations.
angular motion: The type of motion where a body moves in a circular path in the same direction (e.g., giant swing on a high bar).
angular velocity: The measure of angular displacement per unit of time, or how fast a body is rotating.
anorexia nervosa: Condition where individuals fail to eat an adequate amount of food to maintain a reasonable body weight; characterized by severe calorie restriction and starvation.
antagonist: A muscle or group of muscles opposing the action.
anterior: Nearer to the front (e.g., your lips are anterior to your teeth).
anterior cruciate ligament (ACL) tear: Complete rupture of the weaker knee-stabilizing ligament.
antioxidant: A substance, formed from vitamins, that aids in preserving healthy body cells and reacts with free radicals to make them harmless.
apoptosis: Preprogrammed muscle cell loss that occurs with aging.
appendicular skeleton: The section of the human skeleton made up of the pectoral and pelvic girdles and the upper and lower limbs that are appended from the girdles.
arterial–venous oxygen (a–v O_2) difference: The difference in the amount of oxygen that is present in the blood as it leaves the lungs and the amount of oxygen that is present in the blood when it returns to the lungs.
arteriole: Smaller branch of an artery.
artery: Type of cardiovascular vessel that carries blood away from the heart.
ATP resynthesis: The metabolic process that results in the recombination of ADP and P_i to form ATP.
auxotonic contraction: A dynamic contraction in which muscle changes tension.
axial skeleton: The section of the human skeleton composed of the skull, vertebrae, ribs, and sternum.
axis of rotation: An imaginary line either through a joint or the total body about which rotational motion occurs.
axon: Exists as a single extension from the cell body and functions to transmit and carry messages to its terminal endings.

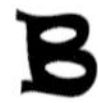

B

balance: The process whereby the body's state of equilibrium is controlled for a given purpose.
ball and socket joint: Type of joint where a rounded bone is fitted into a cuplike receptacle, allowing rotation in all three planes of movement (e.g., joint at the shoulder and the hip).
ballistic stretching: See dynamic stretching.
basal metabolic rate (BMR): The minimum amount of energy the body requires to carry out all vital functions.
bending: Lengthening of a tissue on one side and shortening on the other side caused by a simultaneous tension and compression presented at the respective tissue sides.
Bernoulli's principle: A mathematical relationship expressing an object's motion resulting from a lift force.
bile: A digestive substance secreted by the liver that contains cholesterol, bicarbonate ions, and bile salts and is responsible for digestion and absorption of dietary fats and neutralization of hydrochloric acid in the small intestine.
bile salts: Constituents of bile essential for the digestion and absorption of dietary fats, as they solubilize water-insoluble fats (i.e., convert large fat globules into smaller droplets).
binge eating disorder (BED): Involves ingesting large amounts of food without the purging behavior characteristic of bulimia nervosa.
bioelectrical impedance analysis (BIA): Method of measuring body fat based on differences in electrical conductivity between fat-free mass and mass.
biological adaptation: During strength training, it is the body's adaptation that leads to muscular performance improvements as reflected by the body's increased strength.
biomechanics: The application of mechanics to biology in order to understand the physics underlying various forms of movement.
Bod-Pod: A very expensive but accurate method of measuring body composition that may facilitate measuring very heavy or large individuals.

body composition: The amount of body constituents, such as fat, muscle, bone, and other organs.
body mass index (BMI): An easy alternative for assessing healthy body weight using an individual's weight and height measurements. BMI = weight (kg) / height $(m)^2$; can also be calculated using a nomogram.
Bohr effect: The promotion of oxygen extraction that results from increased body temperature.
boundary layer: A thin layer of air or water molecules surrounding an object moving through fluid. The boundary layer reduces drag.
breath sound check: Monitoring of your volume of breathing in order to establish ventilatory threshold exercise intensity.
bronchiole: The second branch of the trachea.
bronchus: The first branch of the trachea.
bulimia nervosa: Characterized by continual episodes of binge eating followed by purging.
bursitis: Inflammation, weakening, and degeneration of the bursae resulting from overuse and stress.

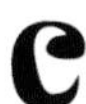

capillary: The smallest cardiovascular vessels, composed of only endothelial cells, which are about the width of one red cell; allow for gas and nutrient exchange.
carbohydrate: One of the essential nutrients and a primary source of energy in the diet.
carbohydrate loading: The nutritional practice of increasing muscle stores before endurance-type competition.
carbon fiber: A strong, lightweight material made of strands of carbon and held together by a resin.
cardiac muscle: The muscle of the heart that has characteristics of both smooth and skeletal muscle and is under involuntary control.
cardiac output: The amount of blood that is pumped into the aorta each minute by the heart (measured in L/min).
cardiorespiratory endurance: The ability to produce energy through an improved delivery of oxygen to the working muscles.
cardiovascular endurance: See cardiorespiratory endurance.
catastrophic failure: A sudden, complete failure of an item, machine, or system.
cell body: Houses the cell nucleus.
center of mass: The point around which the body's mass is equally distributed in all directions.
central nervous system (CNS): The brain and spinal cord; regarded as the body's control center.
cholesterol: A molecule that is synthesized by and is an important constituent of human tissues, but in high levels it has been associated with the development of cardiovascular disease.
circuit training: An exercise program that allows for combination of specific exercises to achieve specific fitness goals.
circumduction: A cone-shaped movement that does not include any rotation; combination of flexion–extension and abduction–adduction.
closed-loop control: A motor control feedback process in which a specific reading is continuously compared with a standard value.
closed skill: Performed under constant, relatively unchanging conditions, so the movement itself is often the goal of the skill.
collagen: The main structural protein in connective tissue.
complementary proteins: Plant-based proteins that supply all of the essential amino acids missing in each other by a careful combination.
complete dislocation: Injury that occurs when the ligaments and other supporting structures of a joint are stretched and torn enough to allow the bony surfaces to completely separate.
complete protein: Type of protein that provides all essential amino acids.
composite diagram: A sequence of stick figures representing either the total body or a portion thereof.
compound fracture: Type of bone fracture that protrudes from the skin.
compression: Shortening of a tissue resulting from a force that presses the ends of a tissue structure.
concentric contraction: Type of contraction in which the muscle shortens as it goes through the range of motion (e.g., flexion).
concussion: An injury to the brain that usually results from a violent shaking or jarring action of the head.
conduction zone: Region that consists of the anatomical structures through which the air passes before reaching the respiratory zone.
conductive segment: Part of the functional region of a neuron that is specialized for the conduction of neural information in the form of nerve impulses.
condyloid joint: Type of joint with oval joint surfaces where one surface is convex and the other is concave (e.g., third metacarpophalangeal joint).
conservation of angular momentum: The phenomenon where an athlete's angular momentum is said to be constant or uniform when airborne.
continuous training: See endurance training.

contusion: Commonly called a bruise, an injury that occurs when a compression force crushes tissue.
Cori cycle: The process of transporting lactic acid from the muscle to the liver and subsequently metabolizing from it pyruvate and then glucose.
coronal plane: See frontal plane.
creeping obesity: A slight change in the energy balance occurring over a period of time causes a gradual increase in fat mass each year.
cross bridge formation: A process during which the heads of the myosin filaments temporarily attach themselves to the actin filaments.
cryotherapy: Application of ice or cold water immersion for 15 to 20 minutes at the site of an injury.
curvilinear motion: Type of linear motion that occurs when the movement path is curved.

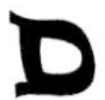

daily value: Label reference value for a nutrient based on a 2,000 kcal per day diet.
database technologies: Computer programs designed to collect and analyze data.
deep: Farther from the surface of the body (e.g., your heart is deep to your rib cage).
deformation: Change in shape caused by a physical load acting on a tissue.
dendrites: Branch-like fibers that extend from the neuron's cell body; serve as centers for stimuli by receiving messages.
depolarization: Action potential that reaches its peak at approximately 40 mV.
diagnosis: The process of identifying deficiencies or weaknesses in subjects.
diaphragm: Large muscle located below the lungs that contracts during inhalation, causing thoracic cavity expansion and lowering of air pressure.
diastole: The pressure in the heart when the ventricles are relaxed and being filled with blood; the second component of blood pressure.
dietary reference intake (DRI): Reference for nutrient intake.
digestion: Process required to dissolve and break down foods into molecules that can be absorbed by the body.
digestive system: Body system composed of numerous structures and organs that work together to process food to produce energy and to transfer energy-rich nutrients, water, and electrolytes to the body's internal environment.
disaccharide: Carbohydrate made of two monosaccharides, of which one is always a glucose molecule.
disordered eating: Refers to a spectrum of poor and unhealthy nutrition behaviors.
displacement: The length and direction of the path an object travels.
distal: Farther from the trunk (e.g., the hands are distal to the arms, or away from the origin).
dorsal: See posterior.
dorsiflexion: Motion of bringing the top of the foot toward the shin, or movement of the ankle so that the dorsal surface of the foot moves superiorly.
drag: Resistance to the movement of an object through a fluid (such as air or water).
drag force: Fluid force always directed parallel to the flow velocity.
dual energy x-ray absorptiometry (DEXA): Indirect method of measuring body fat using x-ray technology; also used to determine bone mineral content.
dynamic contraction: Type of contraction involving movement because the external force is smaller than the internal force generated by the athlete.
dynamic equilibrium: State of a moving system that is not experiencing any change in its direction or speed.
dynamic stretching: Action of rapidly moving a joint through its full range of motion.

E

eccentric contraction: Type of contraction in which the muscle lengthens during movement (e.g., extension).
ectomorph: Body type that exhibits a predominance of linearity, tending to be tall and thin.
efferent neurons: Neurons that carry signals from the brain or spinal cord.
elastic region: The area of a load-deformation curve where tissue has the capacity to return to its original shape after a load is removed.
elastin: Protein in the connective tissue that provides an athlete with stretching ability.
endomorph: Body type that exhibits a predominance of the gut and visceral organs, giving a round appearance.
endurance training: Exercise at approximately 40 to 60 percent of maximal performance ability over a long distance.
energy balance equation: Equation used to relate caloric input and caloric output.
enzyme: Allows breaking down of the chemical bonds of glycogen or glucose during anaerobic glycolysis in the absence of oxygen.
epidural hemorrhage: Bleeding between the skull and the meninges that can result from a severed middle meningeal artery.

equilibrium: The state of a system that is not experiencing any change in its direction or speed.
ergogenic aid: Nutritional, physical, mechanical, psychological, or pharmacological procedures or aids to improve physical work capacity, athletic performance, and responsiveness to exercise training.
erythrocyte: See red blood cell.
erythropoietin (EPO): The circulating hormone that stimulates red blood cell formation.
esophagus: Tube that transports food from the mouth to the stomach through involuntary muscular contractions, or peristalsis.
essential amino acids: Building blocks of proteins that cannot be synthesized by the body.
essential fat (EF): Fat that is required for normal physiological functioning.
essential nutrients: Substances that the body is unable to manufacture, so they must be obtained from outside the body in the form of food or supplements.
eversion: When the sole of the foot is turned outward.
executive program: The overall purpose of an act within a skill hierarchy.
exercise: A subset of physical activities that are planned, structured, and designed to improve or maintain physical fitness.
exercise physiology: The study of how exercise affects the functioning of various tissues and organs of the body, as well as how the body adapts to exercise.
exercise therapy: A health field that aims to develop or restore specific physical capabilities (e.g., strength, neuromuscular coordination) through habilitative and rehabilitative programs, respectively.
expiration: Movement of air out of the lungs.
explosive training load increase: A substantial increase in volume or intensity of training from one training cycle to another.
extension: Sagittal plane motion that increases the angle between two bones at a joint.
external rotation: See lateral rotation.

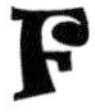

Fartlek: An endurance training method used by runners during the preparatory season.
fat: See lipid.
fat-soluble vitamins: Vitamins that dissolve in lipids; when taken in excess, they are able to be stored in the body's fat tissue.
fast-twitch fiber: Type of muscle fiber that is white in appearance, anaerobic, large, fatigable, and has high contraction speed.
feedback: A continuous reception of information that is related to our movements during a motor skills practice.
female athlete triad (FAT): Medical syndrome of extreme dieting and overtraining to which young women are susceptible because of unrealistic body goals; includes disordered eating, osteoporosis, and amenorrhea.
fibroblastic repair phase: Second phase of the healing process, leading to scar formation and repair of the injured tissue.
field test: Simple and practical tests performed outside of the laboratory setting in an everyday environment.
first class lever: Type of lever where the applied force and the resistance are located on opposite sides.
fixator: Steadies the joint closer to the body axis so that the desired action can occur.
flat bone: Type of bone that largely protects underlying organs and provides areas for muscle attachment (e.g., scapula).
flexibility: The ability of a joint to move through its full range of motion.
flexion: Sagittal plane motion that reduces the angle between two bones at a joint.
form drag: See profile drag.
free radicals: Compounds formed during fat breakdown and oxygen use by the body; responsible for damaging cell membranes and mutating genes.
frontal plane: Any vertical plane at right angles to the median plane.
fulcrum: The axis of rotation on a lever.

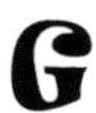

gallbladder: Organ that serves as a storage site for bile secreted from the liver.
gas diffusion: The movement of gases from a higher concentration to a lower concentration.
gastrointestinal tract: The portion of the digestive system that includes the mouth, pharynx, esophagus, stomach, small and large intestines, rectum, and anus.
general coordination abilities: Includes movement rate, motor timing, perceptual timing, and force control.
general motion: A combination of general and angular motion (i.e., body moving linearly and rotating simultaneously; e.g., wrestling).
generalized (dynamic) motor program (GMP): Stored pattern of movements with abstract structure; when well established, they require little or no attention or mental effort, and with experience, their execution becomes fully automatic.

ginglymus joint: See hinge joint.
gliding joint: See plane joint.
gluconeogenesis: The process of forming glycogen from glucose.
glycogen: The form in which glucose is stored in the liver and muscles.
glycolytic system: See lactic acid system.
gradual training load increase: Increasing training load in small steps from one training cycle to another; recommended for beginners and recreational trainees. **[I added this term; it's in the list of key terms for chapter 12, unless you later removed it as a key term (in which case, you should also remove "explosive training load increase").]**
gravity: External force that attracts a physical body with a mass to the center of the earth.
grip dynamometer: Equipment used to measure isometric strength.

H

health and fitness industry: One of the fastest-growing sectors in North America, spurred on by the demands of an increasingly health conscious population.
heart rate: The number of times the heart beats in one minute (measured in beats per minute).
heat stroke: See hyperthermia.
hematocrit: The percentage of the blood that is made up of red blood cells.
hemoglobin: Oxygen-binding substance found in the red blood cells.
high energy phosphate system: Energy production for muscular activity fueled by immediate ATP and creatine phosphate muscle stores.
hinge joint: Type of joint that has one articulating surface that is convex and another that is concave (e.g., humeroulnar joint).
horizontal plane: See transverse plane.
human anatomy: The study of the structures that make up the human body and how those structures relate to each other.
hydrochloric acid: Strongly acidic substance that dissolves the particulate matter in food (except fat) and also kills bacteria that may have entered along with the food.
hydrodynamics: Fluid forces acting in the water.
hydrogenation: Process whereby double bonds in unsaturated fats are converted to single bonds, yielding a more solid fat from oil.
hydrostatic weighing: Indirect method of measuring body fat based on Archimedes' principle of water displacement: When an object is submerged in water, there is a buoyant force equal to the weight of the water displaced. \
hyperthermia: Life-threatening condition resulting from an increase in body core temperature.
hyperventilation: Higher than normal breathing frequency and deepness.

I

immediate phosphate system: See high energy phosphate system.
impact: The application of an external force over a period of time that leads to a loss of momentum.
impulse: The application of an internal force over a period of time that leads to generation of momentum.
incomplete protein: Type of protein that provides some but not all essential amino acids.
inertia: Property of objects where because of their mass, they are reluctant to change their state of motion.
inferior: Nearer to the feet (e.g., the stomach is inferior to the heart).
inferior vena cava: Large vein delivering blood to the right atrium from the lower body.
inflammatory response phase: First phase of the healing process, characterized by tissue inflammation that presents itself as redness, swelling, pain, increased temperature, and loss of function.
information processing: Information input through several stages of processing, which then leads to an output of some desired action or movement.
insertion: A muscle's attachment away from the center of the body; also known as its distal attachment.
insoluble fiber: Important element in our diet that absorbs water from the intestinal tract, thereby aiding in making feces softer and bulkier.
inspiration: Movement of air into the lungs.
intermuscle coordination: The capacity to activate various muscles or muscle groups simultaneously to produce action.
internal rotation: See medial rotation.
interneuron: Neurons that originate or terminate in the brain or spinal cord.
intramuscle coordination: The capacity to activate motor units simultaneously.
inversion: When the sole of the foot is turned inward.
involuntary muscle: Type of muscle that is under the control of the autonomic nervous system and cannot be contracted when a person wants to (e.g., cardiac and smooth muscle).

irregular bone: Type of bone that performs a special function (e.g., the vertebrae).
isokinetic contraction: Type of contraction in which the neuromuscular system works at a constant speed.
isometric contraction: Type of contraction in which there is no visible change in muscle length, even though the muscle has undergone muscle contraction.
isotonic contraction: Type of contraction in which the muscle changes length but not tension.

J

K

kilocalorie: The amount of heat or energy it takes to raise the temperature of 1 kg of water by 1 degree Celsius.
kinematics: The study that describes spatial and timing characteristics of motion.
kinesiology: The cross-disciplinary and dynamic field of study focusing on human movement.
kinetics: The study that focuses on the various forces that cause a movement (i.e., the forces that produce the movement and the resulting motion).
knuckle joint: See condyloid joint.
Kreb's cycle: A metabolic process in which pyruvic acid is metabolized, as are other fuel sources including glucose, fat, and protein.

L

laboratory test: Rigorous and time-consuming tests performed in a laboratory setting.
lactic acid: The by-product of anaerobic glycolysis; it is produced from pyruvate when the rate of work is high.
lactic acid system: Energy system that uses a complex biochemical process called anaerobic glycolysis to release energy in the form of ATP through a stepwise breakdown of glucose and glycogen.
laminar flow: Smooth, layered flow with no disturbances that occurs within the boundary layer.
large intestine: Gastrointestinal tract structure following the small intestine that temporarily stores water, salts, and undigested material and concentrates them for defecation.
lateral: Farther from the medial plane (e.g., your ears are lateral to your cheeks).
lateral ankle sprain: Stretch or tear of the lateral ankle ligaments that occurs during excessive foot inversion.
lateral epicondylitis: Commonly known as tennis elbow, a tendonitis that affects tendons of the forearm extensor/supinator muscles.
lateral rotation: Rotating a body part away from the median plane.
lean body mass (LBM): The nonfat or fat-free component of the human body; generally consists of skeletal muscle, bone, and water.
left atrium: Heart chamber that receives blood from the lungs and then pumps it into the left ventricle.
left ventricle: Heart compartment that pumps blood through the entire body.
lever: A simple mechanical device that augments the amount of work done by an applied force.
lift: An upward force generated by an object as it moves through a fluid.
lift force: Fluid force always directed perpendicular to the flow velocity.
linear motion: Type of motion that occurs when all parts of the body move the same distance, in the same direction, and at the same time (e.g., a skater's glide).
lipid: One of the essential nutrients that is a source of usable energy, insulates our bodies, cushions our organs, is involved in the synthesis of many hormones, and aids in the absorption of fat-soluble vitamins.
liver: Glandular organ that secretes bile.
load: The forces an object is subjected to.
long bone: Type of bone that has proximal and distal enlargements (e.g., the femur).

M

Magnus effect: The whole mechanism involving Magnus force.
Magnus force: Type of force that generates changes in the flight of an object that is spinning about an axis not aligned with the flow velocity vector.
mass: The measure of how much matter an object has.
maturation-remodeling phase: The third phase of the healing process, involving long-term scar tissue remodeling and realigning.
maximal aerobic power: The measure of the maximal volume of oxygen that can be consumed in a given amount of time during maximal effort (units of L/min), providing an evaluation of the maximal power of the aerobic system.
maximal oxygen consumption: See $\dot{V}O_2$max.
maximal strength: The ability to perform maximal voluntary muscular contractions in order to overcome powerful external resistance.

medial: Nearer to the medial plane (e.g., your nose is medial to your eyes).
medial epicondylitis: Commonly known as golfer's or little league elbow, tendonitis that affects tendons of the forearm flexors/pronators.
medial rotation: Rotating a body part toward the median plane.
median plane: A vertical plane that bisects the body into right and left halves.
membrane potential: An imbalance of charges across the nerve cell membrane.
mesomorph: Body type that exhibits a predominance of muscle.
midsagittal plane: See median plane.
minerals: One of the essential nutrients that do not provide calories; instead they are inorganic substances required in small amounts to function as structural elements, regulate body functions, aid in the growth and maintenance of body tissues, and act as catalysts in the release of energy.
mitochondria: Cell organelles in which phosphorylation takes place.
moment arm: The shortest perpendicular distance from the axis of rotation or fulcrum to the line of action of the force.
moment of force: Type of force that causes angular motion.
moment of inertia: The measure of inertia of rotating objects.
momentum: The product of a body's mass and velocity.
monosaccharide: The simplest of sugars, namely glucose, fructose, and galactose.
monounsaturated fat: Type of fat, commonly found in plants, that contains fatty acids with one double carbon-to-carbon bond; not linked to cardiovascular disease.
motility: The muscular contractions that move the contents of the digestive tract forward.
motivation: Psychological entity required by most individuals in order to put forth their full effort.
motor development: The growth and development of the muscular system and the motor neurons that innervate it.
motor end plate: Ending of a motor nerve at a muscle fiber that delivers neural impulses and in turn activates the fiber.
motor learning: The process of encoding, storing, retrieving, and improving motor skills.
motor neuron: See efferent neurons.
motor program: Movement plans that are eventually stored in memory when learning new skills.
motor unit: A group of fibers activated via the same nerve; the basic functional entity of muscular activity.
movement intelligence: An aggregate or vast repertoire of movement experiences developed since birth.
movement technologies: Devices and procedures that are designed to assess the form and efficiency of an athlete's body.
muscle biopsy: A procedure during which a small piece of tissue is cut and removed from the muscle and then analyzed under a microscope.
muscle fiber: A cylinder-shaped cell that makes up skeletal muscle.
muscle force deficit: The difference between assisted and voluntarily generated maximal force during muscle contraction.
muscular endurance: The ability of a muscle or muscle group to sustain a given level of force or contract and relax repeatedly at a given resistance.
muscular endurance cross training: Type of training that involves participating in several different endurance activities to provide variety.
muscular strength: The ability of a muscle or muscle group to exert force against resistance.
myelin sheath: The fatty covering that wraps around the axon.
myofibril: Individual threadlike fibers that run lengthwise and parallel to one another within a muscle fiber and contain contractile units, or sarcomeres.
myofilament: Proteins that make up the sarcomere (i.e., actin and myosin).
myosin: The thick myofilament that makes up the sarcomere.
MyPyramid: Pyramid system used to reflect the diverse nutrition needs of the American population.

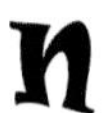

net force: The sum of all the forces acting on a mass.
neuron: The fundamental functional and structural units of the nervous system that allow information to travel throughout the body to various destinations.
Newton's first law: States that objects will not change their state of motion unless acted on by an unbalanced force.
Newton's second law: States that for linear movements, the acceleration a body experiences is directly proportional to the force causing it and takes place in the same direction as the force.
Newton's third law: States that every action has an equal and opposite reaction.
nodes of Ranvier: Gaps that separate myelin sheaths.

norms: Referenced standards established after numerous trials and used for results comparison.
nutrition: The science of food and how the body uses it in health and disease.

obesity: Having an excess of body fat beyond some particular standard that is usually based on age and sex.
one repetition maximum: The greatest force an athlete can exert for a given contraction of muscles, or the highest load the athlete can lift in one attempt.
open-loop control: A motor control feedback process in which the motor program defines the essential details of a skilled action before a movement begins.
open skill: Demand that performers adapt, anticipate, and remain flexible in their responses.
origin: A muscle's attachment that is closer to the center of the body; also known as its proximal attachment.
osteoporosis: Refers to low bone mass; bones become weak and brittle, which in turn increases the risk of fracture.
overload principle: See progressive resistance principle.
oxidative phosphorylation: Breakdown of glucose, glycogen, fat, or protein in the presence of oxygen to produce ATP.
oxygen system: Energy system that utilizes oxidative phosphorylation to produce ATP.

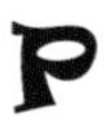

parabolic path: Shape of a path followed by the center of mass of a projectile whenever gravity is the only external force acting on the object.
parameter: Specify the order of events or subroutines, the overall duration of the movement, the overall force needed to accomplish the movement, the temporal patterning, and the spatial and temporal order in which the components of the movement are to be executed.
partial dislocation: See subluxation.
particle model: A simple dot used to represent the center of mass of a body or object.
passive flexibility: The range of movement achieved with the help of external forces.
patellar tendonitis: Also known as jumper's knee, a tendonitis of the infrapatellar ligament caused by repetitive eccentric knee action.
pepsin: An enzyme that begins protein digestion in the stomach.
percent body fat: The proportion of an individual's total mass made up of fat.
perceptual motor abilities: Include reaction time, dexterity, speed of movement, and coordination.
periodization of training principle: States that the training year needs to be divided into periods that allow a coach to prepare players to perform at their optimum during competition.
peripheral nervous system (PNS): Nerve cells and fibers that lie outside the central nervous system; connects the central nervous system to the rest of the body.
peristalsis: Involuntary muscular contractions of the esophagus that are responsible for moving the food down from mouth to stomach.
physical activity: Any movement carried out by the skeletal muscles requiring energy.
physical education: Another name for the study of human movement; considered a less appropriate title than kinesiology because it implies a single mission and a narrower scope of inquiry.
physical fitness: The ability of the body to adjust to demands and stresses of physical effort; a measure of one's physical health.
physical proficiency abilities: Include flexibility, strength, endurance, and balance.
pivot joint: Type of joint where one bone rotates around one axis (e.g., radioulnar joint during pronation and supination).
placement: Grouping individuals on the basis of their skill level measured with a testing tool.
plane joint: Type of joint where both bone surfaces are flat, so the only movement allowed is a gliding action (e.g., bones of the wrist).
plantar flexion: Motion of bringing the top of the foot away from the shin, or movement of the ankle so that the dorsal surface of the foot moves inferiorly.
plasma: A clear fluid found in blood.
plastic region: The area of a load-deformation curve where loads cause permanent tissue deformation, resulting in micro-failure or injury to the tissue.
plyocentric contraction: A hybrid contraction in which muscle performs an isotonic concentric contraction, but from a stretched position.
polarization: Resting membrane potential of a nerve cell of approximately –70 mV.
polysaccharide: Complex carbohydrates composed of extended chains of many sugar units.
polyunsaturated fat: Type of fat, commonly found in plants, that contains fatty acids with two or more double carbon-to-carbon bonds; not linked to cardiovascular disease.

positive training effect: Muscle response under training loads that are at or near a tissue's yield-level point where cells adapt to improve the mechanical properties of the tissue.
posterior: Nearer to the back (e.g., your back is posterior to your abdomen).
power: The ability of an athlete to overcome external resistance by developing a high rate of muscular contraction.
prediction: The process of predicting future events from specialized tests.
PRICE: Injury treatment steps during the inflammatory-response phase that include protection, rest, ice, compression, and elevation.
prime mover: See agonist.
proactive health: A focus on preventive measures to minimize the risk of illness and disease.
profile drag: Resistance to movement that occurs as a result of the shape of an object.
program evaluation: Process that allows superiors to determine, according to established standards, whether or not a particular program has successfully achieved its objectives.
progressive resistance principle: States that in order to ensure the muscles/systems experience a positive training effect, resistance should be periodically increased.
projectile: Any airborne object.
pronation: When the palm is moved to face posteriorly.
prone: Lying face down.
proprioception: The ability to sense the position of a joint in space.
proprioceptive neuromuscular facilitation (PNF) stretching: The most effective stretching method; it exploits the natural protective reflex of the muscle and its tendon sensors.
protein: One of the essential nutrients that serves as a structural component for muscles, bones, blood, enzymes, some hormones, and cell membranes, as well as an energy source.
proximal: Nearer to the trunk (e.g., the arms are proximal to the hands, or toward the origin).
psychomotor ability: Mental functioning that integrates the workings of the central nervous system with the more physical components of fitness and allows athletes to complete exercise-related tasks quickly and accurately.
pyruvate: The last product in the series of breakdowns during anaerobic glycolysis.

qualitative analysis: Type of biomechanical analysis that assesses biomechanical variables visually or aurally; utilized mostly by coaches or teachers.
quantitative analysis: Type of biomechanical analysis that involves techniques to quantitatively or numerically measure biomechanical variables; utilized mostly by researchers.

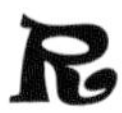

range: Horizontal distance that an object following a parabolic path travels.
reactive health: An approach that centers on the treatment of injury and disease.
receptive segment: Part of the functional region of a neuron that receives a continuous bombardment of synaptic input from numerous other neurons on the receptor site.
recommended daily intake (RDI): The highest RNI that exists for a nutrient; expressed on labels as a percentage of the nutrient's RDI.
recommended nutrient intake (RNI): Established nutrient intake values based on age, sex, body size, and activity level.
rectilinear motion: Type of linear motion that occurs when the movement follows a straight line.
red blood cell: Specialized cells present in the blood that transport oxygen and carbon dioxide.
rehabilitation: A therapist's physical restoration of the injured tissue along with the patient's active participation by following prescribed guidelines on his or her own.
relative refractory period: Several milliseconds during which a neuron can be fired only by a very strong synaptic transmission.
relative strength: A measure of strength that depends on a person's body mass.
relative $\dot{V}O_2max$: An aerobic power measurement that is not related to muscle mass, as it is expressed relative to muscle mass or in ml/kg/min.
reliability: The consistency or repeatability of test scores, data, or observations.
repetition maximum: The maximum feasible number of repetitions of a particular load.
respiratory zone: The region where gas exchange occurs.
response programming stage: Organizes the selected movement during information processing.
response selection stage: Generates a response to one's perception of the stimulus in the form of a motor program during information processing.

response uncertainty: The inability to use the same movement response on two successive attempts when responding to an opponent's intensions.
reticulocytes: New red blood cells.
reversibility principle: States that long interruptions in training have a negative effect and result in stagnation of or even decline in performance.
right atrium: Heart chamber that receives blood from the body and then pumps it into the right ventricle.
right ventricle: Heart compartment that pumps blood to the lungs.
rigid body segment model: Represents each body segment as an irregularly shaped 3D volume.
rotation: See angular motion.

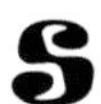

saddle joint: Type of joint where the bones are set together as in sitting on a horse (e.g., carpometacarpal joint of the thumb).
sagittal plane: Any plane parallel to the median plane.
saliva: Fluid that contains mucus to moisten and lubricate food, as well as a digestive enzyme, amylase.
sarcolemma: A connective tissue sheath that surrounds each muscle fiber or cell.
sarcomere: Contractile unit of a skeletal muscle that is organized within a myofibril in series (i.e., attached with other sarcomeres end to end).
sarcopenia: Medical condition of muscle loss in the elderly population.
saturated fat: Type of fat, commonly found in animal products, that contains fatty acids with single carbon-to-carbon bonds; closely associated with cardiovascular diseases.
scalar quantity: Type of quantity that has only magnitude (e.g., time).
second class lever: Type of lever where the applied force and the resistance are on the same side of the axis and the resistance is closer to the axis.
secretion: Production of substances that assist in digestion by various glandular organs and introduction of these substances into the gastrointestinal tract (e.g., production and introduction of bile from the liver).
self-technologies: Methods used by individual athletes to improve their performance, ranging from sport psychology to performance-enhancing drugs to surgical procedures.
sensory neuron: See afferent neurons.
sesamoid bone: Type of bone shaped like a pea and found in tendons (e.g., patella).
shear: Deformation of a tissue that occurs internally as a result of a force that is applied parallel to the surface within an object.
shin splints: Pain and inflammation along the inner surface of the tibia without a disruption of cortical bone, resulting from repeated low-magnitude forces.
short bone: Type of bone shaped to serve as a good shock absorber (e.g., wrist bones).
shoulder impingement: Inflammation in the bursae or rotator cuff tendon in the shoulder, resulting from excessive movement of the humeral head combined with lack of space between the humeral head and acromion.
simple fracture: Type of bone fracture that stays within the surrounding soft tissue.
sinus node: A small bundle of nerve fibers that generates automatic action potentials that govern the beating of the heart.
skeletal muscle: Muscle that is attached to bone; its contraction is responsible for supporting and moving the skeleton, and it is under voluntary control.
skill: The observable side of motor programs; represents movements we perform.
skill as a task: "An action or task that requires voluntary body and/or limb movement to achieve a goal."
skill as quality of performance: The ability to bring about some end result with maximum certainty and minimum outlay of energy, or of time and energy.
skinfold calipers: An instrument that uses two flattened prongs to exert constant tension on a skinfold and measure its thickness.
skinfold measurement: One of the most feasible, reliable, and valid methods of estimating body composition; involves measuring skinfolds at particular sites on the body.
skin-friction drag: Type of fluid drag caused by the roughness of an object as it moves through a fluid.
sliding filament theory: The phenomenon of muscle contraction, during which the sliding of the actin filaments over the myosin filaments causes shortening of the muscle to create movement.
slow long distance (SLD) training: See endurance training.
slow-twitch fiber: Type of muscle fiber that is red in appearance, aerobic, small, fatigue resistant, and has a slow speed of contraction.
small intestine: Gastrointestinal tract structure following the stomach, where digestion is completed and most absorption occurs.
smooth muscle: Forms the walls of blood vessels and body organs; under the control of the autonomic nervous system.

soluble fiber: Important element in our diet that binds cholesterol-containing compounds in the intestine, thus lowering blood cholesterol levels by clearing cholesterol from the intestinal tract.
somatotype: Various body types that become more evident during adolescence.
spatial uncertainty: Occurs with open skills that take place in a temporally and spatially changing environment.
specificity of exercise principle: States that the response to exercise is specific to the nature or type of exercise performed.
speed-strength: See power.
sport management: A field that applies business principles (e.g., accounting, marketing, human resources, law) to the sport industry.
sprain: Injury that occurs when a ligament or the joint capsule is stretched or torn.
stability: A relative measure of the ease or difficulty with which equilibrium can be disturbed.
static contraction: A contraction in which the muscle tension or force exerted against an external object is equal or weaker, so no visible movement of load occurs.
static equilibrium: State of a resting system that is not experiencing any change in its direction or speed.
static stretching: Action of holding a fully stretched position.
station training: The completion of all sets of one exercise before moving to the next exercise.
stick figure model: Represents body segments by rigid bars (sticks) linked together at the joints.
stimulus identification stage: Stage of information processing important for providing information about the nature of the environmental stimuli, including patterns of movement, direction, and speed of movement.
stomach: A sac-like organ that serves as a storage site, dissolves and partially digests food, and prepares food for optimal digestion and absorption in the small intestine.
storage fat (SF): Fat that accumulates as adipose tissue, serves as an energy reserve, and protects internal organs by cushioning them.
strain: Injury that occurs when muscle or tendon tissue is stretched or torn.
streamlining: The process of changing an object's shape to decrease the amount of profile drag.
strength endurance: See muscular endurance.
stress: The "non-specific response of the body to any demand made upon it"; an unemotional bodily response to some type of stressor.
stress fracture: Type of bone fracture that results from repeated low-magnitude training loads.
striated muscle: Another term for skeletal muscle because of the alternating light and dark bands that appear when viewed under a light microscope.
stroke volume: The amount of blood that is pumped out of the left ventricle with each heartbeat (measured in ml per heart beat).
subluxation: Injury that occurs when the ligaments and other supporting structures of a joint are stretched and torn enough to allow the bony surfaces to partially separate.
submaximal static contraction: A contraction in which the low to submaximal muscle tension or force exerted against an external object produces no visible movement of the load (e.g., shooting).
subroutine: Components or units of movement located at lower levels of organization in a skill hierarchy.
superficial: Nearer to the surface of the body (e.g., your skin lies superficial to your muscles).
superior: Nearer to the top of the head (e.g., your lips are superior to your chin).
superior vena cava: Large vein delivering blood to the right atrium from the upper body.
supination: When the palm is moved to face anteriorly.
supine: Lying on your back.
surface drag: Resistance to movement that occurs as a result of the surface of an object.
synapse: A junction at terminal endings of one neuron with dendrites of another nerve cell.
synergist: The muscle that supports or complements the action of a prime mover.
synovial joint: Joints that allow the greatest amount of motion.
systole: The pressure in the ventricles when they are contracting and pushing blood out into the body; the first component of blood pressure.

T

tactical uncertainty: Occurs because of the unpredictability associated with open skill environments.
talk test: Principle stating that you should be able to carry on a conversation while exercising in order to ensure that you are not exercising above the ventilatory threshold.
teaching and coaching: Instructional professions that develop and maintain fitness and motor skill performance in various settings (e.g., schools, community centers, professional sports organizations)

technology: Any tangible, conceptual, or procedural element of modern sport and exercise science aimed at progress.
temporal patterning: The capacity of the performer to integrate the sequential organization of a movement pattern.
temporal uncertainty: Occurs in a temporally changing environment.
tendon: Collagen fibers that link the skeletal muscle to bone.
tendonitis: Injury that occurs when a tendon becomes inflamed initially, then weakened and degenerative; usually caused by excessive repetitive motion.
tension: Lengthening of a tissue resulting from a pulling force.
terminal bronchiole: The smallest branch of the trachea.
terminal endings: The terminal structures of an axon, numbering in the thousands.
third class lever: Type of lever where the applied force and the resistance are on the same side of the axis and the applied force is closer to the axis.
torque: See moment of force.
torsion: Tension and compression of a tissue at an angle across the structure, caused by a twisting force.
total body fat (TBF): Calculated by multiplying total body mass or weight by percent body fat divided by 100.
total body mass (TBM): The total weight of an individual.
trachea: The windpipe responsible for adjusting the air-to-body temperature before the air gets to the lungs.
training frequency: The number of training sessions per week.
training intensity: The degree of stimulation intensity of exercise per unit of time.
training time: The total time devoted to developing fitness.
training volume: The sum total of work performed during a training session or phase of training, measured in various units.
trans fatty acid: Fatty molecule produced during hydrogenation; thought to increase blood cholesterol levels.
translation: Type of linear motion where the body moves as a unit without individual segment parts of the body moving in relation to one another.
transmissive segment: Part of the functional region of a neuron where axon terminals convert the stimulation of the nerve impulse to release chemical neurotransmitters at its synapses.
transverse plane: Any plane at right angles to both the median and frontal planes.
treatment: The administration of care to a patient, usually by a health care professional.
triglyceride: Form of fat in food composed of groupings of a glycerol and three fatty acid molecules.
turbulent flow: Flow with visible disturbances that is produced by large, rough bodies and occurs within the boundary layer.

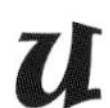

ultimate failure: A tissue response that occurs at the ultimate yield point and results in a bone fracture or ligament tear and a complete unresponsiveness to loads.

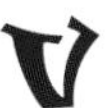

validity: The degree of truthfulness of a test score, referring to the extent to which a test measures what it proposes to measure.
valve: Vein structures that facilitate the return of blood to the heart by preventing the backflow of the blood.
vector: Arrows representing vector quantities.
vector quantity: Type of quantity that has both magnitude and direction (e.g., gravity).
vein: Cardiovascular vessel that carries blood toward the heart.
vegetarian: Relating to diets that eliminate or restrict animal-derived foods.
velocity: The measure of distance traveled per unit time.
ventilation: Breathing.
ventilatory threshold: The point at which breathing becomes just audible, corresponding to one's anaerobic threshold.
ventral: See anterior.
venule: Smaller branch of a vein.
vitamins: One of the essential nutrients that do not provide calories; instead they are organic substances required in small amounts for normal growth, reproduction, and maintenance of health.
voluntary muscle: Type of muscle that can be voluntarily contracted when a person wants to (e.g., quadriceps muscles).
$\dot{V}O_2max$: Maximal rate of aerobic metabolism; the single most important criterion of physical fitness.

W

water-soluble vitamins: Vitamins that are able to dissolve in water and are not readily stored, so that any excess is usually eliminated from the body during urination.

wellness: The combination of health and happiness in a balanced state of well-being.

white blood cell: A specialized type of cell found in the blood.

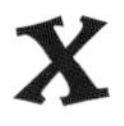

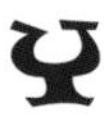

yield-level point: Point on a load-deformation curve that signals the elastic limit of the tissue, where the plastic region begins.

References and Suggested Readings

CHAPTER 1
Introduction to Kinesiology

American Academy of Physical Education. (1990). Resolution on kinesiology. *The Academy Papers, 23*, 104. Champaign, IL: Human Kinetics.

Charles, J. M. (2002). *Contemporary kinesiology* (2nd ed.). Champaign, IL: Stipes Publishing.

Henry, F. M. (1964). Physical education: An academic discipline. *Journal of Health, Physical Education and Recreation, 35*(7), 32-33.

Kretchmar, S. (2007). What to do with meaning? A research conundrum for the 21st century. *Quest, 59*, 373-383.

Lawson, H. (2007). Renewing the core curriculum. *Quest, 59*, 2, 219-243.

National Institutes of Health. (Nov. 2006). NIH roadmap for medical research. Available: http://nihroadmap.nih.gov/interdisciplinary/index.asp.

Wood, T. D. (1894). Some unsolved problems in physical education. *Proceedings of the International Congress of Education of the World: Columbian Exposition*, p. 621. New York, NY: National Education Association.

CHAPTER 2
Human Anatomy: The Pieces of the Body Puzzle

Akesson, E. J., Loeb, J. A., & Wilson-Pauwels, L. (1990). *Core textbook of anatomy* (2nd ed.). Philadelphia, PA: J.B. Lippincott Company.

Moore, K. L., & Dalley, A. F. (1999). *Clinically oriented anatomy* (4th ed.). New York, NY: Lippincott Williams & Wilkins.

Williams, P. L., & Warwick, R. (1986). *Gray's anatomy* (36th ed.). Edinburgh: Churchill Livingstone.

CHAPTER 3
Out of Harm's Way: Sports Injuries

Anderson, M., & Hall, S. J. (1997). *Fundamentals of sports injury management.* Baltimore, MD: Williams & Wilkins.
Hall, S. J. (1999). *Basic biomechanics.* Boston, MA: McGraw-Hill Publishing.

Hammer, W. I. (1999). *Functional soft tissue examination and treatment.* Baltimore, MD: Aspen Publications.

Magee, D. J. (1997). *Orthopedic physical assessment.* Toronto, ON: W.B. Saunders Company.

CHAPTER 4
Muscle Structure and Function

Bompa, T. O. (1999). *Periodization: Theory and methodology of training* (4th ed.). Champaign, IL: Human Kinetics.

Hartmann, J., & Tunnemann, H. (2001). *Fitness and strength training for all sports.* Toronto, ON: Sport Books Publisher.
McArdle, W. D., Katch, F. I., & Katch, V. L. (1991). *Exercise physiology: Energy, nutrition, and human performance* (3rd ed.). Philadelphia, PA: Lea & Febiger.

Shea, C. H., & Wright, D. L. (1997). *An introduction to human movement: The sciences of physical education.* Needham Heights, MA: Allyn & Bacon.

Vander, A. J., Sherman, J. H., & Luciano, D. S. (1994). *Human physiology* (6th ed.). New York, NY: McGraw-Hill Inc.

CHAPTER 5
Muscles at Work

Baechle, T. R., & Earle, R. W. (2000). *Essentials of strength training and conditioning.* Champaign, IL: Human Kinetics.

Bompa, T. O. (1999). *Periodization: Theory and methodology of training* (4th ed.). Champaign, IL: Human Kinetics.

Hartmann, J., & Tunnemann, H. (2001). *Fitness and strength training for all sports.* Toronto, ON: Sport Books Publisher.

Scholich, M. (1999). *Circuit training for all sports.* Toronto: Sport Books Publisher.

Shea, C. H., & Wright, D. L. (1997). *An introduction to human movement: The sciences of physical education.* Needham Heights, MA: Allyn & Bacon.

CHAPTER 6
Energy for Muscular Activity

Baechle, T. R., & Earle, R. W. (2000). *Essentials of strength training and conditioning.* Champaign, IL: Human Kinetics.

Bompa, T. O. (1999). *Periodization: Theory and methodology of training* (4th ed.). Champaign, IL: Human Kinetics.

McArdle, W. D., Katch, F. I., & Katch, V. L. (1991). *Exercise physiology: Energy, nutrition, and human performance* (3rd ed.). Philadelphia, PA: Lea & Febiger.

Shea, C. H., & Wright, D. L. (1997). *An introduction to human movement: The sciences of physical education.* Needham Heights, MA: Allyn & Bacon.

CHAPTER 7
The Heart and Lungs at Work

Guyton, A. C. H. (1998). *Textbook of medical physiology – Pocket companion* (1st ed.). Philadelphia, PA: W.B. Saunders Company.

McArdle, W. D., Katch, F.I., & Katch, V.L. (1991). *Exercise physiology: Energy, nutrition, and human performance* (3rd ed.). Philadelphia, PA: Lea & Febiger.

Oscai, L. B., Williams, B. T., & Hertig, B. A. (1968). Effect of exercise on blood volume. *J Appl Physiol, 24,* 622-624.

Suter, E., Hoppeler, H., Claassen, H., Billeter, R., Aebi, U., Horber, F., Jaeger, P., & Marti, B. (1995). Ultrastructural modification of human skeletal muscle tissue with 6-month moderate-intensity exercise training. *International Journal of Sports Medicine, 16,* 160-166.

CHAPTER 8
How Do I Move? The Science of Biomechanics

Coh, M., & Jost, B. (2000). *Biomechanical characteristics of selected sports.* Faculty of Sport, University of Ljubljana, Ljubljana: Institute of Kinesiology.

Ecker, T. (1996). *Basic track and field biomechanics* (2nd ed.). Mountain View, CA: Tafnews Press.

Hall, S. J. (1999). *Basic biomechanics.* Boston, MA: McGraw-Hill Publishing.

Kreighbaum, E., & Barthels, K. M. (1996). *Biomechanics: A qualitative approach for studying human movement* (3rd ed.). New York, NY: Macmillan Publishing Company.

Winter, D. A. (1990). *Biomechanics and motor control of human movement* (2nd ed.). Toronto, ON: John Wiley & Sons.

CHAPTER 9
Technology and Sport

Martin, J., & Cobb, J. (2002). Bicycle frame, wheels and tires. In A. E. Jeukendrup (Ed.), *High performance cycling,* 113-127. Champaign, IL: Human Kinetics.

Terauds, J. (1985). *Biomechanics of javelin throw.* Del Mar, CA: Academic Publishers.
Vaughan, C. L. (1989). Biomechanics of sport. Boca Raton, FL: CRC Press.

deKonig, J. J., Houdjik, H., deGroot, G., & Borbert, M. F. (2000). From biomechanical theory to application in top sports: The klapskate stroy. *Journal of Biomechanics, 33*(10), 1224-1229.

CHAPTER 10
Information Processing in Human Movement

Adams, J. A. (1971). A closed-loop theory of motor learning. *Journal of Motor Behavior, 3,* 111-150.

Carola, R., Harley, J. P., & Noback, C. R. (1992). *Human anatomy.* New York, NY: McGraw-Hill.

Reilly, R. (1996, February 19). I was just a pawn! *Sports Illustrated,* 96.

Schmidt, R. A. (1991). *Motor learning and performance.* Champaign, IL: Human Kinetics.

Schubert, F. (1988). *Psychology from start to finish.* Toronto, ON: Sport Books Publisher.

Shea, C. H., Shebilske, W. L., & Worchel, S. (1993). *Motor learning and control.* Englewood Cliffs, NJ: Prentice Hall.

CHAPTER 11
Movement Intelligence: A Vast Store of Motor Programs

Fleishman, E. A. (1972). On the relation between abilities, learning, and human performance. *American Psychologist, 27,* 1017-1032.

Guthrie, E. R. (1952). *The psychology of learning.* New York, NY: Harper & Row.

Magill, R. A. (1993). *Motor learning: Concepts and applications.* Madison, WI: WCB Brown and Benchmark Publishers.

Robb, M. D. (1972). *The dynamics of motor-skill acquisition.* Englewood Cliffs, NJ: Prentice Hall.

Schmidt, R. A., & Wrisberg, C. A. (2000). *Motor learning and performance.* Champaign, IL: Human Kinetics.

Shea, C. H., Shebilske, W. L., & Worchel, S. (1993). *Motor learning and control.* Englewood Cliffs, NJ: Prentice Hall.

CHAPTER 12
Physical Fitness

Baechle, T. R., & Earle, R. W. (2000). *Essentials of strength training and conditioning*. Champaign, IL: Human Kinetics.

Bompa, T. O. (1999). *Periodization: Theory and methodology of training*. Champaign, IL: Human Kinetics.

Hartmann, J., & Tunnemann, H. (2001). *Fitness and strength training for all sports*. Toronto, ON: Sport Books Publisher.
Scholich, M. (1999). *Circuit training for all sports*. Toronto, ON: Sport Books Publisher.

CHAPTER 13
Evaluation in Kinesiology

Berg, K. E., & Latin, R. W. (1994). *Essentials of modern research methods in health, physical education, and recreation*. Englewood Cliffs, NJ: Prentice Hall.

The Canadian physical activity, fitness & lifestyle appraisal. (1996). Ottawa: Canadian Society for Exercise Physiology.

Johnson, B. L., & Nelson, J. K. (1986). *Practical measurements for evaluation in physical education* (4th ed.). New York, NY: Macmillan Publishing Company.

Morrow, Jr., J. R., Jackson, A. W., Disch, J. G., & Mood, D. P. (1995). *Measurement and evaluation in human performance*. Champaign, IL: Human Kinetics.

CHAPTER 14
The Nutrition Connection

Gastelu, D., & Hatfield, F. (1997). *Dynamic nutrition for maximum performance: A complex nutritional guide for peak sports performance*. Garden City, NY: Avery Publishing.

Guthrie, H. (1989). *Introductory nutrition* (7th ed.). St. Louis, MO: Mosby-Year Book.

Health and Welfare Canada. (1990). *Action towards healthy eating – Canada's guidelines for healthy eating and recommended strategies for implementation*. Report of the Communications/Implementation Committee. Health and Welfare Canada.

Health and Welfare Canada. (1990). *Nutrition recommendations: Report of the scientific review committee*. Health and Welfare Canada, Cat. No. H49-42/199E.

Health and Welfare Canada. (1992). *Canada's food guide to healthy eating*. Ministry of Supply Services Canada, ISBN 0-662-19648-1.

Insel, P. M., & Roth, W. T. (1994). *Core concepts in health* (7th ed.). Mountain View, CA: Mayfield Publishing Company.

Payne, W. A., & Hahn, D. B. (1992). *Understanding your health* (3rd ed.). St. Louis, MO: Mosby-Year Book.

CHAPTER 15
Weight Management: Finding a Healthy Balance

Fedyck, H., Nadolny, D., & Cremasco, J. (1985). Eat well, live well. *Ontario Dietetic Association*.

Insel, P. M., & Roth, W. T. (1994). *Core concepts in health* (7th ed.). Mountain View, CA: Mayfield Publishing Company.

Payne, W. A., & Hahn, D. B. (1992). *Understanding your health* (3rd ed.). St. Louis, MO: Mosby-Year Book.

Woodside, D. B., & Garfinkel, P. E. (1989). An overview of the eating disorders: Anorexia nervosa and bulimia nervosa, *N.I.N. Review*, *8*, 1-4.

CHAPTER 16 – Appendix
Career Opportunities in Kinesiology

Karoly, L. A., & Panis, C. W. A. (2004). *The 21st century at work: Forces shaping the future workplace in the United States*. Santa Monica: Rand Corporation Press.

Koplan, J. P., et al. (2005). *Preventing childhood obesity: Health in the balance*. Washington, DC: National Academic Press.

Settersten, Jr., R. A. et al. (2005). *On the frontier of adulthood: Theory, research, and public policy*. Chicago, IL: University of Chicago Press.

The United States Bureau of the Census. *Journey to Work: 2000*. U.S. Bureau of the Census, http://www.census.gov/prod2004pubs/c2kbr-33.pdf.

The United States Bureau of Labor Statistics. *Tomorrow's Jobs*. United States Bureau of Labor Statistics, http://www.bls.gov/oco/print/oco2003.htm.

Key Terms Index

A

B

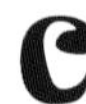

m

n

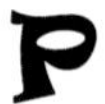

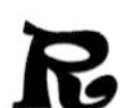

S

T

U

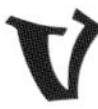

W

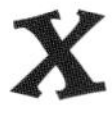

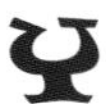

Credits

Source	Pages
Canadian Press	ix, 101 (weightlifter), 112, 116 (weightlifter), 161 (Figure 8.1 B, C, D), 168 (bobsled), 171, 183 (speedskater), 191 (Figure 8.20 C), 209 (Figure 9.7), 230 (Figure 10.7 B), 267 (weightlifter), 322 (Bailey)
Maifith Design Inc.	21, 23, 24, 36 (joint types), 37, 91, 94, 139 (heart), 142, 143, 148, 158, 164 (Figure 8.2 C), 166, 168 (3D images), 169, 181, 184 (Figure 8.15), 187, 219, 220, 278-279, 323, 359
Corbis/Magma Photo Inc.	i, 30 (soccer), 48 (butterfly swimmer), 51 (biceps curl), 79 (baseball pitcher), 82 (swimmer), 85 (Figure 3.12), 88, 107 (tug of war), 120 (Figure 6.12), 813 (cyclists), 228, 229, 230 (Figure 10.7 E, F, G), 232, 233, 257, 259 (muscular strength), 350, 357, 361 (students walking, housecleaning), 366 (background image), 373
Firstlight	44 (boy eating chocolate), 330, 343, 347, 353, 356, 358 (Figure 15.1 right image), 369 (Figure 15.7)
Niko Slana	20, 46 (kayaker), 52 (pole vaulter), 55 (sprint start), 58, 59, 62, 71 (tennis), 75 (Figure 3.7), 77 (tennis player), 83 (runner), 84 (rollerblader), 93 (gymnast), 96 (background images), 99 (high jumper), 107 (gymnast, skier, judo athlete, shooter), 118, 119, 120 (Figure 6.13), 123, 125, 130 (rower), 147 (biathlete), 167 (Figure 8.6 C), 178, 183 (skier), 184 (ski jumper), 188 (Figure 8.18 B, D, F), 189, 195, 196, 205 (pole vaulter), 226, 234, 236, 240, 241, 242, 248 (dancers, rhythmic gymnast, equestrian), 250 (judo), 252 (Figure 11.11), 259 (psychomotor ability), 261, 265 (Figure 12.7), 268, 270, 351 (gymnast), 352 (tennis player), 375
PK Photo	68 (drugs), 69, 96 (arm flexion angles), 109, 141 (Figure 7.4), 153, 156, 170, 225, 230 (Figure 10.7 A), 243, 259 (muscular endurance, body composition), 262, 264 (right image), 266, 267 (top image in box), 285, 286 (rower), 295, 300, 301, 303 (Table 13.5 background image), 305 (Table 13.6 background images), 307, 309, 310 (Figure 13.12 A), 311 (Figure 13.14), 312 (Table 13.13 background images), 315 (Table 13.16 background image), 316 (Table 13.17 background image), 349, 364 (Figure 15.4 B), 380, 391, 394, 395
PhotoDisc	x, 1, 19, 53 (walker), 63, 70, 79 (golfer), 80 (basketball), 84 (stretching), 89, 104, 105, 110, 122, 136, 137, 145 (Figure 7.8), 151 (cyclist), 152, 157, 162, 188 (Figure 8.18 E), 214, 237 (activities), 248 (swimmers, darts), 250 (football, baseball, rugby), 259 (flexibility), 272, 290, 291, 292, 293, 294, 297, 308 (Table 13.8 background image), 361 (skiing, cycling, tennis), 362, 374 (runner)
Stan J. Czerniec	72 (exercises), 73 (basketball), 74 (one-legged balance, ankle strengthening exercises), 77 (exercises), 79 (exercises), 80 (exercises), 82 (exercises), 83 (exercises), 141 (Figure 7.3), 267 (Figure 12.9), 271, 299, 302, 303 (grip strength), 305 (Figure 13.8), 306, 308 (Figure 13.11), 310 (Figure 13.12 B), 311 (Figure 13.13), 312 (Figure 13.15), 313, 314, 315 (Figure 13.18), 316 (Figure 13.19)
Sports Illustrated	vii, 173, 177, 192, 263 (cross-country skiing)
Sportverlag	28, 29, 101 (exercises), 304
VEB Georg Thieme	26, 30 (Figure 2.8: skulls), 31, 32, 33, 34, 35, 36 (background image box), 38, 39, 40, 41, 42, 43 (bones and joints of the foot), 45, 46, 47, 48 (muscles of pectoral girdle), 49, 50 (lateral muscles of the scapulohumeral region), 51 (muscles of the right arm and forearm), 52 (muscles of the pelvic girdle), 53 (posterior muscles of the pelvic girdle), 54, 55 (muscles of the leg), 56, 57 (deep muscles of the abdomen), 71-83 (anatomical images)

Every effort has been made to acknowledge correctly and contact the source and/or copyright holder of each picture, and Sport Books Publisher apologizes for any unintentional errors or omissions, which will be corrected in future editions of this book.

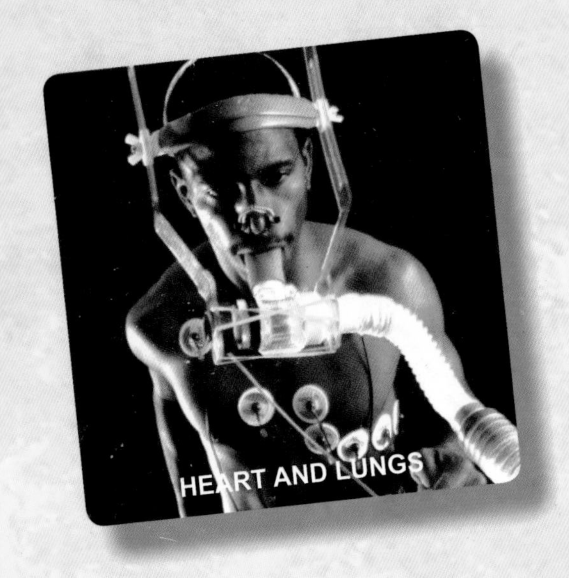
HEART AND LUNGS

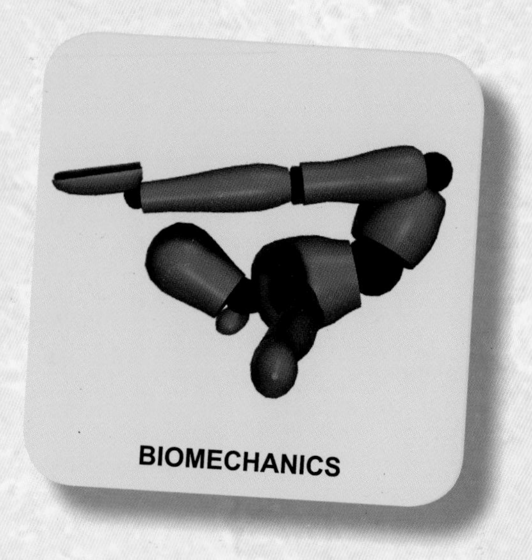
BIOMECHANICS

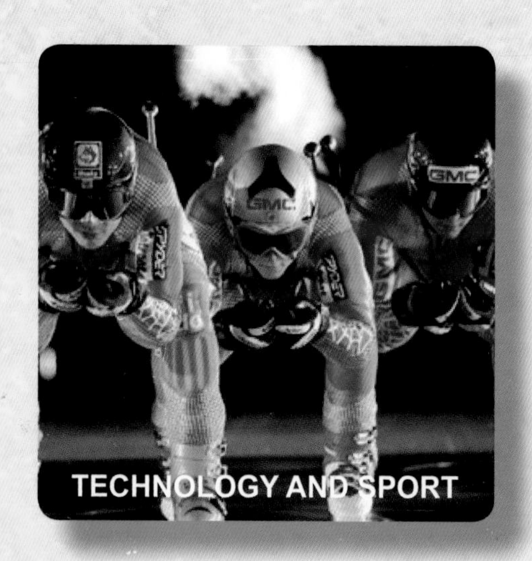
TECHNOLOGY AND SPORT

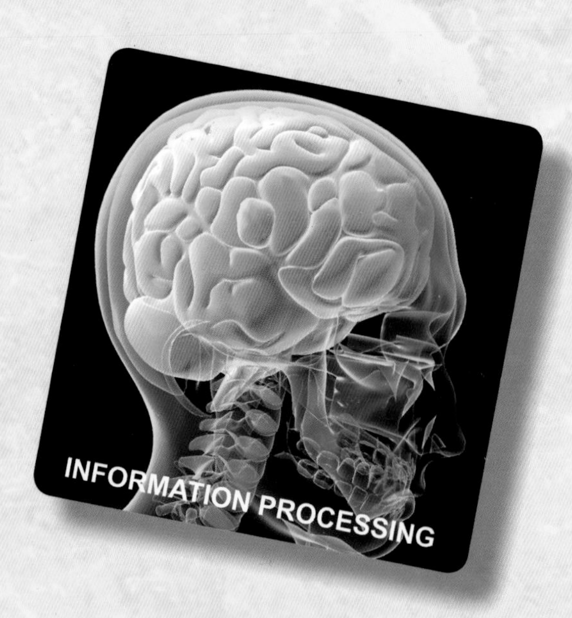
INFORMATION PROCESSING

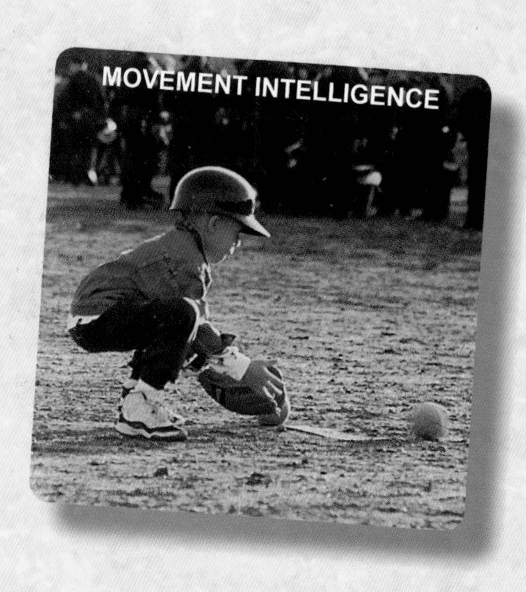
MOVEMENT INTELLIGENCE